Principles and Practice of Botanicals as an Integrative Therapy

Clinical Pharmacognosy Series

Series Editors
Navindra P. Seeram and Luigi Antonio Morrone

Botanical medicines are rapidly increasing in global recognition with significant public health and economic implications. For instance, in developing countries, a vast majority of the indigenous populations use medicinal plants as a major form of healthcare. Also, in industrialized nations, including Europe and North America, consumers are increasingly using herbs and botanical dietary supplements as part of integrative health and complementary and alternative therapies. Moreover, the paradigm shifts occurring in modern medicine, from mono-drug to multi-drug and poly-pharmaceutical therapies, has led to renewed interest in botanical medicines and botanical drugs.

Principles and Practice of Botanicals as an Integrative Therapy

Edited by
Anne Hume
Katherine Kelly Orr

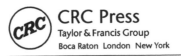

CRC Press
Taylor & Francis Group
Boca Raton London New York

CRC Press is an imprint of the
Taylor & Francis Group, an **informa** business

CRC Press
Taylor & Francis Group
6000 Broken Sound Parkway NW, Suite 300
Boca Raton, FL 33487-2742

First issued in paperback 2021

ISBN 13: 978-0-367-78016-6 (pbk)
ISBN 13: 978-1-4987-7114-6 (hbk)

Library of Congress Cataloging-in-Publication Data

Names: Hume, Anne, editor. | Orr, Katherine Kelly, editor.
Title: Principles and practice of botanicals as an integrative therapy / Anne Hume, Katherine Kelly Orr.
Description: Boca Raton, Florida : CRC Press, [2019] | Series: Clinical pharmacognosy series |
Includes bibliographical references and index.
Identifiers: LCCN 2018047185| ISBN 9781498771146 (hardback : alk. paper) |
ISBN 9781498771160 (ebook)
Subjects: LCSH: Herbs--Therapeutic use. | Integrative medicine.
Classification: LCC RM666.H33 H84 2019 | DDC 615.3/21--dc23
LC record available at https://lccn.loc.gov/2018047185

Visit the Taylor & Francis Web site at
http://www.taylorandfrancis.com

and the CRC Press Web site at
http://www.crcpress.com

Contents

Section I Patient Care Approach

Section II Botanical Integrative Medicine

Introduction

Worldwide, the use of botanicals is a key component of healthcare. In the era of patient-centered and evidence-based care, a solid knowledge of botanicals and other natural products, as well as additional components of integrative healthcare is essential for clinicians. This is especially true in primary care, where clinicians commonly work with diverse individuals, as well as with their families and communities. Recognition and understanding of an individual's interest in the use of botanicals is important in particular, as many chronic conditions, for example, are related to lifestyle choices. The incorporation of botanicals, in addition to behavior changes, may better encourage a person's engagement in their own healthcare.

Many people routinely use botanicals and other natural products as part of one's self-care for general health and wellness across their lifespan. Our focus in this book has been to go beyond this. In addition to briefly reviewing the background, pharmacognosy, dosing and product issues, and safety, the chapter authors review the published clinical trial data on the use of botanicals in common diseases and health conditions in humans and conclude with a brief summary of the clinical application. Of note, similar to prescription and nonprescription drugs, clinical trials with botanicals commonly have issues related to their study methodology and thus their resulting application to patient care. The chapter authors have selected what they consider to provide the best evidence evaluating safety and efficacy in humans, especially as an integrative therapy.

An important consideration is that the individual botanical products studied in clinical trials may differ significantly from those products commonly available in a specific country. Given the complexity of the specific components in a botanical product, the results may not reflect those identified in the clinical trials. Caution should be exercised in extrapolating the results to specific individuals. A final point is that clinicians and researchers should be committed to reviewing the current and emerging evidence of botanicals and other aspects of integrative healthcare in an open, unbiased manner.

Anne Hume, PharmD, FCCP, BCPS

Katherine Kelly Orr, PharmD

Editors

Anne Hume, PharmD, has had an interest in dietary supplements and integrative medicine for the past 20 years, writing extensively on clinical research using dietary supplements including a long-running column in *Pharmacy Today*. She is a published author and more recently the editor of the Complementary Medicine chapters in the *Handbook of Nonprescription Drugs* for the past 4 editions.

Katherine Kelly Orr, PharmD, has presented and published on the evidence based use of natural products, nonprescription medications, and other related self-care topics. She is a current co-author of the Natural Products chapter in the *Handbook of Nonprescription Drugs* for the past 4 editions.

Contributors

Thamer Almangour
Eshelman School of Pharmacy
Division of Pharmacotherapy and Experimental
    Therapeutics
The University of North Carolina
Chapel Hill, North Carolina

and

Department of Clinical Pharmacy
King Saud University
Riyadh, Saudi Arabia

Emily M. Ambizas
Department of Clinical Health Professions
College of Pharmacy and Health Sciences
St. John's University
New York, New York

Gary N. Asher
Department of Family Medicine
School of Medicine
The University of North Carolina
Chapel Hill, North Carolina

Renee A. Bellanger
Department of Pharmacy Practice
Feik School of Pharmacy
University of the Incarnate Word
San Antonio, Texas

Jacintha S. Cauffield
Department of Pharmacy Practice
The Lloyd L. Gregory School of Pharmacy
Palm Beach Atlantic University
West Palm Beach, Florida

Margaret M. Charpentier
Department of Pharmacy Practice
College of Pharmacy
University of Rhode Island
Kingston, Rhode Island

Mary Chavez
Associate Dean for Academic Affairs
University of Texas at El Paso
El Paso, Texas

Pedro Chavez
Department of Biomedical Sciences
Midwestern University at Glendale
Glendale, Arizona

Jack J. Chen
Department of Clinical and Administrative
    Sciences
School of Pharmacy
American University of Health Sciences
Signal Hill, California

Robin Lane Cooke
Department of Clinical Sciences
Fred Wilson School of Pharmacy
High Point, North Carolina

Amanda Corbett
Eshelman School of Pharmacy
Division of Pharmacotherapy and Experimental
    Therapeutics
The University of North Carolina
Chapel Hill, North Carolina

Aimee Dawson
Department of Pharmacy Practice
School of Pharmacy
MCPHS University
Worcester, Massachusetts

Sara E. Dugan
Department of Pharmacy Practice
College of Pharmacy
Northeast Ohio Medical University
Rootstown, Ohio

Kaelen Dunican
Department of Pharmacy Practice
School of Pharmacy
MCPHS University
Worcester, Massachusetts

Christine Eisenhower
Department of Pharmacy Practice
College of Pharmacy
University of Rhode Island
Kingston, Rhode Island

Lana Gettman
Department of Pharmacy Practice
College of Pharmacy
Harding University
Searcy, Arkansas

Oliver Grundmann
Department of Medicinal Chemistry
College of Pharmacy
University of Florida
Gainesville, Florida

Jessica L. Gören
Cambridge Health Alliance
Harvard Medical School
Cambridge, Massachusetts

Arno Hazekamp
Hazekamp Herbal Consulting B.V.
Leiden, The Netherlands

Cheryl Horlen
Assistant Dean and Chair, Pharmacy Practice
Feik School of Pharmacy
University of the Incarnate Word
San Antonio, Texas

Anne Hume
Department of Pharmacy Practice
College of Pharmacy
University of Rhode Island
Kingston, Rhode Island

Lauren M. Hynicka
Department of Pharmacy Practice and Science
School of Pharmacy
University of Maryland
College Park, Maryland

Marina Kawaguchi-Suzuki
Office of Global Pharmacy Education and Research
College of Health Professions
Pacific University School of Pharmacy
Hillsboro, Oregon

Linda E. Klumpers
Tomori Pharmacology Inc.
and
Verdient Science LLC
Denver, Colorado

and

BIRD Life Sciences Consulting B.V.
Delft, The Netherlands

Eunji Ko
Department of Quality and Safety
Brigham and Women's Hospital
Boston, Massachusetts

Ann Lynch
Department of Pharmacy Practice
School of Pharmacy
MCPHS University
Worcester, Massachusetts

Celia P. MacDonnell
Department of Pharmacy Practice
College of Pharmacy
University of Rhode Island
Kingston, Rhode Island

and

Family Medicine
Alpert Medical School
Brown University
Providence, Rhode Island

Kelly L. Matson
Department of Pharmacy Practice
College of Pharmacy
University of Rhode Island
Kingston, Rhode Island

Melissa Max
Department of Pharmacy Practice
College of Pharmacy
Harding University
Searcy, Arkansas

Cydney E. McQueen
Department of Pharmacy Practice and
    Administration
School of Pharmacy
University of Missouri-Kansas City
Kansas City, Missouri

Monika Nuffer
Department of Clinical Pharmacy
Skaggs School of Pharmacy and Pharmaceutical
    Sciences
and
Department of Family Medicine
School of Medicine
University of Colorado
Aurora, Colorado

Wesley Nuffer
Department of Clinical Pharmacy
Skaggs School of Pharmacy and Pharmaceutical
  Sciences
University of Colorado
Aurora, Colorado

LaDonna M. Oelschlaeger
Department of Pharmacy Practice
College of Pharmacy
Marshall B. Ketchum University
Fullerton, California

Jordan O'Leary
PGY1 Resident
College of Pharmacy
University of Rhode Island
Kingston, Rhode Island

Katherine Kelly Orr
Department of Pharmacy Practice
College of Pharmacy
University of Rhode Island
Kingston, Rhode Island

Jennifer Phillips
Department of Pharmacy Practice
Midwestern University
Chicago College of Pharmacy

Britny Rogala
Department of Pharmacy Practice
University of Rhode Island
Kingston, Rhode Island

Rachel Ryu
College of Pharmacy
University of Rhode Island
Kingston, Rhode Island

and

PGY1 Resident
Loma Linda, California

Kelly M. Shields
Associate Dean
Department of Pharmacy Practice
Ohio Northern University
Ada, Ohio

Andrew J. Smith
Department of Pharmacy Practice and
  Administration
School of Pharmacy
University of Missouri-Kansas City
Kansas City, Missouri

Brendan D. Stamper
Pacific University School of Pharmacy
College of Health Professions
Hillsboro, Oregon

Catherine Ulbricht
Department of Quality and Safety
Brigham and Women's Hospital
Boston, Massachusetts

Kristina E. Ward
Director, Drug Information Services
Department of Pharmacy Practice
College of Pharmacy
University of Rhode Island
Kingston, Rhode Island

Gregory Zumach
College of Pharmacy
Oregon State University
Corvallis, Oregon

Section I

Patient Care Approach

1

Evaluating Sources of Information about Botanical Products

Jennifer Phillips and Kristina E. Ward

CONTENTS

1.1 Introduction

Many individuals seek information on botanical products, including consumers, healthcare professionals, and scientists. For all of these individuals, it may be difficult to know where and how to find reliable information on botanical products. The purpose of this chapter is to provide an overview of tools for evaluating the quality and credibility of print and online botanical references. Strategies to use when searching for primary and grey literature will be reviewed. In addition, strategies to use when critically evaluating the reliability of these and other resources will be discussed.

1.2 Tertiary Sources

Tertiary sources, including print books, websites, online databases, or review articles should be used to gather background information on an issue. Tertiary sources interpret and summarize information found in primary and secondary sources (Kee and Duba 2016). Tertiary resources offer the advantage of being easy to use and comprehensive in nature. However, the main disadvantages of use include the potential for author bias and the lag time involved in publishing, which may lead to information being outdated (Kee and Duba 2016). A comprehensive listing of available botanical and other natural product resources, including a description of the content, advantages, disadvantages, and subscription information has been described elsewhere (Gabay et al. 2017). The reader may find this overview helpful in selecting references for various situations. However, the library of botanical references is dynamic and new reference sources

TABLE 1.1

Print Reference Considerations

Content-Related Considerations	Style-Related Considerations
Accuracy	Arrangement
Appropriateness	Durability
Authority	Ease-of-use
Bibliography	Illustrations
Comparability	Index
Completeness	
Content	
Distinction	
Documentation	
Level	
Reliability	
Uniqueness	

are added and retired fairly frequently. Thus, in this era of information abundance, it is prudent to use a systematic approach when analyzing the quality of all reference sources consulted, especially when references are being used by healthcare professionals to make treatment recommendations for patients. Helpful strategies for evaluating different types of tertiary resources are listed below.

1.2.1 Print References

Katz and Kinder identify several qualities to consider when evaluating a reference source (Katz and Kinder 1987). These characteristics can be used to evaluate the quality of print and other resources and can be grouped into style and content-related considerations, as outlined in Table 1.1. In addition, several research studies have evaluated the utility and performance of various botanical reference sources for answering different types of questions; this information may be helpful to scientists and clinicians weighting the merits of each source (Kiefer et al. 2001, Walker 2002, Sweet et al. 2003, Dvorkin et al. 2006, Clauson et al. 2008a,b). Finally, published book reviews may offer additional insight as well.

The DISCERN instrument can also be used to assess the quality of printed consumer health information (British Library and the University of Oxford 2017). It is published as part of the DISCERN project, which is based at the University of Oxford. The instrument consists of 16 components, each ranked on a scale of 1–5. The first part of the instrument helps the end user determine the reliability of the information on the site, the second part helps the reader determine the quality of the information on the treatment choices, and the last question rates the overall quality of the publication. A copy of the assessment and instructions for using it can be found at the following url: http://www.discern.org.uk/discern_instrument.php.

1.2.2 Websites/Online Databases

Much information is available on the Internet and much of it is unregulated. It can be difficult for patients, healthcare professionals, and scientists to discern which information sources are the most reliable and/or useful. A tool specifically designed to evaluate the quality of online websites and databases is the Health on the Net (HON) code (British Library and the University of Oxford 2017, Health on the Net Foundation 2017). Although designed to evaluate only printed resources, the DISCERN instrument has also been applied to evaluate the quality of websites. Results from published studies analyzing the ability of both HON and the DISCERN instrument to predict content quality varies (Khazaal et al. 2012, Nassiri et al. 2016). However, at the present time, these tools remain the most widely used by healthcare professionals, website designers, and patients.

In addition to the use of these tools, healthcare providers and scientists may find it useful to avoid using "general" search engines like Google. Instead, one can try going directly to trusted governmental or healthcare websites to search for information, or using healthcare portals such as the Health on the

TABLE 1.2

The Eight Principles of the HON Code (Health on the Net Foundation Website)

HON Code Principles	Definition
Authority	Qualifications of the authors of the information are provided.
Complementarity	There is a statement on the page indicating that the information on the site is intended to complement, not replace, advice from a healthcare professional.
Confidentiality	Efforts are in place to protect the privacy of users.
Attribution	Information sources are cited.
Justifiability	Information is balanced and objective.
Transparency	Contact details are provided.
Financial disclosure	Funding sources are identified.
Advertising	Advertisement content is clearly differentiated from editorial content.

Net website (www.hon.ch) or Healthfinder (www.healthfinder.gov) to access botanical information on the Internet.

1.2.3 HON Code

The HON Foundation is a not-for-profit nongovernmental organization based in Geneva, Switzerland. Its goal is to ensure the reliability and credibility of information on the Internet for both healthcare professionals and consumers (Health on the Net Foundation 2017). The owners or webmasters of websites must formally apply for certification via a voluntary process. Approval is based on adherence to the eight principles of the HON code listed in Table 1.2. Once approved, they can display the HON logo on their page. While the content of the page is reassessed annually by the HON Foundation, adherence to the HON principles cannot be guaranteed if the content/structure of the website changes over the course of the year; the HON relies on the vigilance of others to report instances of non-compliance. Thus, it is prudent to independently apply the principles to the page when deciding if the information is reliable.

1.2.4 Apps

Many consumer and healthcare professionals now access information via mobile software applications (apps). Like websites, most of these apps are not regulated. Therefore, information contained within these apps must be evaluated with the same level of diligence that is used to evaluate other tertiary resources. The HON code and the DISCERN instrument are not limited to websites and many of their principles can be used when critiquing medical apps. In addition, the American Society of Health-System Pharmacists (ASHP) has published a guidance document that focuses specifically on evaluating medical apps that includes checklists and additional tools app users may find useful (Hanrahan et al. 2014).

1.3 Primary Sources

Primary literature is written work derived from original thought or discovery and can be obtained directly from conduct of research or from observation (Shields and Blythe 2013, Conrad 2016). Some examples of primary literature include clinical trials, observational studies (e.g., cohort studies, case-control studies), case reports or series, and bench research. Written reports should include a description of the methodology and results.

When evaluating primary literature, readers must assess the study quality to determine whether or not the information is clinically meaningful. One way to assess study quality is to evaluate the study design that was used (Sackett et al. 2000). Figure 1.1 shows a hierarchy of study strength, with the highest strength designs being toward the top of the evidence pyramid. Other important factors to assess include the internal and external study validity. For internal validity, assessment of the study methodology is

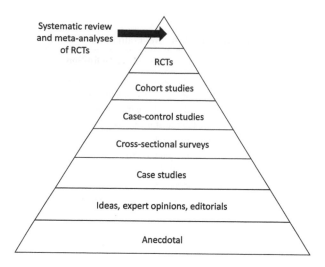

FIGURE 1.1   Evidence pyramid. (Mhaskar, R. et al. *Indian Journal of Sexually Transmitted Diseases* 30; 2009: 112–119.)

crucial and includes review of the inclusion and exclusion criteria, the use of randomization and blinding, and the statistical analysis of the data. External validity involves making an assessment of whether or not the results of the study can be generalized to another population. A full review of critical study evaluation is beyond the scope of this chapter.

1.4 Searching for Primary Literature: Secondary Resources

To locate primary literature regarding the topic of interest (in this case a botanical product), searching secondary resources is essential. These resources broadly encompass searchable databases that either index or abstract primary literature (Shields and Blythe 2013, Brunetti and Hermes DeSantis 2016). Indexing services only provide a citation for the article of interest, while abstracting services provide the citation and the abstract from the article of interest, if available. In the biomedical and health fields, examples include PubMed, Embase, the Cumulated Index to Nursing and Allied Health Literature (CINAHL), and the Cochrane Library. Other secondary resources, such as Scopus and Web of Science, have a broader coverage beyond the biomedical and health fields.

1.4.1 Closed (Controlled) Vocabulary

Each secondary database has its own closed (or controlled) vocabulary; in PubMed, it is the Medical Subject Heading (MeSH) and in Embase it is Emtree (Elsevier B.V. 2017, National Library of Medicine 2012). In a system that uses closed vocabulary, articles included in the database are assigned keywords from the closed vocabulary based on the information and subjects included in the article thus allowing grouping of similar terms. Both MeSH and Emtree are designed as a tree structure with more focused or narrow terms listed below a main term in the tree. For example, when searching natural products in the MeSH database, the term maps to "biological products," but many more specific terms are listed below biologic products in the tree hierarchy, including biological warfare agents, menotropins, plant exudates, plant nectar, and plant preparations to name a few. Therefore, using closed vocabulary allows the terms entered in the search process to be mapped to a common or similar term.

1.4.2 Boolean Operators

Boolean operators are frequently utilized by secondary resources to combine search terms (Shields and Blythe 2013, Brunetti and Hermes DeSantis 2016). When combining search terms with AND, the search results include only those articles that include both of the terms. The use of OR is slightly different; combining two search terms with OR returns articles that contain either term. The use of NOT is less frequent, but can help restrict the number of search results returned by excluding articles that include a specific search term. Boolean operators can be used with or without closed vocabulary.

1.4.3 Explosion, Major Focus, Subheadings, and Limiting

Secondary resources typically contain an enormous amount of information, which can make searching efficiently and successfully challenging. Most secondary resources provide the user with tools within the closed vocabulary to control the breadth of the search which leads to fewer, but more relevant, results for the user to browse (Shields and Blythe 2013, Brunetti and Hermes DeSantis 2016).

The first function that may be provided is explosion. "Exploding" a search means that all subterms in a tree hierarchy are included in the search. Many times, using the explode function results in a large number of results for the researcher to browse through that may not be pertinent to the topic being searched. By choosing to "not explode," only the controlled vocabulary chosen is searched, with the more specific subterms omitted in the search string which should return fewer, more relevant results to browse (Shields and Blythe 2013, Brunetti and Hermes DeSantis 2016).

Another tool is major focus or topic. Limiting a search by major focus/topic, narrows a search to include only articles that have certain closed vocabulary terms assigned as a primary topic or focus of the article. Since it is common for a large number of closed vocabulary terms to be assigned to articles, restricting the search to those lesser number of terms identified as a main focus of the article helps return a smaller number of results that are more relevant (Shields and Blythe 2013, Brunetti and Hermes DeSantis 2016).

Subheadings also allow the user to narrow a search. Subheadings are commonly assigned to each closed vocabulary term, are separate from the tree hierarchy, and are unique to each closed vocabulary term. However, if a subheading is searched and is not assigned to an article of interest, the article will not be returned in the search. Therefore, use of subheadings may be helpful when the user is searching for very specific information or if the user's initial search returned a large number of search results.

For all searches, applying limits to the search can help to further narrow or focus the search. Examples of limits that are frequently used include language of publication, species (e.g., humans, animals), date of publication, and article type (e.g., review article, clinical trial, consensus statement, letter), but many others are available (Shields and Blythe 2013, Brunetti and Hermes DeSantis 2016).

1.5 Searching the Grey Literature

The term "grey literature" was defined at the Fourth International Conference on Grey Literature in 1999 as any literature that "is produced on all levels of government, academics, business, and industry in print and electronic formats, but which is not controlled by commercial publishers" (The New York Academy of Medicine). Grey literature is not accessible though typical secondary resources discussed previously. Examples of grey literature include conference proceedings, technical specifications and standards, preliminary progress and advanced reports, market research reports, statistical reports, theses, and government reports and documents (Alberani et al. 1990). Grey literature does offer potential benefit by presenting alternative viewpoints, limiting the potential effect of publication bias, providing information with less lag time, and providing coverage of trending research (The University of British Columbia).

Two websites specialize in finding and listing grey literature: New York Academy of Medicine Grey Literature Report (Grey Literature Report) and Open Grey (Open Grey). However, the Grey Literature Report publication from the New York Academy of Medicine ceased publication in January 2017 although resources between 1999–2016 remain available. The Canadian Agency for Drugs and Technologies in Health (CADTH) has published a free tool, Grey Matters, to provide guidance for searching the grey literature (Canadian Agency for Drugs and Technologies in Health). The Grey Matters tool provides a checklist of national and international agencies and websites that may publish grey literature. A search of the Internet using Google (or some other Internet search engine) and Google Scholar is also recommended in the guidance, limiting review to the first 50–100 hits of the search. If no results are returned, Grey Matters recommends repeating the search in another search engine.

Searching for grey literature can be challenging and time-consuming, but using the tools presented above can help ensure a systematic search of the grey literature.

1.6 Conclusion

When searching for information on botanical products, a systematic approach should be used to identify reliable primary, secondary, and tertiary sources. In addition, users have the responsibility of discerning the quality of all sources found. Strategies for finding and critiquing information sources on botanical products have been reviewed in this chapter. Utilizing these strategies will help the reader to identify and use appropriate high-quality resources for scientific and medical purposes.

REFERENCES

Alberani, V., Pietrangeli, P. D. C., Mazza, A. M. R. "The use of grey literature in health sciences: A preliminary survey." *Bulletin of the Medical Library Association* 78; 1990: 358–363.

British Library and the University of Oxford. "The discern instrument." Accessed March 2, 2017. http://www. discern.org.uk/discern_instrument.php.

Brunetti, L., Hermes DeSantis, E. R. "Secondary sources of information." In: *The Clinical Practice of Drug Information*. Michael Gabay, (ed.). Burlington, MA: Jones & Bartlett Learning, 2016, pp. 59–69.

Canadian Agency for Drugs and Technologies in Health. "Grey matters: A practical tool for searching health-related grey literature." Last modified December 1, 2015. https://www.cadth.ca/resources/finding-evidence/grey-matters.

Clauson, K. A., Peak, A. S., Marsh, W. A., DiScala, S. L., Bellinger, R. R. "Clinical decision support tools: Focus on dietary supplement databases." *Alternative Therapies in Health and Medicine* 14; 2008b: 36–40.

Clauson, K. A., Polen, H. H., Peak, A. S., Marsh, W. A., DiScala, S. L. "Clinical decision support tools: Personal digital assistant versus online dietary supplement databases." *Annals of Pharmacotherapy* 42; 2008a: 1592–1599.

Conrad, J. L. "Primary sources of information." In: *The Clinical Practice of Drug Information*. Michael Gabay, (ed.). Burlington, MA: Jones & Bartlett Learning, 2016, pp. 71–85.

Dvorkin, L., Whelan, J. S., Timarac, S. "Harvesting the best: Evidence-based analysis of herbal handbooks for clinicians." *Journal of the Medical Library Association* 94; 2006: 442, e208–e213.

Elsevier, B. V. "Getting started with Embase 103 – searching with Emtree." Accessed March 9, 2017. http://help.elsevier.com/app/answers/list/p/9754/c/9540.

Gabay, M., Smith, J. A., Chavez, M. L., Goldwire, M., Walker, S., Coon, S. A., Gosser, R. et al. "White paper on natural products." *Pharmacotherapy* 37; 2017: e1–e15.

Hanrahan, C., Dy Aungst, T., Cole, S. *Evaluating Mobile Medical Applications*. Bethesda, MD: American Society of Health-System Pharmacists, 2014. Accessed March 2, 2017. http://www.ashp.org/DocLibrary/Bookstore/For-Institutions/Mobile-Medical-Apps.pdf.

Health on the Net Foundation. "HONcode section for medical professionals." Accessed March 9, 2017. https://www.hon.ch/HONcode/Pro/intro.html.

Katz, W. A., Kinder, R., (eds.) *The Publishing and Review of Reference Sources*. New York, NY: Haworth Press, 1987.

Kee, V. R., Duba, V. "Tertiary sources of information." In: *The Clinical Practice of Drug Information*. Michael Gabay, (ed.), Burlington, MA: Jones & Bartlett Learning, 2016, pp. 31–58.

Khazaal, Y., Chatton, A., Zullino, D., Khan, R. "HON label and DISCERN as quality indicators of health-related websites." *Psychiatric Quarterly* 83; 2012: 15–27.

Kiefer, D., Shah, S., Gardiner, P., Wechkin, H. "Finding information on herbal therapy: A guide to useful sources for clinicians." *Alternative Therapies in Health and Medicine* 7; 2001: 74–78.

Mhaskar, R., Emmanuel, P., Mishra, S., Patel, S., Naik, E., Kumar, A. "Critical appraisal skills are essential to informed decision-making." *Indian Journal of Sexually Transmitted Diseases* 30; 2009: 112–119.

Nassiri, M., Mohamed, O., Berzins, A., Aljabi, Y., Mahmood, T., Chenouri, S., O'Grady, P. "Surfing behind a boat: Quality and reliability of online resources on scaphoid fractures." *Journal of Hand Surgery (Asian-Pacific Volume)* 21; 2016: 374–381.

National Library of Medicine."Branchingout: TheMeSH®vocabulary," last modified May 2012. https://learn-nlm-nih-gov.uri.idm.oclc.org/rest/training-packets/T0042010P.html.

Open Grey. "System for grey literature in Europe." Accessed March 9, 2017. http://www.opengrey.eu/.

Sackett, D. L., Straus, S. E., Richardson, W. S., Rosenberg, W., Haynes, R. B. *Evidence-Based Medicine. How to Practice and Teach EBM*. 2nd ed. New York, NY: Churchill Livingstone, 2000.

Shields, K. M., Blythe, E. "Drug information resources." In: *Drug Information: A Guide for Pharmacists 5e*. Patrick M. Malone, Karen L. Kier, John E. Stanovich, Meghan J. Malone. (eds.). New York, NY: McGraw-Hill, 2013. Accessed March 08, 2017. http://accesspharmacy.mhmedical.com/content.aspx?bookid=981&sectionid=54480666.

Sweet, B. V., Gay, W. E., Leady, M. A., Stumpf, J. L. "Usefulness of herbal and dietary supplement references." *Annals of Pharmacotherapy* 37; 2003: 494–499.

The New York Academy of Medicine. "*Grey literature report*." Accessed March 9, 2017. http://www.greylit.org/.

The University of British Columbia. "Grey literature for health sciences: Getting started." Last modified March 2, 2017. http://guides.library.ubc.ca/greylitforhealth.

Walker, J. B. "Evaluation of the ability of seven herbal resources to answer questions about herbal products asked in drug information centers." *Pharmacotherapy* 22; 2002: 1611–1615.

2

Pharmacokinetic and Pharmacogenomic Considerations for the Medicinal Use of Botanicals

Marina Kawaguchi-Suzuki and Brendan D. Stamper

CONTENTS

2.1 Fundamental Concepts

Understanding the basic concepts of pharmacokinetics, pharmacodynamics, and pharmacogenomics is essential for clinicians and scientists to evaluate the appropriate use of botanicals in precision medicine. Pharmacokinetics characterizes the processes of drug absorption, distribution, metabolism, and elimination. Pharmacodynamics describes a relationship between drug exposure to a body and the pharmacologic response or effect that is produced. Pharmacogenetics or pharmacogenomics relates genetic information to how an individual responds to drugs. All of these concepts are important to ensure safe and effective use of botanicals, especially in patients receiving concomitant drug therapy.

Botanical-drug interactions may be observed if a botanical affects the pharmacokinetics and/or pharmacodynamics of a drug. A pharmacodynamic interaction occurs when a botanical has an additive, synergistic, or antagonistic effect with concomitant drug therapy. For example, if a patient takes *Ephedra sinica* to lose weight and an antihypertensive drug to lower blood pressure, a pharmacodynamic interaction may be seen due to sympathomimetic effects of ephedrine alkaloids antagonizing the antihypertensive effects of the drug (Gurley 2012). Therefore, it is critical to review the biologic mechanisms of botanicals to help identify potential pharmacodynamic interactions with existing drug therapy for patients.

In addition, consideration has to be given to both botanicals and drugs in terms of determining the "perpetrator" and "victim" of interactions. This is because certain drugs can alter systemic availability of botanical compounds just as botanicals can affect pharmacokinetics of some drugs contrariwise. Exogenous compounds, including both drugs and botanicals, may experience a process called first pass effect, in which they are extensively metabolized by enzymes present in the intestine and/or in the liver, leading to reduced exposure of the parent compounds and potentially increased exposure of metabolites before reaching the systemic circulation. This chapter will focus on how common botanicals may affect drug-metabolizing enzymes called cytochrome P450 (CYP) in humans. More detailed discussions of pharmacokinetics and pharmacogenetics/pharmacogenomics are provided in the following sections.

2.1.1 Pharmacokinetics

Pharmacokinetic interaction may be anticipated with the use of some botanicals. Botanicals may inhibit or induce enzymes or transporters or compete for serum protein binding, resulting in changes to drug's pharmacokinetic profile. Drug-metabolizing enzymes most extensively studied in the context of botanical-drug interactions are CYP enzymes, which are principal enzymes involved in phase I metabolism of many drugs. In general, CYP enzymes catalyze oxidative metabolism of lipophilic xenobiotics and are classified based on how similar their amino acid sequences are. The important CYP enzymes involved in human drug metabolism belong to the subfamilies CYP1A, CYP2B, CYP2C, CYP2D, CYP2E, and CYP3A (Zanger and Schwab 2013; Sprouse and van Breemen 2016). CYP enzymes are primarily expressed in the liver but are also found in other tissues such as the intestines, affecting the amount of systemic exposure after drug administration. More information for each CYP isoform is summarized in Table 2.1.

While oxidative biotransformation by CYP enzymes is responsible for phase I metabolism of most drugs, some substrates undergo glucuronidation, phosphorylation, methylation, sulfonation, acetylation, or glutathione-conjugation reactions during phase II metabolism (Sprouse and van Breemen 2016). Glutathione S-transferase, UDP-glucuronosyltransferase (UGT), and sulfotransferase families are example of enzymes catalyzing these phase II conjugation reactions. The availability or function of transporters may also influence absorption and elimination of compounds, referred to as phase III metabolism. Solute carrier (SLC) and ATP-binding cassette (ABC) proteins are typical influx and efflux transporter families studied in relation to drug disposition. ABC proteins subfamily B member 1 (ABCB1; also referred to as P-glycoprotein or multidrug resistance protein 1 [MDR1]), organic anion-transporting polypeptides (OATP; also referred to as solute carrier organic anion transporters [SLCO], a member of SLC proteins), and organic cation transporters (OCT) are examples of well-known transporters influencing bioavailability of their substrates. Compared to phase I enzymes, the amount of pharmacokinetic evidence is relatively limited, which demonstrates clinically-relevant botanical-drug interactions mediated by phase II enzymes or phase III transporters. However, considering the role of these enzymes and transporters is important when assessing for potential interactions. Additionally, attention should be given to certain genetic factors to understand inter-patient variability in drug- and botanical-response.

TABLE 2.1

Major Drug-Metabolizing Cytochrome P450 (CYP) Enzymes

CYP Isoform	Substrates[a]	Inhibitors[a]	Inducers[a]
CYP1A2	Alosetron, caffeine, clomipramine, clozapine, doxepin, duloxetine, erlotinib, imipramine, lidocaine, melatonin, methadone, mirtazapine, olanzapine, propranolol, ramelteon, rasagiline, theophylline, zolmitriptan (~9% of drugs metabolized by CYP enzymes)	Acyclovir, allopurinol, amiodarone, caffeine, cimetidine, ciprofloxacin, disulfiram, ethinyl estradiol, famotidine, fluvoxamine, isoniazid, kava, norfloxacin, propafenone, propranolol, terbinafine, verapamil, zafirlukast, zileuton	Carbamazepine, montelukast, omeprazole, phenobarbital, phenytoin, rifampin, ritonavir, smoking
CYP2B6	Bupropion, cyclophosphamide, efavirenz, methadone, nevirapine, propofol, selegiline, testosterone, tramadol (~7% of drugs metabolized by CYP enzymes)	Bergamottin, clopidogrel, clotrimazole, raloxifene, sertraline, voriconazole	Carbamazepine, cyclophosphamide, efavirenz, nelfinavir, nevirapine, phenobarbital, phenytoin, rifampin, ritonavir
CYP2C8	Amodiaquine, carbamazepine, dasabuvir, paclitaxel, pioglitazone, repaglinide (~5% of drugs metabolized by CYP enzymes)	Atazanavir, clopidogrel, gemfibrozil, ketoconazole, montelukast, trimethoprim, quercetin	Phenobarbital, rifampin
CYP2C9	Amitriptyline, celecoxib, diclofenac, doxepin, fluvastatin, phenytoin, tolbutamide, voriconazole, (S)-warfarin (~13% of drugs metabolized by CYP enzymes)	Amiodarone, capecitabine, fenofibrate, fluconazole, fluorouracil, fluoxetine, kava, miconazole, naringenin, pomegranate, sulfamethoxazole, tigecycline, valproic acid, voriconazole, zafirlukast	Aprepitant, carbamazepine, phenobarbital, phenytoin, rifampin
CYP2C19	Amitriptyline, citalopram, clomipramine, clopidogrel, diazepam, doxepin, esomeprazole, imipramine, lapatinib, methadone, nelfinavir, omeprazole, phenytoin, thioridazine, voriconazole, (R)-warfarin (~7% of drugs metabolized by CYP enzymes)	Chloramphenicol, cimetidine, efavirenz, esomeprazole, fluconazole, fluoxetine, fluvoxamine, isoniazid, kava, modafinil, naringenin, omeprazole, voriconazole	Aprepitant, carbamazepine, phenobarbital, phenytoin, rifampin
CYP2D6	Amitriptyline, aripiprazole, atomoxetine, chloroquine, chlorpromazine, codeine, desipramine, dextromethorphan, doxepin, doxorubicin, duloxetine, flecainide, fluoxetine, haloperidol, iloperidone, imipramine, metoprolol, nortriptyline, olanzapine, perphenazine, propafenone, propranolol, risperidone, tamoxifen, thioridazine, tramadol, venlafaxine (~20% of drugs metabolized by CYP enzymes)	Amiodarone, amitriptyline, bupropion, chlorpromazine, cimetidine, cinacalcet, darifenacin, duloxetine, fluoxetine, fluphenazine, haloperidol, kava, paroxetine, pomegranate, propafenone, propranolol, quinidine, ritonavir, sertraline, terbinafine	(no significant induction by typical CYP inducers)
CYP2E1	Acetaminophen, chlorzoxazone, ethanol, halothane (~3% of drugs metabolized by CYP enzymes)	Disulfiram	Ethanol, isoniazid

(Continued)

TABLE 2.1 (*Continued*)

Major Drug-Metabolizing Cytochrome P450 (CYP) Enzymes

CYP Isoform	Substrates[a]	Inhibitors[a]	Inducers[a]
CYP3A4/5	Amiodarone, amlodipine, aripiprazole, atazanavir, atorvastatin, budesonide, buspirone, carbamazepine, citalopram, clarithromycin, clozapine, cyclosporine, daclatasvir, darifenacin, dasatinib, dexamethasone, diazepam, diltiazem, docetaxel, doxepin, doxorubicin, efavirenz, eletriptan, erythromycin, estrogens, everolimus, felodipine, fluticasone, haloperidol, indivanir, irinotecan, itraconazole, ketoconazole, lapatinib, lidocaine, lovastatin, midazolam, nefazodone, nifedipine, ondansetron, quinine, sildenafil, simvastatin, triazolam (~30% of drugs metabolized by CYP enzymes)	Aprepitant, atazanavir, ciprofloxacin, clarithromycin, conivaptan, crizotinib, diltiazem, dronedarone, erythromycin, fluconazole, fosamprenavir, grapefruit, indinavir, imatinib, itraconazole, kava, ketoconazole, nefazodone, nelfinavir, pomegranate, posaconazole, ritonavir, saquinavir, telithromycin, verapamil, voriconazole	Carbamazepine, efavirenz, etravirine, nafcillin, phenobarbital, phenytoin, rifampin, topiramate

Source: Sprouse, A. A., and R. B. van Breemen. 2016. *Drug Metab Dispos* 44 (2):162–71. doi: 10.1124/dmd.115.066902; Zanger, U. M., and M. Schwab. 2013. *Pharmacol Ther* 138 (1):103–41. doi: 10.1016/j.pharmthera.2012.12.007; Therapeutic Research Center. 2016. In *Pharmacist's letter*. Stockton, CA.

[a] This is not a comprehensive list of substrates, inhibitors, and inducers but shows common examples.

2.1.2 Pharmacogenetics/Pharmacogenomics

In the late 1800s, the Canadian physician William Osler said, "If it were not for the great variability among individuals, medicine might as well be a science and not an art" (Roses 2000). Over time, we have gained a better understanding of the complexities that surround inter-patient variability in the response to drugs and botanicals, and that numerous factors such as race, sex, diet, disease state age, and genetics all contribute. The field of pharmacogenomics (also commonly referred to as pharmacogenetics) is a specific scientific field concerned with how genetic variation gives rise to variability in drug response. Gaining a better understanding of how genetic variation impacts drug metabolism and disposition may lead to more appropriate drug selection and dosing that improves therapeutic effect and limits toxicity.

The human genome contains approximately 3 billion nucleotides, of which ~1% contribute to approximately 20,000 genes that may code for up to 100,000 different proteins (Venter et al. 2001). Generally speaking, the genomes of any two individuals are quite similar; however, genetic variation does exist and can manifest in different ways, including nucleotide insertions, deletions, duplications, translocations, and single nucleotide polymorphisms (SNPs). SNPs occur when one nucleotide in a specific position is exchanged for another; for example, if a cytosine (C) base is replaced with a guanine (G) base. SNPs within the protein-coding region of a gene have the potential to alter protein function. If that protein is known to interact with a specific drug or botanical, the pharmacokinetic profile for that agent might change leading to clinically relevant differences in efficacy or toxicity in a patient with that variant allele.

Early work in the field of pharmacogenetics focused on polymorphisms associated with proteins involved in drug metabolism and disposition including those that catalyze phase I and phase II reactions such as CYP enzymes and UGTs (Evans and Relling 1999). This approach has expanded to investigate genetic variation in drug transporters, drug targets, and even non-coding regions of deoxyribonucleic acid (DNA) (Rukov and Shomron 2011). The star allele nomenclature is typically used to identify commonly inherited variants implicated as pharmacogenomic markers. The star allele nomenclature uses an asterisk to separate the gene symbol from the genetic variant with the one allele corresponding to the wild-type or consensus allele. For example, *CYP2C9*1* is the wild-type allele, whereas *CYP2C9*2* is a genetic variant in which a cytosine is replaced with a thymine at genomic position 430 (expressed as 430C>T) that leads to an amino acid substitution from arginine to cysteine at position 144 (expressed as R144C). The *CYP2C9*2* allele is associated with impaired metabolism and individuals with this genotype are often deemed as "poor metabolizers" based on the catalytic activity of their variant (Rettie et al. 1994). "Extensive metabolizers" are those individuals who carry alleles with increased activity or multiple copies of the functional allele. *CYP2C9* mutations and their effect on the anticoagulant effect of warfarin are classic examples of how pharmacogenetics may be used clinically. Warfarin is a substrate for CYP2C9 and poor metabolizers (e.g., *CYP2C9*2* or *CYP2C9*3* carriers) may require a lower dose of warfarin than individuals with the *CYP2C9*1* allele (Flockhart et al. 2008). Databases such as the "The Human Cytochrome P450 (CYP) Allele Nomenclature Database" have been developed and provide information on allelic variants in 29 CYP enzymes (Sim and Ingelman-Sundberg 2013). Significant efforts to bring pharmacogenetics into the clinic have resulted in the development of various genotyping technologies to inform better clinical decision making when it comes to choosing a safe and effective dose for a drug or botanical (Deeken 2009).

2.2 Botanicals and Implication for Precision Medicine

This section reviews pharmacokinetic, pharmacodynamic, and/or pharmacogenomic evidence for eight botanicals: black cohosh, echinacea, garlic, ginkgo, ginseng, milk thistle, saw palmetto, and St. John's wort. General information regarding these eight botanicals can be found in Table 2.2.

2.2.1 Black Cohosh

2.2.1.1 Background

Black cohosh is a wildflower found in temperate northern climates. Historically, Native Americans used the rhizomes of black cohosh to treat general malaise, inflammation, sore throat, and gynecopathic applications (McKenna et al. 2001). Current uses of black cohosh include arthritis pain, breast cancer, and most notably, menopausal symptoms. Black cohosh extracts contain alkaloids, flavonoids, and terpenoid glycosides (Liske 1998; Johnson and van Breemen 2003). The terpenoid glycosides are thought to be the pharmacologically active constituents, and commercial products are often standardized based on triterpene glycoside content. The British Herbal Compendium recommends 40–200 mg dried rhizome of 0.4–2 mL of a 1:10 60% ethanol tincture daily (Bradley and British Herbal Medicine Association. Scientific Committee. 2010).

Mixed evidence exists as to whether estrogenic compounds in black cohosh contribute to its pharmacologic effects (Bodinet and Freudenstein 2002; Seidlova-Wuttke et al. 2003). Most studies have found insignificant interactions between the estrogen receptor and black cohosh constituents and their metabolites (Onorato and Henion 2001; Lupu et al. 2003). In rats, a methanol extract was capable of reducing serum levels of luteinizing hormone (Jarry and Harnischfeger 1985; Jarry et al. 1985); however, this effect can vary based on the extract fraction, and has not yet been seen in humans (Duker et al. 1991; Liske et al. 2002). Other evidence suggests that modulation of neurotransmitter action and not hormonal changes may be central to the pharmacologic effects of black cohosh (Reame et al. 2008). Due to uncertain mechanism of action, determining potential implications for pharmacodynamic interactions is challenging. *See Chapter 8 Women's Health for further discussion.*

Significant work has been performed screening for drug interactions with black cohosh based on CYP activity. *In vitro*, black cohosh extracts have been found to inhibit CYP1A2, CYP2D6, CYP2C9, and CYP3A4 in a concentration-dependent manner (Huang et al. 2010). Interest in black cohosh metabolism is in part due to reports of the hepatotoxicity associated with its use (Mahady et al. 2008). *In vitro* evidence suggests constituents in black cohosh extracts do not act as direct hepatotoxicants themselves but may induce drug interactions.

2.2.1.2 Evidence

Enzymatic activities of CYP1A2, CYP2D6, CYP2E1, and CYP3A4 were investigated among healthy volunteers by measuring the metabolism of caffeine, debrisoquine, chlorzoxazone, and midazolam as

TABLE 2.2

General Information and the Pharmacologically-Relevant Chemical Constituents of Nine Botanicals

Botanical	Scientific Name	Native Region	Primary Indication (Mechanism of Action)	Primary Active Constituents	Example Structure
Black cohosh	*Actaea racemose*	Eastern North America	Menopausal symptoms (poorly defined: potential estrogenic effects)	Terpenoid glycosides	Actein:
Echinacea	*Echinacea spp.*	North America	Upper respiratory infections (immunomodulating effects)	Alkamides; phenylpropanoids; polysaccharides	Dodeca-2E,4E,8Z,10Z-tetraenoic acid isobutylamide:
Garlic	*Allium sativum*	Central Asia	Hyperlipidemia (poorly defined: potential inhibition of HMG-CoA reductase)	Organosulfur compounds	Allicin:
Ginkgo	*Ginkgo biloba*	China	Dementia, cerebral insufficiency, and claudication (antioxidant)	Flavone glycosides; terpene lactones	Ginkgolide B:
Ginseng	*Panax spp.*	China (*P. ginseng*) & North America (*P. quinquefolius*)	Type 2 diabetes, cardiovascular disease, and immune booster (insulin-mimetic effects)	Ginsenosides (triterpenoid saponins)	Ginsenoside Rg1:
Milk thistle	*Silybum marianum*	Mediterranean	Liver cirrhosis and hepatitis (antioxidant)	Silymarins	Silybin A:
Saw Palmetto	*Serenoa repens*	Gulf Coast of the United States & Mexico	Benign prostatic hyperplasia (poorly defined: potential inhibition of 5α-reductase activity)	liposterolic content (fatty acids & sterols)	β-sitosterol:
St. John's wort	*Hypericum perforatum*	Europe and Asia	Depression (inhibits synaptic neurotransmitter reuptake of serotonin, norepinephrine, and dopamine)	Hypericin; hyperforin	Hyperforin:

probe drugs or prototypical substrates of each enzyme respectively with supplementation of black cohosh 1,090 mg twice daily for 28 days (Gurley et al. 2005b). This long-term use of black cohosh did not affect the activity of CYP1A2, CYP2E1, and CYP3A4; only a mild 7% reduction in CYP2D6 activity was observed (Gurley et al. 2005b). However, a later study showed no significant effect of black cohosh on CYP2D6 after 14-day supplementation in healthy volunteers at a dose of 40 mg twice daily (Gurley et al. 2008a). When 16 healthy volunteers received black cohosh 40 mg daily for 14 days, no significant effect was suggested on ABCB1, based on measured pharmacokinetics of digoxin, a prototypical substrate of the transporter (Gurley et al. 2006b).

While CYP inhibition has been observed *in vitro*, these effects have not been seen in clinical studies using dosing regimens within the range recommended by the British Herbal Compendium. This evidence suggests no clinically significant effect of black cohosh on CYP1A2, CYP2D6, CYP2E1, and CYP3A4 enzymes or on ABCB1.

2.2.2 Echinacea

2.2.2.1 Background

While echinacea has a long tradition of use as an anti-infective agent, current research has been more narrowly focused on its ability to serve as an immunomodulatory agent (Barrett 2003). Good scientific evidence exists for using echinacea in preventing and treating upper respiratory infections in adults, but not necessarily in children (Taylor et al. 2003). Constituents of echinacea have been shown to have many immunomodulatory effects such as the enhancement of macrophage function, elevation natural killer cell levels, and others (Barnes et al. 2005). Phytochemical diversity exists among the echinacea species with the medically relevant components thought to come from three major structural classes including alkamides, phenylpropanoids (e.g., caffeic acid), and polysaccharides. Historically, substantial evidence exists of poor standardization of echinacea supplements especially by using different species and plant parts (Gilroy et al. 2003). *See Chapter 12 Botanicals for Common Infectious for further discussion.*

Insufficient standardization due to multiple echinacea species make predicting the botanical's activity on human metabolism and transport challenging. The majority of studies using *in vitro* and animal models has investigated interactions between echinacea and CYP enzymes, ABCB1, and OATP-B. Echinacea extracts have been shown to inhibit CYP3A to varying degrees in rats and multiple *in vitro* systems including Caco-2 cells and supersomes (Budzinski et al. 2000; Hellum and Nilsen 2008; Mrozikiewicz et al. 2010). When inhibition studies were performed using echinacea-based alkamides specifically, inhibition of CYP3A4 was observed; however, the alkamide content among different extracts was variable up to 1,400-fold (Modarai et al. 2007). In general, greater CYP3A4 inhibition was associated with greater alkamide content. Alkamides in echinacea, and not caffeic acid derivatives, were also shown to be a moderate CYP2E1 inhibitor in two *in vitro* systems (Raner et al. 2007). Interactions with transport mechanisms have also been investigated *in vitro*, with echinacea serving as a weak ABCB1 inhibitor as well as an inhibitor of OATP-B function at potentially physiologically relevant concentrations (Fuchikami et al. 2006; Hellum and Nilsen 2008; Hansen and Nilsen 2009).

2.2.2.2 Evidence

The clinical effects of echinacea has been examined on various CYP enzymes and transporters as well. An 8-day supplementation of echinacea root extract 400 mg four times daily showed differential effects on intestinal and hepatic CYP3A; in healthy volunteers, the pharmacokinetics of midazolam indicated inhibition of CYP3A in the intestine but induction of the hepatic enzyme (Gorski et al. 2004). The exact mechanism for this differential effect has not been fully determined, and these effects on CYP3A are only modest (Gurley et al. 2012). In addition, only a mild inhibitory effect on CYP1A2 and 2C9 was shown (Gorski et al. 2004). While echinacea did not have a significant effect on CYP2D6 in extensive metabolizers, one individual who was a poor metabolizer had 42% increase in dextromethorphan (CYP2D6 substrate) exposure; however, it is impossible to draw any conclusion regarding CYP2D6 metabolizer status based on this single observation (Gorski et al. 2004). In other studies, clinically significant changes were not detected in CYP1A2, 2D6, 2E1, or 3A4 activity when healthy volunteers received echinacea extract either 267 mg (2.2 mg isobutylamides) three times daily for 14 days or 800 mg twice daily for 28 days (Gurley et al. 2004; Gurley et al. 2008a).

In addition to the healthy volunteer study, to further investigate the effect on CYP3A in patients with human immunodeficiency virus (HIV), darunavir/ritonavir (CYP3A substrate/inhibitor) pharmacokinetics were evaluated with co-administration of echinacea root extract 500 mg every 6 hours for 14 days (Molto et al. 2011). In this study, a clinically significant effect was not observed on either darunavir or ritonavir, and it is possible that the inhibitory property of ritonavir masked any potential effect of echinacea on CYP3A (Molto et al. 2011). A clinically prominent effect was also not shown when etravirine (CYP3A substrate and inducer) was also administered with echinacea root extract 500 mg every 8 hours for 14 days in HIV-infected patients (Molto et al. 2012b). Similarly, while modest reductions in midazolam (CYP3A substrate) exposure was noted with echinacea 500 mg three times daily for 28 days in healthy volunteers, no significant effect was observed for the pharmacokinetics of lopinavir/ritonavir (CYP3A substrate/inhibitor) (Penzak et al. 2010).

Potential effect of echinacea on transporters was also investigated, and a significant impact was not observed on the pharmacokinetics of fexofenadine (ABCB1 and OATP substrate) (Penzak et al. 2010). The pharmacokinetics of digoxin, a more ABCB1-specific substrate, were not significantly affected after 14-day supplementation of echinacea 267 mg three times daily (Gurley et al. 2008b).

The collective clinical evidence suggests that recommended doses of echinacea supplementation are unlikely to produce clinically relevant interaction with CYP1A2, 2C9, 2D6, or 2E1 enzyme or ABCB1 or OATP transporter. However, based on the fact that alkylamides are capable of inhibiting CYP3A and that standardization of alkylamide content in echinacea extracts is generally poor, caution should be exercised with the concomitant use of echinacea with a narrow therapeutic index drug extensively metabolized by intestinal CYP3A.

2.2.3 Garlic

2.2.3.1 Background

Garlic is a ubiquitous bulbous plant that has been cultivated by humans for thousands of years for culinary and medicinal uses. In ancient civilizations, garlic was used to treat infections, pulmonary conditions, digestive disorders, heart disease, and arthritis (Rivlin 2001). Garlic products are now used to treat hyperlipidemia, and its utility in cancer and infectious disease are still being studied. The organosulfur compounds in garlic, such as allicin, diallyl sulfides, and S-allylcysteine are thought to contribute to its pharmacologic activity in hyperlipidemia (Yeh and Liu 2001). The mechanisms by which these compounds act have been proposed include inhibition of HMG-CoA reductase, the rate-limiting enzyme for cholesterol synthesis (Ulbricht and Natural Standard 2010). *See Chapter 5 Cardiovascular Disease for further discussion.*

As with many botanical supplements, the potency and bioavailability of garlic constituents changes based on the extraction method (Amagase 2006). Many garlic supplements are standardized to allicin content and both the World Health Organization and the European Scientific Cooperative on Phytotherapy recommend sources that provide approximately 2–5 mg allicin daily for the treatment of atherosclerosis. Since the structural and physical properties of the organosulfur components of garlic vary, studies have been performed investigating their effects on CYP enzymes. In rats and rat-based models, exposure to various diallyl sulfides was shown to alter hepatic CYP protein levels, including reducing levels of CYP2E1 and increasing CYP1A and CYP2B levels (Pan et al. 1993; Davenport and Wargovich 2005). In human hepatocytes exposed to garlic extracts, dose-dependent decreases in CYP2C9 activity (greater than 90%) were observed (Ho et al. 2010). Interestingly, fresh garlic extracts were shown to have inhibitory effects on *CYP2C9*1*-mediated metabolism, yet stimulate *CYP2C9*2*-based metabolism *in vitro* (Foster et al. 2001). With respect to phase II metabolism, diallyl sulfide led to a 3200-fold induction of *Sult1e1* messenger ribonucleic acid (mRNA) in mice (Sueyoshi et al. 2011).

2.2.3.2 Evidence

Clinical studies have investigated effects of various garlic products on CYP enzymes as well. When healthy volunteers took garlic extract 1,800 mg (approximately 1,800 mcg allicin) twice daily for 14 days, a significant effect was not observed on the activity of CYP2D6 and CYP3A4 based on pharmacokinetics of dextromethorphan and alprazolam, respectively (Markowitz et al. 2003a). A clinically relevant interaction with warfarin was not observed, suggesting the lack of a significant alternation in CYP2C9 and CYP3A4 activities (Macan et al. 2006; Mohammed Abdul et al. 2008). An absence of alteration in CYP2D6 and CYP3A4 activities also aligns with findings of other studies while no change in CYP1A2 activity was similarly reported (Gurley et al. 2002; Gurley et al. 2005a; Gurley et al. 2012). Pharmacokinetics of acetaminophen, a CYP2E1 substrate, did not significantly change after men received garlic extract equivalent to 6–7 cloves of garlic daily for 3 months (Gwilt et al. 1994). However, 31% reduction of metabolite-to-chlorzoxazone ratios, a measure of CYP2E1 activity, was observed with the administration of garlic oil extract containing diallyl sulfide and with dietary levels of ethanol in healthy volunteers (Loizou and Cocker 2001). This finding confirms a previous murine study suggesting CYP2E1 inhibitors are lipophilic, not hydrophilic, organosulfur compounds (Gurley et al. 2012). Long-term supplementation of garlic oil 500 mg three times daily for 28 days similarly demonstrated 39% and 22% inhibition of CYP2E1 activity in healthy young and elderly adults (age 25 ± 3.9 and 67 ± 5.2 years [mean $\pm$ standard deviation]), respectively (Gurley et al. 2002; Gurley et al. 2005a). Among healthy Chinese men, large-dose supplementation of garlic (180 mg allicin) for 14 days was associated with increased peak concentration and exposure of omeprazole, indicating inhibition of CYP2C19 activity, in rapid and intermediate metabolizers (*1/*1, *1/*2, and *1/*3 genotypes) but not in poor metabolizers (*2 homozygotes) (Yang et al. 2009).

Altered pharmacokinetics of saquinavir and ritonavir were reported with garlic powder supplementation. These alterations were considered to be attributable to upregulation of intestinal ABCB1 or ABCC2 activity due to a lack of significant effect on CYP3A4 and *in vitro* findings (Piscitelli et al. 2002a; Gallicano et al. 2003; Gurley et al. 2012). In healthy volunteers, a garlic extract 600 mg (allicin 3,600 mcg) twice daily for 21 days induced duodenal expression of ABCB1 by 31% and was associated with 15% reduction in single-dose saquinavir exposure (a substrate for both ABCB1 and CYP3A4) (Hajda et al. 2010); the larger effect, 51% exposure reduction, was previously noted after multiple dosing of saquinavir (Piscitelli et al. 2002a). A significant effect was not shown on CYP3A4 or OATP1B1 measured by simvastatin and pravastatin pharmacokinetics, respectively (Hajda et al. 2010).

In summary, clinical studies suggest that CYP2E1 activity is inhibited by garlic oil and that ABCB1 is modestly induced by long-term use of garlic extract. The decreased CYP2E1 activity observed in these clinical studies correlate with the reduction in CYP2E1 protein seen in studies using animal studies. However, other than chlorzoxazone, drugs relying solely on CYP2E1 for metabolism are rare and therapeutic indices of CYP2E1 substrates are relatively wide. Therefore, the effect of garlic supplement on CYP enzymes is unlikely to pose a concern. The prolonged use of high-dose garlic extract containing 180 mg allicin should be cautioned for drugs highly subject to ABCB1 efflux since systemic availability may be reduced, potentially resulting in less efficacy.

2.2.4 Ginkgo Biloba

2.2.4.1 Background

Fossil records indicate that ginkgo trees have persisted on earth for the past 270 million years (Isah 2015). Heterogeneous preparations from ginkgo leaf, nut, and fruit have been used in traditional Chinese medicine for centuries to treat a wide range of medical conditions. The development of standardized ginkgo biloba extract products typically are composed of at least 24% flavone glycosides and 6% terpene lactones. Constituents within these two pharmacognostic structural classes include quercetin, kaempferol and various ginkgolides. Based on its high flavonoid content, the mechanisms by which ginkgo is thought to exert its medicinal effects is primarily through antioxidant and free-radical scavenging activity (Marcocci et al. 1994a; Marcocci et al. 1994b). Evidence that ginkgo protects against oxidative stress has been demonstrated through its ability to act as both a neuroprotective and cardioprotective agent (Nash and Shah 2015). *See Chapters 5 Cardiovascular Disease and 10 Neurologic Conditions for further discussion.*

A concerted effort has been spent quantifying ginkgo's ability to effect CYP enzymes; however, conclusive results have been elusive due to the numerous molecular compounds within ginkgo extracts. In studies using rat models, ginkgo appears to induce the content and activity of multiple CYP enzymes with conflicting results for CYP3A4 activity (Ohnishi et al. 2003; Yoshioka et al. 2004; Shord et al. 2009). Compared to rat-based studies, contrary results have been observed using *in vitro* human models. The *in vitro* inhibition of multiple human CYP enzymes has been observed following exposure to various fractions of ginkgo extract such as those containing ginkgolic acids, terpenes, and flavonoids (Gaudineau et al. 2004; von Moltke et al. 2004). Human *in vitro* studies have led to the generalization that exposure to ginkgo extract is associated with broad CYP inhibition (Shord et al. 2009). The role of transporters in ginkgo absorption and bioavailability has also been investigated *in vitro*. One study determined that flavonols such as quercetin, kaempferol, and isorhamnetin were substrates of ABCB1 (Wang et al. 2005), whereas another study concluded that ginkgo may alter intestinal OATP-B function thereby limiting OATP-B-mediated drug transport in humans (Fuchikami et al. 2006). Results from these animal and *in vitro* studies suggest that interpatient variability with respect to both drug metabolizing enzymes and drug transport should be taken into account with ginseng exposure.

2.2.4.2 Evidence

Exposure to tolbutamide (CYP2C9 substrate) decreased by 16% in healthy men who received ginkgo biloba extract 120 mg three times daily for 28 days while midazolam (CYP3A substrate) exposure increased by 25% (Uchida et al. 2006). Modest reductions in the beta-1 selective beta-blocker talinolol (ABCB1 substrate) exposure by 20%–25% are reported with the same dose of ginkgo biloba extract for 14 days in Chinese men (Fan et al. 2009a,b). The majority of human evidence suggests an absence of clinically important drug interactions with ginkgo; these studies examined various drugs, including caffeine, bupropion, flurbiprofen, debrisoquine, dextromethorphan, chlorzoxazone, alprazolam, nifedipine, donepezil, warfarin, ritonavir-boosted lopinavir, diazepam, digoxin, ticlopidine, fexofenadine, metformin, clopidogrel, cilostazol, and aspirin (Engelsen et al. 2002; Gurley et al. 2002; Mauro et al. 2003; Markowitz et al. 2003c; Yoshioka et al. 2004; Yasui-Furukori et al. 2004; Jiang et al. 2005; Mohutsky et al. 2006; Greenblatt et al. 2006; Lu et al. 2006; Wolf 2006; Kudolo et al. 2006; Aruna and Naidu 2007; Robertson et al. 2008; Lei et al. 2009a; Kim et al. 2010; Zuo et al. 2010; Gurley et al. 2012; Hermann and von Richter 2012; Wanwimolruk and Prachayasittikul 2014). This absence of clinically relevant interaction is especially true at doses of 240 mg/day or less and even with chronic supplementation, whereas higher doses may potentiate drug interactions.

Pharmacogenomic data is also available from clinical studies with ginkgo supplementation. One study described a *CYP2C19* genotype-dependent increase in omeprazole hydroxylation. The reduction in the index of omeprazole hydroxylase activity, measured as omeprazole-to-metabolite ratio of areas under the curve, was 42.3% with *1/*1 genotype, 50.3% with *1/*2 or *1/*3 genotype, and 70.6% with *2/*2 or *2/*3 genotype after 12-day supplementation of ginkgo biloba 140 mg twice daily (Yin et al. 2004). However, significant difference in voriconazole pharmacokinetics was not demonstrated between *CYP2C19* *1/*1 extensive metabolizers and *2/*2 poor metabolizers with the same regimen (Lei et al. 2009b). Due to limited available evidence, the significance of *CYP2C19* genotypes remains unclear with ginkgo supplementation.

Taken together, the evidence from *in vitro*, animal models, and clinical studies provide mixed results. In general, ginkgo appears to generally induce CYPs in rats, whereas CYP inhibition is largely seen in human *in vitro* models. It is worth noting that some conflicting rat data, human *in vitro* data, and one clinical study have observed CYP3A inhibition with ginkgo extracts. However, a lack of consistently strong correlations between ginkgo exposure and significant changes in specific CYP activities highlights the challenge in making a definitive clinical recommendation.

2.2.5 Ginseng

2.2.5.1 Background

Native Americans, as well as traditional Chinese medicine practices have utilized ginseng as a whole body tonic, with documented verification of its use in China dating back approximately 2,000 years (Hu 1977; Borchers et al. 2000). The genus name, *Panax*, is derived from the Greek roots *pan* and *akos* meaning "all" and "cure," respectively. American and Asian ginseng belong to the same genus (*Panax*) and generally have similar chemical content, whereas Siberian ginseng refers to a different plant entirely that is distantly related (*Eleutherococcus senticosus*). The best evidence for ginseng's use is for the treatment of Type 2 diabetes, certain cardiovascular conditions, and as an immune booster. In Type 2 diabetes, ginseng mimics insulin activity eliciting a blood glucose lowering effect (Ng and Yeung 1985). In addition to its hypoglycemic effect, many constituents in ginseng have been shown to counteract oxidative stress, induce nitric oxide release, and alter calcium transport, lipid metabolism and platelet adhesiveness, all of which may contribute to the effects of ginseng on the cardiovascular system (Zhou et al. 2004). Ginsenosides are the primary active constituents in ginseng extract. Typically, ginseng extracts are standardized to at least 4% ginsenoside content; however, the content of specific ginsenosides (e.g., Rb1, Rg1, etc.) can vary quite dramatically depending on the extract (Harkey et al. 2001). An examination of 50 commercial ginseng products found ginsenoside content varied between 0% and 9% (w/w) depending on the product (Cui et al. 1994). *Ginseng is further discussed throughout several chapters in this text.*

Ginsenosides themselves are poorly absorbed, but undergo deglycosylation by a diverse set of intestinal micoflora. Metabolism leads to improved absorption, greater bioavailability, and perhaps greater biological effects than the parent compounds (Leung and Wong 2010). This mode of metabolism has interesting implications in regards to precision medicine as both environmental and genetic factors are capable of altering microflora in the gastrointestinal tract. Experiments using human and murine models have both found differences between individuals in their ability to hydrolyze ginsenosides (Hasegawa et al. 1997; Hasegawa and Benno 2000). *In vitro* studies using human liver microsomes found major ginsenoside metabolites are capable of inhibiting CYP2C9 and CYP3A4 activity, suggesting a potential for botanical-drug interactions (Liu et al. 2006). Furthermore, with the exception of the ginsenoside Rd, it is worth noting that limited to no inhibitory effects on CYP enzyme activities were seen with parent ginsenosides (He and Edeki 2004; Liu et al. 2006). Lastly, ginsenoside Rg3 has been shown to serve as a ligand for ABCB1 and is capable of altering the efflux of co-administered drugs (Kim et al. 2003).

2.2.5.2 Evidence

Drug interactions with ginseng first received attention when cases of reduced anticoagulation from warfarin with concurrent ginseng use were reported (Janetzky and Morreale 1997; Rosado 2003; Gurley et al. 2012). A prospective study showed reduced international normalized ratios (a measurement of anticoagulation) with lowered warfarin peak concentrations and exposure when healthy volunteers took American ginseng (Yuan et al. 2004). The findings of this study were limited due to the short-term three-day use of warfarin, the healthy study population, potentially inadequate sampling for the pharmacokinetic determination, and a non-stereoselective assay (Yuan et al. 2004; Gurley et al. 2012). Subsequent studies failed to replicate pharmacokinetic or pharmacodynamic effects of ginseng on warfarin (Jiang et al. 2004; Jiang et al. 2006; Lee et al. 2008b; Gurley et al. 2012). The administration of 500 mg Asian ginseng three times daily did not alter pharmacokinetics of caffeine, debrisoquine, midazolam, chlorzoxazone, suggesting no effect on CYP1A2, 2D6, 3A4, and 2E1 (Gurley et al. 2002; Gurley et al. 2005a). Siberian ginseng in a dosage of 485 mg twice daily did not affect pharmacokinetics of dextromethorphan (CYP2D6 substrate) and alprazolam (CYP3A4 substrate) (Donovan et al. 2003). American ginseng 1 g three times daily, containing dried whole root 500 mg, did not change indinavir (CYP3A4) pharmacokinetics (Andrade et al. 2008). Zidovudine is eliminated via glucuronidation by UGT2B7, and its pharmacokinetics was not affected by supplementation of 200 mg American ginseng twice daily (Lee et al. 2008a).

Overall, while discrepancy exists between results from clinical studies and *in vitro* observations, clinical evidence does not support an inhibitory or inductive action of ginseng administered at recommended standard dosages.

2.2.6 Milk Thistle

2.2.6.1 Background

Recorded use of milk thistle to treat liver disorders and as an antidote dates back to ancient Greek and Roman civilizations (Abenavoli et al. 2010). Its use as a hepatic protectant continues to this day. The pharmacologically active components of milk thistle include silymarin and silybinin (a component of silymarin containing two diastereomers, silybin A and silybin B), which have both been extensively studied based on their hepatoprotective and anti-inflammatory effects. The mechanism of action by which these flavonolignans exert their effect is believed to occur through their antioxidant activities. A wealth of information exists on silymarin's ability to attenuate oxidative stress and act as a free radical scavenger (Surai 2015). Milk thistle extracts are generally standardized to contain at least 70% silymarin content. *See Chapters 7 and 8 for further discussion.*

In humans, silymarin extracts are rapidly absorbed and eliminated with the majority of the dose undergoing extensive glucuronidation and sulfation (Wen et al. 2008). This metabolic profile is thought to limit the utility of *in vitro* studies investigating milk thistle extracts since the concentrations of unconjugated derivatives of silymarin used in these studies are unlikely to be reached in humans. For example, many *in vitro* studies found silybinin capable of inhibiting multiple UGTs and CYP enzymes, yet the concentrations needed for inhibition are typically not enough to be physiologically meaningful (Shord et al. 2009). One exception might be the *in vitro* evidence suggesting that a clinically significant interaction exists between warfarin and silymarin for *CYP2C9**3 carriers (an allele with lower catalytic activity) (Brantley et al. 2010). This observation is in agreement with an earlier clinical study that found altered losartan metabolism among individuals with different *CYP2C9* genotypes (Han et al. 2009a). With respect to transporters, specific flavonolignans have been shown to inhibit ABCB1 activity as well as multiple OATP isoforms to varying degrees (Zhang and Morris 2003; Kock et al. 2013). While the findings from these studies suggest potential pharmacogenetic implications with milk thistle, the *in vivo* relevance is not well established.

2.2.6.2 Evidence

Clinical effect of milk thistle on CYP enzymes has been studied using aminopyrine, phenylbutazone, caffeine, chlorzoxazone, debrisoquine, midazolam, nifedipine, ranitidine, and dextromethorphan (Leber and Knauff 1976; Gurley et al. 2004; Gurley et al. 2006a; Fuhr et al. 2007; Rao et al. 2007; Gurley et al. 2008a; Kawaguchi-Suzuki et al. 2014). Significantly altered effect has not been observed on the pharmacokinetics of these drugs among healthy volunteers, indicating a negligible influence on CYP1A2, 2D6, 2E1, and 3A4 activities (Leber and Knauff 1976; Gurley et al. 2004; Gurley et al. 2006a; Fuhr et al. 2007; Gurley et al. 2008a; Kawaguchi-Suzuki et al. 2014). Significant changes in the pharmacokinetics of ritonavir-boosted darunavir did not occur when patients with HIV infection received milk thistle supplementation (Molto et al. 2012a).

With regard to CYP2C9, the pharmacokinetics of metronidazole (substrate of both CYP3A4 and 2C9) were altered by the use of relatively low-dose 140 mg/day silymarin for 9 days (Rajnarayana et al. 2004). Losartan, another CYP2C9 substrate, was studied in healthy Chinese men, who were *1/*1 extensive metabolizers or *1/*3 intermediate metabolizers, with 14-day treatment with silymarin 140 mg three times daily (Han et al. 2009a). The carriers of *CYP2C9* *1/*1 genotype showed $\geq$2-fold differences in the peak concentration and exposure of losartan between placebo and the silymarin treatments whereas no significant changes in losartan pharmacokinetics were seen in the carriers of *1/*3 genotype (Han et al. 2009a). As an *in vitro* study identified silybin A and silybin B were the most potent constituents inhibiting CYP2C9, a clinical study corroborated that silybin B concentrations attained in healthy volunteers were correlated with peak concentrations of tolbutamide (CYP2C9 substrate) (Brantley et al. 2010; Kawaguchi-Suzuki et al. 2014). Achievement of higher concentrations of silymarin flavonolignans was also reported in patients with hepatitis C infection or nonalcoholic fatty liver disease, suggesting its use needs to be carefully evaluated even though studies in healthy volunteers did not demonstrate alternation of CYP enzyme activities (Schrieber et al. 2008; Hawke et al. 2010; Schrieber et al. 2011). Further investigations are warranted for the effect of milk thistle on CYP2C9 activity for carriers of different metabolizer statuses and with varying concentrations of key constituents.

Milk thistle supplementation has been clinically investigated with various transporter substrates. When indinavir, a substrate of ABCB1 and CYP3A4, was examined with chronic supplementation of milk thistle, a significant effect was not observed (Piscitelli et al. 2002b; DiCenzo et al. 2003). Similarly, changes were not evident with the prototypic ABCB1 substrate, digoxin (Gurley et al. 2006b). Talinolol, which is primarily eliminated to the intestine by ABCB1, showed increase in the exposure by 36% with silymarin administration; however, this was unrelated to the *ABCB1* C3435 T polymorphism, suggesting that the effect is not likely clinically relevant nor ABCB1-mediated (Han et al. 2009b; Hermann and von Richter 2012). Among cancer patients who received milk thistle 200 mg three times daily for 14 days, important changes in irinotecan pharmacokinetics were not observed, indicating no substantial alteration in UGT1A1 and carboxylesterase 2 (van Erp et al. 2005). The pharmacokinetics of rosuvastatin, a multitransporter substrate (intestinal ABCB1, ABCG2, and OATP1A2 and hepatic OATP1B1, 1B3, and 2B1), were not significantly affected in healthy Korean men with silymarin treatment (Deng et al. 2008; Hermann and von Richter 2012).

The clinical studies indicate that milk thistle is unlikely to modulate the activity of CYP1A2, 2D6, 2E1, and 3A4 enzymes and ABC and OATP transporters. The evidence is consistent especially for lack of CYP3A4- or ABCB1-mediated interactions.

2.2.7 Saw Palmetto

2.2.7.1 Background

Historically, Native Americans used saw palmetto to treat urological disorders. Today, its primary use is for the treatment of benign prostatic hyperplasia, which is discussed in the Men's Health chapter (Chua et al. 2014). In spite of saw palmetto's efficacy, its mechanism is poorly understood. Standardized extracts containing greater than 80% liposteric content are recommended and contain multiple sterols and fatty acids. Its mechanisms may include inhibition of 5α-reductase activity, increased metabolism and excretion of dihydrotestosterone, antiandrogen effects, antiestrogen effects, and anti-inflammatory activity (Bonnar-Pizzorno et al. 2006). Overall, saw palmetto is a safe supplement as limited evidence of adverse effects has been reported in patients taking it concomitantly with other agents (Wanwimolruk et al. 2014). *In vitro* data from one source found that a commercially available saw palmetto extract was capable of inhibiting CYP3A4, CYP2D6, and CYP2C9 metabolic activities to a greater extent than other popular botanical products (Yale and Glurich 2005). *See Chapter 9 Men's Health for further discussion.*

2.2.7.2 Evidence

The number of clinical studies with saw palmetto is limited compared to other botanicals covered in this chapter. Saw palmetto administered to healthy volunteers at a dose of 160 mg (standardized to 85%–90% fatty acids and sterols) twice daily for 28 days did not significantly affect CYP1A2, 2D6, 2E1, and 3A4 activities measured by the metabolic ratios of caffeine, debrisoquine, chlorzoxazone, and midazolam respectively (Gurley et al. 2004). In addition, saw palmetto 320 mg daily for 14 days did not alter pharmacokinetics of dextromethorphan (CYP2D6 substrate) and alprazolam (CYP3A4 substrate) in healthy volunteers (Markowitz et al. 2003b). Overall, the impact of saw palmetto supplementation on drug metabolism and disposition is poorly defined based on limited clinical studies.

2.2.8 St. John's Wort

2.2.8.1 Background

St. John's wort contains a variety of chemical structures that contribute to its activity as an antidepressant; however, the most active pharmacologic compounds are hypericin and hyperforin, as well as several flavonoids. Standardization of St. John's wort extract is typically based on hypericin content (0.3%), but may alternatively be standardized to 2%–5% hyperforin (Ulbricht and Natural Standard 2010). *See Chapters 11, 13, and 15 for further discussion.*

Both *in vitro* and *in vivo* studies suggest that St. John's wort alters the metabolism and transport of co-administered drugs. These changes are often attributed to hyperforin as reports of botanical-drug interactions with St. John's wort began appearing after 1998, once a modified extraction method led to a 10–20 fold increase in hyperforin content (Madabushi et al. 2006). The human pregnane X receptor (PXR) plays an important role in the regulation of both CYP3A4 and ABCB1 expression (Wang et al. 2009). This is of particular interest as hyperforin has been shown to not only complex with PXR (Watkins et al. 2003), but also activate it in a concentration-dependent manner *in vitro* (Godtel-Armbrust et al. 2007). Both hyperforin and St. John's wort extract have been shown to increase CYP3A4, CYP2C9, and ABCB1 expression and activity in various human *in vitro* models (Moore et al. 2000; Komoroski et al. 2004; Gutmann et al. 2006; Godtel-Armbrust et al. 2007). This inductive effect on CYP3A and ABCB1 has also been observed in *in vivo* studies using mice (Matheny et al. 2004).

2.2.8.2 Evidence

Because hyperforin was a potent inducer of CYP3A4 and ABCB1 both *in vitro* and in animal studies, botanical-drug interactions can be a clinical concern. The first documentation of clinically significant St. John's wort-drug interaction was in 1999–2000; clinics reported remarkable reductions of cyclosporine concentrations with the concomitant use of St. John's wort in organ transplant recipients, resulting in graft rejection (Gurley et al. 2012).

Clinical studies have demonstrated altered pharmacokinetics of midazolam, cyclosporine, fexofenadine, alprazolam, omeprazole, mephenytoin, nifedipine, and digoxin, indicating induction of CYP3A4, 2E1, and 2C19 and ABCB1, with chronic administration of St. John's wort 300 mg three times daily (Dresser et al. 2003; Markowitz et al. 2003a; Wang et al. 2004a,b; Gurley et al. 2005a; Xie et al. 2005; Gurley et al. 2008b; Wang et al. 2009; Hafner et al. 2010). The pharmacokinetics of dextromethorphan and debrisoquine were not affected, suggesting no modulatory effect on 2D6 (Roby et al. 2001; Markowitz et al. 2003c; Wenk et al. 2004; Gurley et al. 2005a; Gurley et al. 2008a). Evidence is conflicting on the effect of St. John's wort on CYP1A2 activity. Previously, decreased plasma concentrations of theophylline were reported with St. John's wort, but this interaction was not confirmed by a subsequent pharmacokinetic study (Nebel et al. 1999; Morimoto et al. 2004). In a psychiatric patient, a decreased clozapine level was reported, possibly due to CYP1A2 induction (Van Strater and Bogers 2012). However, clinical studies did not show that the pharmacokinetics of caffeine, a CYP1A2 probe, were significantly affected by St. John's wort (Wang et al. 2004a; Gurley et al. 2005a). Similarly, conflicting evidence exists for CYP2C9. While clearance of warfarin was induced by St. John's wort, the pharmacokinetics of other CYP2C9 substrates, ibuprofen and carbamazepine, were not influenced (Burstein et al. 2000; Jiang et al. 2004; Bell et al. 2007).

The severity of drug interaction with St. John's wort appears to depend on hyperfoin content and duration of supplementation. A hyperforin content of 0.2 mg three times daily for 14 days did not significantly affect cyclosporine pharmacokinetics (Mai et al. 2004). Similarly, pharmacokinetics of alprazolam, caffeine, tolbutamide, and digoxin were not significantly affected by low hyperforin content of 3.5 mg daily (Arold et al. 2005). In addition, CYP3A4 was not induced by the 3-day administration of St. John's wort, while a supplementation for 10 days or longer resulted in the induction (Markowitz et al. 2000; Markowitz et al. 2003a). It takes approximately one week for the induced CYP3A activity to return to basal levels after discontinuing St. John's wort treatment (Imai et al. 2008).

Multiple episodes of CYP3A and ABCB1 induction caused by St. John's wort have been reported. As reduced cyclosporine levels were reported in transplant recipients, tacrolimus trough levels were also decreased in renal transplant patients (Bolley et al. 2002). Reductions in the level of immunosuppression may lead to graft loss, so this type of interaction is particularly concerning. Several cases of breakthrough bleeding and unintentional pregnancy have also been reported among women who used St. John's wort with combined oral contraceptives due to induced CYP3A metabolism (Murphy 2002; Hall et al. 2003). Women taking combined oral contraceptives should be warned about potential breakthrough bleeding before using St. John's wort and to recommend the use of additional barrier method of contraception. The CYP3A4-medicated interactions with antiretroviral drugs, such as indinavir and nevirapine, and with anticancer drugs, for example imatinib and irinotecan, should also be avoided (Piscitelli et al. 2000; de Maat et al. 2001; Izzo 2012; Wanwimolruk and Prachayasittikul 2014). In a patient receiving methadone, St. John's wort induced withdrawal symptoms due to decreased drug levels (Eich-Hochli et al. 2003). Since patients may experience discomfort, they should be cautioned about using St. John's wort with methadone. For drugs that have a wide therapeutic index but undergo extensive CYP3A metabolism such as simvastatin, the therapeutic effect should be monitored if patients are using St. John's wort comcomitantly (Sugimoto et al. 2001).

Genetic factors have been extensively studied for St. John's wort-drug interactions than for other botanicals covered in this chapter. As mentioned earlier, PXR is involved in regulating *CYP3A4* gene transcription and the *PXR* gene haplotype, H1/H1, has been associated with weaker basal transcriptional activity (Wang et al. 2009). However, study participants with *PXR* H1/H1 haplotype had significantly attenuated exposure to nifedipine (CYP3A4 substrate); greater induction of CYP3A4 transcription was observed in these participants, compared to those with *PXR* H1/H2 and H2/H2 haplotypes (Wang et al. 2009). CYP2C19-mediated interactions with St. John's wort may also be genotype-dependent. *CYP2C19* extensive metabolizers with *1/*1 genotype had significantly higher induction of mephenytoin metabolism, compared to poor metabolizers carrying *2/*2 or *2/*3 genotype (Wang et al. 2004b). This greater induction of CYP2C19 activity in extensive metabolizers, compared to *2/*2 or *2/*3 carriers, was confirmed with omeprazole (Wang et al. 2004a). In addition, the higher risk of voriconazole treatment failure has been suggested with use of St. John's wort in *CYP2C19* *1/*1 genotype carriers due to the greater induction of the enzyme than in individuals with *1/*2 or *2/*2 genotype (Rengelshausen et al. 2005). Clinical evidence is conflicting on CYP2C9, slightly and not statistically significant decrease in clearance of gliclazide was reported in *CYP2C9* *1/*2 or *2/*2 carriers than in *1/*1 or *1/*3 carriers (Xu et al. 2008). St. John's wort is known to induce ABCB1, and *ABCB1* haplotype comprising 1236C > T, 2677G > T/A, and 3435C > T was associated with the degree of ABCB1 induction by St. John's wort (Schwarz et al. 2007). Study participants with the *ABCB1* variant haplotype had smaller changes in talinolol exposure and duodenal *ABCB1* mRNA expression levels after chronic St. John's wort administration, compared to those with *ABCB1* wild-type haplotype; the variant haplotype carriers had blunted induction in response to the supplementation (Schwarz et al. 2007).

Overall, inductive effect of St. John's wort on CYP2E1 and CYP3A was clinically shown and consistent with *in vitro* and animal models. Limited evidence suggests that induction of CYP2C9, CYP2C19, and ABCB1 may be genotype-dependent. St. John's wort is not likely affect CYP2D6 significantly, but mixed observations have been reported with regard to CYP1A2.

2.3 Conclusions

The clinical effects of botanicals on CYP enzymes and transporters are summarized in Table 2.3. Overall, black cohosh, garlic, ginkgo ($\leq$240 mg/day), ginseng, echinacea, milk thistle, and saw palmetto generally have low risk for drug interactions. On the other hand, St. John's wort may cause a drug interaction if its use is not carefully evaluated in each patient with concomitant drug therapy. A major limitation has been that the clinical data with botanical use were commonly obtained among healthy volunteers. If botanicals are to be used in a population with multiple diseases, especially among those with hepatic or renal dysfunction, caution should be exercised since the active constituents may accumulate. In addition, pharmacokinetic evidence related to botanical use is limited in the elderly and pediatric population. Since CYP expression is age-dependent, the age of the patient is another important factor to consider. (Zanger and Schwab 2013) Based on limited clinical evidence, capacity for CYP-mediated metabolism may change as patients age, potentially making the elderly more susceptible to certain botanical-drug interactions such as St. John's wort (Gurley et al. 2005a).

Clinical evidence does not necessarily corroborate *in vitro* and animal data as reviewed in this chapter. Various factors can be considered for this reason such as constituent concentrations attained *in vivo* at sites of action, where enzymes and transporters are located, and extent of variability inherent among study

TABLE 2.3

Summary of Findings from Clinical Studies on Drug-Metabolizing Enzymes and Transporters

Botanical	Findings
Black cohosh	• No effect on CYP1A2, CYP2D6, CYP2E1, CYP3A, and ABCB1
Echinacea	• No effect on CYP1A2, CYP2C9, CYP2D6, CYP2E1, CYP3A, ABCB1, and OATP
Garlic	• No effect on CYP1A2, CYP2C9, CYP2D6, CYP3A, and OATP1B1 • Mild inhibitory effect on CYP2E1 by garlic oil • Mild inductive effect on ABCB1 • Potentially genotype-dependent effect inhibition of CYP2C19
Ginkgo	• No effect on CYP1A2, CYP2B6, CYP2C9, CYP2D6, CYP2E1, OATP, and OCT • Mixed observations on CYP3A and ABCB1 • Potentially genotype-dependent induction of CYP2C19
Ginseng	• No effect on CYP1A2, CYP2C9, CYP2D6, CYP3A, CYP2E1, and UGT2B7
Milk thistle	• No effect on CYP1A2, CYP2D6, CYP2E1, CYP3A, ABC, OATP, UGT1A1, and carboxylesterase 2 • Potentially genotype-dependent inhibition of CYP2C9
Saw Palmetto	• No effect on CYP1A2, CYP2D6, CYP2E1, and CYP3A
St. John's wort	• Inductive effect on CYP2E1 and CYP3A • Potentially genotype-dependent induction of CYP2C9, CYP2C19, and ABCB1 • No effect on CYP2D6 • Mixed observation on CYP1A2

participants including sex, ethnicity, and genetic variation. In addition, serious consideration needs to be given for different commercial preparations, which may vary in terms of constituent types and amounts and how they are formulated.

Studies conducted with garlic, ginkgo, echinacea, milk thistle, and St. John's wort have provided pharmacogenetic data. However, the only genotype-dependent effect verified by an independent study is CYP2C19 induction by St. John's wort, where *1/*1 carriers had more pronounced induction, compared to *2 or *3 variant carriers. Patients with *CYP2C19* *1/*1 genotype may be more susceptible to St. John's wort-drug interaction; therefore, it should be carefully evaluated whether St. John's wort is appropriate and necessary when a concomitant drug extensively metabolized by CYP2C19 is present. Pharmacogenomic information is limited or lacking for the other botanicals and presents a serious gap in our knowledge considering the ubiquitous use of these products. In order to predict patient's response based on genomic data, further investigation is warranted.

REFERENCES

Abenavoli, L., R. Capasso, N. Milic, and F. Capasso. 2010. "Milk thistle in liver diseases: past, present, future." *Phytother Res* 24 (10):1423–32. doi: 10.1002/ptr.3207.

Amagase, H. 2006. "Clarifying the real bioactive constituents of garlic." *J Nutr* 136 (3 Suppl):716S–25S.

Andrade, A. S., C. Hendrix, T. L. Parsons, B. Caballero, C. S. Yuan, C. W. Flexner, A. S. Dobs, and T. T. Brown. 2008. "Pharmacokinetic and metabolic effects of American ginseng (Panax quinquefolius) in healthy volunteers receiving the HIV protease inhibitor indinavir." *BMC Complement Altern Med* 8:50. doi: 10.1186/1472–6882-8-50.

Arold, G., F. Donath, A. Maurer, K. Diefenbach, S. Bauer, H. H. Henneicke-von Zepelin, M. Friede, and I. Roots. 2005. "No relevant interaction with alprazolam, caffeine, tolbutamide, and digoxin by treatment with a low-hyperforin St John's wort extract." *Planta Med* 71 (4):331–7. doi: 10.1055/s-2005-864099.

Aruna, D., and M. U. Naidu. 2007. "Pharmacodynamic interaction studies of Ginkgo biloba with cilostazol and clopidogrel in healthy human subjects." *Br J Clin Pharmacol* 63 (3):333–8. doi: 10.1111/j.1365-2125.2006.02759.x.

Barnes, J., L. A. Anderson, S. Gibbons, and J. D. Phillipson. 2005. "Echinacea species (Echinacea angustifolia (DC.) Hell., Echinacea pallida (Nutt.) Nutt., Echinacea purpurea (L.) Moench): A review of their chemistry, pharmacology and clinical properties." *J Pharm Pharmacol* 57 (8):929–54. doi: 10.1211/0022357056127.

Barrett, B. 2003. "Medicinal properties of Echinacea: A critical review." *Phytomedicine* 10 (1):66–86. doi: 10.1078/094471103321648692.

Bell, E. C., W. R. Ravis, K. B. Lloyd, and T. J. Stokes. 2007. "Effects of St. John's wort supplementation on ibuprofen pharmacokinetics." *Ann Pharmacother* 41 (2):229–34. doi: 10.1345/aph.1H602.

Bodinet, C., and J. Freudenstein. 2002. "Influence of Cimicifuga racemosa on the proliferation of estrogen receptor-positive human breast cancer cells." *Breast Cancer Res Treat* 76 (1):1–10.

Bolley, R., C. Zulke, M. Kammerl, M. Fischereder, and B. K. Kramer. 2002. "Tacrolimus-induced nephrotoxicity unmasked by induction of the CYP3A4 system with St John's wort." *Transplantation* 73 (6):1009.

Bonnar-Pizzorno, R. M., A. J. Littman, M. Kestin, and E. White. 2006. "Saw palmetto supplement use and prostate cancer risk." *Nutr Cancer* 55 (1):21–7. doi: 10.1207/s15327914nc5501_3.

Borchers, A. T., C. L. Keen, J. S. Stern, and M. E. Gershwin. 2000. "Inflammation and Native American medicine: The role of botanicals." *Am J Clin Nutr* 72 (2):339–47.

Bradley, P. R., and British Herbal Medicine Association. Scientific Committee. 2010. *British herbal compendium: A handbook of scientific information on widely used plant drugs.* British Herbal Medicine Association: Exeter.

Brantley, S. J., N. H. Oberlies, D. J. Kroll, and M. F. Paine. 2010. "Two flavonolignans from milk thistle (Silybum marianum) inhibit CYP2C9-mediated warfarin metabolism at clinically achievable concentrations." *J Pharmacol Exp Ther* 332 (3):1081–7. doi: 10.1124/jpet.109.161927.

Budzinski, J. W., B. C. Foster, S. Vandenhoek, and J. T. Arnason. 2000. "An *in vitro* evaluation of human cytochrome P450 3A4 inhibition by selected commercial herbal extracts and tinctures." *Phytomedicine* 7 (4):273–82. doi: 10.1016/S0944-7113(00)80044-6.

Burstein, A. H., R. L. Horton, T. Dunn, R. M. Alfaro, S. C. Piscitelli, and W. Theodore. 2000. "Lack of effect of St John's Wort on carbamazepine pharmacokinetics in healthy volunteers." *Clin Pharmacol Ther* 68 (6):605–12. doi: 10.1067/mcp.2000.111530.

Chua, T., N. T. Eise, J. S. Simpson, and S. Ventura. 2014. "Pharmacological characterization and chemical fractionation of a liposterolic extract of saw palmetto (Serenoa repens): effects on rat prostate contractility." *J Ethnopharmacol* 152 (2):283–91. doi: 10.1016/j.jep.2013.12.030.

Cui, J., M. Garle, P. Eneroth, and I. Bjorkhem. 1994. "What do commercial ginseng preparations contain?" *Lancet* 344 (8915):134.

Davenport, D. M., and M. J. Wargovich. 2005. "Modulation of cytochrome P450 enzymes by organosulfur compounds from garlic." *Food Chem Toxicol* 43 (12):1753–62. doi: 10.1016/j.fct.2005.05.018.

de Maat, M. M., R. M. Hoetelmans, R. A. Math t, E. C. van Gorp, P. L. Meenhorst, J. W. Mulder, and J. H. Beijnen. 2001. "Drug interaction between St John's wort and nevirapine." *AIDS* 15 (3):420–1.

Deeken, J. 2009. "The Affymetrix DMET platform and pharmacogenetics in drug development." *Curr Opin Mol Ther* 11 (3):260–8.

Deng, J. W., J. H. Shon, H. J. Shin, S. J. Park, C. W. Yeo, H. H. Zhou, I. S. Song, and J. G. Shin. 2008. "Effect of silymarin supplement on the pharmacokinetics of rosuvastatin." *Pharm Res* 25 (8):1807–14. doi: 10.1007/s11095-007-9492-0.

DiCenzo, R., M. Shelton, K. Jordan, C. Koval, A. Forrest, R. Reichman, and G. Morse. 2003. "Coadministration of milk thistle and indinavir in healthy subjects." *Pharmacotherapy* 23 (7):866–70.

Donovan, J. L., C. L. DeVane, K. D. Chavin, R. M. Taylor, and J. S. Markowitz. 2003. "Siberian ginseng (Eleutheroccus senticosus) effects on CYP2D6 and CYP3A4 activity in normal volunteers." *Drug Metab Dispos* 31 (5):519–22.

Dresser, G. K., U. I. Schwarz, G. R. Wilkinson, and R. B. Kim. 2003. "Coordinate induction of both cytochrome P4503A and MDR1 by St John's wort in healthy subjects." *Clin Pharmacol Ther* 73 (1):41–50. doi: 10.1067/mcp.2003.10.

Duker, E. M., L. Kopanski, H. Jarry, and W. Wuttke. 1991. "Effects of extracts from Cimicifuga racemosa on gonadotropin release in menopausal women and ovariectomized rats." *Planta Med* 57 (5):420–4. doi: 10.1055/s-2006-960139.

Eich-Hochli, D., R. Oppliger, K. P. Golay, P. Baumann, and C. B. Eap. 2003. "Methadone maintenance treatment and St. John''s Wort—a case report." *Pharmacopsychiatry* 36 (1):35–7. doi: 10.1055/s-2003-38090.

Engelsen, J., J. D. Nielsen, and K. Winther. 2002. "Effect of coenzyme Q10 and Ginkgo biloba on warfarin dosage in stable, long-term warfarin treated outpatients. A randomised, double blind, placebo-crossover trial." *Thromb Haemost* 87 (6):1075–6.

Evans, W. E., and M. V. Relling. 1999. "Pharmacogenomics: translating functional genomics into rational therapeutics." *Science* 286 (5439):487–91.

Fan, L., X. Q. Mao, G. Y. Tao, G. Wang, F. Jiang, Y. Chen, Q. Li et al. 2009a. "Effect of Schisandra chinensis extract and Ginkgo biloba extract on the pharmacokinetics of talinolol in healthy volunteers." *Xenobiotica* 39 (3):249–54. doi: 10.1080/00498250802687657.

Fan, L., G. Y. Tao, G. Wang, Y. Chen, W. Zhang, Y. J. He, Q. Li et al. 2009b. "Effects of Ginkgo biloba extract ingestion on the pharmacokinetics of talinolol in healthy Chinese volunteers." *Ann Pharmacother* 43 (5):944–9. doi: 10.1345/aph.1L656.

Flockhart, D. A., D. O'Kane, M. S. Williams, M. S. Watson, D. A. Flockhart, B. Gage, R. Gandolfi et al. 2008. "Pharmacogenetic testing of CYP2C9 and VKORC1 alleles for warfarin." *Genet Med* 10 (2):139–50. doi: 10.1097/GIM.0b013e318163c35f.

Foster, B. C., M. S. Foster, S. Vandenhoek, A. Krantis, J. W. Budzinski, J. T. Arnason, K. D. Gallicano, and S. Choudri. 2001. "An *in vitro* evaluation of human cytochrome P450 3A4 and P-glycoprotein inhibition by garlic." *J Pharm Pharm Sci* 4 (2):176–84.

Fuchikami, H., H. Satoh, M. Tsujimoto, S. Ohdo, H. Ohtani, and Y. Sawada. 2006. "Effects of herbal extracts on the function of human organic anion-transporting polypeptide OATP-B." *Drug Metab Dispos* 34 (4):577–82. doi: 10.1124/dmd.105.007872.

Fuhr, U., S. Beckmann-Knopp, A. Jetter, H. Luck, and U. Mengs. 2007. "The effect of silymarin on oral nifedipine pharmacokinetics." *Planta Med* 73 (14):1429–35. doi: 10.1055/s-2007-990256.

Gallicano, K., B. Foster, and S. Choudhri. 2003. "Effect of short-term administration of garlic supplements on single-dose ritonavir pharmacokinetics in healthy volunteers." *Br J Clin Pharmacol* 55 (2):199–202.

Gaudineau, C., R. Beckerman, S. Welbourn, and K. Auclair. 2004. "Inhibition of human P450 enzymes by multiple constituents of the Ginkgo biloba extract." *Biochem Biophys Res Commun* 318 (4):1072–8. doi: 10.1016/j.bbrc.2004.04.139.

Gilroy, C. M., J. F. Steiner, T. Byers, H. Shapiro, and W. Georgian. 2003. "Echinacea and truth in labeling." *Arch Intern Med* 163 (6):699–704.

Godtel-Armbrust, U., A. Metzger, U. Kroll, O. Kelber, and L. Wojnowski. 2007. "Variability in PXR-mediated induction of CYP3A4 by commercial preparations and dry extracts of St. John's wort." *Naunyn Schmiedebergs Arch Pharmacol* 375 (6):377–82. doi: 10.1007/s00210-007-0172-8.

Gorski, J. C., S. M. Huang, A. Pinto, M. A. Hamman, J. K. Hilligoss, N. A. Zaheer, M. Desai, M. Miller, and S. D. Hall. 2004. "The effect of echinacea (Echinacea purpurea root) on cytochrome P450 activity *in vivo*." *Clin Pharmacol Ther* 75 (1):89–100. doi: 10.1016/j.clpt.2003.09.013.

Greenblatt, D. J., L. L. von Moltke, Y. Luo, E. S. Perloff, K. A. Horan, A. Bruce, R. C. Reynolds et al. 2006. "Ginkgo biloba does not alter clearance of flurbiprofen, a cytochrome P450-2C9 substrate." *J Clin Pharmacol* 46 (2):214–21. doi: 10.1177/0091270005283465.

Gurley, B., M. A. Hubbard, D. K. Williams, J. Thaden, Y. Tong, W. B. Gentry, P. Breen, D. J. Carrier, and S. Cheboyina. 2006a. "Assessing the clinical significance of botanical supplementation on human cytochrome P450 3A activity: comparison of a milk thistle and black cohosh product to rifampin and clarithromycin." *J Clin Pharmacol* 46 (2):201–13. doi: 10.1177/0091270005284854.

Gurley, B. J. 2012. "Pharmacokinetic herb-drug interactions (part 1): origins, mechanisms, and the impact of botanical dietary supplements." *Planta Med* 78 (13):1478–89. doi: 10.1055/s-0031-1298273.

Gurley, B. J., G. W. Barone, D. K. Williams, J. Carrier, P. Breen, C. R. Yates, P. F. Song, M. A. Hubbard, Y. Tong, and S. Cheboyina. 2006b. "Effect of milk thistle (Silybum marianum) and black cohosh (Cimicifuga racemosa) supplementation on digoxin pharmacokinetics in humans." *Drug Metab Dispos* 34 (1):69–74. doi: 10.1124/dmd.105.006312.

Gurley, B. J., E. K. Fifer, and Z. Gardner. 2012. "Pharmacokinetic herb-drug interactions (part 2): drug interactions involving popular botanical dietary supplements and their clinical relevance." *Planta Med* 78 (13):1490–514. doi: 10.1055/s-0031-1298331.

Gurley, B. J., S. F. Gardner, M. A. Hubbard, D. K. Williams, W. B. Gentry, J. Carrier, I. A. Khan, D. J. Edwards, and A. Shah. 2004. "In vivo assessment of botanical supplementation on human cytochrome P450 phenotypes: Citrus aurantium, Echinacea purpurea, milk thistle, and saw palmetto." *Clin Pharmacol Ther* 76 (5):428–40. doi: 10.1016/j.clpt.2004.07.007.

Gurley, B. J., S. F. Gardner, M. A. Hubbard, D. K. Williams, W. B. Gentry, Y. Cui, and C. Y. Ang. 2002. "Cytochrome P450 phenotypic ratios for predicting herb-drug interactions in humans." *Clin Pharmacol Ther* 72 (3):276–87. doi: 10.1067/mcp.2002.126913.

Gurley, B. J., S. F. Gardner, M. A. Hubbard, D. K. Williams, W. B. Gentry, Y. Cui, and C. Y. Ang. 2005a. "Clinical assessment of effects of botanical supplementation on cytochrome P450 phenotypes in the elderly: St John's wort, garlic oil, Panax ginseng and Ginkgo biloba." *Drugs Aging* 22 (6):525–39.

Gurley, B. J., S. F. Gardner, M. A. Hubbard, D. K. Williams, W. B. Gentry, I. A. Khan, and A. Shah. 2005b. "In vivo effects of goldenseal, kava kava, black cohosh, and valerian on human cytochrome P450 1A2, 2D6, 2E1, and 3A4/5 phenotypes." *Clin Pharmacol Ther* 77 (5):415–26. doi: 10.1016/j. clpt.2005.01.009.

Gurley, B. J., A. Swain, M. A. Hubbard, D. K. Williams, G. Barone, F. Hartsfield, Y. Tong, D. J. Carrier, S. Cheboyina, and S. K. Battu. 2008a. "Clinical assessment of CYP2D6-mediated herb-drug interactions in humans: effects of milk thistle, black cohosh, goldenseal, kava kava, St. John's wort, and Echinacea." *Mol Nutr Food Res* 52 (7):755–63. doi: 10.1002/mnfr.200600300.

Gurley, B. J., A. Swain, D. K. Williams, G. Barone, and S. K. Battu. 2008b. "Gauging the clinical significance of P-glycoprotein-mediated herb-drug interactions: comparative effects of St. John's wort, Echinacea, clarithromycin, and rifampin on digoxin pharmacokinetics." *Mol Nutr Food Res* 52 (7):772–9. doi: 10.1002/mnfr.200700081.

Gutmann, H., B. Poller, K.B. Buter, A. Pfrunder, W. Schaffner, and J. Drewe. 2006. "Hypericum perforatum: Which constituents may induce intestinal MDR1 and CYP3A4 mRNA expression?" *Planta Med* 72 (8):685–90. doi: 10.1055/s-2006-931585.

Gwilt, P. R., C. L. Lear, M. A. Tempero, D. D. Birt, A. C. Grandjean, R. W. Ruddon, and D. L. Nagel. 1994. "The effect of garlic extract on human metabolism of acetaminophen." *Cancer Epidemiol Biomarkers Prev* 3 (2):155–60.

Hafner, V., M. Jager, A. K. Matthee, R. Ding, J. Burhenne, W. E. Haefeli, and G. Mikus. 2010. "Effect of simultaneous induction and inhibition of CYP3A by St John's Wort and ritonavir on CYP3A activity." *Clin Pharmacol Ther* 87 (2):191–6. doi: 10.1038/clpt.2009.206.

Hajda, J., K. M. Rentsch, C. Gubler, H. Steinert, B. Stieger, and K. Fattinger. 2010. "Garlic extract induces intestinal P-glycoprotein, but exhibits no effect on intestinal and hepatic CYP3A4 in humans." *Eur J Pharm Sci* 41 (5):729–35. doi: 10.1016/j.ejps.2010.09.016.

Hall, S. D., Z. Wang, S. M. Huang, M. A. Hamman, N. Vasavada, A. Q. Adigun, J. K. Hilligoss, M. Miller, and J. C. Gorski. 2003. "The interaction between St John's wort and an oral contraceptive." *Clin Pharmacol Ther* 74 (6):525–35. doi: 10.1016/j.clpt.2003.08.009.

Han, Y., D. Guo, Y. Chen, Y. Chen, Z. R. Tan, and H. H. Zhou. 2009a. "Effect of silymarin on the pharmacokinetics of losartan and its active metabolite E-3174 in healthy Chinese volunteers." *Eur J Clin Pharmacol* 65 (6):585–91. doi: 10.1007/s00228-009-0624-9.

Han, Y., D. Guo, Y. Chen, Z. R. Tan, and H. H. Zhou. 2009b. "Effect of continuous silymarin administration on oral talinolol pharmacokinetics in healthy volunteers." *Xenobiotica* 39 (9):694–9. doi: 10.1080/00498250903060077.

Hansen, T. S., and O. G. Nilsen. 2009. "Echinacea purpurea and P-glycoprotein drug transport in Caco-2 cells." *Phytother Res* 23 (1):86–91. doi: 10.1002/ptr.2563.

Harkey, M. R., G. L. Henderson, M. E. Gershwin, J. S. Stern, and R. M. Hackman. 2001. "Variability in commercial ginseng products: an analysis of 25 preparations." *Am J Clin Nutr* 73 (6):1101–6.

Hasegawa, H., and Y. Benno. 2000. "Anticarcinogenesis in mice by Ginseng-Hydrolyzing Colonic bacteria." *Microb Ecol Health D* 12 (2):85–91. doi: 10.1080/089106000435473.

Hasegawa, H., J. H. Sung, and Y. Benno. 1997. "Role of human intestinal Prevotella oris in hydrolyzing ginseng saponins." *Planta Med* 63 (5):436–40. doi: 10.1055/s-2006-957729.

Hawke, R. L., S. J. Schrieber, T. A. Soule, Z. Wen, P. C. Smith, K. R. Reddy, A. S. Wahed et al. 2010. "Silymarin ascending multiple oral dosing phase I study in noncirrhotic patients with chronic hepatitis C." *J Clin Pharmacol* 50 (4):434–49. doi: 10.1177/0091270009347475.

He, N., and T. Edeki. 2004. "The inhibitory effects of herbal components on CYP2C9 and CYP3A4 catalytic activities in human liver microsomes." *Am J Ther* 11 (3):206–12.

Hellum, B. H., and O. G. Nilsen. 2008. "In vitro inhibition of CYP3A4 metabolism and P-glycoprotein-mediated transport by trade herbal products." *Basic Clin Pharmacol Toxicol* 102 (5):466–75. doi: 10.1111/j.1742-7843.2008.00227.x.

Hermann, R., and O. von Richter. 2012. "Clinical evidence of herbal drugs as perpetrators of pharmacokinetic drug interactions." *Planta Med* 78 (13):1458–77. doi: 10.1055/s-0032-1315117.

Ho, B. E., D. D. Shen, J. S. McCune, T. Bui, L. Risler, Z. Yang, and R. J. Ho. 2010. "Effects of garlic on cytochromes P450 2C9- and 3A4-mediated drug metabolism in human hepatocytes." *Sci Pharm* 78 (3):473–81. doi: 10.3797/scipharm.1002-11.

Hu, S. Y. 1977. "A contribution to our knowledge of ginseng." *Am J Chin Med (Gard City N Y)* 5 (1):1–23.

Huang, Y., B. Jiang, P. Nuntanakorn, E. J. Kennelly, S. Shord, T. O. Lawal, and G. B. Mahady. 2010. "Fukinolic acid derivatives and triterpene glycosides from black cohosh inhibit CYP isozymes, but are not cytotoxic to Hep-G2 cells *in vitro*." *Curr Drug Saf* 5 (2):118–24.

Imai, H., T. Kotegawa, K. Tsutsumi, T. Morimoto, N. Eshima, S. Nakano, and K. Ohashi. 2008. "The recovery time-course of CYP3A after induction by St John's wort administration." *Br J Clin Pharmacol* 65 (5):701–7. doi: 10.1111/j.1365-2125.2008.03120.x.

Isah, T. 2015. "Rethinking Ginkgo biloba L.: Medicinal uses and conservation." *Pharmacogn Rev* 9 (18):140–8. doi: 10.4103/0973-7847.162137.

Izzo, A. A. 2012. "Interactions between herbs and conventional drugs: Overview of the clinical data." *Med Princ Pract* 21 (5):404–28. doi: 10.1159/000334488.

Janetzky, K., and A. P. Morreale. 1997. "Probable interaction between warfarin and ginseng." *Am J Health Syst Pharm* 54 (6):692–3.

Jarry, H., and G. Harnischfeger. 1985. "Studies on the endocrine effects of the contents of Cimicifuga racemosa." *Planta Med* 51 (1):46–9. doi: 10.1055/s-2007-969390.

Jarry, H., G. Harnischfeger, and E. Duker. 1985. "Studies on the endocrine effects of the contents of Cimicifuga racemosa 2. In vitro binding of compounds to estrogen receptors." *Planta Med* 51 (4):316–9. doi: 10.1055/s-2007-969500.

Jiang, X., E. Y. Blair, and A. J. McLachlan. 2006. "Investigation of the effects of herbal medicines on warfarin response in healthy subjects: A population pharmacokinetic-pharmacodynamic modeling approach." *J Clin Pharmacol* 46 (11):1370–8. doi: 10.1177/0091270006292124.

Jiang, X., K. M. Williams, W. S. Liauw, A. J. Ammit, B. D. Roufogalis, C. C. Duke, R. O. Day, and A. J. McLachlan. 2004. "Effect of St John's wort and ginseng on the pharmacokinetics and pharmacodynamics of warfarin in healthy subjects." *Br J Clin Pharmacol* 57 (5):592–9. doi: 10.1111/j.1365-2125.2003.02051.x.

Jiang, X., K. M. Williams, W. S. Liauw, A. J. Ammit, B. D. Roufogalis, C. C. Duke, R. O. Day, and A. J. McLachlan. 2005. "Effect of ginkgo and ginger on the pharmacokinetics and pharmacodynamics of warfarin in healthy subjects." *Br J Clin Pharmacol* 59 (4):425–32. doi: 10.1111/j.1365-2125.2005.02322.x.

Johnson, B. M., and R. B. van Breemen. 2003. "In vitro formation of quinoid metabolites of the dietary supplement Cimicifuga racemosa (black cohosh)." *Chem Res Toxicol* 16 (7):838–46. doi: 10.1021/tx020108n.

Kawaguchi-Suzuki, M., R. F. Frye, H. J. Zhu, B. J. Brinda, K. D. Chavin, H. J. Bernstein, and J. S. Markowitz. 2014. "The effects of milk thistle (Silybum marianum) on human cytochrome P450 activity." *Drug Metab Dispos* 42 (10):1611–6. doi: 10.1124/dmd.114.057232.

Kim, B. H., K. P. Kim, K. S. Lim, J. R. Kim, S. H. Yoon, J. Y. Cho, Y. O. Lee et al. 2010. "Influence of Ginkgo biloba extract on the pharmacodynamic effects and pharmacokinetic properties of ticlopidine: an open-label, randomized, two-period, two-treatment, two-sequence, single-dose crossover study in healthy Korean male volunteers." *Clin Ther* 32 (2):380–90. doi: 10.1016/j.clinthera.2010.01.027.

Kim, S. W., H. Y. Kwon, D. W. Chi, J. H. Shim, J. D. Park, Y. H. Lee, S. Pyo, and D. K. Rhee. 2003. "Reversal of P-glycoprotein-mediated multidrug resistance by ginsenoside Rg(3)." *Biochem Pharmacol* 65 (1):75–82.

Kock, K., Y. Xie, R. L. Hawke, N. H. Oberlies, and K. L. Brouwer. 2013. "Interaction of silymarin flavonolignans with organic anion-transporting polypeptides." *Drug Metab Dispos* 41 (5):958–65. doi: 10.1124/dmd.112.048272.

Komoroski, B. J., S. Zhang, H. Cai, J. M. Hutzler, R. Frye, T. S. Tracy, S. C. Strom et al. 2004. "Induction and inhibition of cytochromes P450 by the St. John's wort constituent hyperforin in human hepatocyte cultures." *Drug Metab Dispos* 32 (5):512–8. doi: 10.1124/dmd.32.5.512.

Kudolo, G. B., W. Wang, M. Javors, and J. Blodgett. 2006. "The effect of the ingestion of Ginkgo biloba extract (EGb 761) on the pharmacokinetics of metformin in non-diabetic and type 2 diabetic subjects--a double blind placebo-controlled, crossover study." *Clin Nutr* 25 (4):606–16. doi: 10.1016/j.clnu.2005.12.012.

Leber, H. W., and S. Knauff. 1976. "Influence of silymarin on drug metabolizing enzymes in rat and man." *Arzneimittelforschung* 26 (8):1603–5.

Lee, L. S., S. D. Wise, C. Chan, T. L. Parsons, C. Flexner, and P. S. Lietman. 2008a. "Possible differential induction of phase 2 enzyme and antioxidant pathways by american ginseng, Panax quinquefolius." *J Clin Pharmacol* 48 (5):599–609. doi: 10.1177/0091270008314252.

Lee, S. H., Y. M. Ahn, S. Y. Ahn, H. K. Doo, and B. C. Lee. 2008b. "Interaction between warfarin and Panax ginseng in ischemic stroke patients." *J Altern Complement Med* 14 (6):715–21. doi: 10.1089/acm.2007.0799.

Lei, H. P., W. Ji, J. Lin, H. Chen, Z. R. Tan, D. L. Hu, L. J. Liu, and H. H. Zhou. 2009a. "Effects of Ginkgo biloba extract on the pharmacokinetics of bupropion in healthy volunteers." *Br J Clin Pharmacol* 68 (2):201–6. doi: 10.1111/j.1365-2125.2009.03442.x.

Lei, H. P., G. Wang, L. S. Wang, D. S. Ou-yang, H. Chen, Q. Li, W. Zhang et al. 2009b. "Lack of effect of Ginkgo biloba on voriconazole pharmacokinetics in Chinese volunteers identified as CYP2C19 poor and extensive metabolizers." *Ann Pharmacother* 43 (4):726–31. doi: 10.1345/aph.1L537.

Leung, K. W., and A. S. Wong. 2010. "Pharmacology of ginsenosides: a literature review." *Chin Med* 5:20. doi: 10.1186/1749-8546-5-20.

Liske, E. 1998. "Therapeutic efficacy and safety of Cimicifuga racemosa for gynecologic disorders." *Adv Ther* 15 (1):45–53.

Liske, E., W. Hanggi, H. H. Henneicke-von Zepelin, N. Boblitz, P. Wustenberg, and V. W. Rahlfs. 2002. "Physiological investigation of a unique extract of black cohosh (Cimicifugae racemosae rhizoma): A 6-month clinical study demonstrates no systemic estrogenic effect." *J Womens Health Gend Based Med* 11 (2):163–74. doi: 10.1089/152460902753645308.

Liu, Y., J. W. Zhang, W. Li, H. Ma, J. Sun, M. C. Deng, and L. Yang. 2006. "Ginsenoside metabolites, rather than naturally occurring ginsenosides, lead to inhibition of human cytochrome P450 enzymes." *Toxicol Sci* 91 (2):356–64. doi: 10.1093/toxsci/kfj164.

Loizou, G. D., and J. Cocker. 2001. "The effects of alcohol and diallyl sulphide on CYP2E1 activity in humans: a phenotyping study using chlorzoxazone." *Hum Exp Toxicol* 20 (7):321–7.

Lu, W. J., J. D. Huang, and M. L. Lai. 2006. "The effects of ergoloid mesylates and ginkgo biloba on the pharmacokinetics of ticlopidine." *J Clin Pharmacol* 46 (6):628–34. doi: 10.1177/0091270006287024.

Lupu, R., I. Mehmi, E. Atlas, M. S. Tsai, E. Pisha, H. A. Oketch-Rabah, P. Nuntanakorn, E. J. Kennelly, and F. Kronenberg. 2003. "Black cohosh, a menopausal remedy, does not have estrogenic activity and does not promote breast cancer cell growth." *Int J Oncol* 23 (5):1407–12.

Macan, H., R. Uykimpang, M. Alconcel, J. Takasu, R. Razon, H. Amagase, and Y. Niihara. 2006. "Aged garlic extract may be safe for patients on warfarin therapy." *J Nutr* 136 (3 Suppl):793S–5S.

Madabushi, R., B. Frank, B. Drewelow, H. Derendorf, and V. Butterweck. 2006. "Hyperforin in St. John's wort drug interactions." *Eur J Clin Pharmacol* 62 (3):225–33. doi: 10.1007/s00228-006-0096-0.

Mahady, G. B., T. Low Dog, M. L. Barrett, M. L. Chavez, P. Gardiner, R. Ko, R. J. Marles, L. S. Pellicore, G. I. Giancaspro, and D. N. Sarma. 2008. "United States Pharmacopeia review of the black cohosh case reports of hepatotoxicity." *Menopause* 15 (4 Pt 1):628–38. doi: 10.1097/gme.0b013e31816054bf.

Mai, I., S. Bauer, E. S. Perloff, A. Johne, B. Uehleke, B. Frank, K. Budde, and I. Roots. 2004. "Hyperforin content determines the magnitude of the St John's wort-cyclosporine drug interaction." *Clin Pharmacol Ther* 76 (4):330–40. doi: 10.1016/j.clpt.2004.07.004.

Marcocci, L., J. J. Maguire, M. T. Droy-Lefaix, and L. Packer. 1994a. "The nitric oxide-scavenging properties of Ginkgo biloba extract EGb 761." *Biochem Biophys Res Commun* 201 (2):748–55.

Marcocci, L., L. Packer, M. T. Droy-Lefaix, A. Sekaki, and M. Gardes-Albert. 1994b. "Antioxidant action of Ginkgo biloba extract EGb 761." *Methods Enzymol* 234:462–75.

Markowitz, J. S., C. L. DeVane, D. W. Boulton, S. W. Carson, Z. Nahas, and S. C. Risch. 2000. "Effect of St. John's wort (Hypericum perforatum) on cytochrome P-450 2D6 and 3A4 activity in healthy volunteers." *Life Sci* 66 (9):PL133–9.

Markowitz, J. S., C. L. Devane, K. D. Chavin, R. M. Taylor, Y. Ruan, and J. L. Donovan. 2003a. "Effects of garlic (Allium sativum L.) supplementation on cytochrome P450 2D6 and 3A4 activity in healthy volunteers." *Clin Pharmacol Ther* 74 (2):170–7. doi: 10.1016/S0009-9236(03)00148-6.

Markowitz, J. S., J. L. Donovan, C. L. DeVane, R. M. Taylor, Y. Ruan, J. S. Wang, and K. D. Chavin. 2003a. "Effect of St John's wort on drug metabolism by induction of cytochrome P450 3A4 enzyme." *JAMA* 290 (11):1500–4. doi: 10.1001/jama.290.11.1500.

Markowitz, J. S., J. L. Donovan, C. L. DeVane, R. M. Taylor, Y. Ruan, J. S. Wang, and K. D. Chavin. 2003b. "Multiple doses of saw palmetto (Serenoa repens) did not alter cytochrome P450 2D6 and 3A4 activity in normal volunteers." *Clin Pharmacol Ther* 74 (6):536–42. doi: 10.1016/j.clpt.2003.08.010.

Markowitz, J. S., J. L. Donovan, C. L. DeVane, L. Sipkes, and K. D. Chavin. 2003c. "Multiple-dose administration of Ginkgo biloba did not affect cytochrome P-450 2D6 or 3A4 activity in normal volunteers." *J Clin Psychopharmacol* 23 (6):576–81. doi: 10.1097/01.jcp.0000095340.32154.c6.

Matheny, C. J., R. Y. Ali, X. Yang, and G. M. Pollack. 2004. "Effect of prototypical inducing agents on P-glycoprotein and CYP3A expression in mouse tissues." *Drug Metab Dispos* 32 (9):1008–14.

Mauro, V. F., L. S. Mauro, J. F. Kleshinski, S. A. Khuder, Y. Wang, and P. W. Erhardt. 2003. "Impact of ginkgo biloba on the pharmacokinetics of digoxin." *Am J Ther* 10 (4):247–51.

McKenna, D. J., K. Jones, S. Humphrey, and K. Hughes. 2001. "Black cohosh: Efficacy, safety, and use in clinical and preclinical applications." *Altern Ther Health Med* 7 (3):93–100.

Modarai, M., J. Gertsch, A. Suter, M. Heinrich, and A. Kortenkamp. 2007. "Cytochrome P450 inhibitory action of Echinacea preparations differs widely and co-varies with alkylamide content." *J Pharm Pharmacol* 59 (4):567–73. doi: 10.1211/jpp.59.4.0012.

Mohammed Abdul, M. I., X. Jiang, K. M. Williams, R. O. Day, B. D. Roufogalis, W. S. Liauw, H. Xu, and A. J. McLachlan. 2008. "Pharmacodynamic interaction of warfarin with cranberry but not with garlic in healthy subjects." *Br J Pharmacol* 154 (8):1691–700. doi: 10.1038/bjp.2008.210.

Mohutsky, M. A., G. D. Anderson, J. W. Miller, and G. W. Elmer. 2006. "Ginkgo biloba: evaluation of CYP2C9 drug interactions *in vitro* and *in vivo*." *Am J Ther* 13 (1):24–31.

Molto, J., M. Valle, C. Miranda, S. Cedeno, E. Negredo, M. J. Barbanoj, and B. Clotet. 2011. "Herb-drug interaction between Echinacea purpurea and darunavir-ritonavir in HIV-infected patients." *Antimicrob Agents Chemother* 55 (1):326–30. doi: 10.1128/AAC.01082-10.

Molto, J., M. Valle, C. Miranda, S. Cedeno, E. Negredo, and B. Clotet. 2012a. "Effect of milk thistle on the pharmacokinetics of darunavir-ritonavir in HIV-infected patients." *Antimicrob Agents Chemother* 56 (6):2837–41. doi: 10.1128/AAC.00025-12.

Molto, J., M. Valle, C. Miranda, S. Cedeno, E. Negredo, and B. Clotet. 2012b. "Herb-drug interaction between Echinacea purpurea and etravirine in HIV-infected patients." *Antimicrob Agents Chemother* 56 (10):5328–31. doi: 10.1128/AAC.01205-12.

Moore, L. B., B. Goodwin, S. A. Jones, G. B. Wisely, C. J. Serabjit-Singh, T. M. Willson, J. L. Collins, and S. A. Kliewer. 2000. "St. John's wort induces hepatic drug metabolism through activation of the pregnane X receptor." *Proc Natl Acad Sci U S A* 97 (13):7500–2. doi: 10.1073/pnas.130155097.

Morimoto, T., T. Kotegawa, K. Tsutsumi, Y. Ohtani, H. Imai, and S. Nakano. 2004. "Effect of St. John's wort on the pharmacokinetics of theophylline in healthy volunteers." *J Clin Pharmacol* 44 (1):95–101. doi: 10.1177/0091270003261496.

Mrozikiewicz, P. M., A. Bogacz, M. Karasiewicz, P. L. Mikolajczak, M. Ozarowski, A. Seremak-Mrozikiewicz, B. Czerny, T. Bobkiewicz-Kozlowska, and E. Grzeskowiak. 2010. "The effect of standardized Echinacea purpurea extract on rat cytochrome P450 expression level." *Phytomedicine* 17 (10):830–3. doi: 10.1016/j.phymed.2010.02.007.

Murphy, P. A. 2002. "St. John's wort and oral contraceptives: reasons for concern?" *J Midwifery Womens Health* 47 (6):447–50.

Nash, K. M., and Z. A. Shah. 2015. "Current perspectives on the beneficial role of Ginkgo biloba in neurological and cerebrovascular disorders." *Integr Med Insights* 10:1–9. doi: 10.4137/IMI.S25054.

Nebel, A., B. J. Schneider, R. K. Baker, and D. J. Kroll. 1999. "Potential metabolic interaction between St. John's wort and theophylline." *Ann Pharmacother* 33 (4):502.

Ng, T. B., and H. W. Yeung. 1985. "Hypoglycemic constituents of Panax ginseng." *Gen Pharmacol* 16 (6):549–52.

Ohnishi, N., M. Kusuhara, M. Yoshioka, K. Kuroda, A. Soga, F. Nishikawa, T. Koishi et al. 2003. "Studies on interactions between functional foods or dietary supplements and medicines. I. Effects of Ginkgo biloba leaf extract on the pharmacokinetics of diltiazem in rats." *Biol Pharm Bull* 26 (9):1315–20.

Onorato, J., and J. D. Henion. 2001. "Evaluation of triterpene glycoside estrogenic activity using LC/MS and immunoaffinity extraction." *Anal Chem* 73 (19):4704–10.

Pan, J., J. Y. Hong, B. L. Ma, S. M. Ning, S. R. Paranawithana, and C. S. Yang. 1993. "Transcriptional activation of cytochrome P450 2B1/2 genes in rat liver by diallyl sulfide, a compound derived from garlic." *Arch Biochem Biophys* 302 (2):337–42.

Penzak, S. R., S. M. Robertson, J. D. Hunt, C. Chairez, C. Y. Malati, R. M. Alfaro, J. M. Stevenson, and J. A. Kovacs. 2010. "Echinacea purpurea significantly induces cytochrome P450 3A activity but does not alter lopinavir-ritonavir exposure in healthy subjects." *Pharmacotherapy* 30 (8):797–805. doi: 10.1592/phco.30.8.797.

Piscitelli, S. C., A. H. Burstein, D. Chaitt, R. M. Alfaro, and J. Falloon. 2000. "Indinavir concentrations and St John's wort." *Lancet* 355 (9203):547–8. doi: 10.1016/S0140-6736(99)05712-8.

Piscitelli, S. C., A. H. Burstein, N. Welden, K. D. Gallicano, and J. Falloon. 2002a. "The effect of garlic supplements on the pharmacokinetics of saquinavir." *Clin Infect Dis* 34 (2):234–8. doi: 10.1086/324351.

Piscitelli, S. C., E. Formentini, A. H. Burstein, R. Alfaro, S. Jagannatha, and J. Falloon. 2002b. "Effect of milk thistle on the pharmacokinetics of indinavir in healthy volunteers." *Pharmacotherapy* 22 (5):551–6.

Rajnarayana, K., M. S. Reddy, J. Vidyasagar, and D. R. Krishna. 2004. "Study on the influence of silymarin pretreatment on metabolism and disposition of metronidazole." *Arzneimittelforschung* 54 (2):109–13. doi: 10.1055/s-0031-1296944.

Raner, G. M., S. Cornelious, K. Moulick, Y. Wang, A. Mortenson, and N. B. Cech. 2007. "Effects of herbal products and their constituents on human cytochrome P450(2E1) activity." *Food Chem Toxicol* 45 (12):2359–65. doi: 10.1016/j.fct.2007.06.012.

Rao, B. N., M. Srinivas, Y. S. Kumar, and Y. M. Rao. 2007. "Effect of silymarin on the oral bioavailability of ranitidine in healthy human volunteers." *Drug Metabol Drug Interact* 22 (2-3):175–85.

Reame, N. E., J. L. Lukacs, V. Padmanabhan, A. D. Eyvazzadeh, Y. R. Smith, and J. K. Zubieta. 2008. "Black cohosh has central opioid activity in postmenopausal women: Evidence from naloxone blockade and positron emission tomography neuroimaging." *Menopause* 15 (5):832–40. doi: 10.1097/gme.0b013e318169332a.

Rengelshausen, J., M. Banfield, K. D. Riedel, J. Burhenne, J. Weiss, T. Thomsen, I. Walter-Sack, W. E. Haefeli, and G. Mikus. 2005. "Opposite effects of short-term and long-term St John's wort intake on voriconazole pharmacokinetics." *Clin Pharmacol Ther* 78 (1):25–33. doi: 10.1016/j.clpt.2005.01.024.

Rettie, A. E., L. C. Wienkers, F. J. Gonzalez, W. F. Trager, and K. R. Korzekwa. 1994. "Impaired (S)-warfarin metabolism catalysed by the R144C allelic variant of CYP2C9." *Pharmacogenetics* 4 (1):39–42.

Rivlin, R. S. 2001. "Historical perspective on the use of garlic." *J Nutr* 131 (3s):951S–4S.

Robertson, S. M., R. T. Davey, J. Voell, E. Formentini, R. M. Alfaro, and S. R. Penzak. 2008. "Effect of Ginkgo biloba extract on lopinavir, midazolam and fexofenadine pharmacokinetics in healthy subjects." *Curr Med Res Opin* 24 (2):591–9. doi: 10.1185/030079908X260871.

Roby, C. A., D. A. Dryer, and A. H. Burstein. 2001. "St. John's wort: effect on CYP2D6 activity using dextromethorphan-dextrorphan ratios." *J Clin Psychopharmacol* 21 (5):530–2.

Rosado, M. F. 2003. "Thrombosis of a prosthetic aortic valve disclosing a hazardous interaction between warfarin and a commercial ginseng product." *Cardiology* 99 (2):111. doi: 69720.

Roses, A. D. 2000. "Pharmacogenetics and the practice of medicine." *Nature* 405 (6788):857–65. doi: 10.1038/35015728.

Rukov, J. L., and N. Shomron. 2011. "MicroRNA pharmacogenomics: Post-transcriptional regulation of drug response." *Trends Mol Med* 17 (8):412–23. doi: 10.1016/j.molmed.2011.04.003.

Schrieber, S. J., R. L. Hawke, Z. Wen, P. C. Smith, K. R. Reddy, A. S. Wahed, S. H. Belle et al. 2011. "Differences in the disposition of silymarin between patients with nonalcoholic fatty liver disease and chronic hepatitis C." *Drug Metab Dispos* 39 (12):2182–90. doi: 10.1124/dmd.111.040212.

Schrieber, S. J., Z. Wen, M. Vourvahis, P. C. Smith, M. W. Fried, A. D. Kashuba, and R. L. Hawke. 2008. "The pharmacokinetics of silymarin is altered in patients with hepatitis C virus and nonalcoholic Fatty liver disease and correlates with plasma caspase-3/7 activity." *Drug Metab Dispos* 36 (9):1909–16. doi: 10.1124/dmd.107.019604.

Schwarz, U. I., H. Hanso, R. Oertel, S. Miehlke, E. Kuhlisch, H. Glaeser, M. Hitzl, G. K. Dresser, R. B. Kim, and W. Kirch. 2007. "Induction of intestinal P-glycoprotein by St John's wort reduces the oral bioavailability of talinolol." *Clin Pharmacol Ther* 81 (5):669–78. doi: 10.1038/sj.clpt.6100191.

Seidlova-Wuttke, D., O. Hesse, H. Jarry, V. Christoffel, B. Spengler, T. Becker, and W. Wuttke. 2003. "Evidence for selective estrogen receptor modulator activity in a black cohosh (Cimicifuga racemosa) extract: Comparison with estradiol-17beta." *Eur J Endocrinol* 149 (4):351–62.

Shord, S. S., K. Shah, and A. Lukose. 2009. "Drug-botanical interactions: A review of the laboratory, animal, and human data for 8 common botanicals." *Integr Cancer Ther* 8 (3):208–27. doi: 10.1177/1534735409340900.

Sim, S. C., and M. Ingelman-Sundberg. 2013. "Update on allele nomenclature for human cytochromes P450 and the Human Cytochrome P450 Allele (CYP-allele) Nomenclature Database." *Methods Mol Biol* 987:251–9. doi: 10.1007/978-1-62703-321-3_21.

Sprouse, A. A., and R. B. van Breemen. 2016. "Pharmacokinetic interactions between drugs and botanical dietary supplements." *Drug Metab Dispos* 44 (2):162–71. doi: 10.1124/dmd.115.066902.

Sueyoshi, T., W. D. Green, K. Vinal, T. S. Woodrum, R. Moore, and M. Negishi. 2011. "Garlic extract diallyl sulfide (DAS) activates nuclear receptor CAR to induce the Sult1e1 gene in mouse liver." *PLoS One* 6 (6):e21229. doi: 10.1371/journal.pone.0021229.

Sugimoto, K., M. Ohmori, S. Tsuruoka, K. Nishiki, A. Kawaguchi, K. Harada, M. Arakawa et al. 2001. "Different effects of St John's wort on the pharmacokinetics of simvastatin and pravastatin." *Clin Pharmacol Ther* 70 (6):518–24.

Surai, P. F. 2015. "Silymarin as a natural antioxidant: An overview of the current evidence and perspectives." *Antioxidants (Basel)* 4 (1):204–47. doi: 10.3390/antiox4010204.

Taylor, J. A., W. Weber, L. Standish, H. Quinn, J. Goesling, M. McGann, and C. Calabrese. 2003. "Efficacy and safety of echinacea in treating upper respiratory tract infections in children: a randomized controlled trial." *JAMA* 290 (21):2824–30. doi: 10.1001/jama.290.21.2824.

Therapeutic Research Center. 2016. "Cytochrome P450 Drug Interactions (PL Detail-Document #320506)." In *Pharmacist's letter.* Stockton, CA.

Uchida, S., H. Yamada, X. D. Li, S. Maruyama, Y. Ohmori, T. Oki, H. Watanabe, K. Umegaki, K. Ohashi, and S. Yamada. 2006. "Effects of Ginkgo biloba extract on pharmacokinetics and pharmacodynamics of tolbutamide and midazolam in healthy volunteers." *J Clin Pharmacol* 46 (11):1290–8. doi: 10.1177/0091270006292628.

Ulbricht, C. E., and Natural Standard. 2010. *Natural Standard herb & supplement guide: An evidence-based reference.* 1st ed. Maryland Heights, Mo.: Elsevier/Mosby.

van Erp, N. P., S. D. Baker, M. Zhao, M. A. Rudek, H. J. Guchelaar, J. W. Nortier, A. Sparreboom, and H. Gelderblom. 2005. "Effect of milk thistle (Silybum marianum) on the pharmacokinetics of irinotecan." *Clin Cancer Res* 11 (21):7800–6. doi: 10.1158/1078-0432.CCR-05-1288.

Van Strater, A. C., and J. P. Bogers. 2012. "Interaction of St John's wort (Hypericum perforatum) with clozapine." *Int Clin Psychopharmacol* 27 (2):121–4. doi: 10.1097/YIC.0b013e32834e8afd.

Venter, J. C., M. D. Adams, E. W. Myers, P. W. Li, R. J. Mural, G. G. Sutton, H. O. Smith et al. 2001. "The sequence of the human genome." *Science* 291 (5507):1304–51. doi: 10.1126/science.1058040.

von Moltke, L. L., J. L. Weemhoff, E. Bedir, I. A. Khan, J. S. Harmatz, P. Goldman, and D. J. Greenblatt. 2004. "Inhibition of human cytochromes P450 by components of Ginkgo biloba." *J Pharm Pharmacol* 56 (8):1039–44. doi: 10.1211/0022357044021.

Wang, L. S., G. Zhou, B. Zhu, J. Wu, J. G. Wang, A. M. Abd El-Aty, T. Li et al. 2004a. "St John's wort induces both cytochrome P450 3A4-catalyzed sulfoxidation and 2C19-dependent hydroxylation of omeprazole." *Clin Pharmacol Ther* 75 (3):191–7. doi: 10.1016/j.clpt.2003.09.014.

Wang, L. S., B. Zhu, A. M. Abd El-Aty, G. Zhou, Z. Li, J. Wu, G. L. Chen et al. 2004b. "The influence of St John's Wort on CYP2C19 activity with respect to genotype." *J Clin Pharmacol* 44 (6):577–81. doi: 10.1177/0091270004265642.

Wang, X. D., J. L. Li, Q. B. Su, S. Guan, J. Chen, J. Du, Y. W. He et al. 2009. "Impact of the haplotypes of the human pregnane X receptor gene on the basal and St John's wort-induced activity of cytochrome P450 3A4 enzyme." *Br J Clin Pharmacol* 67 (2):255–61. doi: 10.1111/j.1365-2125.2008.03344.x.

Wang, Y., J. Cao, and S. Zeng. 2005. "Involvement of P-glycoprotein in regulating cellular levels of Ginkgo flavonols: quercetin, kaempferol, and isorhamnetin." *J Pharm Pharmacol* 57 (6):751–8. doi: 10.1211/0022357056299.

Wanwimolruk, S., K. Phopin, and V. Prachayasittikul. 2014. "Cytochrome P450 enzyme mediated herbal drug interactions (Part 2)." *EXCLI J* 13:869–96.

Wanwimolruk, S., and V. Prachayasittikul. 2014. "Cytochrome P450 enzyme mediated herbal drug interactions (Part 1)." *EXCLI J* 13:347–91.

Watkins, R. E., J. M. Maglich, L. B. Moore, G. B. Wisely, S. M. Noble, P. R. Davis-Searles, M. H. Lambert, S. A. Kliewer, and M. R. Redinbo. 2003. "2.1 A crystal structure of human PXR in complex with the St. John's wort compound hyperforin." *Biochemistry* 42 (6):1430–8. doi: 10.1021/bi0268753.

Wen, Z., T. E. Dumas, S. J. Schrieber, R. L. Hawke, M. W. Fried, and P. C. Smith. 2008. "Pharmacokinetics and metabolic profile of free, conjugated, and total silymarin flavonolignans in human plasma after oral administration of milk thistle extract." *Drug Metab Dispos* 36 (1):65–72. doi: 10.1124/dmd.107.017566.

Wenk, M., L. Todesco, and S. Krahenbuhl. 2004. "Effect of St John's wort on the activities of CYP1A2, CYP3A4, CYP2D6, N-acetyltransferase 2, and xanthine oxidase in healthy males and females." *Br J Clin Pharmacol* 57 (4):495–9. doi: 10.1111/j.1365-2125.2003.02049.x.

Wolf, H. R. 2006. "Does Ginkgo biloba special extract EGb 761 provide additional effects on coagulation and bleeding when added to acetylsalicylic acid 500 mg daily?" *Drugs R D* 7 (3):163–72.

Xie, R., L. H. Tan, E. C. Polasek, C. Hong, M. Teillol-Foo, T. Gordi, A. Sharma et al. 2005. "CYP3A and P-glycoprotein activity induction with St. John's Wort in healthy volunteers from 6 ethnic populations." *J Clin Pharmacol* 45 (3):352–6. doi: 10.1177/0091270004273320.

Xu, H., K. M. Williams, W. S. Liauw, M. Murray, R. O. Day, and A. J. McLachlan. 2008. "Effects of St John's wort and CYP2C9 genotype on the pharmacokinetics and pharmacodynamics of gliclazide." *Br J Pharmacol* 153 (7):1579–86. doi: 10.1038/sj.bjp.0707685.

Yale, S. H., and I. Glurich. 2005. "Analysis of the inhibitory potential of Ginkgo biloba, Echinacea purpurea, and Serenoa repens on the metabolic activity of cytochrome P450 3A4, 2D6, and 2C9." *J Altern Complement Med* 11 (3):433–9. doi: 10.1089/acm.2005.11.433.

Yang, L. J., L. Fan, Z. Q. Liu, Y. M. Mao, D. Guo, L. H. Liu, Z. R. Tan et al. 2009. "Effects of allicin on CYP2C19 and CYP3A4 activity in healthy volunteers with different CYP2C19 genotypes." *Eur J Clin Pharmacol* 65 (6):601–8. doi: 10.1007/s00228-008-0608-1.

Yasui-Furukori, N., H. Furukori, A. Kaneda, S. Kaneko, and T. Tateishi. 2004. "The effects of Ginkgo biloba extracts on the pharmacokinetics and pharmacodynamics of donepezil." *J Clin Pharmacol* 44 (5):538–42. doi: 10.1177/0091270004264161.

Yeh, Y. Y., and L. Liu. 2001. "Cholesterol-lowering effect of garlic extracts and organosulfur compounds: human and animal studies." *J Nutr* 131 (3s):989S–93S.

Yin, O. Q., B. Tomlinson, M. M. Waye, A. H. Chow, and M. S. Chow. 2004. "Pharmacogenetics and herb-drug interactions: experience with Ginkgo biloba and omeprazole." *Pharmacogenetics* 14 (12):841–50.

Yoshioka, M., N. Ohnishi, N. Sone, S. Egami, K. Takara, T. Yokoyama, and K. Kuroda. 2004. "Studies on interactions between functional foods or dietary supplements and medicines. III. Effects of ginkgo biloba leaf extract on the pharmacokinetics of nifedipine in rats." *Biol Pharm Bull* 27 (12):2042–5.

Yuan, C. S., G. Wei, L. Dey, T. Karrison, L. Nahlik, S. Malecar, K. Kasza, M. Ang-Lee, and J. Moss. 2004. "Brief communication: American ginseng reduces warfarin's effect in healthy patients: A randomized, controlled Trial." *Ann Intern Med* 141 (1):23–7.

Zanger, U. M., and M. Schwab. 2013. "Cytochrome P450 enzymes in drug metabolism: Regulation of gene expression, enzyme activities, and impact of genetic variation." *Pharmacol Ther* 138 (1):103–41. doi: 10.1016/j.pharmthera.2012.12.007.

Zhang, S., and M. E. Morris. 2003. "Effects of the flavonoids biochanin A, morin, phloretin, and silymarin on P-glycoprotein-mediated transport." *J Pharmacol Exp Ther* 304 (3):1258–67. doi: 10.1124/jpet.102.044412.

Zhou, W., H. Chai, P. H. Lin, A. B. Lumsden, Q. Yao, and C. J. Chen. 2004. "Molecular mechanisms and clinical applications of ginseng root for cardiovascular disease." *Med Sci Monit* 10 (8):RA187–92.

Zuo, X. C., B. K. Zhang, S. J. Jia, S. K. Liu, L. Y. Zhou, J. Li, J. Zhang et al. 2010. "Effects of Ginkgo biloba extracts on diazepam metabolism: a pharmacokinetic study in healthy Chinese male subjects." *Eur J Clin Pharmacol* 66 (5):503–9. doi: 10.1007/s00228-010-0795-4.

3

Patient Safety

Oliver Grundmann, Eunji Ko, and Catherine Ulbricht

CONTENTS

3.1 Introduction

The use of botanicals for medicinal purposes has been part of healthcare throughout documented history and across different cultures in the world. Botanicals continue to be used by patients for medical and health-related reasons, both with or without guidance from healthcare providers. The use of botanicals for therapeutic purposes is included as a domain of complementary and alternative medicine (CAM) or integrative medicine.

Complementary medicine refers to unconventional practices used with mainstream medicine, while alternative medicine refers to unconventional practices used instead of mainstream medicine (NCCIH 2017). Complementary medicine is valuable as long as adverse effects or interactions are not likely; alternative medicine can be detrimental if it replaces an existing and necessary drug therapy. The combination of standard care and complementary medicine are now referred to as integrative therapy which is used by patients and healthcare providers alike (NCCIH 2017).

Botanicals refer to a plant or plant part valued for its medicinal or therapeutic properties, flavor, and/or scent. Herbs, commonly used for both medicinal and dietary purposes, are a subset of botanicals (NCCIH 2017). To be classified as a dietary supplement in the United States, a botanical must meet the definition established by the Dietary Supplement Health and Education Act (DSHEA) of 1994. Botanicals are considered to be dietary supplements when they contain "one or more of the following dietary ingredients for oral administration: a vitamin, a mineral, an herb or other botanicals, or an amino acid." Concentrates, metabolites, constituents, extracts, or combinations of the dietary ingredients are also considered dietary supplements (NIH Office of Dietary Supplements 2018).

Botanicals may be available as "fresh or dried products, liquid or solid extracts, tablets, tea bags" and many others (ODS—Botanical Dietary Spple). While many botanical formulations are available, there are currently no standardization requirements for botanical dietary supplement manufacturing in the United States. As a result, "standardization" can mean different things among manufacturers and it is important to note that following a specific preparation method alone is not sufficient for a product to be called standardized. However, evidence is insufficient on the exact components that are responsible for the therapeutic effect of most botanicals, ideal standardization that includes chemical markers remains a challenge and is rarely used.

As botanical supplements are comprised of plant components, patients may assume that they are safe to take. However, "natural" and "safe" are not synonymous. Consumers and patients may be unaware of the importance of disclosing the use of supplements to their healthcare providers and the implications of taking botanical supplements and their prescription medications concurrently. Interactions between medications and certain botanicals may occur resulting in serious adverse effects. In addition, the safety of botanical use depends on many factors such as the botanical extract preparation, pharmacokinetics, pharmacodynamics, genetics, dosage, and formulation. Each factor may have an effect on the potency and outcomes with the botanical. As an example, the quantity of botanicals found in extracts, tinctures, or teas varies due to the differences in extraction methods.

Healthcare providers can play an essential role in helping patients manage the potential risks associated with the use of botanicals. Therefore, healthcare providers must be able to evaluate patient safety risks, collect comprehensive medication histories, communicate effectively with the patient, and identify and prevent adverse events associated with botanical use.

3.2 Framework for Evaluating Botanical Use

In the United States, botanical supplements do not follow the same regulations and standards as prescription drugs. Manufacturers do not have to seek approval from the Food and Drug Administration (FDA) before marketing their product. As a result, ensuring the quality and safety of the botanical products is the responsibility of the manufacturer. The FDA will not intervene until there is suggestion that a product might be unsafe.

3.2.1 Food Safety Modernization Act (FSMA)

The Food Safety Modernization Act (FSMA) of 2011 has enabled the FDA to have some oversight on dietary supplement manufacturers. The FSMA provision gives the FDA the authority to mandate product recalls, investigate or detain products if the FDA believes that products are adulterated or misbranded (FSMA 2012). The FSMA also requires the FDA to issue the New Dietary Ingredients (NDI) guidance as manufacturers have to demonstrate safety data and methods to identify the NDI for new botanical supplements before they enter the market (FDA 2011/44).

3.2.2 Dietary Supplement and Nonprescription Drug Consumer Protection Act

Under the Dietary Supplement and Nonprescription Drug Consumer Protection Act, distributors and manufacturers are required to report serious adverse reactions caused by botanicals and other dietary supplements using MedWatch forms issued by the FDA. They can use the safety reporting portal which can be accessed at www.safetyreporting.hhs.gov. This portal is an extension of the FDA's MedWatch reporting system, which combines diverse methods that the agency has established in order to streamline the reporting process (HHS 2018).

The adverse reaction must be reported in detail along with a summary of relevant clinical information, which includes tests, laboratory data, preexisting medical conditions, signs, and symptoms both before and after the possible event. In addition, they need to describe information on how and why the product was used by the patient. If more than one patient experienced the event, manufacturers and distributors should file a separate report for each patient within 15 business days if it occurred within the past 12 months. This portal can also be used by healthcare providers and patients if they establish a reasonable link between botanical supplement use and the adverse effect.

The United States Pharmacopeia and National Formulary (USP-NF) was named by DSHEA as the official compendia for dietary supplements (USP 2018). USP writes reference standards to help manufacturers ensure the identity, strength, quality, and purity of dietary supplements (USP 2018).

TABLE 3.1

DSHEA Definition of Dietary Supplement Adulteration

1. Presents a significant or unreasonable risk of illness or injury when used in accordance with the suggested labeling
2. Is a new entity and lacks adequate evidence to ensure its safety of use
3. Has been declared an imminent hazard by the Secretary of the Department of Health and Human Services
4. Contains a dietary ingredient that is present in sufficient quantity to render the product poisonous or deleterious to human health

Note: Definition of Dietary Supplement adulteration as defined by DSHEA.

Internationally, manufacturers can seek USP verification in order to establish adherence to Good Manufacturing Practice (GMP). This is known as the USP Dietary Supplement Verification Program. This verification process involves product and ingredient testing. The manufacturing documentations are also reviewed during this process (De Smet 2002). Successful verification by the USP will allow manufacturers to earn a distinctive USP Verified Mark for their tested product. Despite the opportunity to acquire USP Verification, few manufacturers have undergone this voluntary process which requires additional quality control testing.

Many botanical supplements are composed of multiple constituents. There are also many factors that affect quality of the supplements, such as intrinsic properties, environmental conditions, agricultural practices respective to each constituent and the extraction process itself (Ekor 2014). Thus, isolating each ingredient for testing would be tedious. The World Health Organization (WHO) defines food adulteration "as unethical and often criminal malpractice, where prohibited substances are either added or used to partially or wholly substitute healthy ingredients or artificially create the impression of freshness of old food" (WHO 2015). The DSHEA defines adulteration of a dietary supplement, and the criterion are noted in Table 3.1 (Tsourounis and Dennehy 2017).

On the contrary, food contamination is not an intended process and it refers to "any substances not intentionally added to food, which are present to such food as a result of the production, manufacture, processing, preparation, treatment, packing, packaging, transport, or holding of such food as a result of environmental contamination" (WHO 2015). In a similar fashion, these two processes affect quality of botanicals as well. Botanical collection in the wild may be contaminated by other species or plants through accidental contamination or intentional adulteration, which may have unsafe consequences (WHO 2004).

In an analysis of 230 Ayurvedic medicines purchased over the Internet, 21% of the Indian-manufactured medicines and 22% of the U.S.-manufactured medicines contained lead, mercury, or arsenic (Saper et al. 2008). Over 700 supplement products have been identified as being adulterated with drugs such as sildenafil, corticosteroids, and stimulants (Basch et al. 2005).

Contaminants and adulterants introduced during the manufacturing process may contribute to multiple potential adverse effects associated with dietary supplements. A survey of FDA recalls between 2004 and 2012 found that 50% of all product recalls involved dietary supplements containing a drug that is likely to result in serious health consequences or death (Harel et al. 2013). In 2002, PC-SPES, a botanical formula for the treatment of prostate cancer was removed from the market by the FDA because some lots were found to contain warfarin, indomethacin, and diethylstilbestrol (Reynolds 2002).

In addition to impurities, a concern also exists about the lack of consistency between manufacturers for the same botanical product. Since regulations for manufacturing botanical supplements is limited, potential inconsistencies in the quality further complicate the ability to discern efficacy of these supplements. For example, goldenseal is often combined with echinacea for its potential additive effects in supporting and promoting immune function (Rehman et al. 1999). However, this type of combination product may not have any clinical activity due to low echinacea concentrations (Basch et al. 2005).

Patients and consumers should be aware that supplement manufacturers do not perform the same rigorous trials and manufacturing standards that drugs are subjected to. Therefore, healthcare providers should have conversations with their patients to clarify that although botanical supplements may potentially have therapeutic effects, these products are not necessarily well understood due to the limited studies supporting their safety and efficacy. Healthcare providers should be able to discuss the risks and benefits of botanical supplements with their patients in order to ensure the appropriateness of their use.

3.3 Adverse Effects in the Clinical Setting

Interactions may involve pharmacokinetic or pharmacodynamic pathways of either the drug or the botanical constituents in the body. Pharmacokinetic interactions involve absorption, distribution, metabolism, and excretion, and all can be associated with treatment failure and toxicity. Pharmacodynamic interactions may be represented as a direct effect at receptor function, may interfere with a biological or physiological control process, or may have additive or opposing pharmacological effects (Palleria et al. 2013). As an example, St. John's Wort possesses both pharmacokinetic and pharmacodynamic interactions due to its potential of affecting enzymatic processes of drug metabolism (pharmacokinetic) and also potentiating serotonin effects of drugs such as the selective serotonin reuptake inhibitors (pharmacodynamic) (Henderson et al. 2002). *See Chapter 2 Pharmacokinetic and Pharmacodynamic Considerations for further discussion.*

Although patients may use botanical supplements for their supposed therapeutic benefits, healthcare providers should counsel patients on their potential risks for a given individual especially the person with a complex drug regimen and multiple comorbid conditions. These risks include drug-botanical interactions, such as St. John's Wort being taken by an individual prescribed warfarin for a pulmonary embolism or atrial fibrillation. Co-administration of this botanical may result in the loss of anticoagulant activity and, potentially, a life threatening event such as a stroke (Jiang et al. 2004).

Some botanical supplements can contribute to the worsening of medical conditions or in causing supplement-induced disease such as hepatotoxicity. For example, black cohosh products have been linked to more than 50 cases of clinically-apparent liver injury that range from a simple enzyme elevation to acute liver failure requiring transplantation. The mechanism is unknown, but there may be an immunological component (NIH, LiverTox 2018a). In addition, another possible explanation is connected to the use of unknown adulterants or botanical products mislabeled as black cohosh, which may be the actual cause of hepatic injury. Several prospective clinical trials have been conducted and according to their results, black cohosh was not associated with serum liver enzyme elevations. Also, another supplement called ma huang (ephedra) can destroy hepatocytes and induce liver injury requiring transplantation, so this botanical would be especially harmful when being used by an individual with hepatitis (Neff et al. 2004). As there are no specific markers for botanical induced liver injury coupled with the difficulty in establishing causality, this further complicates the evaluation process (NIH, LiverTox 2018b). To investigate any possible risks of liver toxicity, a good reference is LiverTox, an online database which may be accessed via the National Institutes of Health (NIH) website. LiverTox is a unique database that incorporates a variety of resources and presents drug and supplement information related to liver toxicity in a convenient and publicly accessible format.

Botanical use has also been associated with the development of nephrotoxicity. Yohimbine, willow bark, and germanium are among 17 supplements discussed in a review by the American Society of Nephrology (Gabardi et al. 2012). The authors also noted that nephrolithiasis is associated with the use of ephedra which, although it has been banned by the FDA since 2004, can be purchased through Internet sources. Concentrated cranberry tablets also increase the risk for calcium-oxalate stone formation due to their oxalate content. Several cases of rhabdomyolysis have been reported related to the use of creatine, wormwood oil, and licorice. Much of the evidence on botanical-induced nephrotoxicity has been from individual case reports which makes establishing actual causality often impossible.

Table 3.2 highlights a few adverse effects and potential interactions associated with the top-selling botanical supplements in the United States in 2011 (Blumenthal et al. 2012). The data is based on purchases from chain drug and food stores, but does not include sales data from other sources such as Wal-Mart, warehouse buying clubs, or convenience stores. The sales statistics were generated by SymphonyIRI, a Chicago-based research firm. As shown in the table, many common botanicals potentially have antiplatelet effects which might increase the risk of bleeding if the patient was also taking drugs such as warfarin, rivaroxaban, and nonsteroidal anti-inflammatory drugs such as ibuprofen.

Despite their common usage, patients and caregivers may still underestimate the potential for adverse effects. One study of botanical use indicated that in a pediatric emergency department, 77% of patients/caregivers were aware that the products carried adverse effects (Lanski et al. 2003). However, only 27% were able to identify a potential adverse effect, and up to 66% believed that supplements do not interact with drugs. Awareness that botanical products can potentially be risky is limited in the general population.

TABLE 3.2

Adverse Reactions and Drug Interactions of Top Herbal Supplements

Supplement Name	Adverse Reactions	Example Potential Interactions
Cranberry	Diarrhea, GI upset Risk for causing calcium oxalate kidney stones	Warfarin
Soy	Hypothyroidism, hypersensitivity	Levothyroxine, warfarin, estrogen derivatives
Saw Palmetto	GI upset and headache	Warfarin
Garlic	GI upset (bloating, flatulence, nausea), spontaneous bleeding, hypersensitivity	Warfarin, antihypertensive agents, saquinavir
Ginkgo Biloba	GI upset, headache, dizziness, heart palpitations, dermatologic reactions	Omeprazole, efavirenz, fluoxetine, St. John's wort, ibuprofen, risperidone, trazodone, warfarin, aspirin, cilostazol
Milk Thistle	GI upset (abdominal bloating, fullness, or pain; anorexia; changes in bowel habits; diarrhea; dyspepsia; flatulence; nausea), headache, impotence, and skin reactions	Metronidazole
Echinacea	Allergic reactions, facial edema, and mild transient GI complaints	Caffeine, midazolam
Black Cohosh Root	Hepatotoxicity, GI upset, dizziness, headaches, tremor	Atorvastatin, azathioprine, cyclosporine, tamoxifen
St. John's Wort	GI upset (dry mouth, nausea, change in bowel habits), itching, photosensitivity, fatigue, dizziness, jitteriness, insomnia, sleep disorders, and headache	Alprazolam, midazolam, buproprion, buspirone, cyclosporine, efavirenz, exemestane, finasteride, nevirapine, voriconazole, zolpidem, digoxin, nifedipine, tacrolimus, venlafaxine, verapamil, all P450 3A4 substrates
Ginseng	Hypertension, diarrhea, sleeplessness, hypersensitivity	Phenelzine, warfarin, imatinib
Valerian Root	Hepatotoxicity, headache, diarrhea	Benzodiazepines
Green Tea	Headache, dizziness, GI upset (nausea, vomiting, constipation, diarrhea), dry mouth, heartburn, fatigue, palpitation, lightheadedness, nocturia, sore throat, insomnia, increased appetite, abdominal discomfort	Antithrombotic agents, bortezomib, folic acid, nadolol, nonsteroidal anti-inflammatory agents (NSAIDS), salicylates, simvastatin
Evening Primrose	Limited information regarding adverse reactions is available. Itchiness, acne, skin rash, GI upset	Antithrombotic agents, NSAIDs, salicylates
Horny Goat Weed	Sweating, tachyarrhythmia, hypomania, rash	Limited information regarding interactions is available.
Bilberry	Limited information regarding adverse reactions is available	Anticoagulants, NSAIDS, hypoglycemic agents, salicylates
Ginger	Abdominal discomfort, heartburn, diarrhea, irritant effect in the mouth and throat	Antithrombotic agents, nifedipine
Grape Seed	Contraindicated in patients with known hypersensitivity	Antithrombotic agents, NSAIDs, salicylates
Elderberry	Nausea, vomiting, diarrhea (especially when raw)	None well documented
Aloe Vera	Burning, itching, oral aloe vera: cramps, abdominal pain, diarrhea, potassium depletion	Diuretics
Yohimbe	Rash, lupus-like syndromes, bronchospasm, arrhythmias, anxiety, irritability, excitability	Antianxiety agents, antihypertensives, aripiprazole, monoamine oxidase inhibitors, tricyclic antidepressants

Note: The 20 Top-Selling Herbal Supplements from Blumenthal et al. 2012. All other data from Lexi-comp, Micromedex, Clinical Pharmacology, and Natural Medicine (Lexi-comp 2016, Natural Medicines 2018).

TABLE 3.3

Prescription Drugs Derived from Botanical Products

Drugs	Uses	Botanical Source	Common Side Effects
Aspirin	Pain relief, anti-platelet	White willow bark	Gastrointestinal ulcer
Digoxin	Atrial fibrillation, heart failure	Foxglove	Dizziness, mental disturbances, headache, nausea, vomiting, diarrhea
Paclitaxel	Various cancers	Bark of the yew tree	Leukopenia, anemia, thrombocytopenia, hypersensitivity, peripheral neuropathy, arthralgias, nausea, vomiting, diarrhea, and mucositis
Yohimbine	Erectile dysfunction, syncope/ orthostatic hypotension	Bark of the yohimbe tree	Few reported with clinical trials
Oseltamivir	Influenza treatment and prophylaxis	Chinese star anise	Nausea, vomiting, diarrhea, abdominal pain
Sinecatechins	External genital and perianal warts	Green tea leaves	Erythema, pruritus, edema, burning, pain/discomfort

Note: All data from Lexi-comp (Lexi-comp 2016).

Reporting adverse effects of botanical supplements is a critical step in improving their safe use. Patients should report adverse effects via the Safety Reporting Portal discussed previously, FDA's MedWatch program, or Natural MedWatch (HHS Safety Reporting Portal 2018, FDA Medwatch 2018, Natural Medicines 2018). These voluntary reports are anonymous and do not constitute a legal claim. They can be accessed via the FDA (http://www.fda.gov/Safety/MedWatch/) or Natural Medicines (https://naturalmedicines.therapeuticresearch.com/) websites. Despite their availability, programs such as MedWatch are not extensively used (Cohen 2014). Dissemination of information through voluntary reporting or case reports regarding adverse events is essential in order to heighten awareness of safety concerns that may be associated with use of supplements.

An important point about supplements and adverse effects that should be shared with patients and consumers is that many prescription drugs have been derived from botanicals. Prescription drugs derived from natural sources still have a range of adverse effects, as indicated in Table 3.3 (Tatti et al. 2008, Ulbricht 2017). Regulated by the FDA, these drugs have undergone extensive research to establish safety and efficacy profiles.

3.4 How to Assess Causality

Adverse effects attributed to botanicals have been identified mostly through case reports which frequently lack critical information for establishing the actual causality. It has been challenging to establish an association between a specific plant and the clinical event (Restani et al. 2016). When botanicals are taken with drug products, determining the exact causative agent(s) of the adverse reaction is difficult, especially in a medically complex patient.

A systematic review involving 66 botanicals concluded that the adverse effects due to botanical ingredients were relatively infrequent and the number of severe clinical reactions was limited when assessed for causality using WHO Causality Assessment Criteria (Di Lorenzo et al. 2015). Although this is encouraging, healthcare providers should remain vigilant and not rule out supplements as a factor in adverse events. Botanical use is often the patient's choice and many individuals may not mention their usage to healthcare providers. The possibility of a serious adverse reaction must always be considered, even when literature suggests that the event is rare.

Key points in establishing causality include *temporality* as one necessary criterion, *consistency of association,* and searching for *alternative explanations* as adding credibility (Lai et al. 2010). A case report of serious thrombocytopenia as part of a clinical trial involving botanicals using the criteria above concluded that the event developed after concomitant use with conventional drugs and as a result may not be attributed to the botanicals alone (Lai et al. 2010). Evaluation of this event gave a general framework of causal criteria establishment. The authors noted that to determine if botanicals are the cause of an adverse reaction, the association between the time of use and the time of the unwanted effect must be established. The consistency of the event should also be established in other settings, different times, and participants. Finally, other possible explanations must be ruled out, such as the event being explained with other drugs that the patient may be taking concomitantly with the supplement (Lai et al. 2010). Given the frequent use of polypharmacy in conjunction with multiple dietary supplements, the complexity of establishing causality between one supplement and the adverse effect can be challenging in the clinical setting. This will often require at least the temporary discontinuation of supplements with stepwise reintroduction if the patient desires to continue taking them. Healthcare providers are advised to work with the patient to choose a supplement that is known to not interfere with concomitant drug therapy.

3.5 Framework for Patient Work Up

A patient workup is a process that must be utilized for every patient, in order to achieve a complete patient evaluation. A patient workup follows a plan, which proposes topics and questions for the healthcare providers to discuss with the patient. It is recommended that the clinician comprehensively explore the patient's medical history, which will promote a better assessment of the patient and help set optimal goals.

Part of the patient workup activity involves detailing current and past medical history, as well as obtaining a comprehensive drug history including prescription and nonprescription drugs, vitamins, and dietary supplements. The 2007–2010 National Health and Nutrition Examination Survey (NHANES) revealed some top reasons for use of dietary supplements by adult patients such as improving overall health, maintaining health, and promoting bone health (Bailey et al. 2013).

In order to help healthcare providers extract accurate, detailed information from patients, it is recommended that they refer to the questions listed in Table 3.4. These questions can be used in developing better patient-provider communication, while allowing for a more accurate patient workup. These questions may help healthcare providers better understand the motivations a patient has for using a particular supplement.

Healthcare providers should be aware of commonly used botanical supplements and inquire about their use when obtaining the history. For example, when a patient reveals that he is taking a green tea supplement believing that it promotes good sleep, the healthcare provider can address the misconception and explain that green tea supplement is used for mental alertness and may actually cause wakefulness.

A useful mnemonic device to guide a clinician's initial encounter with a patient is *SCHOLAR-MAC* (Lauster and Srivastava 2014). The letters of *SCHOLAR-MAC* respectively represent: Symptoms, Characteristics, History of Complaint, Onset, Location, Aggravating Factors, Remitting Factors, Medications, Allergies, and Conditions (Table 3.5). This mnemonic guides healthcare providers through the initial steps of a patient encounter. To maximize the value of *SCHOLAR-MAC,* healthcare providers need to incorporate additional input. The provider may need to explain to the patient that allergies are not limited to just medications. Allergies can also include foods or other substances, such as latex.

The drug history from the patient is not always accurate and may need to be compared against a medical record. When discussing the drug and supplement history with a patient, one asks *how* and *when* they are taking this medication. For example, a patient pursuing additional treatment with a botanical for

TABLE 3.4

Questions to Ask for Effective Patient Communication

- What are you taking this supplement for?
- What other medications are you taking?
- Who is the patient and how old is s/he?
- Are you pregnant or breastfeeding?
- What other underlying co-morbid conditions do you have?
- What has been done to treat it (current or past)?

TABLE 3.5

SCHOLAR-MAC Mnemonic and Workup Examples

S	Symptoms	What symptoms have you noticed?
C	Characteristics	Can you describe the symptoms to me?
H	History of Complaint	Have you had these symptoms in the past?
O	Onset	When did the symptoms first start?
L	Location	Where is the problem?
A	Aggravating Factors	What makes the problem worse?
R	Remitting Factors	What makes the problem better?
M	Medications (past and present)	What prescription medications, over the counter medications, vitamins, or herbal supplements are you taking? What medications or supplements have you taken in the past? Did they help, were not effective, or made the condition worse?
A	Allergies	What allergies do you have?
C	Conditions (past and present)	What other medical conditions do you have?

Source: Modified with permission from Lauster, C. D. and S. B. Srivastava. 2014. *Fundamental Skills for Patient Care in Pharmacy Practice.* Burlington, MA: Jones & Bartlett Learning, 28–32. Print.

lethargy and weight gain may be incorrectly spacing their levothyroxine doses away from their meals. *SCHOLAR-MAC* is a useful starting point when trying to capture relevant information about a patient (*see case studies 3.1 and 3.2*). *Following the case study examples, there is a SCHOLAR-MAC example for each case.*

CASE STUDY 3.1

A 53-year-old female presented to her primary care physician with complaints of rapid heartbeat from time to time, associated with a sudden feeling of warmth mostly in her upper body, including the face, which has been going on for several weeks. After her physician explained that her symptoms might be related to post-menopausal syndrome, she was interested in learning if any natural product might be appropriate in her case. The physician recommended soy isoflavone capsules and a check up a week later if symptoms persist, improve, or get worse. Three weeks later, during her yearly physical appointment, the patient stated she was feeling better while continuing her soy supplements.

Phytoestrogens such as soy isoflavones can be used by women with post-menopausal symptoms, such as hot flashes or vaginal dryness. A recent systematic review based on 62 studies concluded that dietary supplemental soy isoflavones were associated with improvement in some menopausal symptoms, including reductions, even though modest, in hot flashes and vaginal dryness, but not a significant reduction in night sweats (Franco et al. 2016).

SCHOLAR-MAC EXAMPLE:

- S: The healthcare provider should ask the patient what symptoms they are experiencing. For this example, the patient would talk about the complaints of rapid heartbeat associated with a sudden feeling of warmth in the upper body.
- C: The healthcare provider should inquire further about the symptoms and ask for more detail. An example of this would be asking the patient if there is sweating associated with the warmth, how severe, etc. In this case, this depth of information is not provided to us.
- H: The healthcare provider should inquire if the patient has experienced these symptoms in the past. This information was not provided in this case.
- O: The healthcare provider should ask the patient when these symptoms first started. In this example, the patient told us that the symptoms started several weeks ago.

L: The healthcare provider should inquire where the patient is experiencing these symptoms. In this example, for the sudden feeling of warmth, it would have been in the upper body. However, you could try to get the patient to be more specific, if possible. This information could concurrently be gathered through physical examination.

A: The healthcare provider should inquire with the patient what makes the symptoms worse.

R: The healthcare provider should inquire with the patient what makes the symptoms better.

M: The healthcare provider should review the medication list with the patient and ask them what medications they are taking, including OTCs, herbals, and vitamins. Also, they should ask what medications or supplements they have taken in the past, including if they helped, were not effective, or made the condition worse.

A: The healthcare provider should inquire about what allergies the patient has. This would mean asking about medication allergies and food allergies.

C: The healthcare provider should inquire what medical conditions the patient has, including past and present conditions.

CASE STUDY 3.2

A 20-year-old college student presented to her local pharmacy with complaints of a persistent cough and sore throat. She has been having these symptoms for 2 weeks. Upon further questioning, she reports use of Echinacea, St. John's Wort, and Gingko biloba. Her friend told her that Gingko biloba helps with immune function. She also read an article about a study that showed St. John's Wort inhibits the growth of fungi and viruses, as well as an article claiming that Echinacea helps balance her hormones, reduces her monthly cramps, and fights acne. After evaluation with *SCHOLAR-MAC*, the pharmacist suggests that she visit her PCP for antibiotics, as this resembles strep throat. The student stated that she did not want to take antibiotics, which she views as "just chemicals" that will "poison her body." She refuses to "support some big drug company." She would rather take something "natural" (Braude et al. 2011).

This type of encounter is an opportunity for healthcare providers to open a dialogue with the patient and recognize differences in the way people define and value health and illness. It is important for healthcare providers to listen with empathy and understand what the patient's perception of the problem is. Having these qualities in a conversation will yield a productive conversation to optimize a provider's ability to care for his patient. Echinacea is widely used for the prevention and treatment of the cold. However, a randomized, controlled trial reported that Echinacea is not effective in reducing symptoms of the common cold. Therefore, the therapeutic benefit of a conventional drug compared to the use of a natural product should be explained to the patient (Barrett et al. 2002).

SCHOLAR-MAC EXAMPLE:

S: The healthcare provider should inquire about what symptoms she is experiencing. For this example, the patient is complaining of a persistent cough and sore throat.

C: The healthcare provider should ask further about the symptoms and ask for more detail. An example of this would be asking if the cough is dry or wet. In this case, this depth of information is not provided to us.

H: The healthcare provider should inquire if the patient has experienced these symptoms in the past. Again, this information is not provided to us with this case scenario.

O: The healthcare provider should ask the patient when these symptoms first started. In this case, the patient stated the symptoms started 2 weeks ago.

L: The healthcare provider should inquire where the patient is experiencing these symptoms. In this case scenario, the patient has a sore throat.

A: The healthcare provider should inquire about what makes the symptoms worse.

R: The healthcare provider should inquire about what makes the symptoms better.

M: The healthcare provider should review the medication list with the patient and ask them what medications they are taking, including OTCs, herbals, and vitamins. Also, they should ask what medications or supplements have been taken in the past. In this case scenario, the patient mentions several herbal products she has tried, including Echinacea, St. John's Wort, and Gingko biloba.

A: The healthcare provider should inquire about what allergies the patient has. This would include asking about medication allergies, as well as food allergies. This information is not provided to us in the case.

C: The healthcare provider should inquire about what medical conditions the patient has, including past and present conditions.

3.6 Communicating with the Patient

Communication is an important component of patient-provider relationship, as care has evolved into a patient centered model and the individual has an increasing influence in treatment decisions. Patients assess the quality of their care mostly through the experiences of talking with their healthcare providers (Levinson 2011). The healthcare provider should aim to find out if the patient is using botanicals with or instead of conventional drug therapy.

First, studies have found deficiencies in patient-provider communication with patients failing to report drugs, discuss their concerns, and disclose the use of non-prescribed and complementary therapies (Serper et al. 2013). Different observations have shown that patients prefer not to reveal use of botanicals as a complementary medicine, especially if that is their own choice and not the provider's suggestion. For example, cancer patients may not feel confident disclosing that they are taking echinacea to boost their immunity, or milk thistle to protect their liver from toxicity of chemotherapy. A systematic review of 21 studies that reported CAM use revealed that 77% of participants did not disclose this information during their interactions with healthcare providers (Davis et al. 2012). Healthcare providers have an essential role in educating patients about safe botanical use, although proper counseling depends on the patient's disclosure and open communication.

Second, in other cases, where patients acknowledge using botanicals for their diagnosis, full assessment may be lacking. SCHOLAR-MAC does not provide a complete framework and other aspects should be taken into consideration. To improve patient-provider interactions regarding botanicals, the factors influencing that communication must be recognized. In the Western health system, the usage of botanical supplements might seem unconventional and related to patient's cultural background which premises that the physician would not understand or approve of such use. A clinician should seek to hold an open dialogue with their patients to uncover any factors motivating the patients' health decisions, and in the process, be sensitive to any differences that might be unveiled. The following steps outline an approach to developing effective cross-cultural communication (Schrefer 1994). They are:

- Acknowledge that diversity exists
- Understand that culture makes individuals unique
- Respect people/cultures that may be unfamiliar/different from one's own
- Conduct a self-assessment to identify one's own cultural beliefs/biases
- Recognize differences in the way people define and value health and illness
- Be patient, flexible, and willing to modify healthcare delivery to meet patients' cultural needs
- Allow for differences among members of the same cultural group
- Appreciate the richness of culture
- Embrace diversity
- Understand that cultural beliefs and values are difficult to change and may be learned from birth

Furthermore, an open dialogue serves as an opportunity to identify concerns, such as if a patient is experiencing hypotensive symptoms as a consequence of the additive effect with the concomitant use of a botanical supplement. For example, garlic, together with antihypertensive medications, may cause dizziness and fainting due to the additive hypotensive effect. Many healthcare providers consider discussions about complementary medicine as important in communicating respect for patient autonomy and culture and also as a mechanism to enhance the patient-clinician relationship (Shelley et al. 2009). One of the main themes that determine how the communication takes place between patients and their healthcare providers is acceptance / nonjudgement. Data collected to study communication between patients and their healthcare providers about CAM use suggested that when this communication is carried out in a nonjudgmental manner, can demonstrate openness and help the patient overcome anticipated negative interactions during discussion about botanicals (Shelley et al. 2009).

Embracing a patient's choice in such way would ultimately lead to a less formal communication. This way the conversation would be carried in a more open manner, allowing the patient to better inform their provider, who then takes on the role as the patient's advisor on risks and benefits involving the use of botanicals as complementary to existing drug therapy When recommending against use of a botanical, the provider must recommend a reasonable alternative, while making sure to keep the patient feeling valued and involved in their own well-being. Supporting and working with the patient regarding their concerns is essential, as the patient may otherwise continue the use of a detrimental supplement or practices without the clinician's knowledge.

3.7 Conclusion

Use of botanicals alone or in combination with conventional drugs is an increasingly common occurrence observed in the course of healthcare practice. This chapter is a reflection on how botanicals are classified and evaluated, their potential risks, and providing a communication framework for healthcare providers and patients in regards to their use. It is crucial to completely understand patients and the underlying cultural backgrounds that guide their choices. Constant efforts must be made to remain free of judgment and respectful toward the personal motivations and philosophies of each patient. Benefits and risks must be weighed carefully when considering use of a botanical supplement. A clinician's reasoning for or against the use should be clearly communicated to their patients, as patients may have misconceptions about the use of supplements. Patients' motivations for using botanicals should be assessed, as they may be trying to self-treat a problem that requires the healthcare provider's attention.

Acknowledgments

The authors would like to acknowledge the invaluable contributions of pharmacy students from Massachusetts College of Pharmacy and Health Sciences, Northeastern University, and the University of New England: Michael J. Hayes, Jr., Kaitlyn Zheng, Haley T. Duong, Stephanie Lock, Odeta Kulenica, Jay Ketkar, Jaime Patel, Perry Frink, Jennifer Wagner, and Beongick Woo.

REFERENCES

Basch, E., C. Ulbricht, S. Basch et al. 2005. An evidence-based systematic review of Echinacea (E. angustifolia DC, E. pallida, E. purpurea) by the Natural Standard Research Collaboration. *Journal of Herbal Pharmacotherapy* 5, no. 2: 57–88.

Bailey R. L., J. Gahche, P. Miller et al. 2013. Why US adults use dietary supplements. *Journal of the American Medical Association Internal Medicine* 173, no. 5 (Mar): 355–361. doi: 10.1001/jamainternmed.2013.2299.

Barrett, B. P., L. R. Brown, K. Locken, R. Maberry, J. A. Bobula, and D. D'Allessio. 2002. Treatment of the Common cold with unrefined echinacea: A eandomized, double-blind, Placebo-controlled trial. *Annals of Internal Medicine* 137, no. 12 (Dec): 939–946.

Blumenthal, M., A. Lindstrom, C. Ooyen, and M. E. Lynch. 2012. Herb supplement sales increase 4.5% in 2011. *HerbalGram* 95: 60–64.

Braude, S., D. Goran, and A. Miceli. 2011. *Case Studies for Understanding the Human Body.* Jones & Bartlett Publishers.

Cohen, P. A. 2014. Hazards of hindsight: Monitoring the safety of nutritional supplements. *New England Journal of Medicine* 370, no. 14 (Apr): 1277–1280.

Davis, E. L., B. Oh, P. N. Butow, B. A. Mullan, and S. Clarke. 2012. Cancer patient disclosure and patient-doctor communication of complementary and alternative medicine use: A systematic review. *Oncologist.* 2012 17(11): 1475–1481.

De Smet, P. A. 2002. Herbal remedies. *New England Journal of Medicine* 347, no. 25 (Dec): 2046–2056.

Di Lorenzo, C., A. Ceschi, H. Kupferschmidt et al. 2015. Adverse effects of plant food supplements and botanical preparations: A systematic review with critical evaluation of causality. *British Journal of Clinical Pharmacology* 79, no. 4 (Apr):578–92. doi: 10.1111/bcp.12519.

Ekor, M. 2014. The growing use of herbal medicines: Issues relating to adverse reactions and challenges in monitoring safety. *Frontiers in Pharmacology* 4 (Jan):177. doi: 10.3389/fphar.2013.00177.

FDA. 2011/44. https://www.fda.gov/Food/GuidanceRegulation/GuidanceDocumentsRegulatoryInformation/ucm257563.htm (Accessed September 12, 2017).

Franco, OH., R. Chowdhury, J. Troup et al. 2016. Use of plant-based therapies and menopausal symptoms: A systematic review and meta-analysis. *Journal of the American Medical Association* 315, no. 23 (Jun): 2554–2563. doi: 10.1001/jama.2016.8012.

FSMA. 2012. website: https://www.fda.gov/food/guidanceregulation/fsma/ (Accessed September 12, 2017).

Gabardi, S., K. Munz, and C. Ulbricht. 2012. A review of dietary supplement-induced renal dysfunction. *Clinical Journal of the American Society of Nephrology* 2, no. 4 (Apr): 757–65. doi: 10.2215/CJN.00500107.

Harel, Z., S. Harel, R. Wald et al. 2013. The frequency and characteristics of dietary supplement recalls in the United States. *Journal of the American Medical Association Internal Medicine* 173, no. 10 (May): 926–8.

Henderson, L., Q. Y. Yue, C. Bergquist. 2002. St John's wort (Hypericum perforatum): Drug interactions and clinical outcomes. *British Journal of Clinical Pharmacology* 54, no. 4 (Oct):349–56. doi: 10.1046/j.1365-2125.2002.01683.x.

Jiang, X., K. M. Williams, W. S. Liauw et al. 2004. Effect of St John's wort and ginseng on the pharmacokinetics and pharmacodynamics of warfarin in healthy subjects. *British Journal of Clinical Pharmacology* 57, no. 5 (Jul): 592–9.

Lai, J. N., S. C. Hsieh, P. C. Chen, H. J. Chen, and J. D. Wang. 2010. Should herbs take all the blame? Causality assessment of a serious thrombocytopenia event. *Journal of Alternative and Complementary Medicine* 16, no. 11 (Oct): 1221–1224.

Lanski, S. L., M. Greenwald, A. Perkins et al. 2003. Herbal use in a pediatric emergency department population: Expect the unexpected. *Pediatrics* 111, no. 5 pt 1 (May):981–5.

Levinson W. 2011. Patient-centered communication: A sophisticated procedure. *BMJ Quality and Safety* 20, no. 10 (Aug):823–825. doi: 10.1136/bmjqs-2011-000323.

Lexi-comp. 2016. Wolters Kluwer Health, Inc. Riverwoods, IL. Available at: http://online.lexi.com (Accessed July 8, 2016).

Lauster, C. D., and S. B. Srivastava. 2014. *Fundamental Skills for Patient Care in Pharmacy Practice.* Burlington, MA: Jones & Bartlett Learning, 28–32. Print.

National Institutes of Health (NIH), LiverTox. 2018a. Black cohosh. https://livertox.nlm.nih.gov/BlackCohosh. htm (Accessed June 14, 2018).

National Institutes of Health (NIH), LiverTox. 2018b. Ephedra. https://livertox.nlm.nih.gov/Ephedra.htm (Accessed June 14, 2018).

National Institutes of Health (NIH), Office of Dietary Supplements. 2018. Dietary Supplement Health and Education Act of 1994. https://ods.od.nih.gov/About/DSHEA_Wording.aspx (Accessed February 16, 2018).

Natural Medicines. 2018. Natural MedWatch: Adverse Event Reporting Form. https://naturaldatabase. therapeuticresearch.com/nd/adverseevent.aspx (Accessed June 13, 2018).

Neff, G. W., K. R. Reddy, F. A. Durazo, D. Meyer, R. Marrero, and N. Kaplowitz. 2004. Severe hepatotoxicity associated with the use of weight loss diet supplements containing ma huang or usnic acid. *Journal of Hepatology* 41, no. 6: 1062–1064.

NCCIH. 2017. website: https://nccih.nih.gov/health/integrative-health (Accessed September 13, 2017).

Palleria, C., A. Di Paolo, C. Giofre. 2013. Pharmacokinetic drug-drug interaction and their implication in clinical management. *Journal of Research in Medical Sciences* 18, no. 7 (July): 601–610.

Rehman, J., J. M. Dillow, S. M. Carter, J. Chou, B. Le, and A. S. Maisel. 1999. Increased production of antigen-specific immunoglobulins G and M following in vivo treatment with the medicinal plants Echinacea angustifolia and Hydrastis canadensis. *Immunology Letters* 68, no. 2: 391–395.

Restani, P., C. DiLorenzo, A. Garcia-Alvares et al. 2016. Adverse effects of plant food supplements self-reported by consumers in the PlantLIBRA survey involving six European countries. *PLOS One* 11, no. 2 (Feb): e0150089. doi: 10.1371/journal.pone.0150089.

Reynolds, T. 2002. Contamination of PC-SPES remains a mystery. *Journal of the National Cancer Institute* 94, no. 17 (Sep):1266–1268.

Saper, R. B., R. S. Phillips, A. Sehgal et al. 2008. Lead, mercury, and arsenic in U.S. and Indian manufactured Ayurvedic medicines sold via the internet. *Journal of the American Medical Association* 300, no. 8 (Aug): 915–923.

Serper, M., D. M. McCarthy, R. E. Patzer et al. 2013. What patients think doctors know: Beliefs about provider knowledge as barriers to safe medication use. *Patient Education and Counseling* 93, no. 2 (Nov): 306–11. doi: 10.1016/j.pec.2013.06.030.

Schrefer, S. 1994. *Quick Reference to Cultural Assessment.* St. Louis, MO: Mosby; 1994:IV.

Shelley, B. M., A. L. Sussman, R. L. Williams et al. 2009. "They don't ask me so I don't tell them': Patient clinician communication about traditional, complementary and alternative medicine. *Annals of Family Medicine* 7, no. 2 (Mar): 139–147.

Tatti, S., J. M. Swinehart, C. Thielert, H. Tawfik, A. Mescheder, and K. R. Beutner. 2008. Sinecatechins, a defined green tea extract, in the treatment of external anogenital warts: A randomized controlled trial. *Obstetrics & Gynecology* 111. no. 6 (Jun): 1371–1379.

Tsourounis, C. and C. Dennehy. 2017. Chapter 50. Introduction to Dietary Supplements. In Krinsky, D., Ferreri, S., Hemstreet, B. et al. (eds.) *Handbook of nonprescription drugs: An interactive approach to self-care.* 19th Edition. Washington, D.C: American Pharmacists Association.

Ulbricht, C. 2017. Chapter 52. Common Complementary and Alternative Medicine Health Systems. In Krinsky, D., Ferreri, S., Hemstreet, B. et al. (eds.) *Handbook of nonprescription drugs: An interactive approach to self-care.* 19th Edition. Washington, D.C: American Pharmacists Association.

U.S. Department of Health and Human Services (HHS). 2018. The safety reporting portal. Safety Reporting Portal. www.safetyreporting.hhs.gov (Accessed February 16, 2018).

U.S. Food and Drug Administration. 2018. MedWatch: The FDA safety information and adverse event reporting program. http://www.fda.gov/Safety/MedWatch/ (Accessed June 15, 2018).

U.S. Pharmacopeia Convention (USP). 2018. Legal recognition – Standards Categories. http://www.usp.org/about-usp/legal-recognition/usp-us-law#dietSupRegUS (Accessed June 14, 2018).

World Health Organization (WHO). 2004. Medicinal plants – guidelines to promote patient safety and plant conservation for a US$ 60 billion industry. http://www.who.int/mediacentre/news/notes/2004/np3/en/ (Accessed June 14, 2018).

World Health Organization (WHO). 2015. Food safety: What should you know? http://www.searo.who.int/entity/world_health_day/2015/whd-what-you-should-know/en/ (Accessed June 14, 2018).

4

Botanical Use in Special Populations

Margaret M. Charpentier, Kelly L. Matson, Katherine Kelly Orr, and Anne Hume

CONTENTS

4.1 Introduction

The use of botanicals as an integrative therapy for health and wellness, as well as for the treatment of acute and chronic diseases is common worldwide. Unfortunately, healthcare providers continue to overlook or ignore the use of botanicals and other forms of integrative medicine by many individuals. This is especially important in populations such as older adults. Special populations may have unique considerations related to the use of botanicals. This chapter presents a brief overview of a few key issues related to the use of botanicals in selected special populations.

4.2 Pediatrics

4.2.1 Prevalence

An estimated 2% of children were reported using complementary and alternative medicine (CAM) in a 1996 survey (Kemper et al. 2008). Since that time, usage has increased substantially, as shown in a 2012 National Health interview survey of 10,000 children ages 4 to 17 years old, where 11.6% of children surveyed reported using a CAM practice in the past year (NCCIH 2012). The use of nonvitamin nonmineral dietary supplements were reported by about 5% and special diets by another 0.7% of respondents (NCCIH 2012). An estimated 9% of infants under one year of age have been given dietary supplements and teas by their mothers. Infant usage was more common among mothers who also used botanicals and among Hispanic individuals (Zhang et al. 2011). Overall, American families spent $1.9 billion on CAM for their children in 2012 (Nahin et al. 2016).

4.2.2 Clinical Considerations

4.2.2.1 PK/PD Issues

Multiple physiologic changes occur from birth through adolescence which result in pharmacokinetic (PK) and pharmacodynamic (PD) changes for many drugs. In pediatric populations, these changes are potentially most important in the neonate and infant. Some of the physiologic changes include reduced activity of intestinal cytpchrome 3A4 and drug transporters, as well as hepatic phase I enzyme systems (Lu and Rosenbaum 2014). In addition, the glomerular filtration rate, tubular reabsorption, and tubular secretion may also be reduced in the first year of life. Although many botanicals may have been used in neonates and infants, little information is available, especially among premature infants or those with comorbid onditions.

4.2.2.2 Chronic Diseases

Unlike the use of botanicals and other dietary supplements in adults for health maintenance, much of the use in pediatrics is for the treatment of chronic diseases. These conditions include pain, anxiety, attention-deficit hyperactive disorder (ADHD), autism, asthma, allergies, cystic fibrosis, irritable bowel disease, and insomnia (Kemper et al. 2008; NCCIH 2012; McClafferty et al. 2017). These conditions, especially autism and ADHD, can be difficult to treat pharmacologically. As a result, frustrated caregivers may want to explore all options, including botanicals and other supplements, as well as special diets such as the ketogenic diet for epilepsy. The supplements frequently used in children include fish oil/omega-3 fatty acids, melatonin, and pre- and probiotics (McClafferty et al. 2017). Among botanicals specifically, echinacea and flaxseed continue to be commonly reported.

Although data is available for fish oil/omega-3 fatty acids, melatonin, and pre- and probiotics in chronic conditions in children, alternative medicine practices such as the use of secretin or N, N-dimethylglycine for autism spectrum disorder are not supported by published evidence. Overall, autism and other challenging pediatric diseases are potential targets for dangerous interventions and fraud.

4.2.2.3 Safety Issues

Safety is a priority in considering the use of botanicals in children. One study evaluating the use of echinacea in 407 children for upper respiratory tract infections reported the development of rash in 7.1% in the echinacea group compared to 2.7% in the placebo group (Taylor et al. 2003). Whether this simply reflects the higher prevalence of atopic diseases in children is unclear, but this is of potential concern with plant-based therapies. In addition, since much of the use of botanicals in children is for the treatment of chronic disease, the potential for clinically relevant drug interactions is significant especially when the botanical is St. John's wort.

Adverse reactions from CAM products resulted in an estimated 4,965 pediatric emergency departments visits annually (Geller et al. 2015). Child resistant packaging is not required for supplements and the accidental ingestion by unsupervised young children is a unique concern in this population. Among children ages 5 to 18, weight loss and energy supplements were responsible for over 50% of the adverse events, with cardiac symptoms attributed to these products in adolescents (Geller et al. 2015). A report from U.S. Poison Control Centers on dietary supplement exposures between 2000 and 2012 similarly reported acute accidental ingestion of energy, yohimbine, and ma huang supplements in children under 6 years of age (Rao et al. 2017).

Selected botanicals used in children and adolescents are discussed in the Chapters 8 Women's Health, 11 Psychiatric Disorders, and 13 Dermatological Conditions.

4.3 Pregnancy and Lactation

The goal of every pregnancy is a healthy full term infant and a positive maternal experience. In addition, following the infant's birth, an increasing number of women are choosing to breastfeed with the World Health Organization (WHO) now recommending the practice exclusively for at least the first 6 months of life (WHO 2014).

4.3.1 Prevalence

An estimated 13%–78% of pregnant women use some form of CAM or integrative medicine, with this broad range likely due to varied study designs and definitions. For studies assessing botanical use, between 9% and 16% of pregnant women reported use and the actual usage might be significantly higher. Characteristics which predict the use of botanicals include a higher level of education and a history of use prior to becoming pregnant. Motivations vary, although many pregnant women use botanicals and integrative medicine as an adjunct to conventional care. Of note, many pregnant women do not discuss their botanical use with their healthcare providers due to fears of negative feedback or the provider not specifically asking about use (Hall et al. 2011).

4.3.2 Clinical Considerations

4.3.2.1 PK/PD Issues

Pregnancy and the postpartum period are known to have significant effects on the pharmacokinetic parameters of many drugs; these parameters include the volume of distribution, protein binding, and renal clearance (Feghali et al. 2015; Tasnif et al. 2016). Little evidence exists on the physiologic effects of pregnancy on botanical pharmacokinetics.

4.3.2.2 Safety Issues

Special considerations regarding the use of botanicals in pregnancy focuses on ensuring the product is safe without teratogenic or other adverse effects on the developing fetus. In addition, the risk of miscarriage or premature birth should be minimal with the supplement. Since most of the use of botanicals in pregnancy is based on historical use or cultural traditions, the available safety data is often limited, with the exception of ginger (Holst et al. 2011). As with most studies of botanicals in special populations, the literature is difficult to evaluate due to small populations, patient perception of risk and benefits of botanicals, influence and use due to one's cultural background, patterns of use over time during a pregnancy, and the role of the healthcare provider in guiding patient decisions (Adams et al. 2009).

Healthcare providers differ in their perspectives on the use of botanicals in pregnancy. Although some recommend avoidance of botanicals due to insufficient data and the potential for adulteration, other providers with experience and comfort in advising women on botanicals not only evaluate limited safety trials, but also include animal data, pharmacology, and historical use (Marcus and Snodgrass 2005; Low Dog 2009).

4.3.2.3 Lactation

Among breastfeeding women, the production of an adequate milk supply is common concern, with 78% reporting this in an online survey of 188 women. (Bazzano et al. 2017) Galactagogues such as fenugreek are recommended and used to address this concern. Many women have learned about these types of botanicals primarily through friends and lactation consultations, as well as the internet (Bazzano et al. 2017).

Use of botanicals during lactation also provides challenges in evaluating their ability to cross into breast milk and whether or not the infant will have a significant exposure. A systematic review of botanicals and breastfeeding found only 32 studies from the previous 40 years, types varying from safety, efficacy, and survey studies. Quality of safety and efficacy data was overall low, further demonstrating the lack of data (Budzynska et al. 2012).

Botanicals commonly used in pregnancy and lactation are discussed in Chapter 8 Women's Health.

4.4 Geriatrics

Older adults are a heterogeneous group. They range from healthy, independently living individuals even into their late 90s to much younger, but frail patients with multiple comorbid conditions and polypharmacy.

4.4.1 Prevalence

In 2015, 8.5% of the global population, or 617.1 million, were estimated to be over the age 65 years. By 2030, the number will likely increase to 12% of the world's population or about 1 billion people (He et al. 2015).

The reported use of dietary supplements has continued to increase among American adults age 65 and older based on longitudinal data from the 2012 National Health and Nutrition Examination Survey (NHANES), unlike younger age groups (Kantor et al. 2016). Data from the Ginkgo Evaluation of Memory (GEM) study involving over 3,000 independently living adults 75 years and older identified that 27.4% of the cohort were taking a nonvitamin, nonmineral dietary supplement at baseline (Nahin et al. 2009). Among the botanicals commonly reported were ginkgo, garlic, Echinacea, and saw palmetto in this study; use of botanical supplements was associated with having problems with muscle strength and with reading senior health magazines (Nahin et al. 2009). More recent population-based data on the use of specific botanical supplements in older adults is not available, but *Bacopa monnieri* and vinpocetine, for example, are present in many memory products promoted for use by older adults.

4.4.2 Clinical Considerations

4.4.2.1 PK/PD Issues

Two broad issues should be considered with the use of botanicals in older adults. The first is related to the potential PK and PD changes that have been associated with aging in many older adults. These changes may affect both the safety and potential efficacy of a given botanical. For example, renal function declines in manyolder adults especially if the individual has had poorly controlled hypertension or diabetes for a prolonged time. This might result in the botanical and its constituents potentially having reduced clearance resulting in higher concentrations. When this is combined with PD changes such as increased central nervous system sensitivity, more pronounced adverse effects may occur and the safety profile may be reduced.

The PK/PD changes might also increase the potential risk for clinically relevant botanical-drug interactions. As many older adults may have a significant burden of chronic diseases treated with multiple drugs, a potential for interactions may be possible. St. John's wort is well known to induce the metabolism of many drugs such as warfarin, generally resulting in less efficacy of the prescription drug. In terms of PD interactions, concern about an increased risk of bleeding is frequently raised about garlic and ginkgo if the older adult is also taking aspirin, nonsteroidal anti-inflammatory drugs (NSAIDs), and other agents with antithrombotic properties. Of note, in the GEM study, an increased risk of bleeding was not identified with ginkgo compared with placebo (DeKosky et al. 2008).

4.4.2.2 Botanicals and Cognition

An additional concern with botanicals in older adults is that given their burden of chronic disease, their use may be promoted when limited, if any, clinical trial data exist. The best example is in the treatment of Alzheimer's disease and related disorders of cognition. Although huperzine and ginkgo have mixed efficacy data from clinical trials, other botanicals have much more limited data. These botanicals, however, are commonly included in proprietary blends for cognition.

4.5 Liver Disease

Liver disease encompasses a diverse group of conditions including, cirrhosis, alcohol-related hepatitis, nonalcoholic steatohepatitis, viral hepatitis, hepatocellular carcinoma, cholestatic, and autoimmune hepatitis, as well as drug-induced liver disease. In addition, metabolic liver diseases such as Wilson's disease exist among many others.

4.5.1 Prevalence

Precise statistics on the prevalence of cirrhosis, as one example, have been estimated to be between 4.5% and 9.5% of the global population (Sarin and Maiwall 2017). Unfortunately, many liver diseases are unreported and the available estimates may be low. In a population-based surveillance study of 1,040 individuals with newly diagnosed chronic liver disease, 16.8% reported the use of botanicals (Ferrucci et al. 2010). Predictors of botanical use in this study were the presence of alcohol-related liver disease and/or hepatitis C, as well as higher education and family income (Ferrucci et al. 2010). In a substudy of the population, milk thistle, St. John's wort, Echinacea and valerian were most commonly used by 43.8%, 10.7%, 8.9% and 4.5%, respectively (Ferrucci et al. 2010).

4.5.2 Clinical Considerations

Until recently, few safe and effective antiviral treatments were available for hepatitis C. The management of alcohol-related liver disease most importantly stressed alcohol abstinence, avoidance of hepatotoxins, and prevention of complications. Botanicals such as milk thistle and *Phyllanthus amarus* have been used by individuals with diverse liver diseases including specifically for the treatment of their liver disease. Constituents such as silymarin, catechins, glycyrrhizin, and phytosterols have been used worldwide. *Refer to Chapter 7 on Gastrointestinal Disease for further discussion.*

4.5.2.1 PK/PD Changes

Two broad issues should be considered with the use of botanicals in individuals with chronic liver diseases. The first is related to the PK changes in terms of reduced hepatic metabolism of many drugs and botanicals in end stage liver disease. Relatedly, botanicals that induce or inhibit hepatic enzyme systems may be expected to have fewer clinically significant effects on concomitant drugs and botanicals. The precise outcomes are difficult to predict given contributing factors such as polymorphisms in hepatic enzymes, physiologic, and environmental factors, as well as the severity of the liver disease (Palatini and DeMartin 2016). In addition, estimating how well the liver is functioning is challenging and is dependent on using multiple measures such as with the Child-Pugh classification.

4.5.2.2 Botanical-Induced Hepatotoxicity

Another consideration is the potential for botanical-induced hepatotoxicity. This is a complex topic for many reasons, as the evidence is usually from case reports such as with kava, black cohosh, and green tea. These are frequently missing important information such as presence or absence of underlying liver disease or other common causes of liver injury.

Data from the United States Drug Induced Liver Injury Network (DILIN) have suggested 15.5% of reported cases are due to botanicals and other dietary supplements (Navarro et al. 2014). The reporting of cases due to botanicals and other supplements increased from 7% to 20% over the first 10 years of the DILIN (Navarro et al. 2014). In some instances, the wrong plant may have been included in the supplement, either accidentally or for economic adulteration, and now case reports suggest the botanical as hepatotoxic when it may actually be due to a different plant. In addition, supplements may be formulated as proprietary blends so that if liver injury is suspected, the actual causative component may be difficult to establish especially if a mechanism for the adverse reaction has not been previously identified.

Pyrrolizidine alkaloids (PA) may be the compounds in botanicals associated with liver injury and their presence an indicator of a poor quality product. PAs have demonstrated hepatotoxicity by causing veno-occlusive disease and may also be carcinogenic. Butterbur products, for example, may contain unacceptable levels of PAs when raw material is not processed appropriately to remove them. Only products specifically certified ast *PA-free* should be administered (Sutherland and Sweet 2010).

One common botanical that has been associated with hepatotoxicity is green tea. While drinking green tea is safe, concerns have been raised about the use of concentrated green tea extracts. The reported pattern is typically hepatocellular and is apparent around 3 months (LiverTox). Green tea extracts contain widely variable concentrations of catechins such as epigallocatechin-3-gallate (EGCG) which have been implicated in causing mitochondrial injury in an animal model (LiverTox). Women may be at increased risk, although this may also reflect higher usage in this subgroup. In addition, fasting has been identified as a risk factor for the development of liver injury in a safety review by the U.S. Pharmacopeia (Sarma et al. 2008).

Kava was identified as a potential hepatoxin almost 20 years ago. Several countries have restricted the sale of products containing kava due to risks of severe liver injury and case reports of liver failure associated with use. Several factors are still in question as to the origin of liver injury including aqueous versus acetone or ethanol extracts, continuous high doses, inappropriate raw products, and potential contaminants (Teschke and Lebot 2011). Since the initial consumer advisory report warning in the United States in 2002, there have been no updates issued.

4.6 Kidney Disease

Similar to liver disease, kidney diseases encompass diverse conditions affecting glomeruli, tubules and renal interstitium, as well as the renal vasculature. Causes can include genetic, immunologic, metabolic, neoplastic, or pharmacologic mechanisms among others.

4.6.1 Prevalence

An estimated 11%–13% of the global population has chronic kidney disease (CKD), with stage 3 CKD being the most common (Hill et al. 2016). Published estimates of botanical use in CKD, hemodialysis, and in people who have received renal transplants have varied widely. A study of Swiss renal transplant recipients reported 11.8% used some form of CAM, particularly homeopathy and Chinese medicine (Hess et al. 2009). An Egyptian study reported CAM use by 52% of patients with end stage renal disease (ESRD) or a renal transplant, with 78% of this comprised of botanicals and other natural products (Osman et al. 2015).

4.6.2 Clinical Considerations

4.6.2.1 PK/PD Changes

Multiple issues should be considered with the use of botanicals in individuals with CKD, patients receiving hemodialysis, and renal transplant recipients. Pharmacokinetic changes resulting in reduced renal clearance of botanicals especially in CKD and potentially in hemodialysis may be possible. Patients with ESRD receiving hemodialysis are particularly sensitive to CNS effects of drugs and possibly by botanicals, although data is limited.

4.6.2.2 Electrolyte Abnormalities and Other Complications

Electrolyte and mineral disorders occur as CKD progresses and ESRD develops. Both hyperkalemia and hyperphosphatemia are common and require careful management in ESRD and while the patient is on hemodialysis. Some botanicals may contain potassium or phosphorus and should be avoided. Botanicals that contain potassium include dandelion root and turmeric rhizome among many others (NKF 2015). Phosphorus-containing botanicals include milk thistle, borage leaf, evening primrose, feverfew, flaxseed seed, and stinging nettle leaf among many others (NKF 2015). In addition, botanicals that possess antithrombotic or hypertensive effects might theoretically increase the risk of bleeding or cardiovascular events in patients with CKD.

4.6.2.3 Botanical-Induced Nephrotoxicity

Various renal syndromes have been reported after the use of medicinal plants including tubular necrosis, acute interstitial nephritis, Fanconi's syndrome, hyperkalemia/hypokalemia, hypertension, papillary necrosis, chronic interstitial nephritis, nephrolithiasis, and cancer of urinary tract.

The nephropathy associated with the use of aristolochic acid (AA) from plants in the Aristolochia genus is perhaps the best known example. The first reports of AA nephropathy consisted of previously healthy young women who had used a Chinese slimming formula for weight loss which resulted in the rapid development of ESRD. It was later determined that *Aristolochia fangchi* had been substituted for *Stephania tetranda* in the formulation. The mechanisms for developing AA nephropathy are unclear, but acute proximal tubular necrosis develops followed by interstitial and tubular fibrosis (Luciano and Perazella 2015). The presentation, diagnosis, prognosis, treatment and link to urinary tract cancers has been discussed in an excellent review (Luciano and Perazella 2015).

4.6.2.4 Botanical-Drug Interactions in Renal Transplants

An estimated 70,000 renal transplants were performed globally in 2008 (WHO). A major component of a successful transplant is the use of immunosuppressive therapy such as tacrolimus, cyclosporine, mycophenolate, and sirolimus, among other agents. Many of these drugs are metabolized through CYP 3A4 and pharmacogenetic differences are well established for this isoenzyme. Concomitant use of botanicals that are CYP 3 A4 inducers such as St. John's wort might result in rejection of the transplanted organ, while inhibitors might significantly increase the risk of toxicity (Moschella and Jaber 2001; Columbo et al. 2014).

4.7 Cancer

Cancer is a diverse collection of diseases in which genetic changes alter the normal functioning of cells. The changes may be due to many factors including environmental causes such as from cigarette smoking and radiation exposure. The treatment of diverse cancers has undergone fundamental changes in recent years to focus on the underlying genetic mutation instead of solely on the type or location of the cancer (NCI).

4.7.1 Prevalence

CAM is widely used by cancer patients both in the United States and globally. A 1998 survey revealed that greater than 95% of patients had heard of CAM, and over 2/3 were using some form of CAM to treat their cancer, or symptoms related to cancer. Almost 40% were using a botanical product (Dy et al. 2004). The rationale for using CAM includes seeking more control over their disease and relief of cancer symptoms (Richardson et al. 2000; Dy et al. 2004).

4.7.2 Clinical Considerations

4.7.2.1 PK/PD Issues

Three major areas should be considered with the use of botanicals in oncology. Similar to other sections in this chapter, PK-related drug interactions may be important since many of the new targeted therapies are metabolized through cytochrome P450 enzymes, most notably 3A4. A botanical that interferes with this may affect the drug efficacy and/or toxicity. The lack of information on drug interactions is concerning, especially since a higher toxicity is accepted with cancer therapy, and higher dosages experienced due to inhibition of metabolism, may increase toxicity which can be life-threatening or even potentially fatal.

4.7.2.2 Considerations as Adjunctive Therapy

One of the most common uses for botanicals and other natural products in oncology is as adjunctive therapy to decrease the frequency and severity of chemotherapy or radiation therapy induced adverse events. Of note, multiple studies on this role have been published over the years with mixed outcomes. The interpretation of these studies requires the consideration of several factors. Studies evaluating decreased adverse events with botanicals as an adjunct require fewer patients than trials determining if the botanical interferes with the efficacy of the chemotherapy. As an example, a drug may cause an adverse event in 30% of patients, yet the difference in cancer recurrence maybe only 5%–10% from the chemotherapy agent. To investigate this, assuming an absolute survival benefit of 5% from chemotherapy, and assuming that the botanical interferes in this drug completely, a total of 2000 patients would need to be enrolled to determine this (Lawenda et al. 2008). Further, the chemotherapy agent is administered for a few cycles over a few months, while cancer recurrence is measured in years, requiring a long duration of follow up to determine the outcome of the botanical agent on the efficacy of the chemotherapy regimen.

4.7.2.3 Considerations in Prevention and Treatment of Cancer

4.7.2.3.1 Therapy-Related Issues

Experience from the cancer prevention trials illustrates another concern with use of some botanicals. While consumption of dietary levels of a supplement may be beneficial in prevention of cancer, in clinical trials where larger quantities may be used, an increase in cancer risk has been identified in the worst case or a lack of any benefit in the best case (Bairati et al. 2005; Ferreira et al. 2004; Bairati et al. 2006).

Complex tumor physiology makes interpretation of the risks and benefits of botanicals and other dietary supplements frequently challenging. As an example, tumors express a higher level of reactive oxygen species (ROS), relying on higher ROS activity for survival. Decreasing ROS through the use of dietary supplement with antioxidant properties has been proposed to prevent and treat cancer. However, the data has demonstrated a complex interplay of the balance of ROS and cancer progression and survival (Kasiappan and Safe 2016). In addition, radiation therapy and some chemotherapy agents increase ROS activity, tipping this balance to increase apoptosis (Lawenda et al. 2008). In these cases, botanicals with antioxidant properties might potentially decrease the benefit of chemotherapy agents.

In addition to the potential interference of botanicals with established cancer treatments, clinical evidence indicating a benefit with botanicals is often based on comparators that are either no longer in use or do not include a comparator. The available cancer treatments have expanded exponentially during the past decade, with improvements in survival observed for many cancers. Older studies of botanicals demonstrating benefit may not be reflective of current practice.

4.7.2.3.2 Disease-Related Issues

Another consideration with botanicals is which cancers to use an agent. As mentioned, cancer is a general term that encompasses many different diseases. Cancer of the breast is a completely different disease than cancer of the lung. Within each specific tumor type, for example lung cancer, the aggressiveness of the cancer and the response to treatment will vary based on tumor pathophysiology and other markers for disease, such as tumor markers for Epidermal Growth Factor, or Anaplase Lymphoma Kinase.

An additional consideration is the stage of the disease. Early cancers such as stages I, II, and III are often treated differently than advanced, stage IV cancers. Therapies demonstrating efficacy in one stage may not confer a benefit in an earlier stage such as with the use of bevacizumab in colorectal cancer. Therefore, when a treatment is studied for cancer, clear definitions of cancer type, including identified tumor markers, staging, previous treatments, time since diagnosis, patient characteristics such as organ function, age and performance status, are required to evaluate the investigational regimen for efficacy and safety. Since many studies evaluating botanicals are small trials of short durations, information regarding these parameters is often not available, and even if described, the study lacks the power to determine significance. Finally, botanical studies may use outcomes that are of unclear clinical relevance and not in routine use.

Botanicals used in cancer therapy and supportive care are discussed in Chapters 16 Cancer Prevention and 17 Treatment and Supportive and Palliative Care for Cancer.

4.8 Summary

Botanicals and other dietary supplements are used by an increasingly diverse population including those with significant comorbid conditions. Their usage may be both for health maintenance as well as treatment of underlying conditions or mitigation of adverse effects from conventional therapies. An essential element in using botanicals in special populations is open communication between healthcare providers and patients.

REFERENCES

Adams, J., C.-W. Lui, D. Sibbritt, A. Broom, J. Wardle, C. Homer, and S. Beck. 2009. "Women's use of complementary and alternative medicine during pregnancy: A critical review of the literature." *Birth.* 36:237–245.

Bairati, I., F. Meyer, M. Gelinas et al. 2005. "Randomized trial of antioxidant vitamins to prevent acute adverse effects of radiation therapy in head and neck cancer patients." *Journal of Clinical Oncology.* 23(4):5805–5813.

Bairati, I., F. Meyer, E. Jobin, M. Gélinas, A. Fortin, A. Nabid, F. Brochet, and B. Têtu. 2006. "Antioxidant vitamins supplementation and mortality: A randomized trial in head and neck cancer patients." *International Journal of Cancer.* 119(9):2221–2224. doi:10.1002/ijc.22042.

Bazzano, A. N., L. Cenac, A. J. Brandt, J. Barnett, S. Thibeau, and K. P. Theall. 2017. "Maternal experiences with and sources of information on galactagogues to support lactation: A cross-sectional study." *International Journal of Womens Health.* 9:105–113.

Budzynska, K., Z. E. Gardner, J. J. Dugoua, T. Low Dog, and P. Gardiner. 2012. "Systematic review of breastfeeding and herbs." *Breastfeed Med.* 7(6):489–503.

Columbo, D., L. Lunardon, and G. Bellia. 2014. "Cyclosporine and herbal supplement interactions." *Journal Toxicology* 2014, Article ID 145325, 6 pages, doi: 10.1155/2014/145325.

DeKosky, S. T., J. D. Williamson, A. L. Fitzpatrick, R. A. Kronmal, D. G. Ives, J. A. Saxton, O. L. Lopez, G. Burke, M. C. Carlson, L. P. Fried, L. H. Kuller, J. A. Robbins, R. P. Tracy, N. F. Woolard, L. Dunn, B. E. Snitz, R. L. Nahin, C. D. Furberg and the ginkgo evaluation of memory (GEM) study investigators. 2008. "*Ginkgo biloba* for Prevention of Dementia." *JAMA*. 300(19):2253–2262.

Dy, G. K., L. Bekele, L. J. Hanson, A. Furth, S. Mandrekar, J. A. Sloan, and A. A. Adjei. 2004. "Complementary and alternative medicine use by patients enrolled onto phase I clinical trials." *Journal of Clinical Oncology*. 22(23):4810–4815. doi:10.1200/JCO.2004.03.121.

Feghali, M., R. Venkataramanan, S. Caritis. 2015. "Pharmacokinetics of drugs in pregnancy." *Seminars in Perinatol*. 39(7):512–519.

Ferreira, P. R., J. F. Fleck, A. Diehl, D. Barletta, A. Braga-Filho, A. Barletta, and L. Ilha. 2004. "Protective effect of alpha-tocopherol in head and neck cancer radiation-induced mucositis: A double-blind randomized trial." *Head & Neck*. 26(4):313–321. doi:10.1002/hed.10382.

Ferrucci, L. M., B. P. Bell, K. B. Dhotre, M. M. Manos, N. A. Terrault, A. Zaman, R. C. Murphy, G. R. VanNess, A. R. Thomas, S. R. Bialek, M. M. Desai, and A. N. Sofair. 2010. "Complementary and alternative medicine use in chronic liver disease patients." *Journal of Clinical Gastroenterology*. 44(2):e40–e45.

Geller, A.I., N. Shehab, N. J. Weidle, M. C. Lovegrove, B. J. Wolpert, B. B. Timbo, R. P. Mozersky, and D. S. Budnitz. 2015. "Emergency department visits for adverse events related to dietary supplements." *New England Journal of Medicine*. 373:1531–1540.

Hall, H. R., D. L. Griffiths, and L. G. McKenna. 2011. "The use of complementary and alternative medicines by pregnant women: A literature review." *Midwifery*. 27(6):817–824.

He, W., D. Goodkind, and P. Kowal. 2015. U.S. Census Bureau, International Population Reports, P95/16-1, *An Aging World: 2015*. March 2016 U.S. Government Publishing Office, Washington, DC https://www.census.gov/content/dam/Census/library/publications/2016/demo/p95-16-1.pdf

Hess, S., S. De Geest, K. Halter, M. Dickenmann, and K. Denhaerynck. 2009. "Prevalence and correlates of selected alternative and complementary medicine in adult renal transplant patients." *Clinical Transplantation*. 23(1):56–62.

Hill, N. R., S. T. Fatoba, J. L. Oke, J. A. Hirst, C. A. O'Callaghan, and D. S. Lasserson. 2016. "Global prevalence of chronic kidney disease—A systematic review and meta-analysis." *PLOS One*. 11(7):e0158765. doi:10.1371/journal.pone.0158765.

Holst, L., D. Wright, S. Haavik, and H. Nordeng. 2011. "Safety and efficacy of herbal remedies in obstetrics-Review and clinical implications." *Midwifery*. 27(1):80–86.

Kantor, E. D., C. D. Rehm, M. Du, E. White, and E. L. Giovannucci. 2016. "Trends in dietary supplement use among US adults from 1999–2012. *JAMA*. 316(14):1464–1474. doi:10.1001/jama.2016.14403

Kasiappan, R. and S. H. Safe. 2016. "ROS-inducing agents for cancer chemotherapy." *Reactive Oxygen Species*. 1(1):22–37.

Kemper, K. J., S. Vohra, and R. Walls. 2008. "The use of complementary and alternative medicine in pediatrics." *Pediatrics*. 122:1374–1386.

Lawenda, B. D., K. M. Kelly, E. J. Ladas, S. M. Sagar, A. Vickers, and J. B. Blumberg. 2008. "Should supplemental antioxidant administration be avoided during chemotherapy and radiation therapy?" *Journal of the National Cancer Institute*. 100(11):773–783. doi:10.1093/jnci/djn148.

Low Dog, T. 2009. "The use of botanicals in pregnancy and lactation." *Altern Ther Health Med*. 5(1):54–58.

Lu, H. and S. Rosenbaum. 2014. "Developmental pharmacokinetics in pediatric populations." *The Journal of Pediatric Pharmacology and Therapeutics*. 19(4):262–276.

Luciano, R. L. and M. A. Perazella. 2015. "Aristolochic acid nephropathy: Epidemiology, clinical presentation, and treatment." *Drug Safety*. 38(1):55–64. doi: 10.1007/s40264-014-0244-x.

Marcus, D. M. and W. R. Snodgrass. 2005. "Do no harm: Avoidance of herbal medicines during pregnancy." *Obstetrics Gynecology*. 105(5 pt 1):1119–1122.

McClafferty, H., S. Vohra, M. Bailey, M. Brown, A. Esparham, D. Gerstbacher, B. Golianu, A. K. Niemi, E. Sibinga, J. Weydert, and A. M. Yeh. 2017. "Pediatric integrative medicine." *Pediatrics*. 140(3) doi: 10.1542/peds.2017-1961

Moschella, C. and B. L. Jaber. 2001. "Interaction between cyclosporine and hypericum perforatum (St. John's wort) after organ transplantation." *American Journal of Kidney Disease*. 38(5):1105–1107.

Nahin, R. L., M. Pecha, D. B. Welmerink, K. Sink, S. T. DeKosky, and A. L. Fitzpatrick. 2009. Ginkgo evaluation study investigators. "Concomitant use of prescription drugs and dietary supplements in ambulatory elderly people." *Journal of the American Geriatrics Society*. 57(7):1197–1205.

Nahin, R. L., P. M. Barnes, and B. J. Stussman. 2016. "Expenditures on complementary health approaches: United states, 2012." *Natl Health Stat Report.* 95:1–11.

National Center for Complementary and Integrative Health. 2012. Children and the Use of Complementary Health Approaches. URL: https://nccih.nih.gov/health/children#patterns [accessed 2016 Oct 12].

National Kidney Foundation. 2015 https://www.kidney.org/atoz/content/herbalsupp

Navarro, V. J., H. Barnhart, B. L. Bonkovsky, T. Davern, R. J. Fontana, L. Grant, K. R. Reddy, L. B. Seeff, J. Serrano, A. H. Sherker, A. Stolz, J. Talwalkar, M. Vega, and R. Vuppalanchi. 2014. "Liver injury from herbals and dietary supplements in the US drug induced liver injury network." *Hepatology.* 60(4):1399–1408.

Osman, N. A., S. M. Hassanein, M. M. Leil, and M. M. NasrAllah. 2015. "Complementary and alternative medicine use among patients with chronic kidney disease and kidney transplant recipients." *Journal of Renal Nutrition.* 25(6):466–471.

Palatini, P. and S. DeMartin. 2016. "Pharmacokinetic drug interactions in liver disease: An update." *World Journal of Gastroenterology.* 22:1260–1278.

Rao, N., H. A. Spiller, N. L. Hodges, T. Chounthirath, M. J. Casavant, A. K. Kamboj, and G. A. Smith. 2017. "An increase in dietary supplement exposures reported to US poison control centers." *Journal of Medical Toxicology.* 13(3):227–237. doi:10.1007/s13181-017-0623-7.

Richardson, M. A., T. Sanders, J. L. Palmer, A. Greisinger, and S. E. Singletary. 2000. "Complementary/alternative medicine use in a comprehensive cancer center and the implications for oncology." *Journal of Clinical Oncology.* 18(13):2505–2514. doi:10.1200/JCO.2000.18.13.2505.

Sarin, S. K. and R. Maiwall. 2017. *"Global Burden of Liver Disease: A True Burden on Health Sciences and Economies."* World Gastroenterology Organization

Sarma, D. N., M. L. Barrett, M. L. Chavez, P. Gardiner, R. Ko, G. B. Mahady, R. J. Marles, L. S. Pellicore, G. I. Giancaspro, and T. Low Dog. 2008. "Safety of green tea extracts: A systematic review by the US pharmacopeia." *Drug Safety.* 31(6):469–484.

Sutherland, A. and B. V. Sweet. 2010. "Butterbur: An alternative therapy for migraine." *American Journal of Health-System Pharmacy.* 67(9):705–711. doi:10.2146/ajhp090136.

Tasnif, Y., J. Morado, and M. F. Hebert. 2016. "Pregnancy-related pharmacokinetic changes." *Clinical Pharmacology and Therapeutics.* 100(1):53–62.

Taylor, J. A., W. Weber, L. Standish, H. Quinn, J. Goesling, M. McGann, and C. Calabrese. 2003. "Efficacy and safety in treating upper respiratory tract infections in children: A randomized controlled trial." *JAMA.* 290(21):2824–2830.

Teschke, R. and V. Lebot. 2011. "Proposal for a kava quality standardization code." *Food and Chemical Toxicology.* 49(10):2503–2516. doi:10.1016/j.fct.2011.06.075.

World Health Organization, UNICEF, 2014. Global Nutrition Targets 2025: Breastfeeding policy brief. Document WHO/NMH/NHD/14.7. World Health Organization; Geneva. WHO renal transplants http://www.who.int/transplantation/gkt/statistics/en/

Zhang, Y., E. B. Fein, and S. B. Fein. 2011. "Feeding of iedtary botanical supplements and teas to infants in the United States." *Pediatrics.* 127(6):1060–1066.

Section II

Botanical Integrative Medicine

Section II

5

Cardiovascular Disease

Cydney E. McQueen and Andrew J. Smith

CONTENTS

5.1 Introduction

Worldwide, patients with cardiovascular disease have been using supplements such as fish oil for cardiovascular health in increasing numbers for the last several decades. However, the use of botanical medicines for cardiovascular disease treatment is far older. Many botanicals have pharmacologic properties affecting the micro- and macro-vascular systems. Though use is often preventative, many botanicals are taken for treatment effects on blood pressure, lipids, or platelet aggregation. Frequently, this use is in addition to prescription drug therapies, providing opportunity for additive or synergistic benefits, or greater risks of harm.

5.2 Hypertension

Elevated blood pressure is a well-established risk factor of the development of cardiovascular disease such as myocardial infarction, heart failure, and stroke (Kannel 1996). Hypertension is common; risk factors for development include age, race, family history, weight, tobacco use, a high sodium diet, and psychosocial stressors (Mozaffarian et al. 2015, Kantor et al. 2015).

The 2017 treatment guidelines recommend a blood pressure goal of <130/80 mmHg for patients with clinical cardiovascular disease or a high risk of cardiovascular disease defined as a risk score >10% (*see ASCVD risk score in Section 5.4 Dyslipidemia*). Patients without cardiovascular disease and low risk (<10%) have a goal of <140/90 mmHg (Whelton et al. 2017). Lifestyle changes, including exercise and dietary modifications (including sodium restriction), remain the cornerstone of treatment (Eckel et al. 2014). In terms of pharmacological treatment, first line agents for hypertension management are angiotensin converting enzyme (ACE) inhibitors, angiotensin receptor blockers, calcium channel blockers, and thiazide diuretics (Whelton et al. 2017).

5.2.1 Garlic

5.2.1.1 Background

Garlic, *Allium sativum*, is a common food or seasoning ingredient all over the world. In modern years, most usage and research has been focused on cardiovascular benefits on blood pressure and lipids (*See Section 5.4 Dyslipidemia*), influence on the immune system, antimicrobial effects, antioxidant potential, and anti-cancer activities.

5.2.1.2 Pharmacognosy

Only bulbs of the garlic plant are used in the preparation of medicinal products. Garlic plants collect sulfur, which is incorporated first into L-cysteine, then glutathione. Other conversions result in many compounds that utilize and/or store sulfur (Kodera et al. 2017). A major component is allicin, formed when the precursor compound, alliin, is acted upon by the lyase allinase; this occurs when fresh garlic bulbs are crushed or cut and is the primary source of garlic's distinctive pungent aroma. Since allinase is inactivated by heat, no allicin is present in heat-processed garlic products. Odor-free products, whether heat-processed or not, generally contain no allicin. Although allicin was long believed to be the sole active ingredient, many of garlic's compounds contribute to antihypertensive actions. These components include unstable thiosulinates closely related to allicin, *S*-allyl-L-cysteine (SAC), *S*-1-propenyl-l-cysteine (S1PC), and ajoene (Kodera et al. 2017, Shouk et al. 2014).

Raw garlic, garlic powder, garlic extracts, aged garlic extracts (AGE), and the separate components possess multiple activities that lower blood pressure directly or indirectly (Alali et al. 2017, Shouk et al. 2014). Increased nitric oxide causes vasodilation and decreases oxidative stress, while increased hydrogen sulfide causes vasodilation due to increased cystathionine-γ-lyase in vascular smooth muscle. Inhibition of ACE leads to decreased angiotensin II, inhibition of nuclear factor-κB in endothelial cells decreases inflammation and vasoconstriction, and decreased vasoconstriction results from inhibition of vascular smooth muscle cell proliferation.

Various constituents are responsible to different degrees for the activities, which helps to explain why garlic products with different chemical profiles still have antihypertensive action (Alali et al. 2017, Shouk et al. 2014). Additionally, research has demonstrated that when foods are seasoned with garlic, many individuals will preferentially choose food samples containing lower sodium concentrations (Nugrahani and Afifah 2016).

5.2.1.3 Dosing and Preparation

Dosing of garlic for hypertension is dependent upon the type of garlic preparation. Because a wide range of doses was utilized in clinical trials, it is recommended to begin with a low to moderate dose and titrate upwards. The dosage for garlic powder is 400–2,400 mg daily and aged garlic extract is 500–7,200 mg once daily or in divided doses. Garlic oil is not recommended. Products may be standardized to allicin content, 4 to 12 mg daily, or to SAC content, 1.2–2.4 mg daily. Common brands available with evidence to support use are Kwai®, Kyolic®, and Allicor®; however, many "brand extension" products exist that may include additional untested and unnecessary ingredients. One study supports use of timed-release garlic powder tablets over regular release (Sobenin et al. 2009).

5.2.1.4 Safety

Daily *garlic breath* is probably the most common adverse effect associated with its use and a reason for the development of odor-free garlic products. Mild gastrointestinal (GI) symptoms such as nausea, flatulence, and bloating are common and can occur with greater severity, leading to discontinuation in some clinical trials. Allergic reactions, especially pruritis and contact dermatitis, have also been reported with oral and topical use. These are most common with the use of whole raw garlic cloves.

Garlic decreases platelet aggregation and can increase bleeding time; garlic supplements should be stopped 7–10 days prior to any planned surgery or dental procedure. In urgent procedures, increased bleeding is likely. In an interaction study, no pharmacokinetic interaction was noted between warfarin and aged garlic extract, but any concomitant use should be approached cautiously, with additional INR monitoring (Alali et al. 2017). One study of days days of AGE therapy with cilostazol noted no changes in antiplatelet activity.

Cautions about use of garlic with hormonal birth control are common on the internet; despite lack of clinical confirmation of the interaction, it is wise to avoid garlic supplements or use another method of birth control. Garlic use with isoniazid should be avoided as animal studies have noted 65% reductions in AUC and maximum concentration (Dhamija et al. 2006). *See Chapter 2 Pharmacokinetic and Pharmacogenomic Considerations for in-depth discussion of garlic's influence on drug metabolism.*

5.2.1.5 Clinical Evidence

A 2016 meta-analysis included 20 trials comparing garlic supplements to placebo (Ried 2016). All patients, regardless of blood pressure status, showed mean reductions in SBP and DBP of −5.1 mmHg

(P < 0.001) and −2.5 mmHg (P < 0.002), respectively. Hypertensive subjects showed mean reductions of SBP and DBP were −8.7 and −6.1 mmHg (P < 0.001 for each). In subanalyses, both garlic powder and aged garlic extracts provided significant reductions in SBP, −5.8 and −4.1 mmHg, respectively, but DBP reduction, −3.2 mmHg, was only significant for garlic powder. Adverse effects occurred in approximately 1/3 of subjects and included eructation, reflux, and flatulence.

Similar results were seen in an earlier meta-analysis of seven trials conducted in hypertensive patients: mean SBP and DBP reductions were −6.71 and −4.79 mmHg (Xiong et al. 2015). Researchers have stated that blood pressure changes in garlic studies are generally similar to effects seen in an analysis of the five types of prescription antihypertensive agents (Law 2003).

Garlic powder as an additive blood pressure therapy was examined in patients (n = 56) with severe coronary artery disease undergoing angioplasty (Mahdavi-Roshan et al. 2016). Subjects received either 4 m garlic powder containing 1,200 mcg allicin twice daily or placebo tablets, beginning within 3 days after angioplasty. At 3 months, mean SBP and DBP had increased by 6.31 and 4.6 mmHg in the placebo group and 1.11 and 4.11 mmHg in the garlic group. In patients with hypertension at baseline, mean SBP and DBP decreased by −12.1 mmHg (P = 0.001 versus placebo) and −4 mmHg (P = 0.24 versus placebo). Only one patient in the garlic treatment reported GI adverse effects (Mahdavi-Roshan et al. 2016).

5.2.1.6 Clinical Application

Overall, the existing evidence supports garlic's use in patients with mild to moderate hypertension, especially in conjunction with lifestyle and dietary modifications. Garlic's effects are insufficient for patients with modcrate to severe hypertension.

5.2.2 Green Tea (*Camellia sinensis*)

5.2.2.1 Background

After water, tea is the most common beverage in the world. Tea has a rich history globally, but the greatest in China, where tea is consumed not solely as a beverage, but has great social and ceremonial value.

5.2.2.2 Pharmacognosy

All tea comes from the *Camellia sinensis* plant. The green, oolong, and black varieties of tea are developed through processing. Green tea consists of leaves steamed and dried with no fermentation, oolong undergoes a short fermentation period, and black tea is from leaves completely fermented before being dried and packaged (Mazzanti et al. 2015).

Tea contains many constituents; of chief importance are polyphenols and catechins, especially epi-gallocatechin-3-gallate (EGCG), which may provide the greatest bioactivity and makes up half of the catechin content. Flavonoids such as quercetin and kaempferol are also present, along with caffeine (Khan and Mukhtar 2007). Both green and black tea, as well as green tea extracts, possess antioxidant effects, anticancer activities such as induction of apoptosis and inhibition of cell growth and proliferation, cardiovascular and cerebrovascular effects, and anti-obesity actions (Clement 2009). Mechanisms for antihypertensive effects have not been clearly identified, although antioxidant activities may play a role.

5.2.2.3 Dosing and Preparation

Trials of green tea have varied in dosage, dosage form, and amounts of EGCG or other polyphenols. An optimum dosage or form has not been determined. For patients drinking green tea, 2–4 cups per day seems to be the amount associated with the greatest benefits in both epidemiologic studies and in clinical hypertension trials. For green tea extracts, dosages being used range from 250–2,300 mg daily, with EGCG contents of 150–856 mg. However, the highest dosages are associated with greater incidence of adverse effects (Onakpoya et al. 2014a). Until more specific data is available, extract dosages should be limited to 400–1,200 mg daily.

5.2.2.4 Safety

Adverse effects in clinical trials have been limited to GI symptoms and mild rash. With the highest doses of extracts, constipation has been reported. There have been a substantial number of case reports of hepatotoxicity associated with use of green tea extracts or with green tea beverages in "high quantity," although that quantity is undefined in reports (Mazzanti et al. 2015). The majority have resolved after discontinuation of the tea or extract. Patients with liver disease or taking potentially hepatotoxic drugs should avoid green tea extracts and limit beverage consumption to normal dietary amounts to avoid possible additive effects.

Many safety concerns with green tea stem from the caffeine content, which is known to cause short-term increases blood pressure and to act as a diuretic. Green tea should be avoided with stimulant drugs due to additive CNS effects. Patients taking nadolol should avoid green tea completely; daily use of 700 mL of tea (322 mg of EGCG) was shown to decrease nadolol concentration by 85.3% by affecting organic anion transport protein 1A2 (Misaka et al. 2014).

5.2.2.5 Evidence

Epidemiological evidence has demonstrated an inverse relationship between tea or green tea consumption and incidence of hypertension (Clement 2009). Its use is also associated with a reduced risk of stroke. However, findings are not consistent and many studies have been performed in Asia where traditional tea consumption is greater than in the western hemisphere. Other factors may limit effects; a 5-year study in Chinese adults found that greater tea intake was associated with overall lower blood pressure increases over time in non-smokers, but not among smokers (Tong et al. 2014).

Individual interventional trials have had conflicting results. A 2014 meta-analysis of 25 studies noted that green tea had a greater impact on blood pressure, with a mean SBP change of −2.1 mmHg (95% confidence interval [CI]: −2.9, −1.2) and DBP change of −1.7 mmHg (95% CI: −2.9, −0.5), than black tea, mean SBP change of −1.4 mmHg (95% CI: −2.4, −0.4) and DBP change of −1.1 mmHg (95% CI: −1.9, −0.2). (Liu et al. 2014) Benefits were primarily evident in subjects using green tea for at least 12 weeks, with no acute effects discernable; this agrees with the negative findings more common in short duration trials. These results are similar to a 2014 meta-analysis which found a mean SBP reduction of −1.94 mmHg (95% CI: −2.95, −0.93, P = 0.0002) (Onakpoya et al. 2014a). The analysis also noted a dose response effect for EGCG and that doses above 200 mg did not provide additional benefits. No significant reductions were found for DBP.

A meta-analysis analyzed data from 14 green tea or green tea extract studies in overweight or obese adults performed around the world (Li et al. 2015). Researchers noted the great heterogeneity of trial results, but found a statistically significant mean reduction from baseline in SBP and DBP, −1.42 mmHg (95% CI: −2.47, −0.36, P = 0.008) and −1.25 mmHg (95% CI: −2.32, −0.19, P = 0.02). Subgroup analyses revealed that significant effects were only apparent after 12 weeks and that SBP decreases were significant only in trials conducted in non-Asian countries.

A crossover trial compared a green tea extract containing 780 mg of polyphenols daily to placebo for 4 weeks in obese women classified as prehypertensive (Nogueira et al. 2016). Significant decreases from baseline occurred for daytime SBP (−3.61 mmHg, p = 0.04) compared to placebo, but not DBP, (−1.89 mmHg, p = 0.2). The pattern of response was repeated for nighttime blood pressure as well. *See Chapter 15 Obesity and Weight Loss for further discussion.*

5.2.2.6 Clinical Application

Despite mixed results, the overall evidence does support that green tea or green tea extract can reduce blood pressure when used long-term. The extent of reduction is small, so green tea is unlikely to be appropriate as a sole therapy, but could be a useful addition to dietary and lifestyle changes. Patients should understand that higher dosages will not achieve greater blood pressure reductions as the caffeine could possibly work against the benefits provided by the EGCG or other polyphenols.

5.2.3 Green Coffee Bean Extract

5.2.3.1 Background

Coffee beans are roasted when being processed for beverage and food uses. The roasting process both destroys some compounds and creates others. Green coffee bean extract (GCBE) was first investigated for use in weight loss, but blood pressure reductions were noted in animal studies.

5.2.3.2 Pharmacognosy

GCBE's active component is chlorogenic acids (CGA), also common in many fruits, vegetables, and traditional botanical medicines (Tom et al. 2016). One third of the 13 types of CGA undergoes intestinal absorption and is metabolized to quinic, caffeic, and ferulic acids (Stalmach et al. 2014). Ferulic acid increases vasoreactivity, resulting in hypotensive effects, likely through endothelial nitric oxide mechanisms. CGA directly affect the endothelium through three pathways: cyclooxygenase, nitric oxide-synthase, and endothelium-derived hyperpolarizing factors (Tom et al. 2016). Although regular roasted coffee does contain some CGA, it does not have antihypertensive effects because the roasting process creates hydrohydroxyquinone, which counteracts CGA's hypotensive activity (Zhao et al. 2011).

5.2.3.3 Dosing and Preparation

Due to the varied GCBE and CGA dosage forms used in clinical trials, dosing recommendations are preliminary. A GCBE or CGA supplement should supply a minimum of 140 mg of CGA daily with a reasonable upper dosage of 500 mg based on the extent of blood-pressure lowering in clinical trials. Higher dosages undergo decreasing absorption, possibly due to an increase in the speed of intestinal transit (Stalmach et al. 2014). CGA absorption primarily occurs in the large intestine and is reduced by concomitant fat and dairy. Patients with ileostomies or with significant colon disease will have greatly reduced bioavailability (Loader et al. 2017, Stalmach et al. 2014). Patients who already drink coffee may find CGA-enriched coffee drinks an acceptable dosage form; brands used in hypertension trials include Svetol® and Coffee Slender®. Patients who do not drink coffee may be more satisfied with GCBE or CGA tablets or capsules. However, product quality is an issue, as 4 of 8 originally tested supplements failed to meet standards (ConsumerLab.com 2018).

5.2.3.4 Safety

GCBE/CGA is well tolerated with no adverse events reported in clinical trials. However, adverse effects may depend upon the dosage form as GCBE or CGA-containing coffees may have caffeine unless it has been specifically removed.

Most discussions about drug interactions are likewise based on the potential associated with caffeine. One GCBE coffee product has been shown to decrease blood glucose levels slightly in healthy individuals, therefore a caution for extra self-monitoring of blood glucose is advised for patients with diabetes on antihyperglycemic medications (Thom 2007).

5.2.3.5 Evidence

A 2015 meta-analysis included five trials evaluating CGA for blood pressure in 394 total subjects (Onakpoya et al. 2014b). The daily CGA dosages ranged from 25 to 482 mg via coffee, soy soup, fruit, and vegetable juice, or a bottled drink, compared to appropriate placebo controls for 4 to 26 weeks. The mean difference in SBP change compared to placebo was −4.31 mmHg (95% CI: −5.6, −3.01, P < 0.00001). For DBP, the mean difference was −3.68 mmHg (95% CI: −3.91, −3.45, P < 0.00001). Mean differences changed slightly in subanalyses including only patients with hypertension, only parallel-group trials, and only trials with good blinding, but all differences from placebo were significant. Effect size was classified as moderate, with modest clinical relevance (Onakpoya et al. 2014b). The mean SBP reduction in CGA groups ranged from −0.5 to −5.6 mmHg. One caveat to this analysis is inclusion of a trial that was discredited and retracted after publication (Loader et al. 2017).

In 2017, the clinical evidence was reviewed using the requirements for evaluation of dietary ingredient health claims by Health Canada (Loader et al. 2017). The reviewers included four trials not in the 2015 meta-analysis, and did not include the retracted study. Effect size was calculated for 6 of 8 studies; SBP reductions were −1.9 to −4.3 mmHg and DBP reductions were −1.8 to −6.8 mmHg. The other two studies found small SBP and DBP increases which were not different from controls. Evidence was insufficient to support a health claim under the Health Canada guidelines. *See Chapter 15 Obesity and Weight Loss for further discussion.*

5.2.3.6 Clinical Application

The available evidence is insufficient to support a general recommendation for the use of GCBE or CGA in patients diagnosed with hypertension. An optimal dosage or dosage form has not been identified. For patients who are coffee drinkers, the choice to use high-CGA coffee instead of regular coffee may provide slight benefits on blood pressure in addition to other therapies.

5.3 Summary

Of the botanical therapies used for hypertension, garlic supplements have the best evidence of efficacy to support use, while green tea is easily incorporated into daily routines as a beverage. A primary safety consideration may be possible drug interactions, but whether garlic possesses more drug interactions than green tea or green coffee bean extract remains unclear.

5.4 Dyslipidemia

Dyslipidemia is a common condition worldwide and a leading risk factor for the development of coronary artery disease. Total serum cholesterol is composed of three main components: high density lipoprotein (HDL), low-density lipoprotein (LDL), and triglycerides. Elevated LDL-cholesterol and low HDL-cholesterol are risk factors for stroke, coronary artery disease, and peripheral artery disease (Nelson 2013). Elevated triglycerides may increase cardiovascular risk, but levels over 500 mg/dL increase risk of pancreatitis.

The practice guideline for dyslipidemia management focuses on determining a patient's 10-year risk of atherosclerotic cardiovascular disease (ASCVD) (Stone et al. 2013). An ASCVD risk score is determined by demographics, lipid levels, SBP, and comorbid disease states. Treatment is recommended for scores over 7.5% (Stone et al. 2013). Pharmacological treatment primarily focuses on use of statins, with second-line agents used in patients who cannot tolerate a statin or achieve adequate LDL lowering. Nonpharmacological treatment consists of a low-fat diet and exercise. Many patients managing dyslipidemia this way choose to supplement their efforts with botanicals.

5.4.1 Red Yeast Rice

5.4.1.1 Background

Monascus purpureus, a red-colored yeast that grows on fermented rice, has been used for centuries in traditional Chinese medicine for cardiovascular conditions and GI complaints of diarrhea and indigestion (Burke 2015, Ong and Aziz 2016). As a dietary supplement, powdered red yeast rice is used for dyslipidemia.

5.4.1.2 Pharmacognosy

Fermented under controlled conditions, *Monascus purpureus* produces greater quantities of several mevinic acids, also known as monacolins. One of these, monacolin K, is chemically identical to lovastatin, and the names can be used interchangeably (Gordan et al. 2010). Lovastatin inhibits HMG-CoA reductase, serving as a rate-limiting step for hepatic cholesterol synthesis. Additional compounds in red yeast rice, such as isoflavones and phytosterols, also contribute to the cholesterol-lowering activity as the extent of lipid level reduction cannot be fully explained by the small doses of lovastatin present in products used in clinical trials. Animal studies have also demonstrated increased bile acid excretion, but other mechanisms, as yet unidentified, are likely (Ma et al. 2009).

5.4.1.3 Dosing and Preparation

Studies of red yeast rice have commonly used dosages of 1,200–2,400 mg daily, although dosages up to 4,800 mg per day have been used (Gerards et al. 2015). This is generally given twice daily, but once daily dosing has been used in trials. Comparisons between trials must be done cautiously, because different strength products may have similar lovastatin content. For example, in trials using 1,200, 2,400, and 4,800 mg per day of red yeast rice, the monocolin K content was 10–24 mg, 4.8 mg, and 9.96 mg per day, respectively (Gerards et al. 2015).

Purchasing high quality products is essential, not only to ensure the presence of active components, but to ensure the lack of citrinin, a nephrotoxin that can form during an incorrectly performed fermentation process. A 2008 analysis found citrinin in 4 of 12 products purchased from retail stores (Gordan et al. 2010).

5.4.1.4 Safety

In the United States, red yeast rice has been evaluated in trials lasting up to 24 weeks, while a large Chinese trial evaluating cardiovascular outcomes in patients with previous myocardial infarctions evaluated patients for 4.5 years (Li et al. 2009). Red yeast rice is generally well tolerated. Mild side effects reported in clinical trials and postmarketing studies include dizziness, headache, fatigue, bloating, abdominal discomfort, flatulence, and heartburn (Karl et al. 2012). Allergic reactions are possible. Cases of elevated creatinine kinase levels, myalgia, and rhabdomyolysis have occurred, although current data indicates incidence is lower than with statin use. Complicating the issue is contradictory information regarding the true incidence of myalgias associated with statin use; reports range from 0.3% to 33% (Magni et al. 2015).

Additionally, a debated question is whether patients who have experienced rhabdomyolysis or other severe adverse effects with statins can safely take red yeast rice. A 2009 study (N = 62) compared 3600 mg daily of red yeast rice, with total monocolins of 12.96 mg and monocolin K 6.12 mg, to placebo in patients who had discontinued statin therapy due to myalgia (Becker et al. 2009). Two patients taking red yeast rice and one patient taking placebo developed "persistent intolerable myalgias" with normal CPK levels. A second study compared red yeast rice, 9.96 mg monocolin K daily, to pravastatin 40 mg daily in 43 patients with previous statin intolerance due to myalgia (Halbert et al. 2010). Persistent generalized myalgias were reported in 13.6% of pravastatin-treated patients and none with red yeast rice (p = 0.23). When intermittent myalgias were included, reports rose to 23.8% of red yeast rice patients and 36.4% of pravastatin patients (p = 0.10). No patients experienced muscle weakness although two pravastatin-treated patients and one patient taking red yeast rice discontinued due to myalgia.

A patient experiencing myalgias with statin use may still be an appropriate candidate for red yeast rice, although additional caution is recommended. However, patients who have previously developed rhabdomyolysis with the use of a statin or currently taking prescription statins should not take red yeast rice.

5.4.1.5 Evidence

Multiple studies and meta-analyses have examined the efficacy of red yeast rice for lipid reduction against placebo and statins. A 2015 meta-analysis included 20 studies, five from the United States, one in Norway, and the rest in China or Taiwan (Gerards et al. 2015). Average LDL-cholesterol reduction compared to placebo was −39.44 mg/dL, about 1.9 mg/dL less than statin therapy. Average triglyceride reduction was −10.05 mg/dL, while HDL-cholesterol increased 2.71 mg/dL. An additional meta-analysis examined 10 trials comparing red yeast rice, 1–3.6 grams per day, to simvastatin, 10 or 20 mg per day (Ong and Aziz 2016). There were no significant differences in LDL-cholesterol reductions between red yeast rice, −37.51 mg/dL, and simvastatin, −37.9 mg/dL. HDL-cholesterol increases were not significantly different except in two trials which favored simvastatin therapy. The Italian Society for Diabetology and the Italian Society for the Study of Arteriosclerosis issued a joint position paper supporting red yeast rice therapy in patients failing lifestyle modifications who need LDL-cholesterol reductions of less than 25% and with mild to moderate cardiovascular risk (Pirro et al. 2017).

5.4.1.6 Clinical Application

Substantial evidence supports red yeast rice's ability to reduce total cholesterol, LDL-cholesterol, and, to a lesser extent, triglyceride levels. Long-term outcomes data for its effects on cardiovascular morbidity and mortality are not available. Questions remain about adverse effect incidence and the tolerability of red yeast rice in patients unable to tolerate statins. Red yeast rice use should be limited to patients at a lower cardiovascular risk needing no more than a 30 mg/dL reduction in total cholesterol or LDL-cholesterol in order to reach therapeutic goals. Patients with low HDL-cholesterol levels may need other treatment options, as red yeast rice does not consistently nor substantially increase HDL-cholesterol levels. As with other pharmacologic treatments, red yeast rice should be used with appropriate diet and lifestyle modifications.

5.4.2 Green Tea

5.4.2.1 Background

See Hypertension Section 5.2.2 for background discussion.

5.4.2.2 Pharmacognosy

Numerous animal studies demonstrate antilipemic effects of green tea or green tea extracts, which are likely to occur through multiple mechanisms. The EGCG content may reduce dietary fat and cholesterol uptake by decreasing activity of the apical sodium bile acid transporter in the ileum and reducing the solubility and uptake of lipid micelles (Annaba et al. 2010, Koo and Noh 2007). The antioxidant properties of the catechins are important, as these undergo uptake by LDL-cholesterol particles and then remain, reducing LDL-cholesterol oxidation (Suzuki-Sugihara et al. 2016). Both EGCG and linalool, a terpene component of green tea, affect peroxisome proliferator-activated receptor α (PPARα) that aids in regulation of lipid metabolism (Lee and Jia 2015).

5.4.2.3 Dosing and Preparation

As with use for hypertension, the optimum dosage or form of green tea has not been determined. Green tea extracts with standardized amounts of catechins and EGCG are preferred, especially if clinically significant reductions in lipids are needed. Based on results from clinical trials, a reasonable dose range to consider for initial treatment is 400–1,600 mg of catechins daily.

5.4.2.4 Safety

See Hypertension Section 5.2.2 for safety discussion.

5.4.2.5 Evidence

Multiple trials have assessed effects of green tea or green tea catechins on lipid parameters. In pooled data, significant effects included reductions in total cholesterol and LDL-cholesterol, but not HDL-cholesterol or triglycerides. A 2011 meta-analysis of 20 trials concluded that green tea catechins reduced total cholesterol by a mean of -5.46 mg/dL (95% CI: -9.59, -1.32) and LDL-cholesterol by -5.3 mg/dL (95% CI: -9.99, -0.62) (Kim et al. 2011).

Green tea may be less effective in patients with Type 2 diabetes. A meta-analysis of 10 trials of green tea or extracts noted significant changes only in fasting insulin concentrations and waist circumference; mean total cholesterol and LDL-cholesterol levels were reduced, but not significantly, -1.93 mg/dL (95% CI: -1.93, $+7.75$) and -2.71 mg/dL (95% CI: -5.8, $+11.21$) (Li et al. 2016). These reductions are substantially less than in other patient populations.

A study of 1,075 healthy postmenopausal women examined effects of a green tea extract containing 1,315 mg of catechins (843 mg EGCG) daily for a year compared to placebo (Samavat et al. 2016). Similar to other studies, total cholesterol and LDL-cholesterol reductions were significant at -4.35 mg/dL and -4.81 mg/dL, respectively, while no change was seen in HDL-cholesterol. However, triglycerides, significantly lower at baseline in the extract group than the placebo group, were increased by 3.31 mg/dL at one year in the extract group, while the placebo group mean change was -2.6 mg/dL (p = 0.046). As in the previous trial, stratification analysis showed that subjects who had total cholesterol over 240 mg/dL or 200–239 mg/dL, at baseline had greater reductions over placebo than normolipemic subjects: -8.3% versus -2.8% and -3.6% versus -0.2%, respectively. No additive benefits were noted for subjects already on antihyperlipidemic therapies, but this subset of patients was small.

5.4.2.6 Clinical Application

Overall, clinical evidence and the safety profile support the use of green tea and green tea extracts in dyslipidemia. However, the clinical value of green tea is limited. Lipid reductions are generally small and greatest reductions are in those with the highest baseline levels, effects in patients with diabetes may be minimal, and patients with elevated triglycerides as their primary lipid concern are not likely to experience reductions. An additional caveat is the choice of an appropriate green tea product and dose, as these varied widely in clinical trials demonstrating beneficial reductions.

5.4.3 Garlic

5.4.3.1 Background

See Hypertension Section 5.2.1 for background discussion.

5.4.3.2 Pharmacognosy/Mechanism/Plant Part

As with hypertension, garlic constituents have multiple actions that may improve lipid levels. S-allyl cysteine (SAC) and diallyl-di-sulfide are two specific components that inhibit synthesis of cholesterol; cholesterol absorption may also be effected via influence on transport proteins and receptors (Alali et al. 2017). Some inhibition of HMG-CoA reductase is present, but other enzymes, such as fatty acid synthase and glucose-6 phosphate dehydrogenase, are also inhibited (Hosseini and Hosseinzadeh 2015). Garlic's antioxidant effects aid in reducing oxidation of LDL-cholesterol and contribute to anti-atherosclerotic effects such as reduction of endothelial inflammation and formation of atheromatous lesions (Hosseini and Hosseinzadeh 2015).

5.4.3.3 Dosing and Preparation

Both garlic powder and AGE have benefit in reducing total cholesterol, LDL-cholesterol, and triglycerides. For garlic powder, dosage ranges are 0.6–4 grams daily, given in 2–3 divided doses. AGE dosages range from 1–6 grams daily in divided doses. As in use for hypertension, Kwai, Kyolic, and Allicor® are the most clinically tested brands available.

5.4.3.4 Safety

See Hypertension Section 5.2.1 for safety discussion.

5.4.3.5 Evidence

A 2013 meta-analysis of garlic products for reduction of lipids included 39 trials with durations of 2–52 weeks and 2,298 subjects (Ried et al. 2013). Garlic lowered total cholesterol and LDL-cholesterol significantly more than placebo, −15.25 mg/dL (95% CI: −20.72, −9.78) and −6.41 mg/dL (95% CI: −11.77, −1.05), while triglyceride reduction was not significant, −5.45 mg/dL (95% CI: −14.18, 3.27). The mean HDL-cholesterol increase was small, 1.49 mg/dL (95% CI: 0.19, 2.79) and no significant triglyceride effects were noted. For all outcomes, subgroup analyses revealed greater changes in trials longer than 8 weeks and in patients with higher baseline lipid levels. AGE had a greater effect on total cholesterol than garlic powder or oil, while enteric-coated garlic powder interventions had the most impact. Garlic powder had the best results for LDL-cholesterol reduction, although few studies measuring this outcome used other dosage forms. Garlic oil increased HDL-cholesterol by a mean of 5.97 mg/dL.

The question of whether garlic can reduce cardiovascular risk has not been answered, although some study of risk markers has occurred. A placebo-controlled study of AGE, 2400 mg daily, for one year in 55 patients with metabolic syndrome examined effects on coronary plaque (Matsumoto et al. 2016). Plaques with lipid cores are more likely to rupture, causing an acute cardiovascular event; greater core volumes are more unstable and at higher risk of rupture. In the AGE group, cardiac computed tomography angiography at one year noted a significant reduction in the low attenuation plaque percentage, which correlates to greater lipid core volumes, in the patients' coronary arteries. Other outcomes such as total plaque volume were not significantly different from the placebo group (Matsumoto et al. 2016).

5.4.3.6 Clinical Application

The lipid-lowering effects of garlic are clinically significant and few adverse effects exist. Duration of therapy is important, as benefits were often not seen in trials of less than 12 weeks. If garlic is used in dyslipidemia, therapy should continue for a minimum of 3–4 months before efficacy is assessed. Patients who would also benefit from its effects on blood pressure may be better candidates for garlic use.

5.4.4 Psyllium

5.4.4.1 Background

Psyllium comes from *Plantago ovata*, sometimes called isphagula or sand plantain. Psyllium contains both soluble and insoluble fiber and is commonly used for constipation, diarrhea, and various bowel conditions.

5.4.4.2 Pharmacognosy

The active portion of *Plantago ovata* is the seed husk, although occasionally husk and seed are used. The soluble fiber forms a mucilaginous gel in the gut, either binding to bile acids or forming a barrier to reabsorption of bile acids (Eussen et al. 2010). Increased bile acid secretion stimulates up-regulation of cholesterol 7-α-hydroxylase to synthesize more bile acids, depleting hepatic stores of cholesterol, which causes increased expression of LDL receptors, reducing circulating levels of LDL-cholesterol (Anonymous 2002). The soluble and insoluble fiber decreases gut transit time; this, as well as increased viscosity within the gut, leads to decreased glucose and nutrient absorption, reducing overall caloric uptake. General caloric intake may also be decreased as a result of increased feelings of fullness (Eussen et al. 2010).

5.4.4.3 Dosing and Preparation

The dosing of psyllium is variable, but the majority of clinical trials have used at least 10 grams per day, usually given in 2–3 divided doses before meals, with a maximum of 30 gram daily. A 2.5 grams daily dose may be adequate when used as an adjunct to colestipol (Chutkan et al. 2012).

Multiple psyllium dosage forms are marketed, including powder to dissolve into liquid for drinking, capsules, and wafers or cookies. As the powders and wafers can be high in sugar, use of sugar-free versions may be better. Few quality issues have been identified for psyllium, which is widely available.

5.4.4.4 Safety

The greatest safety risk for use of psyllium is lack of adequate water intake, which can lead to constipation or bowel obstruction. Allergic reactions, including anaphylaxis, have been reported (Anonymous 2002). Psyllium fiber undergoes only limited fermentation in the gut, so is generally associated with less bloating than other types of fiber supplements. Titration to the required dose over a period of a few weeks will lessen these GI effects (Uehleke et al. 2008).

Theoretically, psyllium could decrease the absorption of drugs in general, however, this is not a clinically significant issue. There are limited case reports involving lithium and carbamazepine; it is best to use psyllium cautiously with any narrow-therapeutic range drug (Fernandez et al. 2012).

5.4.4.5 Evidence

Multiple studies have shown that psyllium can lower total cholesterol and LDL-cholesterol levels, with greater effects in hypercholesterolemic individuals. In a meta-analysis of 21 studies performed in the U.S., UK, Canada, Australia, and Mexico, psyllium at doses of 3–20.4 g daily was found to reduce total cholesterol by −14.5 mg/dL (95% CI: 9.94–19.1 mg/dL) and LDL-cholesterol by −10.75 mg/dL (95% CI: 8.24–12.06 mg/dL) (Wei et al. 2008). Triglycerides were not significantly reduced and HDL-cholesterol was reduced on average by −1.37 mg/dL. Daily doses of 5, 10, and 15 grams could be expected to lower LDL-cholesterol by 5.6%, 9%, and 12.5%, respectively (Wei et al. 2008). For every 1 g dose increase, a mean 0.84 mg/dL decrease in total cholesterol may be expected (Anonymous 2002).

In patients already treated with statins, adjunctive use of psyllium may have additional benefits. Overall, adding psyllium to a statin regimen resulted in further decreases in lipid levels (Agrawal et al. 2007, Jayaram et al. 2007, Moreyra 2005). Researchers stated that 10 mg of simvastatin plus 15 g daily of psyllium was as effective as the 20 mg daily dose of simvastatin, while 11.2 g daily of psyllium added to 10 mg daily of atorvastatin resulted in LDL-cholesterol reductions of 34.4% versus 22.8% for atorvastatin alone, with fewer adverse events reported (Jayaram et al. 2007, Moreyra 2005). Adjunctive therapy may allow more patients to achieve sufficient lipid-lowering using lower doses of statins with a lower risk of statin-associated adverse effects. However, it is not known if the documented cardiovascular risk reduction associated with statins is still present with the lower doses in combination therapy. *See Chapters 6 Endocrine Disorders, 7 Gastrointestinal Disease, and 15 Obesity and Weight Loss for further discussion of psyllium evidence.*

5.4.4.6 Clinical Application

Although the overall effect size is small and variable, the evidence supports the use of psyllium in dyslipidemia. As psyllium has little to no effect on HDL-cholesterol, patients at increased cardiovascular risk because of low HDL-cholesterol concentrations should not use psyllium alone.

5.4.5 Flaxseed

5.4.5.1 Background

The seeds of the flax plant, *Linum usitatissimum*, also known as linseed, are used for producing oil for foods and for wood finishes. The plant's fibers are used for cloth and paper. Flax has been used both industrially and medicinally for centuries.

5.4.5.2 Pharmacognosy

Flaxseed is one of the few plant sources of omega-3 fatty acids; oil from the seeds is more than 50% α-linolenic acid, which may be responsible for some anti-inflammatory benefits noted in *in vitro* and animal studies (Basch et al. 2007). Secoisolariciresinol diglucoside (SDG), a lignin precursor, is a primary component and usually the marker for standardization of flaxseed extracts. SDG is converted in the gastrointestinal (GI) tract to various lignans, which have phytoestrogenic activities and have been associated with positive effects on lipids, blood pressure, blood glucose, bone health, and possess anticancer activities (Basch et al. 2007). Soluble fiber in the seed husks is believed to be the primary contributor to lipid and glucose lowering effects; increased fat excretion has been demonstrated in both animals and humans (Kristensen et al. 2012). The mucilage formed by the soluble fiber also functions as a stool bulking agent to aid with constipation.

5.4.5.3 Dosing and Preparation

Both whole or ground flaxseed and flaxseed lignin supplements may be used. Flaxseed oil supplements have not demonstrated benefits for dyslipidemia, but may be appropriate for other uses. Doses of 10–50 g of flaxseed daily have been used in dyslipidemia trials, but 30 g daily has been shown to offer clinically relevant results with few adverse effects; titrating doses over the course of 2–3 weeks may help minimize GI effects. Although ingesting flaxseed in food products has provided some benefit, significantly greater cholesterol lowering is demonstrated when ground flaxseed was mixed into liquid for drinking (Kristensen et al. 2012). Providing partially de-fatted flaxseed or flaxseed in baked goods has at times resulted in increases in triglycerides, so would not be appropriate in patients with hypertriglyderidemia (Wong et al. 2013).

Based on the current information, flaxseed lignin products should be standardized to SDG content and provide a daily dose of 500–1,100 mg. Although it is possible to grow and harvest flaxseed in home gardens, raw or unripe seeds may be harmful in some individuals due to the presence of the cyanogenic glycosides, linamarin, neolinustatin, and linustatin (Cunnane et al. 1993). Processed or cooked seeds are safe.

5.4.5.4 Safety

The most common adverse effects are GI in nature and include bloating and gas, nausea, constipation, and diarrhea. Whole flaxseed, whether taken mixed or baked into food or mixed in fluid, should be taken with sufficient water to avoid the possibility of constipation or bowel blockage. Flaxseed should not be used in patients with esophageal or bowel strictures or obstructions of any type. Allergic reactions, including anaphylaxis, have been reported (Basch et al. 2007).

Drug interactions with flaxseed are based on theoretical concerns, primarily due to possible interference with absorption of oral drugs. No clinical reports exist, but to avoid potential problems, patients should separate the dosing of flaxseed and any narrow therapeutic range drugs by 2–3 hours. Pharmacodynamic interactions may result from flaxseed's effects on blood pressure and blood glucose; patients on antihypertensive or antihyperglycemia agents who begin to use flaxseed should be aware of possible additive effects and increase self-monitoring until effects are determined (Basch et al. 2007). *See Chapter 6 Endocrine Disorders for further discussion related to blood glucose.*

5.4.5.5 Evidence

A 2008 meta-analysis included 28 studies of flaxseed or flaxseed extracts, oils, or lignin products (Pan et al. 2009). Although the overall changes in total cholesterol and LDL-cholesterol were statistically significant, −3.87 mg/dL (95% CI: −7.73, 0.0 mg/dL) and −3.09 mg/dL (95% CI: −6.19, 0.0 mg/dL), results differed between products. Whole flaxseed, including crushed/ground, resulted in total cholesterol and LDL-cholesterol reductions of −8.12 and −6.19 mg/dL, while lignans were associated with reductions of −10.83 and −6.19 mg/dL, respectively. Neither significantly affected HDL-cholesterol and triglyceride levels and flaxseed oil did not affect lipid concentrations.

Reductions were greater in women than men, however, other factors such as study size, quality, and type of flaxseed product likely had an impact on those differences. Lipid-lowering responses were greater in studies with subjects with higher baseline lipid concentrations. Good responses were seen in both normoglycemic and diabetic patients.

Dyslipidemia also commonly occurs in patients receiving hemodialysis. A trial of 40 g daily of ground flaxseed added to usual diet for 8 weeks was compared to usual diet only in 30 hemodialysis patients with HDL-cholesterol concentrations less than 40 mg/dL and triglyceride concentrations over 200 mg/dL

(Soltani et al. 2012). Patients were not on any cholesterol-lowering medications. At 8 weeks, significant reductions in total cholesterol, LDL-cholesterol, and triglycerides were reported as −35, −25, and −92 mg/dL, respectively. Mean HDL-cholesterol concentration increased to 6 mg/dL. Additionally, C-reactive protein was reduced from the baseline of 4.8 mg/dL to 3 mg/dL (P < 0.05). The triglyceride response differs significantly from findings in most other patient populations, where flaxseed has little to no impact on triglyceride levels. The HDL-cholesterol increases are likely in response to the triglyceride decreases and the triglyceride exchange process conducted by cholesteryl ester transfer proteins (Soltani et al. 2012).

A 2010 study of flaxseed lignin compared 20 or 100 mg of SDG to placebo in 30 male patients with total cholesterol concentrations of 180–240 mg/dL (Fukumitsu et al. 2010). In the 100 mg group, total cholesterol and LDL-cholesterol levels decreased −6.2% and −8.4% from baseline, a non-significant difference; however, the LDL-cholesterol/HDL-cholesterol ratio at week 12 was −0.43, a significant decrease.

5.4.5.6 Clinical Application

Current evidence supports the use of both flaxseed and flaxseed lignin supplementation for dyslipidemia in both men and women as well as patients receiving hemodialysis. Sufficient water must be consumed with all forms of flaxseed supplements to avoid constipation and bowel blockages. Effects seem greatest effect when ground/milled flaxseed is mixed with liquid and consumed as a drink. Patients who cannot tolerate flaxseed drinks may use ground flaxseed capsules, although the number of capsules required to meet the recommended dosage may be a limiting factor.

5.4.5.7 Summary

Of the botanical supplements discussed, red yeast rice is likely to have the greatest effect for lipid lowering. An exception is in dyslipidemic patients on hemodialysis, for whom flaxseed may well have a greater effect on triglyceride concentrations. For patients with multiple disease states and/or medications, flaxseed may be a better choice due to its safety profile. In patients with colon health concerns, psyllium may provide additional benefits, while garlic may be a better choice in patients who need small to moderate effects on both lipids and blood pressure.

5.5 Heart Failure

Heart failure (HF) is estimated to affect over 8 million adults by 2030 (Mozaffarian et al. 2015). Risk factors for development of HF include coronary artery disease, hypertension, diabetes mellitus, and metabolic syndrome (Yancy et al. 2013).

Heart failure is assessed with the New York Heart Association Functional Class (NYHA-FC), where providers assess patients' symptoms and grade the functional capacity from class I, few to no symptoms, to class IV, symptoms present at rest (Yancy et al. 2013). This assessment helps guide practitioners in treatment decisions (Yancy et al. 2016). Therapy goals vary depending on functional class and stage, but focus on reducing HF hospitalizations, preventing mortality, and improving quality of life. Pharmacological treatment often involves ACE inhibitors, angiotensin receptor blockers, beta-blockers, aldosterone antagonists, diuretics, digoxin, other vasodilators such as hydralazine and nitrates (Yancy et al. 2013). Nonpharmacological treatment focuses on sodium and fluid restrictions. Patients are monitored for symptom improvement, and for functional capacity with a 6-minute walk distance.

5.5.1 Hawthorn

5.5.1.1 Background

Hawthorn is a thorny shrub or tree, native to temperate zones throughout the Northern hemisphere (Wang et al. 2013). Flower and leaf extracts of various *Crataegus* species have been used for cardiovascular conditions for over 1500 years, including HF, arrhythmias, bradycardia, angina, hyperlipidemia, and dyspnea (Koch and Malek 2011). The berries are sometimes used for digestive difficulties, as well as dyspnea and dyslipidemia (Koch and Malek 2011).

5.5.1.2 Pharmacognosy

As with many botanicals, hawthorn has antioxidant and anti-inflammatory effects. *Crataegus* species leaf and flower extracts have been shown to have inotropic effects on cardiac myocytes to improve strength of cardiac muscle contraction (Koch and Malek 2011). Effects on vasculature may be just as essential. The integrity of vascular endothelium is important; hyperpermeability in this barrier can lead to edema and is common in HF. The WS 1442 extract from *Crataegus monogyna/laevigata* has been shown to prevent hyperpermeability by action on pathways disruptive to the endothelium, sarcoplasmic/endoplasmic reticulum Ca^{2+} ATPase and inositol 1,4,5-triphosphate, as well as by stimulation of cortactin to strengthen barrier function (Fuchs et al. 2016, Willer et al. 2012).

Animal studies have shown decreased arterial blood pressure due to actions on muscarinic receptors and possible beta-receptor blockage causing vasodilation (Koch and Malek 2011). Though increased nitric oxide production due to the oligomeric procyanidin (OPC) content is well-documented, negative results of tests of flow-mediated dilation in adults with mild hypertension argue against a nitric oxide-mediated method of activity (Asher et al. 2012, Willer et al. 2012). Extracts also have antiplatelet activity at low doses, but in at least one animal study, opposite effects were seen with higher doses (Shatoor et al. 2012). Anti-arrhythmic effects from hawthorn have been reported with prolongation of the refractory period and the action potential. The components responsible for these activities include the bioflavonoids quercetin, rutin, vitexin, and hyperoside among others (Kumar et al. 2012).

5.5.1.3 Dosing and Preparation

Extracts made from the leaves and flowers are generally standardized to 2.2%–2.5% flavonoids and/or 17.1%–20% OPCs (Koch and Malek 2011). The most clinically tested extracts are WS® 1442, which is standardized to 18.75% OPCs, and LI 132, standardized to 2.2% flavonoids. Both are German products (Crataegutt forte® and Faros 300®, respectively) and are licensed as botanical drugs in some European countries. In the United States, WS 1442 is sold under the brand name HeartCare™ by Nature's Way.

Studies have used doses ranging from 160 to 1,800 mg daily, but clinical trials with positive results have most commonly used 600, 900, or 1,200 mg of standardized extract once daily or in 2–3 divided doses. No differences in adverse event rates exist with once daily versus divided dosing, but direct comparisons have not been completed.

5.5.1.4 Safety

Most trials have reported few adverse effects with use of hawthorn extracts. These were generally mild to moderate and most commonly included GI discomfort, headaches, dizziness, and vertigo (Daniele et al. 2006). Reports have also listed palpitations and arrhythmias, dyspnea, epistaxis, and a rash usually localized to the hands (Holubarsch et al. 2008). Theoretically, uterine tone may be decreased and *Crataegus* should not be used during pregnancy or lactation due to lack of information.

Hawthorn should not be used with nitrates, phosphodiesterase-5 inhibitors, or antihypertensive agents that could result in hypotension. Blood pressure should be monitored closely during therapy initiation or discontinuation of hawthorn.

5.5.1.5 Evidence

A 2008 Cochrane meta-analysis including 14 placebo-controlled and double-blinded trials concluded that the existing evidence supported the use of hawthorn extract as an oral treatment option for chronic heart failure when combined with standard therapy (Guo et al. 2008). The trials most commonly assessed maximal workload and noted a weighted mean difference of 5.35 (95% CI: 0.71, 10.0, P < 0.02) for hawthorn versus placebo. Five additional trials found the outcome of pressure-heart rate product (SBP × heart rate/min ÷ 100) to be reduced 19.22 (95% CI: −30.46, −7.98), and that exercise tolerance, expressed as Watts × minutes, increased 122.76 (95% CI: 32.74, 212.78) (Guo et al. 2008). Since the time of that meta-analysis, trials have had more variable results. This is possibly due to greater use of beta-blockers and ACE inhibitors; patients are now receiving treatment that is more effective in decreasing morbidity and mortality.

The Survival and Prognosis: Investigation of *Crataegus* Extract WS 1442 (SPICE) trial enrolled 2,681 patients with NYHA-FC Class II and III, who were optimally treated with individualized therapy regimens (Holubarsch et al. 2008). Patients received 900 mg/day of WS® 1442 or placebo for up to 24 months. The primary outcome measure was days until the first cardiac event, defined as cardiac death, nonfatal MI, or hospitalization due to heart failure. The average time was similar between the extract and placebo, 620 and 606 days, respectively. The event rates at 6 months were 2.9% and 4.9% for extract and placebo (p = 0.009), but at 24 months, the gap had closed to 13.5% and 14.9% p = 0.269); cardiac mortality was also significantly lower at 6 months in the extract group, but not at 24 months. Rates of sudden cardiac death were similar between the two groups. In a subgroup of patients with ejection fractions of 25%–35%, both cardiac mortality and sudden cardiac death were decreased in the extract group, mortality by a 20% (95% CI: 0.56, 1.10), and sudden cardiac death by 39.7% (95% CI: 0.37, 0.94; P = 0.025).

The HERB-CHF also examined 900 mg daily of WS 1442 or placebo for 6 months in 120 NYHA-FC Class II and III patients on standard medical therapy (Zick et al. 2009). The primary outcome was improvement in the 6-minute walk test. For study inclusion, all subjects had to walk between 150 and 450 meters in two 6-minute walk tests prior to enrollment in the study. The trial had 99% power to detect a 40-meter difference. Secondary outcomes included global assessment by patient and physician, quality of life (QOL), hospitalizations, and other functional assessments and chemical markers. At 6 months, 6-minute walk test results were similar between groups and there were no significant changes from baseline in either group. The patient and physician global assessments, QOL scores, and other chemical marker or functional assessments were also similar in the two groups. Adverse events occurred more commonly in the hawthorn group than the placebo group, 36–23, respectively, but no one type of event was significantly different between groups.

A post-hoc analysis of data from HERB CHF examined the progression of heart failure in the study subjects (Zick et al. 2008). Progression occurred in 43.3% of placebo and 46.6% of extract-treated patients [OR 1.14 (95% CI: 0.56, 2.35; P = 0.86)]. Patients with left ventricular ejection fraction (LVEF) </ = 35% were at greater risk of disease progression in the extract group compared to placebo [OR 3.2 (95% CI: 1.3, 8.3; P = 0.02)]. A limitation recognized by the researchers was that, as the study was not originally designed to examine this outcome, the statistical power for these analyses was less than the original study, 84% or less.

5.5.1.6 *Clinical Application*

The available evidence does support the use of standardized *Crataegus* extracts for treatment of heart failure. However, these extracts are less likely to have a significant clinical benefit in patients who are already on optimized standard treatment regimens or who have more severe disease. This means that *Crataegus* may be more suited to patients who are NYHA-FC I and II, cannot tolerate medications listed in the treatment guidelines, or insist upon treatment options they consider *natural*. The German Federal Institute for Drugs and Medical Devices has recommended that the Committee on Herbal Medicinal Products of the European Medicines Agency re-evaluate *Crataegus* recommendations as current science no longer supports use in NYHA-FC II (Anonymous 2017).

Patients should not use hawthorn without the knowledge and consent of a supervising healthcare provider in order to allow screening for interactions with common heart failure medications and, even more importantly, monitoring of treatment outcomes. The data linking *Crataegus* use to possible worsening of heart failure, although preliminary, must be kept in mind as healthcare practitioners wait for more information to adequately assess the extent of this risk (Table 5.1).

TABLE 5.1

Heart Failure—Foxglove

No information on botanical treatment of heart failure would be complete without mention of foxglove, Digitalis
   purpurea, the original sole medicinal source of the cardiac glycoside digitoxin (Weisse 2010). Foxglove became a
   mainstay of heart failure, or "dropsy," treatment in the 1700s, but had been known to herbalists far longer. Over time,
   various extracts of glycoside mixtures were developed and used until the late 1950s, when the single glycoside, digoxin,
   took precedence (Lesney 2002).

The prescription drug digoxin remained one of the primary treatments of choice for heart failure until the late 1990s, but
   currently, it is given only light mention in treatment guidelines, due to a relatively narrow therapeutic window and
   greater understanding of the subpopulations in which it is most likely to be effective (Weisse 2010; Chaggar et al. 2015).
   More prominent are reports of accidental poisonings, due either to adulterated products or mistakes in distinguishing
   foxglove and comfrey plants by patients collecting their own herbs for use in teas.

Because of narrow therapeutic range and less predictable responses to mixtures of the cardiac glycosides, use of herbal
   formulations of foxglove are not recommended for any conditions.

5.6 Peripheral Artery Disease

Patients with peripheral artery disease (PAD) have an increased risk of both coronary artery disease
development and limb ischemia resulting in amputations (Gerhard-Herman et al. 2017). The classic
symptom of PAD is intermittent claudication (leg cramping with exertion), however, only ~10% of patients
exhibit classic symptoms and 40%–50% have no or nonspecific leg symptoms (Mozaffarian et al. 2015).
Risk factors for PAD development are cigarette smoking, diabetes mellitus, HTN, increasing age, and
dyslipidemia. PAD is diagnosed by an ankle-brachial index (ABI), the ratio of ankle SBP over brachial
artery SBP. An ABI of ≤ 0.90 is abnormal and confirmatory of PAD when paired with symptoms or
physical findings (Gerhard-Herman et al. 2017). Disease progression is monitored by objective measures
of exercise capacity such as 6-minute walk distance or pain free walking distance.

The key nonpharmacological treatment is a supervised exercise program to improve symptoms and
delay the need for intervention (Gerhard-Herman et al. 2017). Pharmacological management aims to
control symptoms and modify risk factors. Cilostazol is the primary drug used to increase walking
distance in patients with claudication. Risk factor modification treatments include antiplatelet agents,
statins, and antihypertensives (Gerhard-Herman et al. 2017).

5.6.1 Ginkgo

5.6.1.1 Background

Ginkgo supplements are extracts from the leaves of the *Ginkgo biloba* tree. Used medicinally in Asia for
at least 2000 years, ginkgo has been well-established in Europe and the Americas for 300 years. The tree
itself is sometimes called "the living fossil," as ginkgo trees have existed for more than 150 million years.

5.6.1.2 Pharmacognosy

The leaf extracts of ginkgo have many components: a variety of flavonoids, including quercetin and
kaempferol, and terpenoids, such as bilobalide and five ginkgolides (Diamond and Bailey 2013). Ginkgo
extracts have anti-inflammatory, antioxidant, antiplatelet, and vasodilatory effects. Some anticancer and
neurologic effects as well as anti-angiogenic activity due to activation of tyrosine phosphatase may exist
(Diamond and Bailey 2013, Koltermann et al. 2008).

In PAD, vascular effects are of primary importance; most benefits are likely to occur through a nitric
oxide (NO) mechanism. The EGb 761® extract increased the NO production by upregulating endothelial
nitric oxide synthase (eNOS) promoters and inducing eNOS phosphorylation (Koltermann et al. 2007).
Up to 48 hours was needed to see maximum effects, which may explain the negative findings in earlier

mechanism studies. Additionally, results were obtained at concentrations comparable to those achieved in humans taking 120–240 mg daily. Aortic tissue studies revealed dose-dependent vascular relaxation up to 50%, while *in vivo* experiments in rats given a 5 mg dose intravenously demonstrated a mean decrease of SBP from 120 to 65 mmHg after 5 minutes.

5.6.1.3 Dosing and Preparation

Extracts are generally standardized to 24%–25% flavonoid glycosides and 6% terpenoids. EGb 761® (Dr. Willmar Schwabe Pharmaceuticals) and LI 1370® (Lichtwer Pharma) are the two extracts primarily used in clinical research and are available worldwide. For PAD, 120–240 mg daily given once or in two divided doses is recommended. One trial supports greater efficacy with the 240 mg daily dosage (Horsch and Walther 2004). Therapeutic use of ginkgo requires at least 24 weeks of treatment to see beneficial effects.

5.6.1.4 Safety

High doses of prepared (usually roasted) seeds or fresh plant material can be toxic, due to the presence of a GABA-inhibiting neurotoxin called ginkgotoxin (4′-O-methylpyridoxine, MPN). In children, fresh and roasted seeds have caused serious injury and death (Kajiyama et al. 2002). Although leaf extracts do contain small quantities of MPN, these are generally below 10 parts per million. To present a risk of harm, leaf extracts would have to be used in amounts vastly above the highest doses used medicinally.

Ginkgo has been well tolerated in clinical trials, with several reporting no adverse effects. The most common are mild GI upset, headache or dizziness, palpitations, and allergic reactions, usually manifesting as rashes (Diamond and Bailey 2013). Patients with life-threatening allergic reactions to poison ivy or poison oak and related plants should avoid ginkgo due to potential cross-reactivity.

Ginkgo has antiplatelet activity, but whether this poses a clinically significant increased bleeding risk has not yet been determined. Meta-analyses and reviews of clinical trials have concluded the risk with doses of 80–480 mg of extract daily is no greater than seen in placebo groups (Kellermann and Kloft 2011). However, multiple case reports exist of increased bleeding time or other bleeding events, alone or in combination with warfarin (Mei et al. 2017, Stoddard et al. 2015). This may be an issue of product quality. Most research is conducted with well-tested, high quality extracts, while the general public may be using products of lower quality or that contain additional ingredients. In any event, caution or avoidance is warranted in patients in whom bleeding consequences could be serious.

The situation for pharmacokinetic drug interactions with ginkgo is similar; case reports suggest clinically significant reductions in drug levels, while interaction studies provide conflicting evidence (Mei et al. 2017). Some of the conflict may be due to the use of different extracts, different durations of study, and widely varying doses (Gurley et al. 2012). *See Chapter 2 Pharmacokinetic and Pharmacogenomic Considerations for further discussion.*

5.6.1.5 Clinical Evidence

A 2004 meta-analysis of nine clinical trials using EGb 761 concluded that ginkgo extract was significantly better than placebo for increasing pain-free walking distance (Horsch and Walther 2004). For each trial, the researchers calculated the ratio of the increase from baseline in pain-free walking distance for EGb 761 and placebo; a ratio of >1.05 represents clinically relevant superiority of one treatment over another. In 6 of the 7 trials with statistically significant increases in walking distance, ratios were >1.05 for EGb 761. When results were pooled from four studies with the most design homogeneity, the ratio increased to 1.18 (95% CI: 1.11, 1.26).

However, conclusions of a later meta-analysis of ginkgo for intermittent claudication were not positive. A 2013 Cochrane Collaboration review included 14 clinical trials conducted between 1984 and 2008 (Nicolaï et al. 2013). Trials lasted from 6–24 weeks, most using the EGb 761 extract. Trials assessed absolute claudication distance (ACD) with effect sizes reported in terms of kilocalories (kcal), translated to meters walked at 3.2 km per hour. As a baseline, exercise therapy assessed at the same speed generally results in an ACD increase of 19.1 kcal. Differences between ginkgo and placebo groups were small and only significant in trials of 24 weeks (321 subjects), where the mean difference in ACD was 4.72 kcal (95% CI: 2.27, 7.16). For a 70 kg individual, this is comparable to an increase of 85.3 meters. Reviewers stated the noted benefits were not clinically significant. *See Chapter 10 Neurological Conditions for further discussion.*

5.6.1.6 Clinical Application

Despite ginkgo's positive effects on the vasculature, the clinical trial results have not always supported expectations. The effect sizes for increases in pain-free walking distance or maximum walking distances are small, 6 months of therapy may be needed before positive benefits are observed, and questions remain about adverse effects. A good candidate for a trial period of ginkgo is a patient without an increased risk of bleeding and not taking multiple medications likely to be affected by ginkgo.

5.7 Coronary Artery Disease

Coronary artery disease (CAD) can present as acute coronary syndrome (ACS) such as a myocardial infarction, or as stable ischemia heart disease (SIHD) with symptoms of angina or chest pain. Risk factors for CAD development and progression include: smoking, diabetes mellitus, HTN, obesity, increasing age, dyslipidemia, and gender (Mozaffarian et al. 2015). CAD monitoring focuses on optimizing risk factors and relieving symptoms such as chest pain (Fihn et al. 2012).

Patients presenting with ACS have aggressive, early invasive treatment to reestablish coronary blood flow. Patients presenting with SIHD are treated with medication management, reserving invasive intervention for persistent symptoms (Fihn et al. 2012). A medically supervised exercise program is the key nonpharmacological treatment for all (Fihn et al. 2012). Patients with CAD should not smoke, and should follow a diet low in saturated fat, cholesterol, *trans* fat, and sodium. Pharmacological management options for symptom control, such as relief of chest pain, include beta blockers, nitrates, calcium channel blockers, and ranolazine. Risk factor modifications are the foundation of CAD management and include optimization of treatments for blood pressure, lipids, and diabetes mellitus. Appropriate antiplatelet therapy is also crucial. Depending on presentation (ACS vs. SIHD), this may consist of clopidogrel, or a similar drug, and/or aspirin for 1–3 years or more (Fihn et al. 2012).

5.7.1 Ginseng (*Panax ginseng* and *Panax quinquefolius*)

5.7.1.1 Background

Though *Panax ginseng* has been used in traditional Asian medical systems for thousands of years, the use of *P. quinquefolius*, American ginseng, is newer. Each species has a slightly different chemical profile, resulting in differences in their clinical effects. American ginseng is used for effects on the immune system and to reduce post-prandial glucose, while *P. ginseng* (panax) is used for cardiovascular and sexual health, as well as for general health and energy.

In traditional Asian medicine, ginseng serves as an *adaptogen*, working to normalize a variety of body functions. Many ginseng constituents occur in pairs; for example, one ginsenoside will increase blood pressure, while another will decrease blood pressure.

5.7.1.2 Pharmacognosy

For medicinal use, roots of the ginseng plant are generally dried, powdered, and encapsulated, or prepared via extraction. Some traditional preparations of *P. ginseng* involve boiling ("red ginseng") or sun-drying ("white ginseng") the root; white ginseng is usually peeled, while red is not. Panax contains a number of constituents; those believed to provide the most medicinal benefit are triterpene saponins, commonly called ginsenosides, and flavonoids (Shin et al. 2000). Of the 30 ginsenosides common to both ginseng types, American ginseng has greater quantities of six - Rb1, Rb2, Rc, Rd, Re, and Rg1 – and also contains polysaccharides with immune stimulating effects and a variety of quinquefolans that affect blood glucose concentrations (Lim et al. 2005).

5.7.1.3 Dosing and Preparation

Optimal doses have not been determined for any cardiovascular indications for *P. ginseng* or *P. quinquefolius*. A dosage range of 0.5 to 3 g daily in divided doses is reasonable, based on the available data and adverse event information. Products are standardized to a wide variety of ginsenoside content; no optimal standardizations can be recommended.

5.7.1.4 Safety

Adverse events for *P. ginseng* may be related to dose and duration of use. Insomnia is the most common adverse effect, with headache, GI complaints of diarrhea or discomfort, hypertension, and hypotension also reported (Coon and Ernst 2002). Effects that suggest estrogenic activity, such as gynecomastia and vaginal bleeding, have been reported, but it is difficult to know whether these were due to *P. ginseng* or to contaminants. Hypersensitivity reactions have occurred, including anaphylaxis and Stevens-Johnson syndrome (Ernst 2002). Doses over 2.5 g daily are associated with tachycardia and palpitations as well as hypertension, and a higher incidence of insomnia (Mancuso and Santangelo 2017).

A number of potential drug interactions have been suggested, but clinical relevance has not been determined and information is contradictory. *See the Chapter 2 Pharmacokinetic and Pharmacogenomic Considerations for further discussion of interactions for P. ginseng and P. quinquefolius.*

P. quinquefolius adverse events are uncommon; headache has been reported (Ernst 2002). It is possible some confusion may exist in that adverse events occurring with use of American ginseng are attributed to *P. ginseng*. Patients using *P. quinquefolius* should be observant for any unusual changes.

5.7.1.5 Evidence

Currently clinical trial data on symptomatic improvement from ginseng is lacking (Buettner et al. 2006). *See Clinical Application section.*

5.7.1.6 Clinical Application

Neither *P. ginseng* nor *P. quinquefolius* can be recommended for treatment of CAD. Patients with concomitant disease states may find these botanicals useful for other reasons such as for blood glucose control.

5.7.2 Terminalia arjuna

5.7.2.1 Background

Terminalia arjuna tree bark, teas, and other bark preparations, have a long history of use in Ayurvedic medicine for cardiovascular conditions (Dwivedi and Chopra 2014). Other traditional uses of arjuna include diabetes, cirrhosis, anemia, earache, and fractures, though most modern research has focused on properties applicable to cardiovascular disorders. The terms *T. bellarica* and *T. chebula* are common synonyms.

5.7.2.2 Pharmacognosy

Arjuna contains flavonoids, terpenoids, glycosides, tannins, and β-sitosterol, and possess antioxidant activities (Kapoor et al. 2014). Animal studies have demonstrated increases in coronary blood flow, hypolipidemic action, decreased platelet activation, both inotropic and chronotropic effects, and protection against ischemic-reperfusion injury to cardiac muscle cells (Dwivedi and Chopra 2014). Inotropic effects may arise from the saponin glycoside components (Kapoor et al. 2014). Alcoholic bark extracts containing a higher percentage of lipophilic constituents have more hypolipidemic and antioxidant effects than other types of extracts (Dwivedi and Chopra 2014). Arjuna inhibits peroxidation of lipids and HMG-CoA reductase, stimulates glutathione peroxidase and catalase, prevents decreases in levels of endogenous antioxidant enzymes, and limits pro-inflammatory cytokines.

5.7.2.3 Dosing and Preparation

Trials in patients with ischemic heart disease have used 500 mg of bark powder, while other dosages have been used: 500 mg of a 90% alcoholic extract three times daily, 500 mg twice daily of a dried aqueous extract, and 500 mg every 8 hours of a dried aqueous and ethanolic extract (Dwivedi and Chopra 2014, Kapoor et al. 2015). Patients should purchase of bark powder or extracts from major companies generally known to offer high quality botanical medicines. At this time, 500 mg two or three times daily of either bark powder or a standardized extract can be recommended.

5.7.2.4 Safety

Adverse events in clinical trials of up to 2 years of use have included nausea, constipation, and stomach upset, headache, insomnia, and generalized body aches (Dwivedi and Chopra 2014). Oral doses of up to 2 g/kg of alcoholic extract were safely tolerated in animal studies, although decreases in thyroid concentrations were observed. Patients with thyroid disorders should only use arjuna with caution and increased monitoring.

Arjuna's potential for drug interactions is unknown, as studies of its effects on metabolic enzymes have not been conducted. Based on known effects in animals and humans, an additive effect with hypoglycemic drugs is possible, so these combinations should be used cautiously. Arjuna has been used in conjunction with standard therapy in several trials. One retrospective study did note increased benefits when arjuna was used with drugs such as ACE inhibitors, beta-blockers, spironolactone or other diuretics, and digoxin (Bhawani et al. 2013).

5.7.2.5 Evidence

Arjuna is believed to improve endothelial function. This was evaluated in a study in young healthy chronic smokers with a mean age of 28 years and age-matched non-smoking controls (Bharani et al. 2004). After baseline measurements of flow-mediated dilation (FMD), subjects took 500 mg of a dried alcoholic and aqueous extract of arjuna bark or placebo every 8 hours for 2 weeks in a crossover design with a 2-week washout. At baseline, mean FMD% was 4.71 in smokers and 11.75 in non-smokers. After treatment, mean FMD% in smokers was increased to 5.17 in the placebo group and to 9.31 in the arjuna group ($P < 0.005$). Researchers stated the benefit was similar to that seen with the antioxidants, vitamins E and C. Vasodilation induced by nitroglycerin, an endothelial-independent reaction, was preserved in both groups.

A 2007 review discussed seven older trials examining anti-ischemic activities, most of which used 500 mg bark powder three times daily, alone or in conjunction with standard treatment (Dwivedi 2007). In general, angina frequency decreased, by 50% in one trial, and improvements were seen in both treadmill test performance and the time until ST changes. Patients with stable angina experienced more benefit than those with unstable angina. Other cardiac benefits observed include improvements in LVEF and NYHA-FC in congestive heart failure, decreases in left ventricular mass, and improvements in lipid profiles.

A trial of arjuna bark powder (500 mg once daily) compared to placebo and vitamin E demonstrated significant ($P < 0.01$) reductions of total cholesterol, LDL-cholesterol, and lipid peroxide of 9.7%, 15.8%, and 29.3%, respectively in the arjuna group, with no significant changes in HDL-cholesterol or triglycerides (Gupta et al. 2001). The only other significant change noted in all subjects was a 36.4% reduction in lipid peroxide in the vitamin E group.

In another study, 116 patients with stable CAD on standard treatment received 500 mg twice daily of a dried aqueous extract of arjuna bark or placebo for 6 months (Kapoor et al. 2015). Researchers evaluated both effects on interleukins 6 and 8, hsCRP, and TNF-α. At 6 months, all inflammatory markers were significantly decreased compared to placebo. Increases in the anti-inflammatory IL-10 were also significant in the arjuna group. Changes in total cholesterol, triglycerides, and HDL-cholesterol were significant at -10.7%, -34.7%, and $+10.4\%$, respectively. LDL-cholesterol decreased by 13% in the arjuna group, while increasing 9.7% in the placebo group, a nonsignificant difference. A review also reports that a 3-month trial of arjuna bark powder along with statin treatment noted results of -15%, -11%, and -16% for total cholesterol, triglycerides, and LDL-cholesterol, respectively (Kapoor et al. 2014).

A study of male patients with chronic stable angina and exercise-provocable ischemia compared arjuna 500 mg every 8 hours of a dried alcoholic and aqueous extract to placebo and isosorbide mononitrate 40 mg daily for one week in a randomized, double-blinded cross-over study. All patients ($n = 58$) used isosorbide dinitrate for acute angina relief. Baseline exercise duration was 4.74 minutes. This was unchanged with placebo, and increased significantly ($P < 0.005$) to 6.14 minutes with arjuna treatment and to 6.45 minutes with isosorbide mononitrate treatment. Improved outcomes were noted for maximal ST depression, recovery time, and the double-product of heart rate $\times$ SBP. Isosorbide dinitrate use was similar between the arjuna and isosorbide mononitrate groups, 5.69 and 5.53 mg/week, respectively, while the placebo group used significantly more at 18.22 mg/week. Adverse effects were mild, although greater with isosorbide mononitrate. Over half of patients improved by at least one NYHA-FC while treated with arjuna or isosorbide mononitrate.

A 2014 systemic review examined five trials in a meta-analysis. However, due to differences in study outcomes, data was either not able to be pooled or was pooled from only two studies (Kaur et al. 2014). No significant differences in any parameters were seen.

5.7.2.6 Clinical Application

Arjuna is an intriguing potential option for CAD and related disorders. The overall evidence and safety picture seems supportive of use, but questions remain. Most clinical trials have been small with methodological limitations and necessary information on effect size, optimal dosage and form, and drug interaction potential is missing. Candidates for use of arjuna should be chosen carefully and monitored frequently. For patients with angina, stable angina may respond more favorably than unstable angina.

5.8 Chronic Venous Insufficiency

Chronic venous insufficiency (CVI) affects many millions worldwide. Varicose veins are the most common presenting symptom, but CVI can progress to skin color changes, ulcer formation, edema, and leg discomfort (Eberhardt and Raffetto 2014). Both a classification and severity scoring system are used. Class 0 (C_0) represents no visible venous disease, C_1 indicates telangiectasis or reticular veins, C_2 signifies varicose veins, C_3 indicates edema, C_4 represents changes in skin color or eczema, and C_5 and C_6 designate presence of either a healed or active ulcer, respectively. The venous clinical severity score assesses ten parameters (pain, varicose veins, ulcers, and others) from absent to severe (0 to 3 points), with a maximum total of 30 points (Eberhardt and Raffetto 2014). Risk factors for CVI development include: age, female gender, obesity, family history, and pregnancy (Committee 2015).

CVI management relies on compression stockings and achievement of a healthy weight (Eberhardt and Raffetto 2014). Wound and skin care are important to prevent infection of compromised skin. Pharmacological treatment options are limited to venoactive drugs such as naftazone and calcium dobesilate, only available in some countries (Committee 2015). Sclerotherapy and surgical intervention is available for patients with poor results with other therapies or unable to comply with compressive treatment (Eberhardt and Raffetto 2014).

5.8.1 Horse Chestnut (*Aesculus hippocastanum*)

5.8.1.1 Background

The horse chestnut tree, *Aesculus hippocastanum*, is native to eastern Europe, but now grows over the world. It is closely related to the Ohio buckeye, *A. glabra*. Horse chestnut seeds have been used for cattle and horse feed. Lime water soaks can remove bitter-tasting components and also reduce toxicity (Ulbricht et al. 2002). Traditional medicinal uses include varicose veins, hemorrhoids, cough, swelling, and diarrhea.

5.8.1.2 Pharmacognosy

The seeds of the horse chestnut tree are the applicable part and only processed and purified seed extracts are used; raw seeds and plant parts contain the toxin aesculin, also known as esculin (Underland et al. 2012). Horse chestnut seed extracts (HCSE) contain flavonoids such as quercetin and proanthocyanidin A_2, coumarins, and 30 or more triterpene saponin glycosides, collectively called aescin or escin (Felixsson et al. 2010). β-aescin may be the most pharmacologically active of these saponins. In bovine veins and arteries, HCSE was shown to cause blood vessel contraction in a dose-dependent manner, although vein response was significantly greater than artery response (Felixsson et al. 2010). Contraction was mediated by 5-HT_{2A} receptors, and was independent of endothelium. Increased gastrointestinal transit speed noted in earlier studies also involves action on 5-HT_{2A} receptors, as does a slight stimulation of platelet aggregation; the overall decreased platelet aggregation seen with HCSE may be a result of the coumarin components and the high flavonoid content. Other tissue and animal studies have demonstrated anti-inflammatory action and a stabilizing effect on capillaries. This causes increased venous tone, decreased permeability, and better blood flow, resulting in reduced edema (Tiffany et al. 2002). Some of the beneficial capillary effects are due to inhibition of elastase and hyaluronidase that degrade proteoglycans in cell walls. Increased prostaglandin F_2 production also reduces blood vessel degradation and increases venous tone (Dudek-Makuch and Studzińska-Sroka 2015, Pittler and Ernst 2012).

5.8.1.3 Dosing and Preparation

Most products are standardized to aescin content of 16%–22%; dosages of aescin used in trials ranged from 50 to 100 mg, given once daily or in 2–3 divided doses. The most common dosage recommendation is 300 mg of HCSE, providing 50 mg of aescin, twice daily (Underland et al. 2012). Of the clinically tested products available for purchase in the U.S., Venastat® (Pharmaton, Ridgefield, CT) is widely available and Venostasin® retard (Klinge Pharma, Berlin, Germany) is available for online purchase. No other extracts have either sufficient clinical evidence or quality testing to be recommended. Topical products are available, generally in a 2% gel form. These products are not recommended unless patients cannot tolerate oral formulations.

5.8.1.4 Safety

HCSE has a favorable safety profile with nausea and stomach upset as the most commonly reported in clinical trials and postmarketing surveillance (Pittler and Ernst 2012). Film-coated or enteric-coated tablets seem to minimize most GI effects. Other adverse effects are headache or dizziness, pruritis, and calf spasms. Although no case reports exist, horse chestnut chitinases have been shown to cause responses in laboratory skin prick tests in patients allergic to latex (Blanco et al. 1999).

HCSE can have antiplatelet activity; one case report exists of a rupture of a renal angiomyolipoma in a woman taking HCSE and no other medications (Snow et al. 2012). Use with anticoagulants or antiplatelet medications is generally not recommended.

Parenteral HCSE products are available in Europe and are associated with a greater incidence of serious adverse events including anaphylaxis and hepatic and renal effects; animal toxicity studies confirm that oral use is safer than parenteral (Dudek-Makuch and Studzińska-Sroka 2015). Although a study of HCSE use in women with pregnancy-induced venous insufficiency noted no adverse effects and animal studies have shown no teratogenic effects, use in pregnancy and lactation is not recommended due to the overall lack of information (Dudek-Makuch and Studzińska-Sroka 2015, Tiffany et al. 2002).

5.8.1.5 Evidence

A 2002 clinical review included 14 randomized controlled trials of HCSE in patients with CVI (Tiffany et al. 2002). Reviewers concluded that HCSE treatment provided greater reduction than placebo in outcome measurements such as leg volume and circumference and leg pain. Additionally, they noted that outcomes in trials comparing HCSE to compression stockings demonstrated similar results. However, an important consideration is compliance; in at least one trial, compression stocking compliance was 90%, which is nearly double the compliance rate seen in real-world use of compression stockings. The trial noted reductions in leg volume of 53.6 and 56.6 mL for HCSE and compression stocking treatments, respectively (Tiffany et al. 2002). In another 4-week study, leg volume decreased by 40 mL from baseline, while ankle circumference decreased by 6.5 mm in the HCSE group and increased 1 mm in the placebo group. Other studies noted much smaller reductions in leg and ankle circumference (Tiffany et al. 2002).

A 2012 Cochrane Collaboration review examined 17 clinical trials of HCSE against placebo, pycnogenol, or compression stockings in the treatment of CVI (Pittler and Ernst 2012). HCSE improved outcomes of pain, edema, pruritis, leg volume, and leg circumference compared to baseline; improvements seen were greater than placebo and generally similar to compression stockings. Despite study limitations, the review concluded that the evidence did support HCSE use for CVI. However, the recommendation was limited to short-term therapy as no trial longer than 16 weeks has been conducted. A consensus statement from German and Swiss vascular medicine and dermatological practitioners also supports use of the HCSE products tested in trials. Combination therapy with compression stockings is recommended if monotherapy does not provide sufficient results, as dual therapy may provide synergistic benefit due to the differing mechanisms of action (Stücker et al. 2016).

An overall issue in meta-analysis of HCSE trials is the variety of outcome measurements and methodologies, which makes result comparisons or calculations of true effect size difficult. Longer, more rigorous controlled trials are needed to strengthen the recommendations possible.

One CVI complication is venous leg ulceration, which can develop into a chronic issue for some patients. One placebo-controlled trial assessed use of HCSE against placebo for 12 weeks in 54 Australian patients with venous leg ulceration (Leach et al. 2006b, *Journal of Wound Care*). Results were mixed and nonsignificant between groups, with the exception of significant differences in wound slough percentages, and decreases in nursing visits, dressing changes, and overall costs. A cost-benefit analysis found that weekly wound management costs were significantly ($P = 0.011$) reduced in the HCSE group (Leach et al. 2006a). The average savings was $101 (Australian dollars) per venous ulcer treated compared to placebo.

5.8.1.6 Clinical Application

HCSE use in mild-to moderate CVI is supported by clinical evidence. Oral extracts can be recommended alone or in conjunction with compression stockings. Although the safety profile is encouraging, the lack of information regarding potential drug interactions other than additive antithrombotic effects must be kept in mind when considering potential candidates for HCSE therapy.

5.9 Summary

Overall, multiple botanical options exist to help patients with cardiovascular disorders. The greatest support may be for red yeast rice for dyslipidemia treatment efficacy, while psyllium and flaxseed have the strongest safety records. Horse chestnut seed extract has added value as a treatment option simply because of the paucity of other pharmacologic therapies for peripheral artery disease. However, a primary consideration for all botanical medicines discussed is the lack of long-term outcomes data. More well-designed research is needed to evaluate how these botanical medicines compare to prescription drug therapies for the reduction of morbidity and mortality.

REFERENCES

Agrawal, A. R., M. Tandon, and P. L. Sharma. "Effect of combining viscous fibre with lovastatin on serum lipids in normal human subjects." *International Journal of Clinical Practice* 61, no. 11 2007: 1812–18. doi:10.1111/j.1742-1241.2007.01512.x.

Alali, F. Q., T. El-Elimat, L. Khalid, R. Hudaib, T. S. Al-Shehabi, and A. H. Eid. "Garlic for cardiovascular disease: Prevention or treatment?" *Current Pharmaceutical Design* 23, no. 7 2017: 1028–41. doi:10.217 4/1381612822666161010124530.

Annaba, F., P. Kumar, A. K. Dudeja, S. Saksena, R. K. Gill, and W. A. Alrefai. "Green tea catechin EGCG inhibits ileal apical sodium bile acid transporter ASBT." *AJP: Gastrointestinal and Liver Physiology* 298, no. 3 2010. doi:10.1152/ajpgi.00360.2009.

Anonymous. "*Plantago ovata.* (Psyllium)." *Alternative Medicine Review* 7, no. 2 2002: 155–9.

Anonymous. "*Pharmazeutische Zeitung online: Herzinsuffizienz: Weidorn nicht mehr empfohlen.*" *Startseite.* Accessed August 04, 2017. http://www.pharmazeutische-zeitung.de/index.php?id=66952. Translation provided by Jesse Reece, University of Missouri-Kansas City School of Pharmacy.

Asher, G. N., A. J. Viera, M. A. Weaver, R. Dominik, M. Caughey, and A. L. Hinderliter. "Effect of hawthorn standardized extract on flow mediated dilation in prehypertensive and mildly hypertensive adults: a randomized, controlled cross-over trial." *BMC Complementary and Alternative Medicine* 12, no. 1 2012. doi:10.1186/1472-6882-12-26.

Basch, E., S. Bent, J. Collins, C. Dacey, P. Hammerness, M. Harrison, M. Smith, P. Szapary, C. Ulbricht, M. Vora, and W. Weissner. "Flax and flaxseed oil (*Linum usitatissimum*): A review by the natural standard research collaboration." *Journal of the Society for Integrative Oncology* 05, no. 03 2007: 92. doi:10.2310/7200.2007.005.

Becker, D. J., R. Y. Gordon, S. C. Halbert, B. French, P. B. Morris, and D. J. Rader. "Red yeast rice for dyslipidemia in statin-intolerant patients." *Annals of Internal Medicine* 150, no. 12 2009: 830–9.

Bharani, A., L. K. Ahirwar, and N. Jain. "*Terminalia arjuna* reverses impaired endothelial function in chronic smokers." *Indian Heart Journal* 56, no. 2 2004: 123–28.

Bhawani, G., A. Kumar, K. S. N. Murthy, N. Kumari, and C. G. Swami. "A retrospective study of effect of *Terminalia arjuna* and evidence based standard therapy on echocardiographic parameters in patients of dilated cardiomyopathy." *Journal of Pharmacy Research* 6, no. 5 2013: 493–98. doi:10.1016/j.jopr.2013.05.006.

Blanco, C., A. Diaz-Perales, C. Collada, R. Sánchez-Monge, C. Aragoncillo, R. Castillo, N. Ortega, M. Alvarez, T. Carrillo, and G. Salcedo. "Class I chitinases as potential panallergens involved in the latex-fruit syndrome." *Journal of Allergy and Clinical Immunology* 103, no. 3 1999: 507–13. doi:10.1016/s0091-6749(99)70478-1.

Buettner, C., G. Y. Yeh, R. S. Phillips, M. A. Mittleman, and T. J. Kaptchuk. "Systematic review of the effects of ginseng on cardiovascular risk factors." *Annals of Pharmacotherapy* 40, no. 1 2006: 83–95. doi:10.1345/aph.1g216.

Burke, F. M. "Red yeast rice for the treatment of dyslipidemia." *Current Atherosclerosis Reports* 17, no. 4 2015: 22. doi: 10.1007/s11883-015-0495-8.

Chaggar, P. S., S. M. Shaw, and S. G. Williams. "Is foxglove effective in heart failure?" *Cardiovascular Therapeutics* 33, no. 4 2015: 236–41. doi:10.1111/1755-5922.12130.

Chutkan, R., G. Fahey, W. L. Wright, and J. McRorie. "Viscous versus nonviscous soluble fiber supplements: Mechanisms and evidence for fiber-specific health benefits." *Journal of the American Academy of Nurse Practitioners* 24, no. 8 2012: 476–87. doi:10.1111/j.1745-7599.2012.00758.x.

Clement, Y. "Can green tea do that? A literature review of the clinical evidence." *Preventive Medicine* 49, no. 2–3 2009: 83–7. doi:10.1016/j.ypmed.2009.05.005.

Coon, J. T., and E. Ernst. "Panax ginseng." *Drug Safety* 25, no. 5 2002: 323–44. doi:10.2165/00002018-200225050-00003.

Cunnane, S. C., S. Ganguli, C. Menard, A. C. Liede, M. J. Hamadeh, Z.-Y. Chen, T. M. S. Wolever, and D. J. A. Jenkins. "High α-linolenic acid flaxseed (*Linum usitatissimum*): Some nutritional properties in humans." *British Journal of Nutrition* 69, no. 02 1993: 443. doi:10.1079/bjn19930046.

Daniele, C., G. Mazzanti, M. H. Pittler, and E. Ernst. "Adverse-event profile of crataegus Spp." *Drug Safety2* 9, no. 6 2006: 523–35. doi:10.2165/00002018-200629060-00005.

Dhamija, P., S. Malhotra, and P. Pandhi. "Effect of oral administration of crude aqueous extract of garlic on pharmacokinetic parameters of isoniazid and rifampicin in rabbits." *Pharmacology* 77, no. 2 2006: 100–4. doi:10.1159/000093285.

Diamond, B. J., and M. R. Bailey. "Ginkgo biloba." *Psychiatric Clinics of North America* 36, no. 1 2013: 73–83. doi:10.1016/j.psc.2012.12.006.

Dudek-Makuch, M., and E. Studzińska-Sroka. "Horse chestnut – efficacy and safety in chronic venous insufficiency: An overview." *Revista Brasileira de Farmacognosia* 25, no. 5 2015: 533–41. doi:10.1016/j.bjp.2015.05.009.

Dwivedi, S. "*Terminalia arjuna* Wight & Arn.—A useful drug for cardiovascular disorders." *Journal of Ethnopharmacology* 114, no. 2 2007: 114–29. doi:10.1016/j.jep.2007.08.003.

Dwivedi, S., and D. Chopra. "Revisiting *Terminalia arjuna* – An ancient cardiovascular drug." *Journal of Traditional and Complementary Medicine* 4, no. 4 2014: 224–31. doi:10.4103/2225-4110.139103.

Eberhardt, R. T., and J. D. Raffetto. "Chronic venous insufficiency." *Circulation* 130, no. 4 2014: 333–46. doi:10.1161/circulationaha.113.006898.

Eckel, R. H., J. M. Jakicic, J. D. Ard, J. M. De Jesus, N. H. Miller, V. S. Hubbard, I-M. Lee et al. "2013 AHA/ACC guideline on lifestyle management to reduce cardiovascular risk." *Circulation* 129, no. 25 suppl 2 2014. doi:10.1161/01.cir.0000437740.48606.d1.

Ernst, E. "The risk–benefit profile of commonly used herbal therapies: Ginkgo, St. Johns Wort, Ginseng, Echinacea, Saw Palmetto, and Kava." *Annals of Internal Medicine* 136, no. 1 2002: 42. doi:10.7326/0003-4819-136-1-200201010-00010.

Eussen, S., O. Klungel, J. Garssen, H. Verhagen, H. Van Kranen, H. Van Loveren, and C. Rompelberg. "Support of drug therapy using functional foods and dietary supplements: Focus on statin therapy." *British Journal of Nutrition* 103, no. 09 2010: 1260–77. doi:10.1017/s0007114509993230.

Felixsson, E., I. A.-L. Persson, A. C. Eriksson, and K. Persson. "Horse chestnut extract contracts bovine vessels and affects human platelet aggregation through 5-HT2A receptors: An in vitro study." *Phytotherapy Research* 24, no. 9 2010: 1297–301. doi:10.1002/ptr.3103.

Fernandez, N., C. Lopez, R. Díez, J. J. Garcia, M. J. Diez, A. Sahagun, and M. Sierra. "Drug interactions with the dietary fiber *Plantago ovata* husk." *Expert Opinion on Drug Metabolism & Toxicology* 8, no. 11 2012: 1377–86. doi:10.1517/17425255.2012.716038.

Fihn, S. D., J. M. Gardin, J. Abrams, K. Berra, J. C. Blankenship, A. P. Dallas, P. S. Douglas et al. "2012 ACCF/AHA/ACP/AATS/PCNA/SCAI/STS guideline for the diagnosis and management of patients with stable Ischemic Heart Disease: A Report of the American College of Cardiology Foundation/American Heart Association Task Force on Practice Guidelines, and the American College of Physicians, American Association for Thoracic Surgery, Preventive Cardiovascular Nurses Association, Society for Cardiovascular Angiography and Interventions, and Society of Thoracic Surgeons." *Circulation* 126, no. 25 2012. doi:10.1161/cir.0b013e318277d6a0.

Fuchs, S., I. Bischoff, E. Willer, J. Bräutigam, M. Bubik, C. Erdelmeier, E. Koch et al. "The dual Edema-Preventing molecular mechanism of the crataegus extract WS 1442 can be assigned to distinct phytochemical fractions." *Planta Medica* 83, no. 08 2016: 701–9. doi:10.1055/s-0042-123388.

Fukumitsu, S., K. Aida, H. Shimizu, and K. Toyoda. "Flaxseed lignan lowers blood cholesterol and decreases liver disease risk factors in moderately hypercholesterolemic men." *Nutrition Research* 30, no. 7 2010: 441–46. doi:10.1016/j.nutres.2010.06.004.

Gerards, M. C., R. J. Terlou, H. Yu, C. H. W. Koks, and V. E. A. Gerdes. "Traditional Chinese lipid-lowering agent red yeast rice results in significant LDL reduction but safety is uncertain – a systematic review and meta-analysis." *Atherosclerosis* 240, no. 2 2015: 415–23. doi: 10.1016/j.atherosclerosis.2015.04.004.

Gerhard-Herman, M. D., H. L. Gornik, C. Barrett, N. R. Barshes, M. A. Corriere, D. E. Drachman, L. A. Fleisher et al. "2016 AHA/ACC guideline on the management of patients with lower extremity peripheral artery disease: Executive summary: A report of the American College of Cardiology/American Heart Association Task Force on Clinical Practice Guidelines." *Circulation* 135, no. 12 2017: e686–e725. doi:10.1161/cir.0000000000000470.

Gordan, R. Y., T. Cooperman, W. Obermeyer, and D. J. Becker. "Marked variability of monacolin levels in commercial red yeast rice products." *Archives of Internal Medicine* 170, no. 19 2010: 1722–27.

Green Coffee Bean Extract Supplement Reviewed by ConsumerLab.com. Accessed December 28, 2018. https://www.consumerlab.com/reviews/green_coffee_%20extract_weight_loss/greencoffee/.

Guo, R., M. H. Pittler, and E. Ernst. "Hawthorn extract for treating chronic heart failure." *Cochrane Database of Systematic Reviews* Jan 23;(1):CD005312 2008. doi:10.1002/14651858.cd005312.pub2.

Gupta, R., S. Singhl, A. Goyle, and V. N. Sharma. "Antioxidant and hypocholesterolaemic effects of *Terminalia arjuna* tree-bark powder: A randomised placebo-controlled trial." *The Journal of the Association of Physicians of India* 49 2001: 231–35.

Gurley, B., E. Fifer, and Z. Gardner. "Pharmacokinetic herb-drug interactions (Part 2): Drug interactions involving popular botanical dietary supplements and their clinical relevance." *Planta Medica* 78, no. 13 2012: 1490–514. doi:10.1055/s-0031-1298331.

Halbert, S. C., B. French, R. Y. Gordon, J. T. Farrar, K. Schmitz, P. B. Morris, P. D. Thompson, D. J. Rader, and D. J. Becker. "Tolerability of red yeast rice (2,400 mg twice daily) versus pravastatin (20 mg twice daily) in patients with previous statin intolerance." *The American Journal of Cardiology* 105, no. 2 2010: 198–204. doi:10.1016/j.amjcard.2009.08.672.

Holubarsch, C. J. F., W. S. Colucci, T. Meinertz, W. Gaus, and M. Tendera. "The efficacy and safety of *Crataegus* extract WS® 1442 in patients with heart failure: The SPICE trial." *European Journal of Heart Failure* 10, no. 12 2008: 1255–63. doi:10.1016/j.ejheart.2008.10.004.

Horsch, S., and C. Walther. "*Ginkgo biloba* special extract EGb 761 in the treatment of peripheral arterial occlusive disease (PAOD)—a review based on randomized, controlled studies." *Int. Journal of Clinical Pharmacology and Therapeutics* 42, no. 02 2004: 63–72. doi:10.5414/cpp42063.

Hosseini, A., and H. Hosseinzadeh. "A review on the effects of Allium sativum (Garlic) in metabolic syndrome." *Journal of Endocrinological Investigation* 38, no. 11 2015: 1147–57. doi:10.1007/s40618-015-0313-8.

Jayaram, S., H. B. Prasad, V. B. Sovani, and P. R. Mane. "Randomised study to compare the efficacy and safety of isapgol plus atorvastatin versus atorvastatin alone in subjects with hypercholesterolaemia." *Journal of the Indian Medical Association* 105, no. 3 2007: 142–45, 150.

Kajiyama, Y., K. Fujii, H. Takeuchi, and Y. Manabe. "Ginkgo seed poisoning." *Pediatrics* 109, no. 2 2002: 325–27. doi:10.1542/peds.109.2.325.

Kannel, W. B. "Blood pressure as a cardiovascular risk factor." *Jama* 275, no. 20 1996: 1571. doi:10.1001/jama.1996.03530440051036.

Kantor, E. D., C. D. Rehm, J. S. Haas, A. T. Chan, and E. L. Giovannucci. "Trends in prescription drug use among adults in the United States From 1999–2012." *Jama* 314, no. 17 2015: 1818. doi:10.1001/jama.2015.13766.

Kapoor, D., D. Trikha, R. Vijayvergiya, K. K. Parashar, D. Kaul, and V. Dhawan. "Short-term adjuvant therapy with *Terminalia arjuna* attenuates ongoing inflammation and immune imbalance in patients with stable coronary artery disease: In vitro and in vivo evidence." *Journal of Cardiovascular Translational Research* 8, no. 3 2015: 173–86. doi:10.1007/s12265-015-9620-x.

Kapoor, D., R. Vijayvergiya, and V. Dhawan. "*Terminalia arjuna* in coronary artery disease: Ethnopharmacology, pre-clinical, clinical & safety evaluation." *Journal of Ethnopharmacology* 155, no. 2 2014: 1029–45. doi:10.1016/j.jep.2014.06.056.

Karl, M., M. Rubenstein, C. Rudnick, and J. Brejda. "A multicenter study of nutraceutical drinks for cholesterol (evaluating effectiveness and tolerability)." *Journal of Clinical Lipidology* 6, no. 2 2012: 150–58. doi:10.1016/j.jacl.2011.09.004.

Kaur, N., N. Shafiq, H. Negi, A. Pandey, S. Reddy, H. Kaur, N. Chadha, and S. Malhotra. "*Terminalia arjuna* in chronic stable angina: Systematic review and meta-analysis." *Cardiology Research and Practice* 2014 2014: 1–7. doi:10.1155/2014/281483.

Kellermann, A. J., and C. Kloft. "Is there a risk of bleeding associated with standardized *Ginkgo biloba* extract therapy? A systematic review and meta-analysis." *Pharmacotherapy* 31, no. 5 2011: 490–502. doi:10.1592/phco.31.5.490.

Khan, N., and H. Mukhtar. "Tea polyphenols for health promotion." *Life Sciences* 81, no. 7 2007: 519–33. doi:10.1016/j.lfs.2007.06.011.

Kim, A., A. Chiu, M. K. Barone, D. Avino, F. Wang, C. I. Coleman, and O. J. Phung. "Green tea catechins decrease total and low-density lipoprotein cholesterol: A systematic review and meta-analysis." *Journal of the American Dietetic Association* 111, no. 11 2011: 1720–29. doi:10.1016/j.jada.2011.08.009.

Koch, E., and F. Malek. "Standardized extracts from hawthorn leaves and flowers in the treatment of cardiovascular disorders – Preclinical and clinical studies." *Planta Medica* 77, no. 11 2011: 1123–28. doi:10.1055/s-0030-1270849.

Kodera, Y., M. Ushijima, H. Amano, J.-I. Suzuki, and T. Matsutomo. "Chemical and biological properties of *S*-1-propenyl-l-cysteine in aged garlic extract." *Molecules* 22, no. 4 2017: 570. doi:10.3390/molecules22040570.

Koltermann, A., A. Hartkorn, E. Koch, R. Fürst, A. M. Vollmar, and S. Zahler. "*Ginkgo biloba* extract EGb® 761 increases endothelial nitric oxide production in vitro and in vivo." *Cellular and Molecular Life Sciences* 64, no. 13 2007: 1715–22. doi:10.1007/s00018-007-7085-z.

Koltermann, A., J. Liebl, R. Fürst, H. Ammer, A. M. Vollmar, and S. Zahler. "*Ginkgo biloba* extract EGb®761 exerts anti-angiogenic effects via activation of tyrosine phosphatases." *Journal of Cellular and Molecular Medicine* 13, no. 8b 2008: 2122–30. doi:10.1111/j.1582-4934.2008.00561.x.

Koo, S., and S. Noh. "Green tea as inhibitor of the intestinal absorption of lipids: Potential mechanism for its lipid-lowering effect." *The Journal of Nutritional Biochemistry* 18, no. 3 2007: 179–83. doi:10.1016/j.jnutbio.2006.12.005.

Kristensen, M., M. G. Jensen, J. Aarestrup, K. E. Petersen, L. Søndergaard, M. S. Mikkelsen, and A. Astrup. "Flaxseed dietary fibers lower cholesterol and increase fecal fat excretion, but magnitude of effect depend [sic] on food type." *Nutrition & Metabolism* 9, no. 1 2012: 8. doi:10.1186/1743-7075-9-8.

Kumar, D., V. Arya, Z. A. Bhat, N. A. Khan, and D. N. Prasad. "The genus *Crataegus*: Chemical and pharmacological perspectives." *Revista Brasileira de Farmacognosia* 22, no. 5 2012: 1187–200. doi:10.1590/s0102-695×2012005000094.

Law, M. R. "Value of low dose combination treatment with blood pressure lowering drugs: analysis of 354 randomised trials." *British Medical Journal* 326, no. 7404 2003: 1427. doi:10.1136/bmj.326.7404.1427.

Leach, M. J., J. Pincombe, and G. Foster. "Using horsechestnut [sic] seed extract in the treatment of venous leg ulcers: A cost-benefit analysis." *Ostomy/Wound Management* 52, no. 4 2006a: 68–78.

Leach, M. J., J. Pincombe, and G.W. Foster. "Clinical efficacy of horse chestnut seed extract in the treatment of venous ulceration." *Journal of Wound Care* 15, no. 4 2006b: 159–67. doi:10.12968/jowc.2006.15.4.26898.

Lee, S.-J., and Y. Jia. "The effect of bioactive compounds in tea on lipid metabolism and obesity through regulation of peroxisome proliferator-activated receptors." *Current Opinion in Lipidology* 26, no. 1 2015: 3–9. doi:10.1097/mol.0000000000000145.

Lesney, M. S. "Flowers for the heart." *Modern Drug Discovery*. March 2002. Accessed December 28, 2018. http://pubs.acs.org/subscribe/archive/mdd/v05/i03/html/03timeline.html. Vol. 5, no. 3, pp 46.

Li, J.-J., Z.-L. Lu, W.-R. Kou, Z. Chen, Y.-F. Wu, X.-H. Yu, and Y.-C. Zhao. "Beneficial impact of Xuezhikang on cardiovascular events and mortality in elderly hypertensive patients with previous myocardial infarction from the China Coronary Secondary Prevention Study (CCSPS)". *Journal of Clinical Pharmacology* 49, no. 8 2009: 947–56. doi:10.1177/0091270009337509.

Li, G., Y. Zhang, L. Thabane, L. Mbuagbaw, A. Liu, M. A. h. Levine, and A. Holbrook. "Effect of green tea supplementation on blood pressure among overweight and obese adults." *Journal of Hypertension* 33, no. 2 2015: 243–54. doi:10.1097/hjh.0000000000000426.

Li, Y., C. Wang, Q. Huai, F. Guo, L. Liu, R. Feng, and C. Sun. Effects of tea or tea extract on metabolic profiles in patients with type-2 diabetes mellitus: a meta-analysis of ten randomized controlled trials. *Diabetes/Metabolism Research and Reviews* 32, no. 1 2016: 2–10. doi:10.1002/dmrr.2641.

Lim, W., K. W. Mudge, and F. Vermeylen. "Effects of population, age, and cultivation methods on ginsenoside content of wild American Ginseng (*Panax quinquefolium*)." *Journal of Agricultural and Food Chemistry* 53, no. 22 2005: 8498–505. doi:10.1021/jf051070y.

Liu, G., X.-N. Mi, X.-X. Zheng, Y.-L. Xu, J. Lu, and X.-H. Huang. "Effects of tea intake on blood pressure: A meta-analysis of randomised controlled trials." *British Journal of Nutrition* 112, no. 07 2014: 1043–54. doi:10.1017/s0007114514001731.

Loader, T. B., C. G. Taylor, P. Zahradka, and P. J. h. Jones. "Chlorogenic acid from coffee beans: Evaluating the evidence for a blood pressure–regulating health claim." *Nutrition Reviews* 75, no. 2 2017. doi:10.1093/nutrit/nuw057.

Ma, K.-Y., Z.-S. Zhang, S.-X. Zhao, Q. Chang, Y.-M. Wong, S. Y. Yeung, Y. Huang, and Z. Y. Chen. "Red yeast rice increases excretion of bile acids in hamsters." *Biomedical and Environmental Sciences* 22 2009: 269–77. doi: 10.1016/S0895-3988(09)60056-8.

Magni, P., C. Macchi, B. Morlotti, C. R. Sirtori, and M. Ruscica. "Risk identification and possible countermeasures for muscle adverse effects during statin therapy." *European Journal of Internal Medicine* 26 2015: 82–8. doi: 10.1016/j.ejim.2015.01.002.

Mahdavi-Roshan, M., J. Nasrollahzadeh, A. M. Zadeh, and A. Zahedmehr. "Does garlic supplementation control blood pressure in patients with severe coronary artery disease? A clinical trial study." *Iranian Red Crescent Medical Journal* 18, no. 11 2016. doi:10.5812/ircmj.23871.

Mancuso, C., and R. Santangelo. "*Panax ginseng* and *Panax quinquefolius*: From pharmacology to toxicology." *Food and Chemical Toxicology* 107 2017: 362–72. doi:10.1016/j.fct.2017.07.019.

Matsumoto, S., R. Nakanishi, D. Li, A. Alani, P. Rezaeian, S. Prabhu, J. Abraham et al. "Aged garlic extract reduces low attenuation plaque in coronary arteries of patients with metabolic syndrome in a prospective randomized double-blind study." *Journal of Nutrition* 146, no. 2 2016. doi:10.3945/jn.114.202424.

Mazzanti, G., A. D. Sotto, and A. Vitalone. "Hepatotoxicity of green tea: An update." *Archives of Toxicology* 89, no. 8 2015: 1175–91. doi:10.1007/s00204-015-1521-x.

Mei, N., X. Guo, Z. Ren, D. Kobayashi, K. Wada, and L. Guo. "Review of Ginkgo biloba-induced toxicity, from experimental studies to human case reports." *Journal of Environmental Science and Health, Part C* 35, no. 1 2017: 1–28. doi:10.1080/10590501.2016.1278298.

Misaka, S., J. Yatabe, F. Müller, K. Takano, K. Kawabe, H. Glaeser, M. S. Yatabe et al. "Green tea ingestion greatly reduces plasma concentrations of nadolol in healthy subjects." *Clinical Pharmacology & Therapeutics* 95, no. 4 2014: 432–38. doi:10.1038/clpt.2013.241.

Moreyra, A. E. "Effect of combining psyllium fiber with simvastatin in lowering cholesterol." *Archives of Internal Medicine* 165, no. 10 2005: 1161. doi:10.1001/archinte.165.10.1161.

Mozaffarian, D., E. J. Benjamin, A. S. Go, D. K. Arnett, M. J. Blaha, M. Cushman, S. R. Das et al. "Heart disease and stroke statistics—2016 update." *Circulation* 133, no. 4 2015. doi:10.1161/cir.0000000000000350.

Nelson, R. H. "Hyperlipidemia as a risk factor for cardiovascular disease." *Primary Care: Clinics in Office Practice* 40, no. 1 2013: 195–211. doi:10.1016/j.pop.2012.11.003

Nicolaï, S. P., L. M. Kruidenier, B. L. Bendermacher, M. H. Prins, R. A. Stokmans, P. P. Broos, and J. A. Teijink. "*Ginkgo biloba* for intermittent claudication." *Cochrane Database of Systematic Reviews* Jun 6; (6): CD006888 2013. doi:10.1002/14651858.cd006888.pub3.

Nogueira, L. D. P., J. F. Nogueira Neto, M. R. S. T. Klein, and A. F. Sanjuliani. "Short-term effects of green tea on blood pressure, endothelial function, and metabolic profile in obese prehypertensive women: A crossover randomized clinical trial." *Journal of the American College of Nutrition* 36, no. 2 2016: 108–15. doi:10.1080/07315724.2016.1194236.

Nugrahani, G., and D. N. Afifah. "Effect of garlic as a spice on salt preferences of hypertensive individuals." *Pakistan Journal of Nutrition* 15, no. 7 2016: 633–8. doi:10.3923/pjn.2016.633.638.

Onakpoya, I., E. Spencer, C. Heneghan, and M. Thompson. "The effect of green tea on blood pressure and lipid profile: A systematic review and meta-analysis of randomized clinical trials." *Nutrition, Metabolism and Cardiovascular Diseases* 24, no. 8 2014a: 823–36. doi:10.1016/j.numecd.2014.01.016.

Onakpoya, I. J., E. A. Spencer, M. J. Thompson, and C. J. Heneghan. "The effect of chlorogenic acid on blood pressure: A systematic review and meta-analysis of randomized clinical trials." *Journal of Human Hypertension* 29, no. 2 2014b: 77–81. doi:10.1038/jhh.2014.46.

Ong, Y. C., and Z. Aziz. "Systematic review of red yeast rice compared with simvastatin in dyslipidemia." *Journal of Clinical Pharmacy and Therapeutics* 42, no. 2 2016: 170–9. doi: 10.1111/jcpt.12374.

Pan, A., D. Yu, W. Demark-Wahnefried, O. H. Franco, and X. Lin. "Meta-analysis of the effects of flaxseed interventions on blood lipids." *American Journal of Clinical Nutrition* 90, no. 2 2009: 288–97. doi:10.3945/ajcn.2009.27469.

Pirro, M., C. Vetrani, C. Bianchi, M. R. Mannarino, F. Bernini, and A. A. Rivellese. "Joint position statement on "Nutraceuticals for the treatment of hypercholesterolemia" of the Italian Society of Diabetology (SID) and of the Italian Society for the Study of Arteriosclerosis (SISA)." *Nutrition, Metabolism and Cardiovascular Diseases* 27, no. 1 2017: 2–17. doi:10.1016/j.numecd.2016.11.122.

Pittler, M. H., and E. Ernst. "Horse chestnut seed extract for chronic venous insufficiency." *Cochrane Database of Systematic Reviews* Nov 14;11:CD003230 2012. doi:10.1002/14651858.cd003230.pub4.

Ried, K. "Garlic lowers blood pressure in hypertensive individuals, regulates serum cholesterol, and stimulates immunity: An updated meta-analysis and review." *Journal of Nutrition* 146, no. 2 2016. doi:10.3945/jn.114.202192.

Ried, K., C. Toben, and P. Fakler. "Effect of garlic on serum lipids: An updated meta-analysis." *Nutrition Reviews* 71, no. 5 2013: 282–99. doi:10.1111/nure.12012.

Samavat, H., A. R. Newman, R. Wang, J.-M. Yuan, A. H. Wu, and M. S. Kurzer. "Effects of green tea catechin extract on serum lipids in postmenopausal women: A randomized, placebo-controlled clinical trial." *American Journal of Clinical Nutrition* 104, no. 6 2016: 1671–82. doi:10.3945/ajcn.116.137075.

Shatoor, A. S., H. Soliman, F. Al-Hashem, B. E. Gamal, A. Othman, and N. El-Menshawy. "Effect of hawthorn (Crataegus aronia syn. Azarolus (L)) on platelet function in albino wistar rats." *Thrombosis Research* 130, no. 1 2012: 75–80. doi:10.1016/j.thromres.2012.01.001.

Shin, H. R., J. Y. Kim, T. K. Yun, G. Morgan, and H. Vainio. "The cancer-preventive potential of Panax ginseng: A review of human and experimental evidence." *Cancer Causes & Control* 11, no. 6 (July 2000): 565–76. UI: 10880039

Shouk, R., A. Abdou, K. Shetty, D. Sarkar, and A. H. Eid. "Mechanisms underlying the antihypertensive effects of garlic bioactives." *Nutrition Research* 34, no. 2 2014: 106–15. doi:10.1016/j.nutres.2013.12.005.

Snow, A., D. Halpenny, G. Mcneill, and W. C. Torreggiani. "Life-threatening rupture of a renal angiomyolipoma in a patient taking over-the-counter horse chestnut seed extract." *The Journal of Emergency Medicine* 43, no. 6 2012. doi:10.1016/j.jemermed.2010.11.044.

Sobenin, I. A., I. V. Andrianova, I. V. Fomchenkov, T. V. Gorchakova, and A. N. Orekhov. "Time-released garlic powder tablets lower systolic and diastolic blood pressure in men with mild and moderate arterial hypertension." *Hypertension Research* 32, no. 6 2009: 433–7. doi:10.1038/hr.2009.36.

Soltani, S. K., R. Jamaluddin, H. Tabibi, B. N. M. Yusof, S. Atabak, S.-P. Loh, and L. Rahmani. "Effects of flaxseed consumption on systemic inflammation and serum lipid profile in hemodialysis patients with lipid abnormalities." *Hemodialysis International* 17, no. 2 2012: 275–81. doi:10.1111/j.1542-4758.2012.00754.x.

Stalmach, A., G. Williamson, and A. Crozier. "Impact of dose on the bioavailability of coffee chlorogenic acids in humans." *Food Functional* 5, no. 8 2014: 1727–737. doi:10.1039/c4fo00316k.

Stoddard, G. J., M. Archer, L. Shane-McWhorter, B. E. Bray, D. F. Redd, J. Proulx, and Q. Zeng-Treitler. "Ginkgo and Warfarin Interaction in a Large Veterans Administration Population." *AMIA … Annual Symposium proceedings. AMIA Symposium2015* 2015: 1173–83. PMC: PMC4765589

Stone, N. J., J. G. Robinson, A. H. Lichtenstein, C. N. Bairey Merz, C. B. Blum, R. H. Eckel, A. C. Goldberg et al. "2013 ACC/AHA guideline on the treatment of blood cholesterol to reduce atherosclerotic cardiovascular risk in adults." *Circulation* 129, no. 25 suppl 2 2013. doi:10.1161/01.cir.0000437738.63853.7a.

Stücker, M., E. S. Debus, J. Hoffmann, M. Jünger, K. Kröger, A. Mumme, A.-A. Ramelet, and E. Rabe. "Consensus statement on the symptom-based treatment of chronic venous diseases." *JDDG: Journal der Deutschen Dermatologischen Gesellschaft* 14, no. 6 2016: 575–83. doi:10.1111/ddg.13006.

Suzuki-Sugihara, N., Y. Kishimoto, E. Saita, C. Taguchi, M. Kobayashi, M. Ichitani, Y. Ukawa, Y. M. Sagesaka, E. Suzuki, and K. Kondo. "Green tea catechins prevent low-density lipoprotein oxidation via their accumulation in low-density lipoprotein particles in humans." *Nutrition Research* 36, no. 1 2016: 16–23. doi:10.1016/j.nutres.2015.10.012.

Thom, E. "The effect of chlorogenic acid enriched coffee on glucose absorption in healthy volunteers and its effect on body mass when used long-term in overweight and obese people." *Journal of International Medical Research* 35, no. 6 2007: 900–8. doi:10.1177/147323000703500620.

Tiffany, N., C. Ulbricht, S. Bent, M. Smith, C. Dennehy, H. Boon, E. Basch, E. P. Barrette, D. Sollars, and P. Szapary. "Horse chestnut: A multidisciplinary clinical review." *Journal of Herbal Pharmacotherapy* 2, no. 1 2002: 71–85.

Tom, E. N. Lemba, C. Girard-Thernier, and C. Demougeot. "The Janus face of chlorogenic acid on vascular reactivity: A study on rat isolated vessels." *Phytomedicine* 23, no. 10 2016: 1037–42. doi:10.1016/j.phymed.2016.06.012.

Tong, X., A. W. Taylor, L. Giles, G. A. Wittert, and Z. Shi. "Tea consumption is inversely related to 5-year blood pressure change among adults in Jiangsu, China: A cross-sectional study." *Nutrition Journal* 13, no. 1 2014. doi:10.1186/1475-2891-13-98.

Uehleke, B., M. Ortiz, and R. Stange. "Cholesterol reduction using psyllium husks – Do gastrointestinal adverse effects limit compliance? Results of a specific observational study." *Zeitschrift für Phytotherapie* 29, no. S 1 2008. doi:10.1055/s-2008-1047842.

Ulbricht, C., N. Tiffany, H. Boon, C. Ulbricht, E. Basch, S. Bent, E. P. Barrette et al. "Horse chestnut: A multidisciplinary clinical review." *Journal of Herbal Pharmacotherapy* 2, no. 1 2002: 71–85. doi:10.1300/j157v02n01_10.

Underland, V., I. Sæterdal, and E. S. Nilsen. "Cochrane summary of findings: Horse chestnut seed extract for chronic venous insufficiency." *Global Advances in Health and Medicine* 1, no. 1 2012: 122–3. doi:10.7453/gahmj.2012.1.1.018.

Wang, J., X. Xiong, and B. Feng. "Effect of *Crataegus* usage in cardiovascular disease prevention: An evidence-based approach." *Evidence-Based Complementary and Alternative Medicine* 2013 2013: 1–16. doi:10.1155/2013/149363.

Wei, Z.-H., H. Wang, X.-Y. Chen, B.-S. Wang, Z.-X. Rong, B.-S. Wang, B.-H. Su, and H.-Z. Chen. "Time- and dose-dependent effect of psyllium on serum lipids in mild-to-moderate hypercholesterolemia: A meta-analysis of controlled clinical trials." *European Journal of Clinical Nutrition* 63, no. 7 2008: 821–7. doi:10.1038/ejcn.2008.49.

Weisse, A. B. "A fond farewell to the foxglove? The decline in the use of digitalis." *Journal of Cardiac Failure* 16, no. 1 2010: 45–8. doi:10.1016/j.cardfail.2009.08.001.

Willer, E. A., R. Malli, A. I. Bondarenko, S. Zahler, A. M. Vollmar, W. F. Graier, and R. Fürst. "The vascular barrier-protecting hawthorn extract WS® 1442 raises endothelial calcium levels by inhibition of SERCA and activation of the IP3 pathway." *Journal of Molecular and Cellular Cardiology* 53, no. 4 2012: 567–77. doi:10.1016/j.yjmcc.2012.07.002.

Whelton, P. K., R. M. Carey, W. S. Aronow, D. E. Casey, K. J. Collins, C. D. Himmelfarb, S. M. Depalma et al. "2017 ACC/AHA/AAPA/ABC/ACPM/AGS/APhA/ASH/ASPC/NMA/PCNA guideline for the prevention, detection, evaluation, and management of high blood pressure in adults: Executive summary." *Journal of the American College of Cardiology* 71(19), 2017: 2199–269. doi:10.1016/j.jacc.2017.11.005.

Wong, H., N. Chahal, C. Manlhiot, E. Niedra, and B. W. McCrindle. "Flaxseed in pediatric hyperlipidemia." *JAMA Pediatrics* 167, no. 8 2013: 708. doi:10.1001/jamapediatrics.2013.1442.

Writing Committee, Wittens, C., A. H. Davies, N. Bækgaard, R. Broholm, A. Cavezzi, S. Chastanet, M. De Wolf et al. "Editors choice – Management of chronic venous disease." *European Journal of Vascular and Endovascular Surgery* 49, no. 6 2015: 678–737. doi:10.1016/j.ejvs.2015.02.007.

Xiong, X. J., P. Q. Wang, S. J. Li, X. K. Li, Y. Q. Zhang, and J. Wang. "Garlic for hypertension: A systematic review and meta-analysis of randomized controlled trials." *Phytomedicine* 22, no. 3 2015: 352–61. doi:10.1016/j.phymed.2014.12.013.

Yancy, C. W., M. Jessup, B. Bozkurt, J. Butler, D. E. Casey, M. M. Colvin, M. H. Drazner et al. "2016 ACC/AHA/HFSA focused update on new pharmacological therapy for heart failure: An update of the 2013 ACCF/AHA guideline for the management of heart failure." *Journal of the American College of Cardiology* 68, no. 13 September 27, 2016: 1476–88. doi:10.1016/j.jacc.2016.05.011.

Yancy, C. W., M. Jessup, B. Bozkurt, J. Butler, D. E. Casey, M. H. Drazner, G. C. Fonarow et al. "2013 ACCF/AHA guideline for the management of heart failure: A report of the American College of Cardiology Foundation/American Heart Association Task Force on Practice Guidelines." *Circulation* 128, no. 16 2013: E240–347. doi:10.1161/cir.0b013e31829e8776.

Zhao, Y., J. Wang, O. Ballevre, H. Luo, and W. Zhang. "Antihypertensive effects and mechanisms of chlorogenic acids." *Hypertension Research* 35, no. 4 2011: 370–74. doi:10.1038/hr.2011.195.

Zick, S. M., B. Gillespie, and K. D. Aaronson. "The effect of *Crataegus oxycantha* [sic] special extract WS 1442 on clinical progression in patients with mild to moderate symptoms of heart failure." *European Journal of Heart Failure* 10, no. 6 2008: 587–93. doi:10.1016/j.ejheart.2008.04.008.

Zick, S. M., B. M. Vautaw, B. Gillespie, and K. D. Aaronson. "Hawthorn Extract Randomized Blinded Chronic Heart Failure (HERB CHF) Trial." *European Journal of Heart Failure* 11, no. 10 2009: 990–9. doi:10.1093/eurjhf/hfp116.

6

Endocrine Disorders

Kaelen Dunican, Aimee Dawson, and Ann Lynch

CONTENTS

6.1 Introduction

The two endocrine disorders with published evidence on botanicals are diabetes mellitus (DM) and thyroid disorders. The American Association of Clinical Endocrinologists (AACE) has recognized the increased demand and desire for the use of dietary supplements, nutraceuticals, and botanical products to treat endocrine disorders and as such, published evidence-based guidelines in 2003 (Mechanick et al. 2003). These guidelines are limited in the scope of botanicals that are included. Additional evidence has also become available since the time of publication. This chapter aims to expand upon the existing guidelines to provide more comprehensive information and evidence regarding botanical use in endocrine disorders.

6.2 Diabetes Mellitus

Diabetes mellitus is a chronic condition affecting 422 million adults globally (World Health Organization 2017). Patients are increasingly seeking natural products for self-care. A survey of patients with DM demonstrated that 31% of the patients reported using integrative medicine for treatment of DM (Ryan et al. 2001). Many patients are using these products in conjunction with their prescription medications to optimize glycemic control. Due to safety, efficacy, and financial considerations for use of botanicals, patients and clinicians should be adequately informed about the evidence of use, benefits, and risks associated with these supplements.

6.2.1 American Ginseng

6.2.1.1 Background

Ginseng refers to both American ginseng (*Panax quinquefolius*) and Asian (Panax or Korean) ginseng (*Panax ginseng*). American ginseng grows mainly in North America, primarily in Ontario, Canada (Mucalo et al. 2013). Similar to Asian or Panax ginseng, American ginseng is made from the light tan-colored ginseng root and the long, thin offshoots called root hairs. The plant from which Asian ginseng is produced is a relative of the North American species. Native Americans historically used the root as a stimulant, as well as a treatment for fever, headaches, indigestion, and infertility. As of today, ginseng continues to be one of the most popular botanicals used for digestive disorders, cancer-related fatigue, preventing respiratory illness and the effects of aging, improving cognitive function and athletic performance, and enhancing the immune system (Biondo et al. 2008, Ichikawa et al. 2009). Additionally, both American and Asian ginseng are used to reduce blood glucose levels in patients with type-2 diabetes mellitus (T2DM).

6.2.1.2 Pharmacognosy

Both ginsengs belong to the genus "Panax," and thus have comparable chemical and medicinal properties exhibited via ginsenosides, saponins, and polysaccharide glycans such as quinquefolans A, B, and C (Kitts et al. 2000, Vuksan et al. 2000b, Mucalo et al. 2013). Each type of ginseng exhibits antioxidant effects via different types and amounts of their inherent ingredients. Ginseng has been labeled as an *adaptogen*.

6.2.1.3 Dosing and Preparation

Taking 3 g within 2 hours of a meal has been shown to produce a desired level of hypoglycemia. It is important to take it only around meal times to avoid an unwanted hypoglycemic event. American ginseng comes in many oral formulations, including capsules, tablets, root powders, teas, and tinctures.

6.2.1.4 Safety

American ginseng appears safe when used in doses 100–3000 mg daily for up to 12 weeks for most commercial preparations (Morris et al. 1996, Vuksan et al. 2000a). A single dose of as much as 10 grams has been administered safely (Vuksan et al. 2000b) and a specific product developed in Canada (CVT-E002) has been given for 64 months without adverse consequences (McElhaney et al. 2011). Administration of American ginseng may be safe in children, however evidence stating its safety seems to be limited to CVT-E002 in doses of 4.5–26 mg daily for 3 days (Vohra et al. 2008). American ginseng should be avoided in pregnancy, as it may be unsafe when taken orally due to the teratogenic effect of American ginseng's ingredient ginsenosides Rb1 in animals (Chan et al. 2003). Evidence is insufficient to establish the safety of American ginseng in breastfeeding and thus should be avoided. Few adverse effects are associated with American ginseng when taken orally at recommended doses. While most adverse effects are associated with Asian ginseng and few have been associated with American ginseng specifically, potential adverse effects could include diarrhea or gastrointestinal upset, itching, insomnia, headache, anxiety, tachycardia, hypertension or hypotension, breast tenderness, and vaginal bleeding (Wiwanitkit and Taungjaruwinai 2004, Stavro et al. 2006).

While American ginseng may be expected to cause pharmacodynamic drug interactions, studies have shown that daily doses of dried whole root have not altered metabolism via CYP3A4 or glucuronidation (Shader and Greenblatt 1985, Janetzky and Morreale 1997, Vuksan et al. 2000a,b, McElhaney et al. 2004). While many natural products including ginseng can cause bleeding on their own and thus possibly contribute to a synergistic bleeding effect with all antithrombotics, American ginseng has been shown to *decrease* the effectiveness of warfarin, resulting in the possibility of an increased risk of clotting. Although the mechanism of this interaction is not well defined, this interaction results in a major potential risk and concomitant use should be avoided (Janetzky and Morreale 1997). There is no data to suggest a similar interaction with direct-acting oral anticoagulants (DOACs). Because American ginseng has the potential to lower blood glucose levels, a potential interaction exists with insulin, glyburide, pioglitazone, fenugreek among others, causing an increase in hypoglycemia (Vuksan et al. 2000a,b). If used together with other hypoglycemic agents, blood glucose levels should be monitored closely. Monoamine oxidase inhibitors (MAOIs) such as phenelzine and tranylcypromine may interact with American ginseng. Because American ginseng may stimulate the body's immune function, it should be used with caution when taken concurrently with immunosuppressants such as cyclosporine, as theoretically it can decrease their effectiveness (McElhaney et al. 2004). *See Chapter 2 Pharmacokinetic and Pharmacogenomic Considerations for further discussion.*

6.2.1.5 Evidence

Human studies have shown that the ginsenosides contained in American ginseng increase insulin levels in the body, resulting in lower postprandial and fasting glucose levels (Vuksan et al. 2000a,b, Mucalo et al. 2012). Oral doses of 3 g of American ginseng, given to patients with T2DM as much as 2 hours before meals, produced a statistically significant reduction of approximately 20% in glucose levels after eating (Vuksan et al. 2000a,b, 2001, Yeh et al. 2003, Wu et al. 2007). Doses greater than 3 g did not show any additional benefit (Vuksan et al. 2000b). While more research is needed, studies have suggested that American ginseng may help to prevent retinal and cardiac complications resulting from DM (Sen et al. 2013). One study confirmed that ginseng berry extract produced a three-fold greater reduction in blood glucose levels than the same concentration of root extract. Reasons for the differences in potency are unclear (Dey et al. 2003).

6.2.1.6 Clinical Application

American ginseng has been shown to reduce glucose levels in T2DM. Adverse effects have been mild and include GI upset, itching, anxiety, increased bleeding, and modest changes in blood pressure. A clinically significant drug interaction with warfarin is important to avoid. American ginseng can be used for up to 12 weeks safely to reduce elevated blood glucose levels. Therapy exceeding 12 weeks should be used with caution and under supervision until further evidence is available.

6.2.2 Asian Ginseng

6.2.2.1 Background

The term *ginseng* is classically associated with Asian (Panax or Korean) ginseng (*Panax ginseng*). Its chemical and medicinal properties are comparable to American ginseng. Historically, it has been in used in traditional Chinese medicine (TCM) in many Asian countries (Shin et al. 2000, Jung et al. 2011). While Asian ginseng is typically promoted as a stimulant in Western medicine, it is also used for purposes similar to American ginseng including T2DM.

6.2.2.2 Pharmacognosy

Similarly, its primary active elements are ginsenosides and saponins with additional constituents including polysaccharide glycans (e.g., panaxans), polysaccharide fraction DPG-3-2, B vitamins, pectin, peptides, flavonoids, and volatile oil (Shin et al. 2000, Jung et al. 2011). *See Chapter 10 Neurological Conditions for more discussion.*

6.2.2.3 Dosing and Preparation

Asian ginseng supplements are made from the ginseng root and the long root hairs from the species Panax ginseng plant that is indigenous to Korea, northeastern China, and eastern Siberia (Shin et al. 2000, Rhee et al. 2014). Dosing regimens for treatment of T2DM include 2.7 grams/day of fermented Panax ginseng for 4 weeks (Oh et al. 2014), 6 g daily of Panax ginseng root in 3 divided doses for 12 weeks given concomitantly with additional antidiabetes therapies (Vuksan et al. 2008), and Panax ginseng 100–200 mg once daily for 8 weeks (Sotaniemi et al. 1995).

6.2.2.4 Safety

Asian or Panax ginseng is generally safe when used appropriately up to 6 months (An et al. 2011, Lee et al. 2012). Oral administration of Asian ginseng in infants is associated with intoxication with the potential for death (Edward 2000). Given this potential and the limited evidence in children of any age, use of Asian ginseng should be avoided (Niederhofer 2009). Asian ginseng should be avoided in pregnancy as it may be unsafe when taken orally due to the teratogenic effect of American ginseng's ingredient ginsenosides Rb1 in animals (Chan et al. 2003). Evidence is insufficient to establish the safety of Asian ginseng in breastfeeding and thus should be avoided.

While Asian ginseng is usually well tolerated when taken orally, adverse effects are possible. Insomnia is the most common adverse effect. Less commonly, diarrhea or gastrointestinal upset, itching, insomnia, headache, anxiety, tachycardia, hypertension or hypotension, edema, decreased appetite, mania, breast tenderness, and vaginal bleeding may occur (Martinez-Mir et al. 2004, Wiwanitkit and Taungjaruwinai 2004, Stavro et al. 2006). Although rare, Stevens-Johnson syndrome, cholestatic hepatitis, and severe allergic reactions are serious side effects that should be reported immediately to healthcare providers (Hamid et al. 1997).

Asian ginseng has many pharmacodynamic and pharmacokinetic drug, food, and botanical interactions (Sotaniemi et al. 1995, Scaglione et al. 1996, Caron et al. 2002, Hao et al. 2011). Asian ginseng can increase the metabolism and clearance of alcohol via the induction of alcohol and aldehyde dehydrogenase (Lee et al. 1987). Asian ginseng may potentially interact with warfarin and other anticoagulants and antiplatelets by decreasing platelet aggregation, causing more bleeding (Hwa-Jin et al. 1996). Conflicting studies suggest that American ginseng does not affect platelet aggregation; therefore, precautions must be taken with concurrent use (Jiang et al. 2004). In theory, Asian ginseng has the potential to either lower, not affect, or raise blood glucose levels, thus close monitoring should be followed if it is used together with other hypoglycemic agents (Sotaniemi et al. 1995). The use of Asian ginseng with stimulants such as caffeine and methylphenidate may cause an increase in the stimulant effect. Caution should be observed with the administration of this combination. *See Chapter 2 Pharmacokinetic and Pharmacogenomic Considerations for discussion of issues related to pharmacokinetic drug interactions.*

6.2.2.5 Evidence

The ability of Asian ginseng to lower blood glucose levels remains controversial. Some studies have shown that daily doses of 200–6000 mg of Asian ginseng may have hypoglycemic effects in people with T2DM, resulting in decreased fasting and postprandial glucose levels (Vuksan et al. 2008, Oh et al. 2014). Other clinical studies suggest that the specific ginsenosides found in Korean Red ginseng in oral doses of 250–500 mg daily might either cause hyperglycemia or result in no significant reduction in postprandial glucose levels (Kim et al. 2011). Until better quality research is done, the use of Asian ginseng in T2DM should either be avoided or used under careful monitoring and supervision (Kim et al. 2011, Reeds et al. 2011).

6.2.2.6 Clinical Application

Asian ginseng may lower glucose levels in patients with T2DM, however studies are conflicting. The hypoglycemic effects compared to American ginseng are less convincing. Asian ginseng can be used in non-pregnant, non-breast feeding adults for up to 6 months. Adverse effects are similar to those of American ginseng with the additional possibility of rare but severe dermatologic effects or cholestatic hepatitis, making monitoring its use important.

6.2.3 Berberine

6.2.3.1 Background

Berberine is an isoquinoline alkaloid that is present in several species of plants including Berberis vulgaris, Coptis chinensis, and Berberis aristata (Pirillo and Catapano 2015). It has been used in botanical medicine for several indications, as it has glucose and cholesterol lowering, antimicrobial, antitumor, and immune-modulatory activities.

6.2.3.2 Pharmacognosy

Berberine itself is the active component providing pharmacologic effect. Two mechanisms have been hypothesized for the hypoglycemic effects, including the upregulation of insulin receptors causing increased glucose uptake and antimicrobial activity modulating gut microbiotic effects on obesity and glycemic control (Pirillo and Catapano 2015).

6.2.3.3 Dosing and Preparations

A limitation to berberine is the wide variety of dosing and preparations that have been studied. Doses range from 0.5 to 1.5 g in 2 to 3 divided doses, with the majority of clinical trials using 0.5 mg of berberine three times daily for up to 18 weeks (Pirillo and Catapano 2015). Berberine is available in oral formulations including capsules, tablets, liquid extracts, or powders. It is also found in combination products. Berberine has a low bioavailability and is often combined with other ingredients that may increase its absorption (Pirillo and Catapano 2015).

6.2.3.4 Safety

Berberine is safe with a meta-analysis concluding that the incidence of adverse effects was similar between berberine and control (Pirillo and Catapano 2015). Individual trials most commonly report mild gastrointestinal symptoms (Di Pierro et al. 2012, Pirillo and Catapano 2015). Some have hypothesized that these GI effects are similar to those of an alpha-glucosidase inhibitor such as acarbose (Di Pierro et al. 2012). The long-term safety of berberine in the diabetic population has not been adequately studied, with the longest trial being 18 weeks (Pirillo and Catapano 2015).

A disadvantage to berberine is its potential for clinically significant drug interactions (Table 6.1) (Pirillo and Catapano 2015). This includes an interaction with metformin, a common medication for T2DM. Berberine can also reduce the concentrations of P-glycoprotein (P-gp) substrates. The effects on P-gp also seem to impair berberine's own bioavailability. Inversely, berberine's concentration can be rapidly increased in the presence of P-gp inhibitors. One study used this drug interaction to its advantage by combining the botanical with milk thistle, another potent inhibitor of P-gp, in an effort to increase the concentration and effects of berberine in patients with DM (Di Pierro et al. 2012). The results were promising, but further research is warranted before recommending this combination. Overall, caution should be used when combining berberine with other drugs that are P-gp substrates, inhibitors, or inducers.

Berberine can also interact with drugs metabolized through the CYP 450 enzymes. Notably, it has been shown to inhibit CYP 3A4 (Pirillo and Catapano 2015). Patients taking berberine should inform their providers and pharmacists so that proper monitoring and therapy adjustments can be made to prevent these drug interactions.

TABLE 6.1

Clinically Significant Drug Interactions with Berberine

Drug	Mechanism for Interaction
Cyclosporine A	P-gp/CYP3A4
Dextromethorphan	CYP2D6
Digoxin	P-gp
HIV Protease inhibitors	P-gp
Losartan	CYP2C9
Metformin	OCT1/OCT2
Midazolam	CYP3A4
Quinidine	OCT/P-gp
Tacrolimus	CYP3A4
Tolbutamide	CYP2C9
Verapamil	P-gp

Source: Pirillo, A. and A. L. Catapano. 2015. *Atherosclerosis* 243 (2): 449–461.

6.2.3.5 Evidence

Multiple clinical trials in humans have shown benefits from the use of berberine in the treatment of DM (Di Pierro et al. 2012, Lan et al. 2015, Pirillo and Catapano 2015). Berberine has consistently demonstrated significant glucose lowering effects. Berberine has been shown to lower hemoglobin A1c (HbA1c) by 0.9%–2% which may be comparable to metformin. Its effects are on fasting and postprandial blood glucose levels. These findings should be balanced with the limitations of the studies, primarily small populations that may limit the generalizability of the findings.

In addition to the beneficial effects on glycemic control, berberine also has favorable effects on a fasting lipid profile (Pirillo and Catapano 2015). Patients diagnosed with T2DM are at high risk of macrovascular complications, including myocardial infarction and stroke, so this beneficial effect on lipids is highly advantageous.

6.2.3.6 Clinical Application

Berberine is effective at reducing HbA1c while improving fasting lipid panel. Safety concerns include minor GI adverse effects and clinically significant drug interactions. T2DM is a chronic condition, but berberine has only been studied for up to 18 weeks. Caution should be used in long-term use until further evidence is available.

6.2.4 Bitter Melon

6.2.4.1 Background

Bitter melon (*Momordica charantia*), also known as bitter gourde, balsam pear, kerala, and wild cucumber, is a climbing vine plant in the Cucurbitaccae family that is native to tropical regions of Asia, India, East Africa, South America, and the Caribbean (Grover and Yadav 2004, Leung et al. 2009). The fruit resembles a cucumber and the characteristic bitter taste is enhanced as the plant ripens. Reported uses for oral bitter melon include DM, gastrointestinal upset, induction of menstruation, intestinal worms, kidney stones, and hepatitis.

6.2.4.2 Pharmacognosy

Several active chemicals are in bitter melon; the hypoglycemic constituents include a mixture of charantin, insulin-like peptides, and vicine (Ooi et al. 2010, Joseph and Jini 2013). Several mechanisms have been proposed including insulin-like activity, decreased hepatic gluconeogenesis, increased hepatic glycogen synthesis, and increased peripheral glucose oxidation, as well as reports of enhanced pancreatic insulin secretion (Ooi et al. 2010, Joseph and Jini 2013).

6.2.4.3 Dosing and Preparation

Bitter melon fruit in doses up to 6 g/day may be consumed as a juice or dry fruit powder or eaten as a vegetable; all components including the leaves, seeds, and stem are used for its medicinal properties (Ooi et al. 2010, Joseph and Jini 2013).

6.2.4.4 Safety

Aside from hypoglycemia, which may be potentiated by antidiabetic drugs, common adverse effects of bitter melon are abdominal discomfort, diarrhea, and headaches (Leung et al. 2009). Bitter melon has been associated with lowered fertility and induced abortion, as well as favism (hemolytic anemia) in patients with glucose-6-phosphate dehydrogenase deficiency. Hypoglycemic coma and death have been reported in children (Leung et al. 2009).

6.2.4.5 Evidence

Human trials have investigated the hypoglycemic effects of bitter melon in patients with type-1 diabetes mellitus (T1DM) and T2DM, as well as patients at increased risk of developing DM (Leung et al. 2009, Joseph and Jini 2013). Many animal studies and small, low quality clinical trials have found that oral and subcutaneous injections of bitter melon decreases glucose levels (Leatherdale et al. 1981, Welihinda et al. 1986, Srivastava et al. 1993). However, a systematic Cochrane review that included four randomized controlled trials with 479 patients failed to demonstrate significant reductions in blood glucose with bitter melon in doses up to 6 g/day for up to 3 months (Ooi et al. 2010).

6.2.4.6 Clinical Application

Given that data is conflicting, additional trials are needed to determine the role of bitter melon in the treatment of DM.

6.2.5 Black and Blond Psyllium

6.2.5.1 Background

Black psyllium (*Plantago psyllium*) and blond psyllium (*Plantago ovata*), also known as ispaghula, ispaghula psyllium, and psyllium husk are viscous soluble dietary fibers (Chutkan et al. 2012). Psyllium is a nonprescription bulk-forming laxative that is commonly used for constipation, and may have other health benefits including cholesterol reduction, glycemic control, lower blood pressure, and weight loss.

6.2.5.2 Pharmacognosy

As a viscous fiber, psyllium works to delay the rate of digestion thereby delaying the absorption of carbohydrates resulting in reduced postprandial blood glucose (Chutkan ct al. 2012). *See Chapter 7 Gastrointestinal Disease for further discussion.*

6.2.5.3 Dosage and Preparations

Psyllium is prepared from the seed of the *Plantago* plant and is administered orally in multiple formulations including a powder to be mixed with water, capsules, and wafers. Psyllium 12–15 g divided three times daily administered with carbohydrates has been reported to reduce glycemic index of foods and HbA1c (Frati et al. 1998, Gibb et al. 2015).

6.2.5.4 Safety

Psyllium is commonly associated with flatulence, abdominal discomfort, dyspepsia, and bloating (Bajorek and Morello 2010). More serious adverse effects include case reports of intestinal obstruction; therefore, patients at increased risk of bowel obstruction should avoid use of psyllium. Esophageal obstruction resulting in choking has also been reported with psyllium; therefore, patients with dysphagia should avoid use of psyllium. Allergic reactions resulting in anaphylaxis have also been reported with psyllium. Psyllium may also delay absorption of other medications due to delayed gastric transit time; therefore, psyllium should also be administered at least 2 hours apart from other medications.

6.2.5.5 Evidence

Several clinical trials have demonstrated metabolic benefits of psyllium in patients with DM including reduction in total and LDL cholesterol, triglycerides, HbA1c, postprandial blood glucose, and fasting blood glucose (Rodriguez-Moran et al. 1998, Anderson et al. 1999, Sierra et al. 2002, Ziai et al. 2005, Clark et al. 2006). The significance of these improvements varied among trials. A meta-analysis including

37 trials in patients with T1DM, T2DM, or euglycemia treated with psyllium 7–12 grams in 2–3 divided doses, showed overall significant reductions in fasting blood glucose (−37 mg/dL) and HbA1c (−0.97%) (Gibb et al. 2015). The degree of glycemic reduction correlated with baseline blood glucose; patients with higher baseline blood glucose experienced the largest reductions whereas patients with euglycemia experienced no reductions in blood glucose.

6.2.5.6 Clinical Application

Given the relative safety and potential health benefits, psyllium may be an adjunctive treatment option for some patients with DM.

6.2.6 Cinnamon

6.2.6.1 Background

Cinnamon is a spice that comes from the inner bark of the *Cinnamomum* tree which is dried and ground into powder or made into an extract. Cinnamon contains essential oils, the significant oil being cinnamaldehyde, providing cinnamon with its unique properties. Cinnamon comes in two different formulations: cassia and ceylon. Cassia, also known as Chinese cinnamon, has the strongest flavor of the varieties and is the most common variety of cinnamon sold in North America. Cassia comes from the *Cinnamomum cassia* tree originating from Southern China. "True" cinnamon, also known as ceylon cinnamon, is made from the inner bark of the *Cinnamomum verum* tree native to southern India and Sri Lanka (Suksomboon et al. 2011).

Cinnamon has been used since ancient Egyptian times, 2000 BC and approximately 4000 years ago in China (Dugoua et al. 2007). Cinnamon has multiple uses which include DM, flatulence and gastrointestinal symptoms, infections, impotence, kidney or menstrual disorders, hypertension, cramps, and as a mosquito repellant.

6.2.6.2 Pharmacognosy

Using cinnamon to lower blood glucose levels is common among patients with T2DM. Polyphenolic polymers (e.g., methylhydroxychalcone) appear to be the active ingredients found in cassia cinnamon and seem to potentiate insulin action by increasing phosphorylation of the insulin receptor, resulting in increased insulin sensitivity and possible improvement in blood glucose and lipid levels (Dugoua et al. 2007). Cinnamon may also increase glucose uptake via activation of glycogen synthetase (Imparl-Radosevich et al. 1998, Jarvill-Taylor et al. 2001, Anderson et al. 2004). While animal studies suggest cassia cinnamon produces no hypoglycemic effects despite a release of insulin, human trials did produce lower blood glucose levels when administered during a glucose tolerance test. Perhaps because it has been studied in humans more, studies seem to confirm that cassia cinnamon is more effective than ceylon cinnamon bark in stimulating insulin's action and lowering blood glucose levels; however, it is not as effective as a sulfonylurea such as glyburide (Verspohl et al. 2005).

6.2.6.3 Dosing and Preparation

Based on the available evidence for cassia cinnamon, it is recommended over ceylon cinnamon and is dosed for adults with T2DM in the range of 120 mg–6 g daily of cassia cinnamon for up to 4 months (Khan et al. 2003). Ceylon cinnamon can also be used in the same doses if desired. Children with T1DM, ages 13–18 only, may use cassia cinnamon in doses of 1 g daily for up to 3 months (Altschuler et al. 2007). Available formulations of cassia and ceylon cinnamon include capsules, powders, tinctures, and oils.

6.2.6.4 Safety

Cassia cinnamon has been rated as generally safe, especially in appropriate doses used up to 4 months (Khan et al. 2003). It can be considered likely safe when used in children ages 13–18 with T1DM in doses of 1 g daily for a maximum of 3 months (Altschuler et al. 2007). When given orally in high doses such as 50–7000 mg per day and for long periods of time, cassia cinnamon, not ceylon cinnamon, may cause reversible hepatotoxicity due to high, innate amounts of coumarin and should be considered possibly unsafe (Choi et al. 2001). Evidence is insufficient on the safety of medicinal doses of cassia cinnamon in pregnancy or breastfeeding and thus should be avoided. When used in dosages of 1–6 g per day in a 40-day randomized controlled trial, cassia cinnamon caused no significant adverse effect (Khan et al. 2003). Two additional but smaller trials at lower doses also did not report any adverse effects (Mang et al. 2006, Vanschoonbeek et al. 2006). Although well tolerated, potential adverse effects include contact irritation and allergic reaction with skin or mucous membranes (Dugoua et al. 2007).

Few drug interactions are of concern with cassia cinnamon. The major interactions occur with other agents that either also lower blood glucose levels or cause hepatotoxicity. Cassia cinnamon in combination with other hypoglycemic agents may cause excessive hypoglycemia, warranting close monitoring of blood glucose level (Khan et al. 2003, Vanschoonbeek et al. 2006). While cassia cinnamon is unlikely to cause hepatotoxicity on its own, it is theoretically possible that its main constituent, coumarin, could increase the risk of developing hepatotoxicity when used concurrently with other hepatotoxic agents (Choi et al. 2001).

6.2.6.5 Evidence

A 10%–29% reduction in fasting blood glucose was demonstrated in two small, randomized clinical trials in patients with T2DM using oral dosages of 1–6 g daily. Despite these positive results, cassia cinnamon was not shown to significantly lower HbA1c after 4 months of use (Khan et al. 2003, Vanschoonbeek et al. 2006). Lower lipid values were reported in one trial but not others (Dugoua et al. 2007).

6.2.6.6 Clinical Application

Until a steady decline in HbA1c and lipid markers are consistently demonstrated, cinnamon should not be recommended as an alternative to prescription drugs for DM. It may, however, be used as an adjunctive therapy if desired.

6.2.7 Fenugreek

6.2.7.1 Background

Fenugreek (*Trigonella foenum-graecum* L. *Leguminosae*) is an annual, clover-like plant, indigenous to the Mediterranean, southern Europe, and western Asia regions that grows leaves and seeds used for various purposes, including medical uses (Reeder et al. 2013). Its maple-like aromatic properties were used in ancient Egypt as incense. It was also used to embalm mummies. Traditional Chinese medicine used fenugreek for treatment of edema of the legs (Smith 2003). Today, fenugreek is used as treatment for DM, in addition to gastroesophageal reflux disease (GERD), kidney disease, male impotence and infertility, polycystic ovary syndrome, obesity, and hyperlipidemia. *See Chapter 8 Women's Health for more discussion.*

6.2.7.2 Pharmacognosy

The possible hypoglycemic and antihyperlipidemic properties of oral fenugreek seed powder have been suggested by the results of animal and human trials. The portion of the fenugreek seed that may exhibit the hypoglycemic effects is the testa, which contains the hallmark smell, while the bitter taste and the amino acid 4-hydroxyisoleucine acts only upon the pancreatic beta cells, stimulating glucose-dependent insulin secretion. A secondary mechanism by which fenugreek may lower blood glucose levels is via its 30% soluble and 20% insoluble fiber content which may slow the rate of glucose absorption following a meal. Saponins, another main ingredient contained in fenugreek, may have a role in lowering key lipid parameters by increasing biliary excretion of cholesterol, contributing to lowering common complications in DM.

108   *Principles and Practice of Botanicals as an Integrative Therapy*

6.2.7.3 Dosing and Preparation

Powdered fenugreek seeds taken as either powder, capsules, or ground seeds can be used to treat T2DM in doses of 5–50 grams/day, added to 1–2 meals per day from 4 days to 24 weeks (Neelakantan et al. 2014). Fenugreek can also be consumed as a hydroalcoholic extract in doses of 1 g/day for 2 months (Gupta et al. 2001). There are no suggested dosages for children.

6.2.7.4 Safety

In the U.S., fenugreek has obtained the status of Generally Recognized as Safe (GRAS) and is likely safe when ingested in amounts most commonly found in foods. Taking fenugreek in medicinal strengths for a maximum of 6 months reduces its safety profile to possibly safe and should be used with caution (Sharma et al. 1996a, Bordia et al. 1997, Singh et al. 1998). Use in children should be avoided due to a potential loss of consciousness for which there is no determined cause (Sewell et al. 1999). Its use in pregnancy should be avoided due to the potential stimulation of oxytocin production and uterine contractions. Doses of 1725 mg three times daily for up to 3 weeks to stimulate lactation has not been associated with adverse effects in either the infant or mother (Reeder et al. 2013). Fenugreek is typically considered well tolerated and not associated with any clinically significant adverse effects. Minor effects include potential allergy, diarrhea, flatulence, dizziness, and excessive hypoglycemia. When taken by pregnant women during labor, fenugreek can cause a maple syrup-like odor in newborn infants which can lead to a false suspicion of maple syrup urine disease (Dugoua et al. 2007).

Drug interactions can occur with fenugreek. Fenugreek can have additive effects when taken with antithrombotic and hypoglycemic agents (Madar et al. 1988, Duke and Beckstrom-Sternberg 1994). Fenugreek can have antagonistic effects to theophylline, reducing its effectiveness, potentially requiring dosage adjustments (Al-Jenoobi et al. 2015). Because fenugreek contains 50% fiber, fenugreek might interfere with the absorption of certain medications. To avoid potential interactions, fenugreek should be taken at least 2 hours apart from other medications (Smith 2003).

6.2.7.5 Evidence

Both animal and human studies have shown that taking doses of 5–50 g of powdered fenugreek seed at 1 or 2 meals per day for 24 weeks can improve fasting blood glucose levels. Reductions in blood glucose levels after glucose tolerance tests have also been documented. Smaller doses resulted in no change in glucose tolerance (Sharma and Raghuram 1990, Raghuram et al. 1994, Sharma et al. 1996b, Neelakantan et al. 2014). Patients with T1DM demonstrated a 54% reduction in a 24-hour urine glucose test after taking 50 grams of fenugreek seed powder twice a day for 10 days (Sharma et al. 1990). Doses of 5–100 g of fenugreek per day for up to 24 weeks have lowered total and low-density lipoprotein (LDL) cholesterol by 2% and 5%, respectively (Sharma et al. 1990, Bordia et al. 1997). Effects on high-density lipoprotein (HDL) cholesterol and triglycerides have been inconsistent (Sharma et al. 1990, Sharma et al. 1996a, Bordia et al. 1997, Singh et al. 1998); however, using 1 g of fenugreek orally per day for 2 months has decreased triglyceride levels and increased HDL cholesterol levels (Gupta et al. 2001).

6.2.7.6 Clinical Application

Taken orally, fenugreek has demonstrated the ability to lower random, fasting, and post-glucose-tolerance-test glucose levels in patients with T2DM. Adverse effects have been seen as mild and include GI upset, allergy, increased bleeding, and excessive hypoglycemia. Caution should be used when administering fenugreek with anticoagulants and hypoglycemic agents due to additive effects. Fenugreek may also antagonize theophylline; thus, close monitoring of symptoms and drug levels should be followed.

6.2.8 Flaxseed

6.2.8.1 Background

Flaxseed, also known as linseed, (Linum usitatissimum L.), is the golden yellow to reddish brown seeds that come from flax which grows in Europe, Asia, and the Mediterranean region (Hall et al. 2006). Similar to other botanicals, flaxseed use can be dated back to ancient Egypt as both a food staple and medicine, primarily as a bulk-forming laxative. Other uses for oral flaxseed or flaxseed oil include bowel disorders, benign prostate hyperplasia (BPH), cancers, menopausal symptoms, depression, DM, and hypercholesterolemia.

6.2.8.2 Pharmacognosy

The seeds contain phytoestrogens, flaxseed oil, and soluble fiber among other components. Both the flaxseed and its oil contain alpha-linoleic acid (ALA), an omega-3 fatty acid, used for heart disease and to decrease total and LDL cholesterol. *See Chapter 5 Cardiovascular Disease for more discussion.* The phytoestrogens found in flaxseed include the specific lignan, secoisolariciresinol, which lowers blood glucose levels.

6.2.8.3 Dosing and Preparation

Ground flaxseed 10–40 grams daily for 4–12 weeks has been used to lower blood glucose levels (Mani et al. 2011). A specific standardized flaxseed lignan extract of 600 mg, providing 360 mg secoisolariciresinol diglucoside, taken three times daily for 12 weeks was also effective in lowering blood glucose levels (Pan et al. 2007). Oral flaxseed products are available as whole flaxseeds, ground flaxseed, softgels containing flaxseed oil, liquid oils, and tinctures/extracts as mentioned above.

6.2.8.4 Safety

When used orally, ground flaxseed is likely safe and has been used in a variety of dosages and intervals in clinical trials (Bierenbaum et al. 1993, Cunnane et al. 1993, Clark et al. 1995, Cunnane et al. 1995, Lucas et al. 2002). When a specific lignin is isolated and used in an extract, flaxseed lignin is possibly safe to use for up to 12 weeks (Pan et al. 2007, 2008). Raw or unripe flaxseed can be potentially toxic due to the potential for cyanogenic glycosides (Cunnane et al. 1993). Flaxseed should be avoided in pregnancy, as it has mild estrogenic effects (Adlercreutz et al. 1986). Flaxseed should be avoided in lactation as evidence on its adverse effects are lacking. Common adverse effects include gas, bloating, feeling of fullness, diarrhea, and constipation, thus use should be avoided in patients with gastrointestinal obstruction or strictures of any kind (Dodin et al. 2005). In some patients, triglycerides may be increased, thus monitoring should be performed. Allergic reactions, including anaphylaxis, have been reported (Jenkins et al. 1999).

Theoretical and pharmacodynamic drug interactions have been reported for flaxseed. As flaxseed may decrease blood glucose levels, caution should be used when combining with other hypoglycemic agents due to the risk of increased hypoglycemia (Cunnane et al. 1993). Since flaxseed's primary component, ALA, can increase the risk of bleeding, antithrombotic agents should be used carefully, monitoring for signs of excess bleeding (Nordström et al. 1995). Proper absorption of other medications, particularly narrow therapeutic index drugs, may be affected by co-administration of flaxseed, thus spacing out doses at least 2 hours is important to avoid this possibility. The lignans contained in flaxseed may compete with and reduce estrogen binding to estrogen receptors resulting in an anti-estrogen effect and thus potentially altering the efficacy of oral contraceptives and hormone therapy (Mousavi and Adlercreutz 1992). Evidence suggests that flaxseed can lower diastolic blood pressure (Cornish et al. 2009). Theoretically, flaxseed can lower diastolic blood pressure and may contribute to the hypotensive effect of antihypertensive agents. Monitoring for drug efficacy and toxicities is important when combining flaxseed with these agents.

6.2.8.5 Evidence

Clinical trials have shown that a standardized extract providing 360 mg of secoisolariciresinol diglucoside three times a day for 12 weeks to patients with T2DM significantly reduced HbA1C levels and inflammatory markers when compared to placebo. Other important parameters such as fasting blood glucose (FBG), inulin or lipid levels were not reduced (Pan et al. 2007, 2008). Other trials indicate that using ground flaxseed daily, in doses of 10–40 grams for 4–12 weeks resulted in a significant reduction in FBG by as much as 20% and HbA1c by as much as 16% in patients withT2DM (Mani et al. 2011, Rhee and Brunt 2011, Hutchins et al. 2013). Doses of 32 grams of milled flaxseed incorporated into baked goods did not produce a significant reduction in the markers of insulin resistance, FBG, or HBA1c when compared to a control group that consumed baked goods without flaxseed (Taylor et al. 2010). *See Chapter 5 Cardiovascular Disease for more discussion in dyslipidemia.*

6.2.8.6 Clinical Application

Oral flaxseed lowers FBG and HbA1c in T2DM. Mild adverse effects include GI effects, increased bleeding, and hypoglycemia; thus, caution should be used in patients taking antithrombotic or hypoglycemic agents due to potential additive effects. Flaxseed should be avoided in pregnancy and lactation due to its estrogenic properties.

6.2.9 Garlic

6.2.9.1 Background

Garlic is a perennial bulb made up of 4–20 cloves that has been used as both a food source and medicine since the Egyptian pyramid times, used by many cultures as an antiseptic to both treat and prevent infection (Mulrow et al. 2000). Garlic supplements are prepared from fresh, dried, aged, and garlic oil, each form potentially having a different effect on the body when ingested. Garlic is used today for many purposes including preventing heart disease and atherosclerosis, hypercholesterolemia, DM, hypertension, and as an immunostimulant. It is also used for its proposed antioxidant properties for the potential prevention of cancer and Alzheimer's disease (Dillon et al. 2003).

6.2.9.2 Pharmacognosy

See Chapter 5 Cardiovascular Disease for discussion.

6.2.9.3 Dosage and Preparation

Garlic doses of 300 mg 2–3 times per day have been used in combination with metformin or an oral sulfonylurea for 4–24 weeks in patients with T2DM. *See Chapter 5 Cardiovascular Disease for more discussion.*

6.2.9.4 Safety

Garlic is safe in amounts found in food as well as in medicinal dosages that have been used up to 7 years in trials with no major toxicities reported. Children ages 8–18 have been safely given garlic orally in doses up to 300 mg three times daily for up to 8 weeks (McCrindle et al. 1998). Doses larger than that may be dangerous or even fatal in children (Edward 2000). Use in pregnancy is likely safe when ingesting amounts of garlic commonly found in food (Bloch 2000). Higher doses for medicinal purposes may not be safe in pregnancy as garlic may have abortifacient activity (Farnsworth et al. 1975) and may be distributed into the amniotic fluid, even after just a single dose (Mennella et al. 1995). Despite this information, evidence is not available to support garlic adversely affecting pregnancy, even when doses reached 800 mg per day in the third trimester (Ziaei et al. 2001, Reza 2005). Garlic ingested in amounts found in medicinal doses, is possibly unsafe in lactation as the components of the garlic bulb do cross over into breast milk (Bloch 2000).

Garlic and all of its constituents and forms, including allicin and oil, respectively, have the potential for clinically significant drug, food, and botanical interactions (Rose et al. 1990, Silagy and Neil 1994, Gurley et al. 2002, Piscitelli et al. 2002, Markowitz et al. 2003, Dhamija et al. 2006). *See Chapter 2 Pharmacokinetic and Pharmacogenomic Considerations for a more detailed discussion related to drug interactions.*

6.2.9.5 Evidence

Evidence for garlic's reduction in FBG, hypercholesterolemia, and hypertension shows conflicting outcomes. While some research reported a significant decrease in FBG, serum fructosamine, and lipid markers, other trials report that garlic provides no significant reduction in glucose or lipid levels. Trials that found a significant outcome were exploring garlic doses of 300 mg 2–3 times per day in combination with metformin or an oral sulfonylurea for 4–24 weeks of treatment in patients with T2DM (Sobenin et al. 2008, Ashraf et al. 2011) compared to the multiple trials that have indicated taking garlic orally has no long-term, significant effect on glucose, blood pressure, antiplatelet, or lipid factors in patients with or without T2DM (Ackermann et al. 2001). Thus, using garlic to reduce blood glucose or reduce the risk of comorbid conditions in patients with T2DM becomes more of a risk versus benefit discussion rather than a strongly supported recommendation. *See Chapter 5 Cardiovascular Disease for discussion related to hypertension.*

6.2.9.6 Clinical Application

Evidence is conflicting as to whether garlic is effective in lowering blood glucose in patients with T2DM. Other than mild GI upset and dyspepsia, doses found in food are typically safe for any age and in pregnancy. Higher doses consumed may result in excessive bleeding, abortifacient activity in pregnancy and cross into breast milk. Due to its potential for hypotension, increased bleeding and effects on the CYP 450 enzyme system, garlic should be used with caution in anyone taking other medications for the respective disease states.

6.2.10 Glucomannan

6.2.10.1 Background

Glucomannan, also known as konjac and konjac mannan, is a soluble viscous fiber derived from the tuberous roots of the *Amorphophallus konjac* plant found in Asia (Vuksan et al. 2001, Sood et al. 2008). Glucomannan has been used for weight loss and as a treatment for constipation, T2DM, and hypercholesterolemia.

6.2.10.2 Pharmacognosy

Glucomannan is reported to have higher viscosity than other polysaccharides including xanthan and psyllium (Kim et al. 1996). When taken orally, glucomannan prolongs gastric emptying which results in delayed glucose absorption and a reduced rise in postprandial glucose; along with increased satiety and possible reduction in body weight (Sood et al. 2008). Shortly after ingestion of glucomannan, ghrelin decreased significantly (Chearskul et al. 2009). Glucomannan may increase excretion of bile acids which may explain the lipid lowering effects.

6.2.10.3 Dosage and Preparation

Glucomannan root is ground to a flour that is then added to food products or made into a gel and eaten. The recommended daily dose is 3 g per day or less and the maximum recommend dose is 10 g/day.

6.2.10.4 Safety

Glucomannan use is commonly associated with loose stools, flatulence, and abdominal discomfort. Serious adverse effects are rare, but there are case reports of esophageal obstruction, acute hepatitis, and gastrointestinal obstruction (Villaverde et al. 2004, Vanderbeek et al. 2007). A drug interaction with glucomannan and glibenclamide has been reported, this may be due to the delay in gastric emptying; therefore, it is recommended to space oral medication at least 1 hour before or 4 hours after the botanical (Shima et al. 1983). Glucomannan may decrease absorption of fat soluble vitamins possibly due to increased bile acid excretion since bile acids aid in the absorption of vitamins A, D, E, and K (Doi 1995).

6.2.10.5 Evidence

Several clinical trials have demonstrated positive cardiovascular and metabolic effects of glucomannan in patients with DM (Vuksan et al. 1999, Trask et al. 2013). A meta-analysis of 14 trials involving 531 patients demonstrated metabolic benefits of glucomannan in patient with and without DM, as well as patients with impaired glucose tolerance. Doses ranging from 2 to 15.1 g for 3 to 16 weeks (mean 5.2 weeks) resulted in significant reductions in total cholesterol (-19.28 mg/dL), LDL cholesterol (-15.99 mg/dL), triglycerides (-11.08 mg/dL), body weight (-0.79 kg), and fasting blood glucose (-7.44 mg/dL) (Sood et al. 2008). Although higher doses were associated with the greater reductions, subanalyses at various doses less than 3 g per day and less than 10 g per day continued to demonstrate positive results. Another subanalysis of the four trials with patients with DM or impaired glucose tolerance also demonstrated these positive findings albeit a lower reduction in FBG by 1.58 mg/dL.

6.2.10.6 Clinical Application

Glucomannan is relatively safe and provides generally positive metabolic effects.

6.2.11 Green and Black Tea

6.2.11.1 Background

Excluding water, tea is the most consumed beverage in the world (Mackenzie et al. 2007, Yang et al. 2014). Both green and black teas have been used for their therapeutic benefits in DM. Tea is made from extracts of *Camellia* leaves that are completely oxidized before drying (Mackenzie et al. 2007). Green tea is made from leaves that have been cut and dried (Mackenzie et al. 2007). Black tea is made from leaves that have been allowed to completely oxidize before desiccation (Mackenzie et al. 2007).

6.2.11.2 Pharmacognosy

Several active substances in tea may act as hypoglycemic agents. This includes the catechins, especially epigallocatechin gallate (EGCG), polyphenols, and theaflavins. It is suggested from in vitro rat models that these may have a role in DM by enhancing insulin activity and possibly preventing cytokine-induced damage to beta-cells (Mackenzie et al. 2007). EGCG is the most abundant catechin and its mechanism is more defined. EGCG has been shown to reduce insulin resistance, enhance pancreatic islet function, prevent beta-cell damage, and have antioxidant properties in rats (Ortsäter et al. 2012).

6.2.11.3 Dosage and Preparation

Beneficial effects have been seen from both tea extracts made into oral supplements, and drinking the tea itself. The recommended dosing for DM is drinking at least 4 cups of tea per day, but there are no sub-analyses on which type of tea (green versus black) is preferred (Yang et al. 2014). *See Chapter 5 Cardiovascular Diseases for additional information on green tea.*

6.2.11.4 Safety

Tea is safe at normal rates of consumption. Adverse effects are not typically reported in trials related to DM. *See Chapter 5 Cardiovascular Disease for additional information on green tea.*

6.2.11.5 Evidence

Cohort studies and a meta-analysis have demonstrated that people who drink at least 3–4 cups of tea per day have a lower incidence of DM compared to their control counterparts, although this evidence is not consistent (Mackenzie et al. 2007, Yang et al. 2014).

The evidence in using tea as a treatment for DM is limited. A randomized controlled trial using capsules containing extracts from both green and black tea was conducted to measure its effects on patients with DM (Mackenzie et al. 2007). Depending on treatment allocation, patients took 1–2 capsules per day of tea capsules containing 150 mg of green tea catechins (equivalent of 7 cups of green tea) and 75 mg of theaflavins (equivalent of 35 cups of black tea). The study did not find a significant change in HbA1c at 3 months of therapy.

6.2.11.6 Clinical Application

For patients who already enjoy drinking tea as their primary beverage, it may confer a lower risk of developing DM and could be encouraged at a rate of 4 cups or more per day. Although it seems to be protective, there is no evidence of beneficial effect to support the use of tea for purposes of treating DM.

6.2.12 Gymnema

6.2.12.1 Background

Gymnema, also known as *Gymnema sylvestre*, gurmur, gurmar (meaning "sugar destroyer" in Hindi), and merasingi, is a woody climbing plant found in India and tropical regions of Africa and Australia (Leach 2007, Nahas and Moher 2009). Both the dried leaves and the dried root are widely used in Ayurvedic medicine to treat DM, elevated cholesterol, and obesity.

6.2.12.2 Pharmacognosy

While the active components of gymnema remain unclear, gymnemic acid, gurmarin, and conduritol are the main constituents. Gymnemic acid is comprised of many saponins of which gymnemmadises one to five play key roles.

Several mechanisms have been proposed by which gymnema may exert its hypoglycemic effects including stimulation of insulin release from pancreatic beta cells (Leach 2007, Tiwari et al. 2014), regeneration of pancreatic beta cells (Leach 2007), inhibition of intestinal glucose absorption (Leach 2007, Tiwari et al. 2014), and increased glycolysis via interaction with glyceraldehyde-3-phosphate dehydrogenase (Tiwari et al. 2014).

The gumarin constituent may interfere with oral taste cells by preventing the taste of sweetness, thereby reducing the consumption of sugar in patients with DM (Cicero et al. 2004, Tiwari et al. 2014). This blockade of sweet taste receptors explains the bitter taste associated with gymnema (Cicero et al. 2004).

6.2.12.3 Dosage and Preparation

Clinical benefit has been demonstrated with gymnema extract, as well as the ground powder in doses ranging from 200 to 500 mg administered twice daily (Baskaran et al. 1990, Kumar et al. 2010, Li et al. 2015).

6.2.12.4 Safety

Common adverse effects of gymnema are the bitter taste and hypoglycemia. Hypoglycemic effects have been reported in patients with and without DM and may result in an additive effect when combined with hypoglycemic drugs (Khare et al. 1983). While serious adverse effects are rare, a case report of gymnema-induced liver injury suggest the need for further investigation on any hepatic effects (Shiyovich et al. 2010).

6.2.12.5 Evidence

Published evidence supporting the hypoglycemic effects of gymnema is limited to four small, open-label trials (Baskaran et al. 1990, Shanmugasundaram et al. 1990, Kumar et al. 2010, Li et al. 2015). Doses ranging from 200 mg of gymnema extract (GS4) to 500 mg of the ground botanical administered twice daily to patients with T2DM for 1one to 20 months resulted in reductions in fasting blood glucose and HbA1C (Baskaran et al. 1990, Kumar et al. 2010, Li et al. 2015). A trial of 27 patients with T1DM demonstrated that 200 mg of an ethanolic acid-precipitated extract of gymnema (GS4) administered twice daily for 6–30 months resulted in a 50% reduction in insulin requirements as well as reduction in HbA1c and fasting blood glucose (Shanmugasundaram et al. 1990).

6.2.12.6 Clinical Application

While preliminary evidence demonstrates the hypoglycemic effects of gymnema, data is limited to small, open label trials and further research is needed.

6.2.13 Ivy Gourd

6.2.13.1 Background

Ivy gourd (*Coccinia grandis, Coccinic cordifolia* and *Coccinia indica*), belongs to the Cucurbitaceae family along with other melons (Medagama and Bandara 2014). Ivy gourd is often known as "baby watermelon" in parts of the Indian subcontinent and Sri Lanka and is cooked as a vegetable in Bengal (Khan et al. 1980, Medagama and Bandara 2014).

6.2.13.2 Pharmacognosy

Despite having been used since ancient times and having clinical trials dating back into the 1980s, the mechanism for ivy gourd as an antidiabetic is still under investigation (Khan et al. 1980). This particular species of the gourd/melon family is thought to be an insulin mimetic (Medagama and Bandara 2014). Evidence suggests three distinct species exist, and all are likely interchangeable in terms of medicinal properties.

6.2.13.3 Dosing and Preparation

Ivy gourd can be prepared into oral supplements with the dose used in studies being 1 g daily (Medagama and Bandara 2014). More commonly, ivy gourd is ingested by eating the leaves within a salad or as a snack (Medagama and Bandara 2014). Patients should consume about 20 g of leaves to elicit its beneficial effects (Medagama and Bandara 2014).

6.2.13.4 Safety

No trials of ivy gourd have documented serious adverse effects (Kuriyan et al. 2008, Munasinghe et al. 2011, Medagama and Bandara 2014). The largest trial in 60 patients with DM reported 59% of patients having mild hypoglycemia, often around midmorning (Kuriyan et al. 2008). Patients were counseled to eat a snack which resolved this adverse effect. Although the long-term effects have not been studied beyond 90 days, ivy gourd has been safely used historically as part of a regular diet in India (Munasinghe et al. 2011).

6.2.13.5 Evidence

A double-blind controlled trial investigated ivy gourd as a treatment for DM (Khan et al. 1980). The study included patients with uncontrolled and untreated T2DM and investigated the effect of tablets made of freeze-dried leaves of *Coccinia indica*. The study showed statistically significant improvements in fasting blood glucose, and glucose levels after 1–2 hours after a 50 g glucose tolerance test. Notably, fasting blood levels in the ivy gourd group improved from 178.8 mg/dL at baseline to 122.1 mg/dL after 6 weeks. Similar effects were observed in the oral glucose tolerance test results. Glucose levels did not improve immediately, but significant effects occurred starting at week 3.

The leaves contain a slow-acting substance that may take at least 3–6 weeks to provide benefit (Medagama and Bandara 2014). In contrast, the most recent trial conducted with ivy gourd was a phase 1 controlled clinical trial conducted in healthy patients using leaves of *Coccinia grandis* prepared as a salad served for breakfast (Munasinghe et al. 2011). The reduction in 1 h and 2 h glucose tolerance tests were significant compared to placebo after just one meal.

The best evidence of the antidiabetic effects of ivy gourd was in newly diagnosed diabetics who received an oral capsule containing extracts of *Coccinia cordifolia* (Kuriyan et al. 2008). Significant reductions in fasting and postprandial blood glucose values were compared to placebo. Importantly, a significant reduction in HbA1c from 6.7% to 6.1% occurred in the ivy gourd group, which was not observed with placebo.

6.2.13.6 Clinical Application

The consistent findings with ivy gourd in randomized control trials using different formulations, species, and patient populations, suggest that this botanical is likely effective in treating patients with DM to help lower their glucose and HbA1c. Additional trials are needed to find the optimal dosage form, dose, and extraction technique.

6.2.14 Red Yeast Rice

6.2.14.1 Background

Red yeast, or red yeast rice (RYR), is a traditional Chinese product used as a dietary staple in cooking, as well as in traditional medicine. Red yeast rice (RYR) is made by growing yeast (Monascus purpureus) on rice. For many years, RYR has been taken orally to maintain healthy lipid levels and reducing lipid levels in patients with hyperlipidemia. It has also been used for overall gastrointestinal health and improving circulation (Becker et al. 2009). Some products contain monacolins which are produced by the yeast. Monacolin K has been reported to be chemically identical to lovastatin. Red yeast rice has also been used to decrease FBG and postprandial glucose levels (Fang and Li 2000).

6.2.14.2 Pharmacognosy

See Chapter 5 Cardiovascular Disease for discussion.

6.2.14.3 Dosage and Preparation

While clinical data supports the use of RYR in the reduction of cholesterol, evidence for its use for lowering FBG in diabetes is weak and lacking (J. Wang et al. 1997, Heber et al. 1999, Fang and Li 2000). Despite the weak evidence, initial research reported some effectiveness of 600 mg of red yeast daily for 8 weeks in the reduction of both FBG and postprandial glucose levels by 33%–56% and decreased levels of total cholesterol (27.1%) and triglycerides (42.3%), in the treatment of type-2 diabetes compared to pretreatment (Fang and Li 2000). *See Chapter 5 Cardiovascular Disease for more discussion.*

6.2.14.4 Safety

Red yeast rice products have been shown to be possibly safe when used in trials for more than 4 years (Robbers and Tyler 1998, Heber et al. 1999). As much as two-thirds of RYR products may contain citrinin, a nephrotoxin that is produced from incorrect rice fermentation (Heber et al. 1999). In vitro and in animal research, citrinin has been reported to cause kidney damage, but no such results have been observed in human research (Liu et al. 2005). All statins are not safe to use in pregnancy due to the potential for fetal skeletal malformations that have shown up in animal studies. Due to insufficient or reliable information, RYR should not be used in lactation. Although data is limited on the adverse effects of red yeast rice, they likely are similar to those reported with low-dose statins. Potential adverse effects are typically dose-related and include rash, myopathy, rhabdomyolysis (rare) and hepatotoxicity, hypo- or hyperglycemia (Chang et al. 2006, Wang et al. 2006), gastrointestinal upset and abdominal bloating (Huang et al. 2011), and dizziness (Wang et al. 1997).

Drug interactions involving red yeast rice can occur through many different mechanisms. As RYR can cause hepatotoxicity and myopathy, it can have an additive effect if administered with other agents that can also cause liver damage (Liu et al. 2006) or myopathy respectively (e.g., cyclosporine, niacin, statins) (Prasad et al. 2002). Substances that inhibit CYP3A4 such as clarithromycin and grapefruit juice will inhibit the metabolism of red yeast rice, potentially leading to increased levels and toxicities of RYR (Kantola et al. 1998). *See Chapter 5 Cardiovascular Disease for more discussion.*

6.2.14.5 Evidence

Initial research reported some effectiveness of 600 mg of red yeast daily for 8 weeks in the reduction of both FBG and postprandial glucose levels by 33%–56% and decreased levels of total cholesterol (27.1%) and triglycerides (42.3%), in the treatment of T2DM compared to pretreatment (Fang and Li 2000) and thus makes a good argument for trying it for glucose-lowering activity.

6.2.14.6 Clinical Application

In addition to its lipid-lowering properties, RYR may have place in hypoglycemic therapy as it can significantly lower FBG and postprandial glucose levels. Adverse effects are typically dose-related and can include GI effects, myopathies and shifts in glucose levels, both up and down. Drug interactions can be both pharmacodynamic and pharmacokinetic in nature and thus should be used with caution when administered concurrently with other medications.

6.2.15 Soy

6.2.15.1 Background

Soybean, *Glycine max*, is an annual legume native to China and is currently grown in many other countries including North America (Hymowitz 1970, Graham and Vance 2003). The primary ingredients in soy are phytoestrogens and isoflavones which have a structure similar to naturally occurring estrogen (Budhathoki et al. 2015). A common use of medicinal soy is to treat premenstrual syndrome and menopausal symptoms including hot flashes and cyclic breast pain. Other uses of oral, medicinal soy administration include preventing or treating cancer, improving memory and cognitive function, fibromyalgia, osteoporosis, hyperlipidemia, and T2DM.

6.2.15.2 Pharmacognosy

See Chapter 8 Women's Health for discussion.

6.2.15.3 Dosage and Preparation

Soy extract 300 mg three times daily with meals has been used for 3–6 months in patients with T2DM (Fujita et al. 2001). Thirty grams of isolated soy protein containing 132 mg of phytoestrogens has been used daily for up to 12 weeks in postmenopausal women with T2DM (Jayagopal et al. 2002). Soy comes as beans, milk, extract, and capsules.

6.2.15.4 Safety

The use of soy is likely safe in all populations (Potter et al. 1998, Scambia et al. 2000), when taken orally at appropriate doses. Although uncommon, allergic reactions can occur when taking soy, including skin rashes and itching (Teixeira et al. 2000). Small children with allergies to other entities may experience allergic reactions to soy as well (Mora et al. 2002). When taken long-term, in high doses, postmenopausal women may experience endometrial hyperplasia (Unfer et al. 2004), as can pregnant and lactating women, when taken in amounts greater than is commonly found in food (Franke et al. 1998, Pino et al. 2000). Soy is typically tolerated well, but some common adverse effects include constipation, diarrhea, bloating, and nausea (Albertazzi et al. 1998, Chen et al. 2003, Kumar et al. 2004). Insomnia has also been experienced by some people taking soy (Jenkins et al. 2002).

Since soy may have inherent hypoglycemic and hypotensive effects, caution should be used with concomitant administration of other hypoglycemic, hypotensive, and diuretic agents to avoid added effects (Gimenez et al. 1998, He et al. 2005, Li et al. 2005). Additional drug interactions can occur via soy's potential induction of CYP2C9 (Wang et al. 2009), decreasing levels of substrates of this isoenzyme. Concurrent use of MAOIs and soy should be avoided due to the theoretical tyramine content of soy and the potentially resulting hypertensive crisis (Shulman and Walker 1999).

6.2.15.5 Evidence

Soybean reduces glucose levels in patients with T2DM. FBG levels were reduced by 3.85 mg/dL in patients with and without DM after following an all-soy diet (Liu et al. 2011). Fasting insulin levels, HbA1c, insulin resistance, and LDL levels were reduced by a dose of 132 mg of isoflavones taken daily for 12 weeks by postmenopausal women (Jayagopal ct al. 2002). Postprandial glucose and triglyceride levels decreased following the ingestion of 10 grams of a soy fiber product with a meal each day (Tsai et al. 1987).

Despite the positive evidence on the effectiveness of soy in the treatment of DM, evidence to the contrary also exists. Some clinical trials have also suggested that compared with control groups, patients with T2DM did not experience a reduction in any DM markers (Yang et al. 2011) Another trial did not result in improving glucose levels or HbA1c after patients took 50 grams of a soy protein product every day for 42 days (Hermansen et al. 2001). An additional study reported no difference in insulin or glucose levels with the addition of 10 grams of soy polysaccharide to a low-carbohydrate diet (Thomas et al. 1988). The formulations have varied from trial to trial and this may contribute to the different results. Soy has not been found to produce clinically significant improvements in treating diabetic nephropathy (Anderson 2008).

6.2.15.6 Clinical Application

Soy has not been shown to consistently reduce glucose levels or HbA1c. It is well tolerated, but can produce various drug interactions and thus should be used with caution in patients taking other medications. Further information is needed to determine if soy is a worthwhile treatment option.

6.2.16 Stevia

6.2.16.1 Background

Stevia (*Stevia rebaudia* Bertoni) is a bushy shrub in the Asterae/Compositae family that is indigenous to Paraguay, Brazil, and Argentina (Curi et al. 1986, Chatsudthipong and Muanprasat 2009). Stevia is a non-caloric sweetener that may have antihyperglycemic and antihypertensive effects. Extracts from the stevia leaves have been used as a sweetener and as traditional medicine for hundreds of years.

6.2.16.2 Pharmacognosy

The major components of stevia leaf are steviol glycosides including stevioside, rebaudioside A, rebaudioside C, and dulcoside; the sweetness of these glycosides are 50–450 times sweeter than sucrose. The antihyperglycemic effects extend beyond caloric reduction, in vitro and animal data demonstrate several potential mechanisms including: stimulation of insulin secretion via direct activity on beta cells, inhibition of intestinal glucose absorption, increased insulin sensitivity, and slowed hepatic gluconeogenesis (Chatsudthipong and Muanprasat 2009). The antihypertensive effects of stevia have been attributed to direct vasodilation and diuresis.

6.2.16.3 Dosing and Preparation

In the U.S., the rebaudioside A component has GRAS status as a food additive sweetener, whereas the leaves and extract are marketed as dietary supplements. The dose of stevia ranges from 250 mg three times daily to 5 g every 6 hours.

6.2.16.4 Safety

Co-administration of stevia with antihyperglycemic and antihypertentive drugs may result in additive effects. Stevia is generally well tolerated with mild adverse effects including abdominal fullness, headache, dizziness, nausea, and asthenia (Barriocanal et al. 2008).

6.2.16.5 Evidence

While animal studies show a clear hypoglycemic effect with stevia, data from clinical trials is conflicting. A small trial with 16 healthy volunteers found that 5 g stevia leaves in an aqueous extract administered every 6 hours for 3 days resulted in decreased plasma glucose (Curi et al. 1986). Another trial showed a single 1 g dose of stevoside administered to 12 patients with T2DM resulted in an 18% reduction in postprandial glucose as compared to a control group (Gregersen et al. 2004). However, benefits were inconsistent in a 3-month pilot study that compared stevia 250 mg administered three times daily to placebo in patients with T1DM and T2DM, and euglycemic patients (Barriocanal et al. 2008). Only patients with T1DM treated with stevia experienced a reduction in blood glucose and blood pressure.

6.2.16.6 Clinical Application

Stevia offers a non-caloric sweetening alternative to sugar for patients with DM. It may result in reduced energy consumption; however, data is insufficient to support that this mechanism results in glycemic control or weight reduction (Gardner 2014). Data supporting the value of stevia in the treatment of DM is inconsistent; further trials are necessary to define the role of stevia for DM.

6.2.17 Miscellaneous Botanicals for Diabetes

Many more botanicals may have hypoglycemic effects. Unlike those previously discussed, evidence is insufficient to recommend the use of these botanicals for patients with DM (Mechanick et al. 2003). Further studies are necessary to establish clinical benefit, optimal dose, and extraction technique or administration method (Table 6.2).

6.3 Thyroid Disorders Overview

Botanicals are most often used to increase or enhance the physiologic effects of the body. It is rare that botanicals suppress a physiologic effect (Yarnell and Abascal 2006). Botanicals for the treatment of thyroid

TABLE 6.2

Botanical Products with Hypoglycemic Effects but Limited Clinical Evidence

Allium cepa
Aloe vera
Azadirachta indica
Brassica juncea
Caesalpinia bonducella
Canjanus cajan
Catharanthus roseus
Eugenia jambolana
Ficus bengalenesis
Jiangtangkang (chrysanthemum)
Mucuna pruriens
Murraya koeingii
Nopalea (prickly pear cactus)
Ocimum sanctum
Opuntia
Pterocarpus marsupium
Swertia chirayita
Syzygium cumini
Tecoma
Tinospora cordifolia

Source: Mechanick, J. I. et al. 2003. *Endocrine Practice: Official Journal of the American College of Endocrinology and the American Association of Clinical Endocrinologists* 9 (5): 417–470.

disorders are an interesting exception. The greatest evidence of effect for botanical products relate to their ability to suppress thyroid function and therefore are being used to treat hyperthyroidism. Despite anecdotal and the internet claims that botanicals can help with hypothyroidism, the available evidence doesn't support this. Hypothyroidism should be treated with thyroid hormone replacement therapies such as levothyroxine (Mechanick et al. 2003). Botanicals may have a role in assisting with some of the symptoms of hypothyroidism such as fatigue or weight gain, but these need to still be coupled with appropriate prescription treatment.

6.3.1 Hyperthyroidism

Graves' disease, an autoimmune disorder, is the most common cause of persistent hyperthyroidism in adults (Burch and Cooper 2015). Botanical products may be appropriately used in hyperthyroidism, but it is recommended that they are combined with prescription treatment (Yarnell and Abascal 2006). Patients with severe Graves' disease should not be treated with botanical products alone and should be referred to both an endocrinologist and a botanical expert.

6.3.1.1 Bugleweed and Gypsywort

6.3.1.1.1 Background

Bugleweed (*Lycopus virginicus*) is a botanical native to North America that has some evidence to support its use in treating hyperthyroidism (Yarnell and Abascal 2006). It is a derivative of the mint (lamiaceae) family and similar to other Lycopus species found throughout the world, including gypsywort (*Lycopus europaeus*) found in Europe. Gypsywort and bugleweed have been found to be equally effective and often sources will use these two species interchangeably.

6.3.1.1.2 Pharmacognosy

The mechanism of action for bugleweed and gypsywort in improving symptoms of hyperthyroidism or Graves' disease is four-fold. Proposed mechanisms include interfering with antibodies binding to thyroid cells in Graves' disease, reducing production of thyroid-stimulating hormone (TSH), reducing peripheral thyroxine (T4) deiodinization, and possibly inhibiting iodine metabolism.

6.3.1.1.3 Dosing and Preparation

A clinical trial for treating hyperthyroidism used an oral supplement containing 20 mg of gypsywort given twice a day (Beer et al. 2008).

6.3.1.1.4 Safety

Bugleweed can interfere with other hormones, notably luteinizing hormone (LH) and follicle-stimulating hormone (FSH). Therefore, it should be avoided in pregnant women (Yarnell and Abascal 2006). It has the potential to worsen hypothyroidism due to its mechanism of action.

6.3.1.1.5 Evidence

A prospective open label study was conducted to investigate the clinical effects of gypsywort compared to placebo for hyperthyroidism (Beer et al. 2008). Gypsywort caused a significant increase in T4 excretion in the urine, but had no effect on triiodothyronine (T3). The authors concluded that this finding may be due to impaired reabsorption of T4 in the renal tubules. The clinical significance of this increased excretion is not clinically meaningful in the treatment of hyperthyroidism. Gypsywort also did not cause any statistically significant changes in free T3/T4 or TSH in the serum. These findings are consistent with other trials which did not find meaningful differences in thyroid markers in humans after administration of gypsywort. It also did not affect quality of life questionnaires (SF12) or clinical symptoms. Despite a lack of difference in any measurable outcomes, most patients reported the efficacy of gypsywort as "good," which may be related to bias often seen in open label studies, especially in a population eager to use natural products.

6.3.1.1.6 Clinical Application

No evidence supports the use of gypsywort, and by similarity bugleweed, for hyperthyroidism; however, patients do report satisfaction with their use. Further studies would be needed before recommending these products for patients.

6.3.1.2 Gromwell

6.3.1.2.1 Background

Gromwell belongs to the Boraginaceae family and is native to North America and Europe.

6.3.1.2.2 Pharmacognosy

Gromwell has been shown to reduce secretion of TSH, inhibit binding of TSH, inhibit iodine transport into thyroid cells, and reduce peripheral T4 deiodinization (Yarnell and Abascal 2006). Therefore, gromwell is considered to work similarly to bugleweed and gypsywort.

6.3.1.2.3 Dosage and Preparation

It is recommended to prepare gromwell as a low-ethanol tincture, using no more than 40% ethanol (Yarnell and Abascal 2006). This will minimize the amount of alkaloids contained within the product and which are responsible for severe adverse effects. The usual dose of this tincture is 1–2 mL three times daily for adults (Yarnell and Abascal 2006).

6.3.1.2.4 Safety

Gromwell is considered to be more potent and dangerous than previous botanicals discussed in this section. Gromwell contains unsaturated pyrrolizidine alkaloids (PAs), which lead to increased adverse effects (Yarnell and Abascal 2006). Animals and humans that have consumed PAs from plants have developed severe liver and kidney damage (Yarnell and Abascal 2006). These effects are considered rare, but caution is warranted (Yarnell and Abascal 2006). Chronic use of gromwell should be avoided

(Yarnell and Abascal 2006). Similarly to bugleweed and gypsywort, gromwell can affect LH and FSH and should not be used in pregnant women (Yarnell and Abascal 2006).

6.3.1.2.5 Evidence

Clinical trials have not evaluated gromwell in humans for hyperthyroidism. Only expert experience, animal studies, and pharmacokinetic studies have supported its use.

6.3.1.2.6 Clinical Application

Evidence demonstrating clinical significant effects in humans on hyperthyroidism is limited. It is likely that the benefits of gromwell do not outweigh the risks. Gromwell should be used with caution.

6.3.1.3 Lemon Balm

6.3.1.3.1 Background

Similar to bugleweed, lemon balm (*Melissa officinalis*) belongs to the mint (lamiaceae) family (Yarnell and Abascal 2006). This botanical is a common component of formulations for hyperthyroidism.

6.3.1.3.2 Pharmacognosy

In vitro and animal studies demonstrate lemon balm works in the same manner as bugleweed to modulate the thyroid (Yarnell 1998, Yarnell and Abascal 2006). *See Chapters 11 Psychiatric Disorders and 12 Botanicals for Common Infections for more discussion on lemon balm. Dosing and Preparation.*

Clinicians familiar with botanical products recommend against using lemon balm as monotherapy, but using it synergistically may boost the effects of bugleweed (Yarnell and Abascal 2006). *See Chapters 11 Psychiatric Disorders and 12 Botanicals for Common Infections for more discussion on lemon balm.*

6.3.1.3.3 Safety

There are no known contraindications to lemon balm and it is considered to have minimal adverse effects. Unlike bugleweed and gromwell, lemon balm is safe to use during pregnancy and lactation (Yarnell 1998). *See Chapter 11 Psychiatric Disorders for more discussion on lemon balm.*

6.3.1.3.4 Evidence

Historical evidence has not shown that lemon balm has a clinical effect on hyperthyroidism, nor is there documentation that euthyroid patients taking it for other indications have ever developed hypothyroidism (Yarnell 1998). There are no published reports discussing its clinical efficacy for the indication of hypothyroidism.

6.3.1.3.5 Clinical Application

The role of lemonbalm would be limited to being used in combination with bugleweed or gypsywort (Yarnell and Abascal 2006).

6.4 Conclusion

Patients are increasingly seeking natural products to treat their chronic health conditions. Several botanicals have demonstrated potential effectiveness in lowering blood glucose and HbA1c including: American ginseng, berberine, fenugreek, flaxseed, ivy gourd, and red yeast rice. Glucomannan and psyllium have also demonstrated a potential role as an adjunct treatment for DM. There is insufficient data to determine if cinnamon, gymnema, and stevia will be helpful in the treatment of DM. Data regarding the utility of Asian ginseng, bitter melon and soy for DM is conflicting. There is limited and at times conflicting evidence supporting the use of gypsywort, bugleweed, and lemon balm for hyperthyroidism. The limited data available for gromwell suggests that the benefits may not outweigh the risks and it should be used in caution.

REFERENCES

Ackermann, R. T., C. D. Mulrow, G. Ramirez, C. D. Gardner, L. Morbidoni, and V. A. Lawrence. 2001. "Garlic shows promise for improving some cardiovascular risk factors." *Archives of Internal Medicine* 161 (6): 813–824.

Adlercreutz, H., T. Fotsis, C. Bannwart, K. Wähälä, T. Mäkelä, G. Brunow, and T. Hase. 1986. "Determination of urinary lignans and phytoestrogen metabolites, potential antiestrogens and anticarcinogens, in urine of women on various habitual diets." *Journal of Steroid Biochemistry* 25 (5): 791–797.

Albertazzi, P., F. Pansini, G. Bonaccorsi, L. Zanotti, E. Forini, and D. De Aloysio. 1998. "The effect of dietary soy supplementation on hot flushes." *Obstetrics & Gynecology* 91 (1): 129–135.

Al-Jenoobi, F. I., A. Ahad, G. M. Mahrous, A. M. Al-Mohizea, K. M. AlKharfy, and S. A. Al-Suwayeh. 2015. "Effects of fenugreek, garden cress, and black seed on theophylline pharmacokinetics in beagle dogs." *Pharmaceutical Biology* 53 (2): 296–300.

Altschuler, J. A., S. J. Casella, T. A. MacKenzie, and K. M. Curtis. 2007. "The effect of cinnamon on A1C among adolescents with type 1 diabetes." *Diabetes Care* 30 (4): 813–816. doi:30/4/813 [pii].

An, X., A. L. Zhang, A. W. Yang, L. Lin, D. Wu, X. Guo, J. L. Shergis, F. C. Kong Thien, C. J. Worsnop, and C. C. Xue. 2011. "Oral ginseng formulae for stable chronic obstructive pulmonary disease: A systematic review." *Respiratory Medicine* 105 (2): 165–176.

Anderson, J. W. 2008. "Beneficial effects of soy protein consumption for renal function." *Asia Pacific Journal of Clinical Nutrition* 17 (S1): 324–328.

Anderson, R. A., C. Leigh Broadhurst, M. M. Polansky, W. F. Schmidt, A. Khan, V. P. Flanagan, N. W. Schoene, and D. J. Graves. 2004. "Isolation and characterization of polyphenol type-A polymers from cinnamon with insulin-like biological activity." *Journal of Agricultural and Food Chemistry* 52 (1): 65–70.

Anderson, J. W., L. D. Allgood, J. Turner, P. R. Oeltgen, and B. P. Daggy. 1999. "Effects of psyllium on glucose and serum lipid responses in men with type 2 diabetes and hypercholesterolemia." *American Journal of Clinical Nutrition* 70 (4): 466–473.

Ashraf, R., R. A. Khan, and I. Ashraf. 2011. "Garlic (allium sativum) supplementation with standard antidiabetic agent provides better diabetic control in type 2 diabetes patients." *Pakistan Journal of Pharmaceutical Sciences* 24 (4): 565–570.

Bajorek, S. A. and C. M. Morello. 2010. "Effects of dietary fiber and low glycemic index diet on glucose control in subjects with type 2 diabetes mellitus." *Annals of Pharmacotherapy* 44 (11): 1786–1792.

Barriocanal, L. A., M. Palacios, G. Benitez, S. Benitez, J. T. Jimenez, N. Jimenez, and V. Rojas. 2008. "Apparent lack of pharmacological effect of steviol glycosides used as sweeteners in humans. A pilot study of repeated exposures in some normotensive and hypotensive individuals and in type 1 and Type 2 diabetics." *Regulatory Toxicology & Pharmacology* 51 (1): 37–41.

Baskaran, K., B. Kizar Ahamath, K. Radha Shanmugasundaram, and E. R. B. Shanmugasundaram. 1990. "Antidiabetic effect of a leaf extract from gymnema sylvestre in non-insulin-dependent diabetes mellitus patients." *Journal of Ethnopharmacology* 30 (3): 295–305.

Becker, D. J., R. Y. Gordon, S. C. Halbert, B. French, P. B. Morris, and D. J. Rader. 2009. "Red yeast rice for dyslipidemia in statin-intolerant patients: A randomized trial." *Annals of Internal Medicine* 150 (12): 830–839.

Beer, A. M., K. R. Wiebelitz, and H. Schmidt-Gayk. 2008. "Lycopus europaeus (gypsywort): Effects on the thyroidal parameters and symptoms associated with thyroid function." *Phytomedicine: International Journal of Phytotherapy and Phytopharmacology* 15 (1–2): 16–22. doi:S0944-7113(07)00273-5 [pii].

Bierenbaum, M. L., R. Reichstein, and T. R. Watkins. 1993. "Reducing atherogenic risk in hyperlipemic humans with flax seed supplementation: A preliminary report." *Journal of the American College of Nutrition* 12 (5): 501–504.

Biondo, P. D., S. J. Robbins, J. D. Walsh, L. J. McCargar, V. J. Harber, and C. J. Field. 2008. "A randomized controlled crossover trial of the effect of ginseng consumption on the immune response to moderate exercise in healthy sedentary men." *Applied Physiology, Nutrition, and Metabolism* 33 (5): 966–975.

Bloch, A. S. 2000. "Pushing the envelope of nutrition support: Complementary therapies." *Nutrition* 16 (3): 236–239.

Bordia, A., S. K. Verma, and K. C. Srivastava. 1997. "Effect of ginger (zingiber officinale rosc.) and fenugreek (trigonella foenumgraecum L.) on blood lipids, blood sugar and platelet aggregation in patients with coronary artery disease." *Prostaglandins, Leukotrienes and Essential Fatty Acids* 56 (5): 379–384.

Budhathoki, S., M. Iwasaki, N. Sawada, T. Yamaji, T. Shimazu, S. Sasazuki, M. Inoue, and S. Tsugane. 2015. "Soy food and isoflavone intake and endometrial cancer risk: The japan public health center-based prospective study." *BJOG: An International Journal of Obstetrics & Gynaecology* 122 (3): 304–311.

Burch, H. B. and D. S. Cooper. 2015. "Management of graves disease: A review." *Jama* 314 (23): 2544–2554. doi:10.1001/jama.2015.16535 [doi].

Caron, M. F., A. L. Hotsko, S. Robertson, L. Mandybur, J. Kluger, and C. M. White. 2002. "Electrocardiographic and hemodynamic effects of panax ginseng." *The Annals of Pharmacotherapy* 36 (5): 758–763. doi:10.1345/aph.1A411 [doi].

Chan, L. Y., P. Y. Chiu, and T. K. Lau. 2003. "An in-vitro study of ginsenoside Rb1-induced teratogenicity using a whole rat embryo culture model." *Human Reproduction (Oxford, England)* 18 (10): 2166–2168.

Chang, J.-C., M. C. Wu, I.-M. Liu, and J.-T. Cheng. 2006. "Plasma glucose-lowering action of hon-chi in streptozotocin-induced diabetic rats." *Hormone and Metabolic Research* 38 (2): 76–81.

Chatsudthipong, V. and C. Muanprasat. 2009. "Stevioside and related compounds: Therapeutic benefits beyond sweetness." *Pharmacology & Therapeutics* 121 (1): 41–54.

Chearskul, S., W. Kriengsinyos, S. Kooptiwut, S. Sangurai, S. Onreabroi, M. Churintaraphan, N. Semprasert, and W. Nitiyanant. 2009. "Immediate and long-term effects of glucomannan on total ghrelin and leptin in type 2 diabetes mellitus." *Diabetes Research and Clinical Practice* 83 (2): e40–e42.

Chen, Y.-M., S. C. Ho, S. S. H. Lam, S. S. S. Ho, and J. L. F. Woo. 2003. "Soy isoflavones have a favorable effect on bone loss in chinese postmenopausal women with lower bone mass: A double-blind, randomized, controlled trial." *The Journal of Clinical Endocrinology & Metabolism* 88 (10): 4740–4747.

Choi, J., K.-T. Lee, H. Ka, W.-T. Jung, H.-J. Jung, and H.-J. Park. 2001. "Constituents of the essential oil of the cinnamomum cassia stem bark and the biological properties." *Archives of Pharmacal Research* 24 (5): 418–423.

Chutkan, R., G. Fahey, W. L. Wright, and J. McRorie. 2012. "Viscous versus nonviscous soluble fiber supplements: Mechanisms and evidence for fiber-specific health benefits." *Journal of the American Academy of Nurse Practitioners* 24 (8): 476–487.

Cicero, A., G. Derosa, and A. Gaddi. 2004. "What do herbalists suggest to diabetic patients in order to improve glycemic control? Evaluation of scientific evidence and potential risks." *Acta Diabetologica* 41 (3): 91–98.

Clark, C. A., J. Gardiner, M. I. McBurney, S. Anderson, L. J. Weatherspoon, D. N. Henry, and N. G. Hord. 2006. "Effects of breakfast meal composition on second meal metabolic responses in adults with type 2 diabetes mellitus." *European Journal of Clinical Nutrition* 60 (9): 1122–1129.

Clark, W. F., A. Parbtani, M. W. Huff, E. Spanner, H. de Salis, I. Chin-Yee, D. J. Philbrick, and B. J. Holub. 1995. "Flaxseed: A potential treatment for lupus nephritis." *Kidney International* 48 (2): 475–480.

Cornish, S. M., P. D. Chilibeck, L. Paus-Jennsen, H. Jay Biem, T. Khozani, V. Senanayake, H. Vatanparast, J. P. Little, S. J. Whiting, and P. Pahwa. 2009. "A randomized controlled trial of the effects of flaxseed lignan complex on metabolic syndrome composite score and bone mineral in older adults." *Applied Physiology, Nutrition, and Metabolism* 34 (2): 89–98.

Cunnane, S. C., S. Ganguli, C. Menard, A. C. Liede, M. J. Hamadeh, Z.-Y. Chen, T. M. S. Wolever, and D. J. A. Jenkins. 1993. "High a-linolenic acid flaxseed (linum usitatissimum): Some nutritional properties in humans." *British Journal of Nutrition* 69 (2): 443–453.

Cunnane, S. C., M. J. Hamadeh, A. C. Liede, L. U. Thompson, T. M. Wolever, and D. J. Jenkins. 1995. "Nutritional attributes of traditional flaxseed in healthy young adults." *The American Journal of Clinical Nutrition* 61 (1): 62–68.

Curi, R., M. Alvarez, R. B. Bazotte, L. M. Botion, J. L. Godoy, and A. Bracht. 1986. "Effect of Stev/a Reba Ud/Ana on glucose tolerance in normal adult humans." *Brazilian Journal of Medical and Biological Research*.

Dey, L., J. T. Xie, A. Wang, J. Wu, S. A. Maleckar, and C.-S. Yuan. 2003. "Anti-hyperglycemic effects of ginseng: Comparison between root and berry." *Phytomedicine* 10 (6–7): 600–605.

Dhamija, P., S. Malhotra, and P. Pandhi. 2006. "Effect of oral administration of crude aqueous extract of garlic on pharmacokinetic parameters of isoniazid and rifampicin in rabbits." *Pharmacology* 77 (2): 100–104. doi:93285 [pii].

Dillon, S. A., R. S. Burmi, G. M. Lowe, D. Billington, and K. Rahman. 2003. "Antioxidant properties of aged garlic extract: An in vitro study incorporating human low density lipoprotein." *Life Sciences* 72 (14): 1583–1594.

Di Pierro, F., N. Villanova, F. Agostini, R. Marzocchi, V. Soverini, and G. Marchesini. 2012. "Pilot study on the additive effects of berberine and oral type 2 diabetes agents for patients with suboptimal glycemic control." *Diabetes, Metabolic Syndrome and Obesity: Targets and Therapy* 5: 213–217. doi:10.2147/DMSO.S33718 [doi].

Dodin, S., A. Lemay, H. Jacques, F. Légaré, J.-C. Forest, and B. Mâsse. 2005. "The effects of flaxseed dietary supplement on lipid profile, bone mineral density, and symptoms in menopausal women: A randomized, double-blind, wheat germ placebo-controlled clinical trial." *The Journal of Clinical Endocrinology & Metabolism* 90 (3): 1390–1397.

Doi, K. 1995. "Effect of konjac fibre (glucomannan) on glucose and lipids." *European Journal of Clinical Nutrition* 49: 190–197.

Dugoua, J.-J., D. Seely, D. Perri, K. Cooley, T. Forelli, E. Mills, and G. Koren. 2007. "From type 2 diabetes to antioxidant activity: A systematic review of the safety and efficacy of common and cassia cinnamon bark this article is one of a selection of papers published in this special issue (part 1 of 2) on the safety and efficacy of natural health products." *Canadian Journal of Physiology and Pharmacology* 85 (9): 837–847.

Duke, J. A. and S. M. Beckstrom-Sternberg. 1994. "Dr. Duke's Phytochemical and Ethnobotanical Databases."

Edward, M. J. 2000. "American herbal products association's botanical safety handbook edited by M. McGuffin, C. Hobbs, R. Upton, and A. Goldberg, CRC Press, Boca Raton, FL, 231 Pages, 1997. 39.95." *Journal of Toxicology: Cutaneous and Ocular Toxicology* 19 (2–3): 167–168.

Fang, Y. and W. Li. 2000. "Effect of xuezhikang on lipid metabolism and islet cell function in type II diabetic patients." *Journal of Capital Medicine* 7 (2): 44–45.

Farnsworth, N. R., A. S. Bingel, G. A. Cordell, F. A. Crane, and H. H. S. Fong. 1975. "Potential value of plants as sources of new antifertility agents I." *Journal of Pharmaceutical Sciences* 64 (4): 535–598.

Franke, A. A., L. J. Custer, and Y. Tanaka. 1998. "Isoflavones in human breast milk and other biological fluids." *The American Journal of Clinical Nutrition* 68 (6 Suppl): 1466S–1473S.

Frati Munari, A.C., W. Benitez Pinto, C. Raul Ariza Andraca, and M. Casarrubias. 1998. "Lowering glycemic index of food by acarbose and plantago psyllium mucilage." *Archives of Medical Research* 29: 137–41.

Fujita, H., Yamagami, T., and Ohshima, K. 2001. "Long-term ingestion of a fermented soybean-derived touchi-extract with alpha-glucosidase inhibitory activity is safe and effective in humans with borderline and mild type-2 diabetes." *The Journal of Nutrition* 131 (8): 2105–2108.

Gardner, C. 2014. "Non-nutritive sweeteners: Evidence for benefit vs. risk." *Current Opinion in Lipidology* 25 (1): 80–84.

Gibb, R. D., J. W. Jr. McRorie, D. A. Russell, V. Hasselblad, and D. A. D'Alessio. 2015. "Psyllium fiber improves glycemic control proportional to loss of glycemic control: A meta-analysis of data in euglycemic subjects, patients at risk of type 2 diabetes mellitus, and patients being treated for type 2 diabetes mellitus." *American Journal of Clinical Nutrition* 102 (6): 1604–1614.

Gimenez, I., R. M. Martinez, M. Lou, J. A. Mayoral, R. P. Garay, and J. O. Alda. 1998. "Salidiuretic action by genistein in the isolated, perfused rat kidney." *Hypertension (Dallas, Tex.: 1979)* 31 (2): 706–711.

Graham, P. H. and C. P. Vance. 2003. "Legumes: Importance and constraints to greater use." *Plant Physiology* 131 (3): 872–877. doi:10.1104/pp.017004 [doi].

Gregersen, S., P. B. Jeppesen, J. J. Holst, and K. Hermansen. 2004. "Antihyperglycemic effects of stevioside in type 2 diabetic subjects." *Metabolism: Clinical & Experimental* 53 (1): 73–76.

Grover, J. K. and S. P. Yadav. 2004. "Pharmacological actions and potential uses of momordica charantia: A review." *Journal of Ethnopharmacology* 93 (1): 123–132.

Gupta, A., R. Gupta, and B. Lal. 2001. "Effect of trigonella foenum-graecum (fenugreek) seeds on glycaemic control and insulin resistance in type 2 diabetes." *Journal of the Association of Physicians India* 49: 1057–1061.

Gurley, B. J., S. F. Gardner, M. A. Hubbard, D. Keith Williams, W. Brooks Gentry, Y. Cui, and C. Y. Ang. 2002. "Cytochrome P450 phenotypic ratios for predicting herb-drug interactions in humans." *Clinical Pharmacology and Therapeutics* 72 (3): 276–287.

Hall, C., M. C. Tulbek, and Y. Xu. 2006. "Flaxseed." *Advances in Food and Nutrition Research* 51: 1–97.

Hamid, S., S. Rojter, and J. Vierling. 1997. "Protracted cholestatic hepatitis after the use of prostata." *Annals of Internal Medicine* 127 (2): 169–170.

Hao, M., Q. Ba, J. Yin, J. Li, Y. Zhao, and H. Wang. 2011. "Deglycosylated ginsenosides are more potent inducers of CYP1A1, CYP1A2 and CYP3A4 expression in HepG2 cells than glycosylated ginsenosides." *Drug Metabolism and Pharmacokinetics* 26 (2): 201–205.

He, J., D. Gu, X. Wu, J. Chen, X. Duan, J. Chen, and P. K. Whelton. 2005. "Effect of soybean protein on blood pressure: A randomized, controlled trial." *Annals of Internal Medicine* 143 (1): 1–9.

Heber, D., I. Yip, J. M. Ashley, D. A. Elashoff, R. M. Elashoff, and V. L. Go. 1999. "Cholesterol-lowering effects of a proprietary chinese red-yeast-rice dietary supplement." *The American Journal of Clinical Nutrition* 69 (2): 231–236.

Hermansen, K., M. Sondergaard, L. Hoie, M. Carstensen, and B. Brock. 2001. "Beneficial effects of a soy-based dietary supplement on lipid levels and cardiovascular risk markers in type 2 diabetic subjects." *Diabetes Care* 24 (2): 228–233.

Huang, J., J. Frohlich, and A. P. Ignaszewski. 2011. "The impact of dietary changes and dietary supplements on lipid profile." *Canadian Journal of Cardiology* 27 (4): 488–505.

Hutchins, A. M., B. D. Brown, S. C. Cunnane, S. G. Domitrovich, E. R. Adams, and C. E. Bobowiec. 2013. "Daily flaxseed consumption improves glycemic control in obese men and women with pre-diabetes: A randomized study." *Nutrition Research* 33 (5): 367–375.

Hwa-Jin, P., L. Jung-Hee, S. Yong-Bum, and P. Ki-Hyun. 1996. "Effects of dietary supplementation of lipophilic fraction from panax ginseng on cGMP and cAMP in rat platelets and on blood coagulation." *Biological and Pharmaceutical Bulletin* 19 (11): 1434–1439.

Hymowitz, T. 1970. "On the domestication of the soybean." *Economic Botany* 24 (4): 408–421.

Ichikawa, T., J. Li, P. Nagarkatti, M. Nagarkatti, L. J. Hofseth, A. Windust, and T. Cui. 2009. "American ginseng preferentially suppresses STAT/iNOS signaling in activated macrophages." *Journal of Ethnopharmacology* 125 (1): 145–150.

Imparl-Radosevich, J., S. Deas, M. M. Polansky, D. A. Baedke, T. S. Ingebritsen, R. A. Anderson, and D. J. Graves. 1998. "Regulation of PTP-1 and insulin receptor kinase by fractions from cinnamon: Implications for cinnamon regulation of insulin signalling." *Hormone Research in Paediatrics* 50 (3): 177–182.

Janetzky, K. and A. P. Morreale. 1997. "Probable interaction between warfarin and ginseng." *American Journal of Health-System Pharmacy: AJHP : Official Journal of the American Society of Health-System Pharmacists* 54 (6): 692–693.

Jarvill-Taylor, K. J., R. A. Anderson, and D. J. Graves. 2001. "A hydroxychalcone derived from cinnamon functions as a mimetic for insulin in 3T3-L1 adipocytes." *Journal of the American College of Nutrition* 20 (4): 327–336.

Jayagopal, V., P. Albertazzi, E. S. Kilpatrick, E. M. Howarth, P. E. Jennings, D. A. Hepburn, and S. L. Atkin. 2002. "Beneficial effects of soy phytoestrogen intake in postmenopausal women with type 2 diabetes." *Diabetes Care* 25 (10): 1709–1714.

Jenkins, D. J. A., C. W. C. Kendall, P. W. Connelly, C.-J. C. Jackson, T. Parker, D. Faulkner, and E. Vidgen. 2002. "Effects of high-and low-isoflavone (phytoestrogen) soy foods on Iiflammatory biomarkers and proinflammatory cytokines in middle-aged men and women." *Metabolism* 51 (7): 919–924.

Jenkins, D. J., C. W. Kendall, E. Vidgen, S. Agarwal, A. V. Rao, R. S. Rosenberg, E. P. Diamandis et al. 1999. "Health aspects of partially defatted flaxseed, including effects on serum lipids, oxidative measures, and ex vivo androgen and arogestin Activity: A controlled crossover trial." *The American Journal of Clinical Nutrition* 69 (3): 395–402.

Jiang, X., K. M. Williams, W. S. Liauw, A. J. Ammit, B. D. Roufogalis, C. C. Duke, R. O. Day, and A. J. McLachlan. 2004. "Effect of St. John's wort and ginseng on the pharmacokinetics and pharmacodynamics of warfarin in healthy subjects." *British Journal of Clinical Pharmacology* 57 (5): 592–599.

Joseph, B. and D. Jini. 2013. "Antidiabetic effects of momordica charantia (bitter melon) and its medicinal potency." *Asian Pacific Journal of Tropical Disease* 3 (2): 93–102.

Jung, H. L., H. E. Kwak, S. S. Kim, Y. C. Kim, C. D. Lee, H. K. Byurn, and H. Y. Kang. 2011. "Effects of panax ginseng supplementation on muscle damage and inflammation after uphill treadmill running in humans." *The American Journal of Chinese Medicine* 39 (3): 441–450.

Kantola, T., K. T. Kivistö, and P. J. Neuvonen. 1998. "Grapefruit juice greatly increases serum concentrations of lovastatin and lovastatin acid." *Clinical Pharmacology and Therapeutics* 63 (4): 397–402.

Khan, A., M. Safdar, M. M. Ali Khan, K. N. Khattak, and R. A. Anderson. 2003. "Cinnamon improves glucose and lipids of people with type 2 diabetes." *Diabetes Care* 26 (12): 3215–3218.

Khan, A. K., S. AKhtar, and H. Mahtab. 1980. "Treatment of diabetes mellitus with coccinia indica." *British Medical Journal* 280 (6220): 1044.

Khare, A. K., R. N. Tondon, and J. P. Tewari. 1983. "Hypoglycaemic activity of an indigenous drug (gymnema sylvestre, 'gurmar') in normal and diabetic persons." *Indian Journal of Physiology and Pharmacology* 27 (3): 257–258.

Kim, E. H., V. Vuksan, and E. Wong. 1996. "The relationship between viscosity of soluble dietary fiber and their hypoglycemic effects." *The Korean Journal of Nutrition (Korea Republic).*

Kim, S., B.-C. Shin, M. S. Lee, H. Lee, and E. Ernst. 2011. "Red ginseng for type 2 diabetes mellitus: A systematic review of randomized controlled trials." *Chinese Journal of Integrative Medicine* 17 (12): 937–944.

Kitts, D. D., A. N. Wijewickreme, and C. Hu. 2000. "Antioxidant properties of a north american ginseng extract." *Molecular and Cellular Biochemistry* 203 (1): 1–10.

Kumar, N. B., A. Cantor, K. Allen, D. Riccardi, K. Besterman-Dahan, J. Seigne, M. Helal, R. Salup, and J. Pow-Sang. 2004. "The specific role of isoflavones in reducing prostate cancer risk." *The Prostate* 59 (2): 141–147.

Kumar, S. N., U. V. Mani, and I. Mani. 2010. "An open label study on the supplementation of gymnema sylvestre in type 2 diabetics." *Journal of Dietary Supplements* 7 (3): 273–282.

Kuriyan, R., R. Rajendran, G. Bantwal, and A. V. Kurpad. 2008. "Effect of supplementation of coccinia cordifolia extract on Newly Detected Diabetic Datients." *Diabetes Care* 31 (2): 216–220. doi:dc07-1591 [pii].

Lan, J., Y. Zhao, F. Dong, Z. Yan, W. Zheng, J. Fan, and G. Sun. 2015. "Meta-analysis of the effect and safety of berberine in the treatment of type 2 diabetes mellitus, hyperlipemia and hypertension." *Journal of Ethnopharmacology* 161: 69–81. doi:10.1016/j.jep.2014.09.049 [doi].

Leach, M. J. 2007. "Gymnema sylvestre for diabetes mellitus: A systematic review." *The Journal of Alternative and Complementary Medicine* 13 (9): 977–983.

Leatherdale, B. A., R. K. Panesar, G. Singh, T. W. Atkins, C. J. Bailey, and A. H. Bignell. 1981. "Improvement in glucose tolerance due to momordica charantia (karela)." *British Medical Journal (Clin Res Ed)* 282 (6279): 1823–1824.

Lee, C.-S., J.-H. Lee, M. Oh, K.-M. Choi, M. R. Jeong, J.-D. Park, D. Y. Kwon, K.-C. Ha, E.-O. Park, and N. Lee. 2012. "Preventive effect of korean red ginseng for acute respiratory illness: A randomized and double-blind clinical trial." *Journal of Korean Medical Science* 27 (12): 1472–1478.

Lee, F. C., J. H. Ko, J. K. Park, and J. S. Lee. 1987. "Effects of panax ginseng on blood alcohol clearance in man." *Clinical and Experimental Pharmacology and Physiology* 14 (6): 543–546.

Leung, L., R. Birtwhistle, J. Kotecha, S. Hannah, and S. Cuthbertson. 2009. "Anti-diabetic and hypoglycaemic effects of momordica charantia (bitter melon): A mini review." *British Journal of Nutrition* 102 (12): 1703–1708.

Li, Y., M. Zheng, X. Zhai, Y. Huang, A. Khalid, A. Malik, P. Shah, S. Karim, S. Azhar, and X. Hou. 2015. "Effect of gymnema sylvestre, citrullus colocynthis and artemisia absinthium on blood gucose and lipid profile in diabetic human." *Acta Poloniae Pharmaceutica* 72 (5): 981–985.

Li, Z., K. Hong, P. Saltsman, S. DeShields, M. Bellman, G. Thames, Y. Liu, H. J. Wang, R. Elashoff, and D. Heber. 2005. "Long-term efficacy of soy-based meal replacements vs. an individualized diet plan in obese type II DM patients: Relative effects on weight loss, metabolic parameters, and c-reactive protein." *European Journal of Clinical Nutrition* 59 (3): 411–418.

Liu, B. H., T. S. Wu, M. C. Su, C. P. Chung, and F. Y. Yu. 1-12-2005. "Evaluation of citrinin occurrence and cytotoxicity in monascus fermentation products." *Journal of Agricultural Food Chemistry* 53 (1): 170–175.

Liu, J., J. Zhang, Y. Shi, S. Grimsgaard, T. Alraek, and V. Fønnebø. 2006. "Chinese red yeast rice (monascus purpureus) for primary hyperlipidemia: A meta-analysis of randomized controlled trials." *Chinese Medicine* 1 (1): 4.

Liu, Z. M., Y. M. Chen, and S. C. Ho. 2011. "Effects of soy intake on glycemic control: A meta-analysis of randomized controlled trials." *The American Journal of Clinical Nutrition* 93 (5): 1092–1101. doi:10.3945/ajcn.110.007187 [doi].

Lucas, E. A., R. D. Wild, L. J. Hammond, D. A. Khalil, S. Juma, B. P. Daggy, B. J. Stoecker, and B. H. Arjmandi. 2002. "Flaxseed improves lipid profile without altering biomarkers of bone metabolism in postmenopausal women." *The Journal of Clinical Endocrinology and Metabolism* 87 (4): 1527–1532.

Mackenzie, T., L. Leary, and W. B. Brooks. 2007. "The effect of an extract of green and black tea on glucose control in adults with type 2 diabetes mellitus: Double-blind randomized study." *Metabolism: Clinical and Experimental* 56 (10): 1340–1344. doi:S0026-0495(07)00190-4 [pii].

Madar, Z., R. Abel, S. Samish, and J. Arad. 1988. "Glucose-lowering effect of fenugreek in non-insulin dependent diabetics." *European Journal of Clinical Nutrition* 42 (1): 51–54.

Mang, B., M. Wolters, B. Schmitt, K. Kelb, R. Lichtinghagen, D. O. Stichtenoth, and A. Hahn. 2006. "Effects of a cinnamon extract on plasma glucose, HbA1c, and serum lipids in diabetes mellitus type 2." *European Journal of Clinical Investigation* 36 (5): 340–344.

Mani, U. V., I. Mani, M. Biswas, and S. N. Kumar. 2011. "An open-label study on the effect of flax seed powder (linum usitatissimum) supplementation in the management of diabetes mellitus." *Journal of Dietary Supplements* 8 (3): 257–265.

Markowitz, J. S., C. Lindsay DeVane, K. D. Chavin, R. M. Taylor, Y. Ruan, and J. L. Donovan. 2003. "Effects of garlic (allium sativum L.) supplementation on cytochrome P450 2D6 and 3A4 activity in healthy volunteers." *Clinical Pharmacology and Therapeutics* 74 (2): 170–177.

Martinez-Mir, I., E. Rubio, F. J. Morales-Olivas, and V. Palop-Larrea. 2004. "Transient ischemic attack secondary to hypertensive crisis related to panax ginseng." *The Annals of Pharmacotherapy* 38 (11): 1970. doi:aph.1E213 [pii].

McCrindle, B. W., E. Helden, and W. T. Conner. 1998. "Garlic extract therapy in children with hypercholesterolemia." *Archives of Pediatrics and Adolescent Medicine* 152 (11): 1089–1094.

Mcelhaney, J. E., S. Gravenstein, S. K. Cole, E. Davidson, D. O'neill, S. Petitjean, B. Rumble, and J. J. Shan. 2004. "A placebo-controlled trial of a proprietary extract of north american ginseng (CVT-E002) to prevent acute respiratory illness in institutionalized older adults." *Journal of the American Geriatrics Society* 52 (1): 13–19.

McElhaney, J. E., A. E. Simor, S. McNeil, and G. N. Predy. 2011. "Efficacy and safety of CVT-E002, a proprietary extract of panax Quinquefolius in the prevention of respiratory infections in influenza-vaccinated community-dwelling adults: A multicenter, randomized, double-blind, and placebo-controlled trial." *Influenza Research and Treatment* 2011: 759051. doi:10.1155/2011/759051 [doi].

Mechanick, J. I., E. M. Brett, A. B. Chausmer, R. A. Dickey, S. Wallach, and American Association of Clinical Endocrinologists. 2003. "American association of clinical endocrinologists medical guidelines for the clinical use of dietary supplements and nutraceuticals." *Endocrine Practice: Official Journal of the American College of Endocrinology and the American Association of Clinical Endocrinologists* 9 (5): 417–470. doi:C7TYMYF9E2MHNWHB [pii].

Medagama, A. B. and R. Bandara. 2014. "The use of complementary and alternative medicines (CAMs) in the treatment of diabetes mellitus: Is continued use safe and effective?" *Nutrition Journal* 13: 102-2891-13-102. doi:10.1186/1475-2891-13-102 [doi].

Mennella, J. A., A. Johnson, and G. K. Beauchamp. 1995. "Garlic ingestion by pregnant women alters the odor of amniotic fluid." *Chemical Senses* 20 (2): 207–209.

Mora, G. E., A. Warm, S. Arslanoglu, and V. Miniello. 2002. "Management of bovine protein allergy: New perspectives and nutritional aspects." *Annals of Allergy, Asthma and Immunology* 89 (6): 91–96.

Morris, A. C., I. Jacobs, T. M. McLellan, A. Klugerman, L. C. H. Wang, and J. Zamecnik. 1996. "No ergogenic effect of ginseng ingestion." *International Journal of Sport Nutrition* 6 (3): 263–271.

Mousavi, Y. and H. Adlercreutz. 1992. "Enterolactone and estradiol inhibit each other's proliferative effect on MCF-7 breast cancer cells in culture." *The Journal of Steroid Biochemistry and Molecular Biology* 41 (3): 615–619.

Mucalo, I., E. Jovanovski, D. Rahelić, V. Božikov, Ž. Romić, and V. Vuksan. 2013. "Effect of american ginseng (panax quinquefolius L.) on arterial stiffness in subjects with type-2 diabetes and concomitant hypertension." *Journal of Ethnopharmacology* 150 (1): 148–153.

Mucalo, I., D. Rahelic, E. Jovanovski, V. Bozikov, Z. Romic, and V. Vuksan. 2012. "Effect of american ginseng (panax quinquefolius L.) on glycemic control in type 2 diabetes." *Collegium Antropologicum* 36 (4): 1435–1440.

Mulrow, C., V. Lawrence, and R. Ackermann. 2000. *Garlic: Effects on cardiovascular risks and disease, protective effects against cancer, and clinical adverse effects.* AHRQ Publication 01-E023. Rockville MD: *Agency for Healthcare Research and Quality, October 2000.*

Munasinghe, M. A., C. Abeysena, I. S. Yaddehige, T. Vidanapathirana, and K. P. Piyumal. 2011. "Blood sugar lowering effect of coccinia grandis (L.) J. Voigt: Path for a new drug for diabetes mellitus." *Experimental Diabetes Research* 2011: 978762. doi:10.1155/2011/978762 [doi].

Nahas, R. and M. Moher. 2009. "Complementary and alternative medicine for the treatment of type 2 diabetes." *Canadian Family Physician Medecin De Famille Canadien* 55 (6): 591–596. doi:55/6/591 [pii].

Neelakantan, N., M. Narayanan, R. J. de Souza, and R. M. van Dam. 2014. "Effect of fenugreek (trigonella foenum-graecum L.) intake on glycemia: A meta-analysis of clinical trials." *Nutrition Journal* 13 (1): 7.

Niederhofer, H. 2009. "Panax ginseng may improve some symptoms of attention-deficit hyperactivity disorder." *Journal of Dietary Supplements* 6 (1): 22–27.

Nordström, D. C. E., C. Friman, Y. T. Konttinen, V. E. A. Honkanen, Y. Nasu, and E. Antila. 1995. "Alpha-linolenic acid in the treatment of rheumatoid arthritis. A double-blind, placebo-controlled and randomized study: Flaxseed vs. safflower seed." *Rheumatology International* 14 (6): 231–234.

Oh, M.-R., S.-H. Park, S.-Y. Kim, H.-I. Back, M.-G. Kim, J.-Y. Jeon, K.-C. Ha, W.-T. Na, Y.-S. Cha, and B.-H. Park. 2014. "Postprandial glucose-lowering effects of fermented red ginseng in subjects with impaired fasting glucose or type 2 diabetes: A randomized, double-blind, placebo-controlled clinical trial." *BMC Complementary and Alternative Medicine* 14 (1): 237.

Ooi, C. P., Z. Yassin, and T.-A. Hamid. 2010. "Momordica charantia for type 2 diabetes mellitus." *The Cochrane Library*. Feb 17;(2) CD007845. doi:10.1002/14651858.CD007845.pub2

Ortsäter, H., N. Grankvist, S. Wolfram, N. Kuehn, and Å. Sjöholm. 2012. "Diet supplementation with green tea extract epigallocatechin gallate prevents progression to glucose intolerance in db/db mice." *Nutrition and Metabolism* 9 (1): 11.

Pan, A., W. Demark-Wahnefried, X. Ye, Z. Yu, H. Li, Q. Qi, J. Sun, Y. Chen, X. Chen, and Y. Liu. 2008. "Effects of a flaxseed-derived lignan supplement on c-reactive protein, IL-6 and retinol-binding protein 4 in type 2 diabetic patients." *British Journal of Nutrition* 101 (8): 1145–1149.

Pan, A., J. Sun, Y. Chen, X. Ye, H. Li, Z. Yu, Y. Wang, W. Gu, X. Zhang, and X. Chen. 2007. "Effects of a Flaxseed-derived lignan supplement in type 2 Diabetic patients: A randomized, double-blind, cross-over trial." *PLoS One* 2 (11): e1148.

Pino, A. M., L. E. Valladares, M. A. Palma, A. M. Mancilla, M. Yáñez, and C. Albala. 2000. "Dietary isoflavones affect sex hormone-binding globulin levels in postmenopausal women 1." *The Journal of Clinical Endocrinology & Metabolism* 85 (8): 2797–2800.

Pirillo, A. and A. L. Catapano. 2015. "Berberine, a plant alkaloid with lipid- and glucose-lowering properties: From in vitro evidence to clinical studies." *Atherosclerosis* 243 (2): 449–461. doi:10.1016/j.atherosclerosis.2015.09.032 [doi].

Piscitelli, S. C., A. H. Burstein, N. Welden, K. D. Gallicano, and J. Falloon. 2002. "The effect of sarlic Supplements on the pharmacokinetics of saquinavir." *Clinical Infectious Diseases: An Official Publication of the Infectious Diseases Society of America* 34 (2): 234–238. doi:CID010586 [pii].

Potter, S. M., J. A. Baum, H. Teng, R. J. Stillman, N. F. Shay, and J. W. Erdman Jr. 1998. "Soy protein and isoflavones: Their effects on blood lipids and bone density in postmenopausal Women." *The American Journal of Clinical Nutrition* 68 (6 Suppl): 1375S–1379S.

Prasad, G. V. R., T. Wong, G. Meliton, and S. Bhaloo. 2002. "Rhabdomyolysis due to red yeast rice (monascus purpureus) in a renal transplant recipient." *Transplantation* 74 (8): 1200–1201.

Raghuram, T. C., R. D. Sharma, B. Sivakumar, and B. K. Sahay. 1994. "Effect of fenugreek seeds on intravenous glucose disposition in non-insulin dependent diabetic patients." *Phytotherapy Research* 8 (2): 83–86.

Reeder, C., A. Legrand, and S. K. O'connor-Von. 2013. "The effect of fenugreek on milk production and prolactin levels in mothers of preterm infants." *Clinical Lactation* 4 (4): 159–165.

Reeds, D. N., B. W. Patterson, A. Okunade, J. O. Holloszy, K. S. Polonsky, and S. Klein. 2011. "Ginseng and ginsenoside re do not improve beta-cell function or insulin sensitivity in overweight and obese subjects with impaired glucose tolerance or diabetes." *Diabetes Care* 34 (5): 1071–1076. doi:10.2337/dc10-2299 [doi].

Reza, S. P. 2005. "Preecamplsia is an Important Complication of Pregnancy which can Result in Morbidity and Mortality in Mother, Fetus and the Neonate."

Rhee, M.-Y., B. Cho, K.-I. Kim, J. Kim, M. K. Kim, E.-K. Lee, H.-J. Kim, and C.-H. Kim. 2014. "Blood pressure lowering effect of korea ginseng derived ginseol K-G1." *The American Journal of Chinese Medicine* 42 (3): 605–618.

Rhee, Y. and A. Brunt. 2011. "Flaxseed supplementation improved insulin resistance in obese glucose intolerant people: A randomized crossover design." *Nutrition Journal* 10 (1): 44.

Robbers, J. E. and V. E. Tyler. 1998. *Tyler's Herbs of Choice: The Therapeutic use of Phytomedicinals.* Routledge.

Rodriguez-Moran, M., F. Guerrero-Romero, and G. Lazcano-Burciaga. 1998. "Lipid- and glucose-lowering efficacy of plantago psyllium in type II diabetes." *Journal of Diabetes and Its Complications* 12 (5): 273–278.

Rose, K. D., P. D. Croissant, C. F. Parliament, and M. B. Levin. 1990. "Spontaneous spinal epidural hematoma with associated platelet dysfunction from excessive garlic ingestion: A case report." *Neurosurgery* 26 (5): 880–882.

Ryan, E. A., M. E. Pick, and C. Marceau. 2001. "Use of alternative medicines in diabetes mellitus." *Diabetic Medicine : A Journal of the British Diabetic Association* 18 (3): 242–245. doi:dme450 [pii].

Scaglione, F., G. Cattaneo, M. Alessandria, and R. Cogo. 1996. "Efficacy and safety of the standardised ginseng extract G115 for potentiating vaccination against the influenza syndrome and protection against the common cold [corrected]." *Drugs Under Experimental and Clinical Research* 22 (2): 65–72.

Scambia, G., D. Mango, P. G. Signorile, R. A. Angeli, C. Palena, D. Gallo, E. Bombardelli, P. Morazzoni, A. Riva, and S. Mancuso. 2000. "Clinical effects of a standardized soy extract in postmenopausal women: A pilot study." *Menopause (New York, N. Y.)* 7 (2): 105–111.

Sen, S., Chen, S., Wu, Y., Feng, B., Lui, E. K. and Chakrabarti, S. 2013. "Preventive effects of aorth American ginseng (*panax quinquefolius*) on diabetic retinopathy and cardiomyopathy." *Phytotherapy Research* 27: 290–298.

Sewell, A. C., A. Mosandl, and H. Böhles. 1999. "False diagnosis of maple syrup urine disease owing to ingestion of herbal tea." *New England Journal of Medicine* 341 (10): 769–769.

Shader, R. I. and D. J. Greenblatt. 1985. *Phenelzine and the Dream Machine-Ramblings and Reflections.*

Shanmugasundaram, E. R. B., G. Rajeswari, K. Baskaran, B. R. Rajesh Kumar, K. Radha Shanmugasundaram, and B. Kizar Ahmath. 1990. "Use of gymnema sylvestre leaf extract in the control of blood glucose in insulin-dependent diabetes mellitus." *Journal of Ethnopharmacology* 30 (3): 281–294.

Sharma, R. D. and T. C. Raghuram. 1990. "Hypoglycaemic effect of fenugreek seeds in non-insulin dependent diabetic subjects." *Nutrition Research* 10 (7): 731–739.

Sharma, R. D., T. C. Raghuram, and N. S. Rao. 1990. "Effect of fenugreek seeds on blood glucose and serum lipids in type I diabetes." *European Journal of Clinical Nutrition* 44 (4): 301–306.

Sharma, R. D., A. Sarkar, D. K. Hazra, B. Misra, J. B. Singh, B. B. Maheshwari, and S. K. Sharma. 1996a. "Hypolipidaemic effect of fenugreek seeds: A chronic study in non-insulin dependent diabetic patients." *Phytotherapy Research* 10 (4): 332–334.

Sharma, R. D., A. Sarkar, D. K. Hazara, B. Mishra, J. B. Singh, S. K. Sharma, B. B. Maheshwari, and P. K. Maheshwari. 1996b. "Use of fenugreek seed powder in the management of non-insulin dependent diabetes mellitus." *Nutrition Research* 16 (8): 1331–1339.

Shima, K., A. Tanaka, H. Ikegami, M. Tabata, N. Sawazaki, and Y. Kumahara. 1983. "Effect of dietary fiber, glucomannan, on absorption of sulfonylurea in man." *Hormone and Metabolic Research* 15 (1): 1–3.

Shin, H. R., J. Y. Kim, T. K. Yun, G. Morgan, and H. Vainio. 2000. "The cancer-preventive potential of panax ginseng: A review of human and experimental evidence." *Cancer Causes and Control* 11 (6): 565–576.

Shiyovich, A., I. Sztarkier, and L. Nesher. 2010. "Toxic hepatitis induced by gymnema sylvestre, a natural remedy for type 2 diabetes mellitus." *The American Journal of the Medical Sciences* 340 (6): 514–517. doi:10.1097/MAJ.0b013e3181f41168 [doi].

Shulman, K. I. and S. E. Walker. 1999. "Refining the MAOI diet: Tyramine content of pizzas and soy products." *The Journal of Clinical Psychiatry* 60 (3): 191–193.

Sierra, M., J. J. Garcia, N. Fernandez, M. J. Diez, and A. P. Calle. 2002. "Therapeutic effects of psyllium in type 2 diabetic patients." *European Journal of Clinical Nutrition* 56 (9): 830–842.

Silagy, C. A. and H. A. W. Neil. 1994. "A meta-analysis of the effect of garlic on blood pressure." *Journal of Hypertension* 12 (4): 463–468.

Singh, R. B., M. A. Niaz, V. Rastogi, N. Singh, A. Postiglione, and S. S. Rastogi. 1998. "Hypolipidemic and antioxidant effects of fenugreek seeds and triphala as adjuncts to dietary therapy in patients with mild to moderate hypercholesterolemia." *Perfusion* 11 (3): 124.

Smith, M. 2003. "Therapeutic applications of fenugreek." *Alternative Medicine Review* 8 (1): 20–27.

Sobenin, I. A., L. V. Nedosugova, L. V. Filatova, M. I. Balabolkin, T. V. Gorchakova, and A. N. Orekhov. 2008. "Metabolic effects of time-released garlic powder tablets in type 2 diabetes mellitus: The results of double-blinded placebo-controlled study." *Acta Diabetologica* 45 (1): 1–6.

Sood, N., W. L. Baker, and C. I. Coleman. 2008. "Effect of glucomannan on plasma lipid and glucose concentrations, body weight, and blood pressure: Systematic review and meta-analysis." *The American Journal of Clinical Nutrition* 88 (4): 1167–1175. doi:88/4/1167 [pii].

Sotaniemi, E. A., E. Haapakoski, and A. Rautio. 1995. "Ginseng therapy in non-insulin-dependent diabetic patients." *Diabetes Care* 18 (10): 1373–1375.

Srivastava, Y., H. Venkatakrishna-Bhatt, Y. Verma, K. Venkaiah, and B. H. Raval. 1993. "Antidiabetic and adaptogenic properties of momordica charantia extract: An experimental and clinical evaluation." *Phytotherapy Research* 7 (4): 285–289.

Stavro, P. M., M. Woo, L. A. Leiter, T. F. Heim, J. L. Sievenpiper, and V. Vuksan. 2006. "Long-term intake of north american ginseng has no effect on 24-hour blood pressure and renal function." *Hypertension (Dallas, Tex.: 1979)* 47 (4): 791–796. doi:01.HYP.0000205150.43169.2c [pii].

Scholey, A., A. Ossoukhova, L. Owen et al. 2010. Effects of american ginseng (panax quinquefolius) on neurocognitive function: An acute, randomised, double-blind, placebo-controlled, crossover study. *Psychopharmacology (Berl)* 212 (3): 345–356.

Suksomboon, N., N. Poolsup, S. Boonkaew, and C. C. Suthisisang. 2011. "Meta-analysis of the effect of herbal supplement on glycemic control in type 2 diabetes." *Journal of Ethnopharmacology* 137 (3): 1328–1333.

Taylor, C. G., A. D. Noto, D. M. Stringer, S. Froese, and L. Malcolmson. 2010. "Dietary milled flaxseed and flaxseed oil improve N-3 fatty acid status and do not affect glycemic control in individuals with well-controlled type 2 diabetes." *Journal of the American College of Nutrition* 29 (1): 72–80.

Teixeira, S. R., S. M. Potter, R. Weigel, S. Hannum, J. W. Erdman Jr., and C. M. Hasler. 2000. "Effects of feeding 4 levels of soy protein for 3 and 6 Wk on blood lipids and apolipoproteins in moderately hypercholesterolemic men." *The American Journal of Clinical Nutrition* 71 (5): 1077–1084.

Thomas, B. L., D. C. Laine, and F. C. Goetz. 1988. "Glucose and insulin response in diabetic subjects: Acute effect of carbohydrate level and the addition of soy polysaccharide in defined-formula diets." *The American Journal of Clinical Nutrition* 48 (4): 1048–1052.

Tiwari, P., B. N. Mishra, and N. S. Sangwan. 2014. "Phytochemical and pharmacological properties of gymnema sylvestre: An important medicinal plant." *BioMed Research International* 2014: 830285. doi:10.1155/2014/830285 [doi].

Trask, L., N. Kasid, K. Homa, and S. Chaidarun. 2013. "Safety and efficacy of the nonsystemic chewable complex carbohydrate dietary supplement PAZ320 on postprandial glycemia when added to oral agents or insulin in patients with type 2 diabetes mellitus." *Endocrine Practice* 19 (4): 627–632.

Tsai, A. C., A. I. Vinik, A. Lasichak, and G. S. Lo. 1987. "Effects of soy polysaccharide on postprandial plasma glucose, insulin, glucagon, pancreatic polypeptide, somatostatin, and triglyceride in obese diabetic patients." *The American Journal of Clinical Nutrition* 45 (3): 596–601.

Unfer, V., M. L. Casini, L. Costabile, M. Mignosa, S. Gerli, and G. C. Di Renzo. 2004. "Endometrial effects of long-term treatment with phytoestrogens: A randomized, double-blind, placebo-controlled study." *Fertility and Sterility* 82 (1): 145–148.

Vanderbeek, P. B., C. Fasano, G. O'Malley, and J. Hornstein. 2007. "Esophageal obstruction from a hygroscopic pharmacobezoar containing glucomannan." *Clinical Toxicology* 45 (1): 80–82.

Vanschoonbeek, K., B. J. Thomassen, J. M. Senden, W. K. Wodzig, and L. J. van Loon. 2006. "Cinnamon supplementation does not improve glycemic control in postmenopausal type 2 diabetes patients." *The Journal of Nutrition* 136 (4): 977–980. doi:136/4/977 [pii].

Verspohl, E. J., K. Bauer, and E. Neddermann. 2005. "Antidiabetic effect of cinnamomum cassia and cinnamomum zeylanicum in vivo and in vitro." *Phytotherapy Research* 19 (3): 203–206.

Villaverde, A. F., S. Benlloch, M. Berenguer, J. M. Rayón, R. Pina, and J. Berenguer. 2004. "Acute hepatitis of cholestatic type possibly associated with the use of glucomannan (amorphophalus konjac)." *Journal of Hepatology* 41 (6): 1061–1062.

Vohra, S., B. C Johnston, K. L. Laycock, W. K. Midodzi, I. Dhunnoo, E. Harris, and L. Baydala. 2008. "Safety and tolerability of north american ginseng extract in the treatment of pediatric upper respiratory tract infection: A phase II randomized, controlled trial of 2 dosing schedules." *Pediatrics* 122 (2): e402–10. doi:10.1542/peds.2007-2186 [doi].

Vuksan, V., D. J. Jenkins, P. Spadafora, J. L. Sievenpiper, R. Owen, E. Vidgen, F. Brighenti, R. Josse, L. A. Leiter, and C. Bruce-Thompson. 1999. "Konjac-mannan (glucomannan) improves glycemia and other associated risk factors for coronary heart disease in type 2 diabetes. A randomized controlled metabolic trial." *Diabetes Care* 22 (6): 913–919.

Vuksan, V., J. L. Sievenpiper, V. Y. Y. Koo, T. Francis, U. Beljan-Zdravkovic, Z. Xu, and E. Vidgen. 2000a. "American ginseng (panax quinquefolius L) reduces postprandial glycemia in nondiabetic subjects and subjects with type 2 diabetes mellitus." *Archives of Internal Medicine* 160 (7): 1009–1013.

Vuksan, V., J. L. Sievenpiper, Z. Xu, E. Y. Y. Wong, A. L. Jenkins, U. Beljan-Zdravkovic, L. A. Leiter, R. G. Josse, and M. P. Stavro. 2001. "Konjac-mannan and american ginsing: Emerging alternative therapies for type 2 diabetes mellitus." *Journal of the American College of Nutrition* 20 (5 Suppl): 370S–380S.

Vuksan, V., M. P. Stavro, J. L. Sievenpiper, U. Beljan-Zdravkovic, L. A. Leiter, R. G. Josse, and Z. Xu. 2000b. "Similar postprandial glycemic reductions with escalation of dose and administration time of american ginseng in type 2 diabetes." *Diabetes Care* 23 (9): 1221–1226.

Vuksan, V., M.-K. Sung, J. L. Sievenpiper, P. Mark Stavro, A. L. Jenkins, M. Di Buono, K.-S. Lee, L. A. Leiter, K. Y. Nam, and J. T. Arnason. 2008. "Korean red ginseng (panax ginseng) improves glucose and insulin regulation in well-controlled, type 2 diabetes: Results of a randomized, double-blind, placebo-controlled study of efficacy and safety." *Nutrition, Metabolism and Cardiovascular Diseases* 18 (1): 46–56.

Wang, G., C. Q. Xiao, Z. Li, D. Guo, Y. Chen, L. Fan, R. H. Qian, X. J. Peng, D. L. Hu, and H. H. Zhou. 2009. "Effect of soy extract administration on losartan pharmacokinetics in healthy female volunteers." *The Annals of Pharmacotherapy* 43 (6): 1045–1049. doi:10.1345/aph.1L690 [doi].

Wang, J., Z. Lu, J. Chi, W. Wang, M. Su, W. Kou, P. Yu, L. Yu, L. Chen, and J.-S. Zhu. 1997. "Multicenter clinical trial of the serum lipid-lowering effects of a monascus purpureus (red yeast) rice preparation from traditional chinese medicine." *Current Therapeutic Research* 58 (12): 964–978.

Wang, J.-J., M.-J. Shieh, S.-L. Kuo, C.-L. Lee, and T.-M. Pan. 2006. "Effect of red mold rice on antifatigue and exercise-related changes in lipid peroxidation in endurance exercise." *Applied Microbiology and Biotechnology* 70 (2): 247–253.

Welihinda, J., E. H. Karunanayake, M.H. H. Sheriff, and K. S. A. Jayasinghe. 1986. "Effect of momordica charantia on the glucose tolerance in maturity onset diabetes." *Journal of Ethnopharmacology* 17 (3): 277–282.

Wiwanitkit, V. and W. Taungjaruwinai. 2004. "A case report of suspect ginseng allergy." *MedGenMed: Medscape General Medicine* 6 (3): 9. doi:482833 [pii].

World Health Organization. "Diabetes." Accessed March 29, 2017, http://www.who.int/diabetes/en/.

Wu, Z., J. Z. Luo, and L. Luo. 2007. "American ginseng modulates pancreatic beta cell activities." *Chinese Medicine* 2 (1): 11.

Yang, B., Y. Chen, T.-C. Xu, Y.-H. Yu, T. Huang, X.-J. Hu, and D. Li. 2011. "Systematic review and meta-analysis of soy products consumption in patients with type 2 diabetes mellitus." *Asia Pacific Journal of Clinical Nutrition* 20 (4): 593–602.

Yang, J., Q. X. Mao, H. X. Xu, X. Ma, and C. Y. Zeng. 2014. "Tea consumption and risk of type 2 diabetes mellitus: A systematic review and meta-analysis apdate." *BMJ Open* 4 (7): e005632-2014-005632. doi:10.1136/bmjopen-2014-005632 [doi].

Yarnell, E. "Lemonbalm: Humble yet potent herb." *Alternative Complementary Therapy* December 1998. 4(6): 417–419.

Yarnell, E. and K. Abascal. "Botanical medicine for thyroid regulation." *Alternative Complemtenary Therapy* June 2006 12(3): 107–112.

Yeh, G. Y., D. M. Eisenberg, T. J. Kaptchuk, and R. S. Phillips. 2003. "Systematic review of herbs and dietary supplements for glycemic control in diabetes." *Diabetes Care* 26 (4): 1277–1294.

Ziaei, S., S. Hantoshzadeh, P. Rezasoltani, and M. Lamyian. 2001. "The effect of garlic tablet on plasma lipids and platelet aggregation in nulliparous pregnants at high risk of preeclampsia." *European Journal of Obstetrics & Gynecology and Reproductive Biology* 99 (2): 201–206.

Ziai, S. A., B. Larijani, S. Akhoondzadeh, H. Fakhrzadeh, A. Dastpak, F. Bandarian, A. Rezai, H. N. Badi, and Tara Emami. 2005. "Psyllium decreased serum glucose and glycosylated hemoglobin significantly in diabetic outpatients." *Journal of Ethnopharmacology* 102 (2): 202–207.

7

Gastrointestinal Disease

Lauren M. Hynicka, LaDonna M. Oelschlaeger, and Gregory Zumach

CONTENTS

7.1 Introduction

The use of complementary and alternative medicine (CAM) has increased significantly in the United States over the past 20 years (Clarke et al. 2015). Data from the 2012 National Health Interview Survey identified CAM use in a sample of 34,525 American adults (Dossett et al. 2014). Of these, 39% of respondents reported at least one gastrointestinal (GI) condition in the past year and 42%, or 5,629, had used CAM. Botanical use ranged from 19.5% to 30.7% for abdominal pain, acid reflux and heartburn, digestive allergy, liver conditions, nausea and vomiting, and ulcers (Dossett et al. 2014). Finally, an important consideration is that gastrointestinal conditions are a key area where multiple botanicals are used in combination, especially for functional dyspepsia and irritable bowel syndrome.

UPPER GASTROINTESTINAL

7.2 Functional Nonulcer Dyspepsia

7.2.1 Caraway (*Carum carvi*)

7.2.1.1 Background

Caraway is a biennial plant in the family of Apliaceae that is native to Northern Africa, Europe, and Asia. The use of caraway may have originated with the ancient Arabs, who called the seeds karawya, a name they still bear in the East, and probably the origin of the modern English word caraway and the Latin name Carvi. Caraway was used in Egypt, in ancient Mesopotamian civilizations, and by the Greeks and Romans (Saller et al. 2001).

7.2.1.2 Pharmacognosy

The caraway seeds and fruit are the plant parts that are predominantly used for health benefits. Leaves and roots are also used in some preparations. The oils extracted from the seeds may be used for medicinal purposes. Human studies have demonstrated an antispasmodic effect attributed to peppermint/caraway oil preparations (Micklefield et al. 2003; Goerg and Spilker 2003; Micklefield et al. 2000). The exact mechanism of action is not well understood and the effects of caraway alone are unclear.

7.2.1.3 Dosing and Preparation

Caraway is used orally for digestive problems. The general dose for adults is 1–6 g of dried caraway fruit daily or ripe caraway fruit crushed directly before use. A tea may be prepared using 1–2 tsp of pressed seeds in 150 mL of boiling water. The tea should be covered and allowed to steep for 10–15 minutes; consume 2–4 cups daily between meals.

The dose for children over 10 years of age has included 1.5–6 g of dried caraway fruit or 3–6 drops of caraway oil daily. For children aged 4–10 years, 1–4 g of dried fruit or 3–6 drops of caraway oil daily has been used. For children aged 1–4 years, 1–2 g of dried fruit or 2–4 drops of caraway oil has been used daily (Dorsch et al. 1998).

7.2.1.4 Safety

The consumption of caraway is likely safe when used orally in medicinal amounts (Madisch et al. 1999). It has been recognized as safe (GRAS) in the U.S. The combination product Enteroplant®, consisting of 90 mg of peppermint oil and 50 mg of caraway, has been well tolerated in studies (Freise and Kohler 1999; May et al. 2000; Micklefield et al. 2000). Adverse effects such as a substernal burning sensation, eructation, flatulence, vomiting, and nausea were observed in response to caraway administration (May et al. 2000; Micklefield et al. 2000). These symptoms may be less frequent in patients treated with enteric-coated capsules containing peppermint and caraway oils.

7.2.1.5 Evidence

In a prospective, randomized, double-blind, controlled multicenter trial, 223 patients with nonulcer dyspepsia compared the safety and efficacy of two preparations of a fixed combination of peppermint oil and caraway oil. The test formulation was an enteric coated capsule containing 90 mg peppermint oil and 50 mg caraway oil, while an enteric soluble formulation containing 36 mg peppermint oil and 20 mg of caraway oil was the reference product. The main outcome was the difference in pain intensity between the beginning and end of therapy, measured by the patient on a visual analogue scale (0 = no pain, 10 = extremely strong pain). Both groups were similar with respect to concomitant variables. The efficacy of the test preparation was significantly better with regard to pain frequency (p = 0.04). Both preparations were well tolerated (Freise and Kohler 1999).

A multi-ingredient combination product, Iberogast, contains caraway among many other components. A meta-analysis of three placebo-controlled studies with this product reported a reduction in gastrointestinal symptoms from functional dyspepsia (Melzer et al. 2004).

7.2.1.6 Clinical Application

Caraway oil is part of many preparations used to treat functional nonulcer dyspepsia. When used with peppermint oil, caraway is effective in treating disorders associated with the gastrointestinal symptoms regardless of their *Helicobacter pylori* (*H. pylori*) status. The effects of caraway alone are unclear.

7.3 Gastritis/Intestinal Ulcers

7.3.1 Licorice (*Glycyrrhiza glabra, Glycyrrhiza glabra var. Glandulifera, Glycyrrhiza uralensis*)

7.3.1.1 Background

Licorice root is a perennial herb native to the Mediterranean region, as well as central and Southwestern Asia. It has been used for more than 4,000 years for the treatment of hepatic protection, Addison's disease, asthma, bronchitis, peptic ulcer disease, and arthritis (Del Prete et al. 2012; Kaur et al. 2013). Licorice is used throughout the food industry as a drink, candy, and sweetener, as well as by the tobacco industry (Isbrucker and Burdock 2006; Jung et al. 2014).

7.3.1.2 Pharmacognosy

Glycyrrhizin is an aqueous extract from the root of the *Glycyrrhizin glabra* plant (Dhiman and Chawla 2005). It contains glycyrrhetic acid, multiple flavonoids, isoflavonoids, hydroxycoumarins, and sterols. Glycyrrhizin is likely beneficial in gastritis and intestinal ulcers secondary to its anti-inflammatory actions.

In laboratory studies, glycyrrhizin has been shown to inhibit production of prostaglandins and nitric oxide. The inhibition of hydrocortisone metabolism by 11 beta-hydroxysteroid dehydrogenase has also been suggested as a potential mechanism of its anti-inflammatory action.

7.3.1.3 Dosing and Preparation

In general, licorice products are standardized to glycyrrhizin content and are available orally, topically, and intravenously.

7.3.1.4 Safety

Licorice is generally safe at a dose of 100 mg per day or less (Isbrucker and Burdock 2006). Clinical studies indicate that licorice may cause edema and Cushing Syndrome secondary to inhibition of 11β-hydroxysteroid dehydrogenase type 2 (Kao et al. 2014). Long-term use may increase the risk of a range of cardiovascular complications, including hypertension and chronic heart failure, especially among people with underlying cardiovascular or renal diseases. Pseudohyperaldosteronism has been attributed to excessive licorice ingestion (Sabbadin and Armanini 2016).

Licorice has the potential for multiple drug interactions including with corticosteroids. Concomitant use of licorice and oral corticosteroids, such as hydrocortisone, has been shown to potentiate the duration of activity, and increase blood levels, of corticosteroids (Armanini et al. 1996; Quinkler and Stewart 2003).

7.3.1.5 Evidence

Many of the published studies on the efficacy of licorice for the treatment of peptic disease are over 40 years old. The studies were conducted before the widespread clinical use of histamine-2 receptor antagonists (H2RAs) and proton pump inhibitors (PPIs) such as omeprazole. Although more recent data in humans is limited, healthcare providers have become aware of the risks of H2RAs and PPIs especially when used inappropriately for prolonged periods of time. Licorice has been suggested as a method for tapering off more these drugs for peptic ulcer disease.

More recently, the use of licorice has been evaluated in multiple studies as part of treatment regimens for patients with *H. pylori* as the likely cause of their peptic ulcer disease. In an Iranian clinical trial of 60 patients with a mean age of about 41 years with confirmed *H. pylori* peptic ulcer disease, participants were randomized to quadruple therapy consisting of amoxicillin, metronidazole, and omeprazole with the addition of either licorice or bismuth as the fourth agent. The urea breath test was repeated in 4 weeks with 67% and 57% of the licorice and bismuth groups, respectively, demonstrating a positive response to treatment (Momeni et al. 2014).

The evidence for its use for hepatic disease is discussed in Section 7.7.

7.3.1.6 Clinical Application

Although older studies have supported its role in peptic ulcer disease, information comparing licorice to standard treatments is limited. Most clinicians however are concerned about the long-term adverse effects of PPIs for peptic ulcer disease. Importantly, several small studies have suggested a potential role in *H. pylori* associated disease.

7.3.2 Mastic (*Pistacia*)

7.3.2.1 Background

Pistacia lentiscus of the family *Anacardiaceae* is grown in the eastern Mediterranean especially in Greece and Turkey. Mastic gum is a resin from the trunk and branches of the shrub. It has been used in Greek medicine for dyspepsia and peptic ulcer disease for over 2,000 years (Paraschos et al. 2007).

7.3.2.2 Pharmacognosy

The mechanism of action of mastic in the healing of gastric and duodenal ulcers has not been identified. Of note, mastic may have antisecretory effects reducing gastric acidity (Huwez et al. 1998; Paraschos et al. 2007). In addition, mastic has antibacterial action against *H. pylori in vitro*. *H. pylori* neutrophil activating protein, a potential virulence factor, has pro-inflammatory and immunomodulating effects and mastic may inter with this protein (Kottakis et al. 2009). *In vitro* and *in vivo* studies have demonstrated that colonization with *H. pylori* is reduced and that triterpenic acids may contribute to this effect (Paraschos et al. 2007). The anti-inflammatory effects of *Pistacia lentiscus* may also involve inhibition of xanthine oxidase (Berboucha et al. 2010).

7.3.2.3 Dosing and Preparation

Dosages of mastic gum have been 350 mg three times daily in studies of *H. pylori* infection and functional dyspepsia. Mastic gum has been added to standard *H. pylori* regimens for a total of 14 days, while dyspepsia studies have been for a duration of 3–4 weeks (Dabos et al. 2010a,b).

7.3.2.4 Safety

Mastic gum is well tolerated (Kartalis et al. 2016).

7.3.2.5 Evidence

A small, open label study of patients with gastric ulcer evaluated the effects of mastic resin on the treatment of the ulcer (Huwez and Al-Habbal 1986). Participants took 1 g of mastic powder twice daily, before breakfast and at bedtime, for 4 weeks. All 6 patients had symptomatic relief with five experiencing ulcer healing.

A double-blind, randomized controlled trial comparing the administration of 1 g of mastic powder versus 1 g of lactose placebo for the treatment of duodenal ulcer (Al Habbal et al. 1984). Sixty patients with duodenal ulcer were assigned to mastic or placebo. Subjects were instructed to ingest 1 g of powder daily with breakfast. Patients were excluded if they had taken any antiulcer medication within 1 month prior to enrollment, were pregnant or lactating, were less than 20 years of age, or had pyloric stenosis. At the end of the 2-week period, patients returned for a clinical examination including a repeat endoscopy. Twenty-two patients were lost to follow-up and were not included in the final analysis. Of patients completing the study, those receiving mastic had at least a three-fold greater ulcer healing, as confirmed by endoscopy. In addition, almost twice as many participants receiving mastic experienced symptomatic relief. This study was limited by a 37% dropout rate and limited information on blinding and randomization (Al Habbal et al. 1984).

7.3.2.6 Clinical Application

Mastic gum is well tolerated. Given the increasing resistance of *H. pylori,* it may be a useful addition to the treatment of peptic ulcer disease due to this bacteria.

7.4 Nausea/Vomiting

7.4.1 Ginger (*Zingiber officinale*)

7.4.1.1 Background

Ginger originated in Southeast Asia and has been used as a spice and medicine for thousands of years (Afzal et al. 2001; Ahmad et al. 2015). The use of ginger can be found in the ancient writings in Chinese, Indian, and Middle Eastern cultures. Common uses for ginger include cough, cold, motion sickness, gastrointestinal, and liver disorders.

7.4.1.2 Pharmacognosy

Ginger is the underground rhizome of the ginger plant. Over 60 active compounds have been found in ginger which are divided into volatile and nonvolatile compounds (Ahmad et al. 2015). The nonvolatile compounds vary depending on the place of origin and whether the rhizomes are fresh or dried (Ali et al. 2008). The nonvolatile compounds, which are responsible for ginger's biological effects include gingerols, shagaols, paradols, and zingerone. Zingerone and shagaols are the dehydrated form of gingerols and develop when ginger is stored. Paradols are the result of the reduction of shogaols (Afzal et al. 2001). Ginger may neutralize gastrointestinal toxins and acids, thereby slowing feedback from the stomach to the nausea centers in the brain (Ahmad et al. 2008). Ginger may also have antagonist activity at the serotonin 5-HT$_3$ receptor, contributing to its antiemetic properties.

7.4.1.3 Dosing and Preparation

Most studies of this botanical have administered the ginger in a capsule formulation. The frequency of administration and dosing of ginger in studies has varied, with the dosages between 167 and 800 mg per capsule. One study investigated the possibility of developing a transdermal patch containing numerous ingredients of which ginger was included. The authors used the volatile component of ginger. It is unclear if the volatile components would have a similar biological effect as the nonvolatile components. No clinical studies have evaluated the efficacy of this dosage form to administer ginger (Saleem and Idris 2016).

A 2006 study evaluated the concentrations of 6-gingerol, 6-shogaol, 8-gingerol, and 10-gingerol, in 10 commercially available ginger root dietary supplements purchased from both local pharmacies and health food stores. A wide variation in concentrations of nonvolatile components was identified between supplements and the suggested serving size ranged from 250 mg to 4.77 g per day (Schwertner et al. 2006).

7.4.1.4 Safety

In a systematic review, the most common adverse events with ginger when used for the treatment of chemotherapy induced nausea and vomiting (CINV) included heartburn, bruising, flushing, rash, and gastrointestinal discomfort (Marx et al. 2013). In terms of drug interactions, concerns have existed about using ginger in combination with antithrombotic agents. In typical dosages, however, ginger does not influence platelet function and case reports have not documented an increased risk of bleeding when used in combination with antithrombotic agents (Vaes and Chyka 2000). *See Chapter 8 Women's Health for further discussion.*

7.4.1.5 Evidence

Ginger has been investigated for the treatment of nausea and vomiting due to motion sickness, pregnancy, chemotherapy, and following surgery. Ginger has been approved by the German Commission E for the prevention of motion sickness. Several small studies have been conducted to determine the efficacy of ginger in the prevention or motion sickness. Doses varied from 500 to 3150 mg but all studies showed an increased time before the patients felt nauseous and decreased the severity of nausea (Abascal and Yarnell 2009). *See Chapters 8 Women's Health, 14 Musculoskeletal Conditions, and 17 Supportive Care for use for other conditions.*

7.4.1.6 Clinical Application

Ginger may be effective in the relief of nausea but has less impact on vomiting. It is well tolerated and has few safety concerns. Significant variability in terms of nonvolatile components has been observed among commercially available ginger products.

LOWER GASTROINTESTINAL CONDITIONS

7.5 Diarrhea

7.5.1 Arrowroot

7.5.1.1 Background

Arrowroot is a starch found in the rootstock or rhizome of several related species, most notably *Maranta arundinacea*. Arrowroot is most commonly found in tropical climates, especially Central and South America, the Caribbean, and the West Indies. The starch found in *Maranta arundinacea* does not contain gluten and is being used increasingly by individuals who have celiac disease, as well as others.

7.5.1.2 Pharmacognosy

The key starch found in arrowroot comes from extraction from the rhizomes. Its mechanism to reduce diarrhea is not well understood. Animal models have provided evidence that arrowroot decreases toxin effects from cholera. It is unclear if the starch is able to block the toxins of any other pathogenic species of bacteria, such as salmonella or shigella (Cooke et al. 2000). This starch product is not completely absorbed in the small intestine with 20% unchanged entering the colon. The greater amounts of starch in diet increase fecal bulking through supply of a larger quantity of unchanged starch to reach the colon and subsequently be broken down by gut bacteria. By providing an increased energy source, more fiber may be able to pass through the colon without being broken down by normal gut flora (Shetty and Kurpad 1986).

7.5.1.3 Dosing and Preparation

Through the starch extraction from the rootstock, arrowroot is able to be ground up and dried into a powder form. Unfortunately, the pure white powder form has a history of unscrupulous mixing with potato flour, while misidentifying the product as pure arrowroot. In powder form, it can be used as a substitute for other starches in baking. Medicinal quantities are not well defined with the only study using 10 milliliters three times daily (Cooke et al. 2000).

7.5.1.4 Safety

Consumption of arrowroot is generally considered safe in amounts found in food and medicinal amounts of 10 milliliters powder three times daily. Adverse effects were primarily gastrointestinal related with the most common being dark stools and constipation (Cooke et al. 2000).

7.5.1.5 Evidence

Arrowroot may be beneficial in patients with diarrhea. In a pilot study, arrowroot was provided with meals to 11 patients who were classified as having irritable bowel syndrome. Each participant was provided 10 milliliters of arrowroot powder three times daily for one month. At the end of the study, patients were given a questionnaire in order to describe symptoms. A reduction in abdominal pain, as well as diarrhea, was reported by participants (Cooke et al. 2000). Of note, the study was small and was not blinded.

7.5.1.6 Clinical Application

The use of arrowroot is predominantly for diarrhea symptoms. Research has also centered on evaluating its usage in gastrointestinal motility disorders such as irritable bowel syndrome.

7.5.2 Carob Fruit

7.5.2.1 Background

The Carob fruit tree, *Ceratonia siliqua*, is a common plant native to the Mediterranean. The seeds are primarily exported to be produced into carob bean gum (CBG) to thicken and flavor foods. In addition, carob pods have been used as a cocoa substitute (Goulas et al. 2016).

7.5.2.2 Pharmacognosy

As a member of the Fabaceae family, carob is related to other legumes such as peas, soybeans, lentils, and peanuts. The fruit of *Ceratonia siliqua* is an elongated pod, which is incorporated into two major components, the pulp (90%) and the seeds (10%). Carob pulp is high in sugars such as sucrose, glucose, and fructose, as well as dietary fibers and, predominantly when ripened, polyphenols.

7.5.2.3 Dosing and Preparation

Carob fiber is removed via water separation where a combination of soluble and insoluble fibers are present. CBG originates from the polysaccharides found in the seed endosperm. Tannins, predominantly phenols, gallotannins, and flavonoids, are abundantly found within the fiber, pulp, and seed (Goulas et al.

2016). When evaluating dosing and potency of carob, products with a high concentration of tannins have been linked to greater control of diarrhea symptoms.

7.5.2.4 Safety

Carob is generally regarded as safe with no adverse effects related to its use in patients aged 3 months and older.

7.5.2.5 Evidence

Research related to the antidiarrheal effects of carob are centered on the activity of tannins. One study used concentrations of 40% tannins from the carob pod extract in infants aged 3–21 months. After 24–48 hours, patients given carob had improvements in bowel movements, body temperature, and body weight. The improvements of GI function may be related to an effect on common gut pathogens, *E.coli* and rotavirus (Loeb et al. 1989). The research in tannins has been validated by an *in vitro* study (Liu et al.2014). The study demonstrated that when the intestines are exposed to tannins, aquaporin expression is decreased, one of the gut's main protein channels responsible for transferring water into the gut leading to GI motility (Liu et al. 2014). A study from Switzerland assessed the efficacy and adverse effects from carob for traveler's diarrhea with no difference in efficacy between those who took the product correctly and those who were noncompliant (Hostettler et al. 1995).

7.5.2.6 Clinical Application

Carob fruit offers an appealing option for patients suffering from diarrhea. It is well tolerated and may offer the benefit of reducing GI motility, especially in infants.

7.6 Constipation

7.6.1 Aloe (*Aloe Vera, Synonyms Aloe barbadensis, Aloe indica, Aloe africana, Aloe arborescens, Synonyms Aloe natalensis*)

7.6.1.1 Background

Aloe is a cactus-like plant in the Liliacaea or Lily family and grows in hot, dry climates (Vogler and Ernst 1999). In the United States, aloe is cultivated in Florida, Texas, and Arizona.

7.6.1.2 Pharmacognosy

The applicable part of aloe is the leaf from which multiple components can be extracted. Most aloe-containing products use aloe gel or aloe latex. The different forms of aloe contain varied active constituents and physiologic effects. Aloe contains strong laxative compounds such as aloin, aloe-emodin, and barbaloin (Reynolds and Dweck 1999; Foster et al. 2011). In colorectal mucosa *in vitro*, aloe gel has an antioxidant effect, decreasing levels of colorectal prostaglandin E2 and interleukin-8 (Langmead et al. 2004).

7.6.1.3 Dosing and Preparation

The typical oral dose for constipation is 100–200 mg aloe or 50 mg aloe extract taken in the evening. A 500 mg capsules containing a formulation of celandine, aloe, and psyllium in a 6:3:1 ratio, starting at a dose of one capsule daily and increasing to three capsules daily as required, has been used (Odes and Madar 1991).

See Chapter 13 Dermatological Conditions for discussion on topical use.

7.6.1.4 Safety

Some evidence has indicated that anthraquinones in aloe latex are carcinogenic or promote tumor growth, although data are conflicting (Cosmetic Ingredient Review Expert Panel 2007). One rat study using nondecolorized whole leaf extract containing aloin demonstrated tumors in the large intestines (NCCIH 2016). An additional study using decolorized extract did not identify a similar carcinogenic risk (NCCIH 2016).

7.6.1.5 Evidence

One study evaluated the effect of a laxative preparation, composed of celandin, aloevera, and psyllium, in patients with chronic constipation (Odes and Madar 1991). Thirty-five men and women were randomized to receive capsules containing celandin-aloevera-psyllium, or placebo, in a double-blind trial lasting 28 days. Symptoms in the last 2 weeks of the treatment period were compared to those in the 14-day pre-trial basal period. In the active treatment group, bowel movements became more frequent, the stools were softer and laxative dependence was reduced. In the placebo group, these parameters were unchanged. Abdominal pain was not reduced in either group. The results of this study show that the preparation is an effective laxative in the treatment of constipation.

See Chapter 13 Dermatological Conditions for discussion on topical use.

7.6.1.6 Clinical Application

Few recent clinical studies have been conducted to evaluate the laxative effect of aloe latex in humans. The question of whether aloe latex may offer a safe approach to treating constipation is unanswered, especially given the other available options.

7.6.2 Barley (*Hordeum vulgare, Hordeum distychum*)

7.6.2.1 Background

Barley is a cereal grain used as a staple food in many countries. It is commonly used as an ingredient in baked products and soup in Europe and the United States. Barley was historically used by the Romans to treat boils and by the Greeks to treat gastrointestinal inflammation. Barley has been used for many gastrointestinal conditions including gastritis and inflammatory bowel disease.

7.6.2.2 Pharmacognosy

Germinated barley foodstuff (GBF) is derived from the aleurone and scutellum fractions of germinated barley. GBF appears to induce proliferation of intestinal epithelial cells and facilitate defecation through bacterial production of short-chain fatty acids, especially butyrate. GBF may facilitate epithelial repair and suppress epithelial NFkB-DNA binding activity through butyrate by the microflora *Bifidobacterium* and *Eubacterium*. GBF has been associated with increased growth of these microflora in the intestinal tract (Kanauchi et al. 2001).

7.6.2.3 Dosing and Preparation

Both GBF, 9 g or 18 g daily for 10 days, and GBF, 9 g daily for 14 days, have been studied for the relief of constipation in humans (Kanauchi et al. 1998).

7.6.2.4 Safety

Barley is generally safe (Fuchs et al. 1999; Alberts et al. 2000; Schatzkin et al. 2000). It is well tolerated in healthy adults in normal doses for short periods of time. Multiple cases of allergy have been reported, and cross-reactivity may occur in individuals with an allergy to grass or wheat. GBF in doses as high as 30 g was tolerated in 10 patients with mild-to-moderate active ulcerative colitis over a 4-week period (Kanauchi et al. 2001).

7.6.2.5 Evidence

Nine healthy volunteers received 9 g of GBF daily for 10 days, after which the dose was increased to 18 grams for an additional 10 days (Kanauchi et al. 1998). Outcome measures included fecal weight and short-chain fatty acid content, which were compared to baseline values. Results indicated that GBF at both doses resulted in increases in fecal butyrate content and fecal weight compared to baseline.

Following this study, a second trial was conducted in 16 volunteers who were chronically constipated (Kanauchi et al. 1998). These subjects were administered 9 g of GBF daily for 14 days. Measured outcomes included frequency and volume of stool, assessed by a subjective questionnaire survey. The GBF significantly improved these measures compared to baseline. Of note, a standardized measurement instrument was not used, long-term outcomes were not assessed, and the results were not compared to a control group.

See Chapter 15 Obesity and Weight Loss for further discussion.

7.6.2.6 Clinical Application

Barley has been used traditionally as a treatment for constipation due to its high fiber content.

7.6.3 Psyllium (*Plantago psyllium, Synonym Psyllium afra, Psyllium indica, Synonym Psyllium arenaria*)

7.6.3.1 Background

Psyllium is a dietary fiber from the seeds of *Plantago* and related species. Psyllium is used commonly for chronic constipation and for softening stools in conditions such as hemorrhoids, anal fissures, anorectal surgery, and pregnancy (NCCIH). In addition, psyllium has been used as an adjunct to improve glycemic control in patients with Type 2 diabetes mellitus.

7.6.3.2 Pharmacognosy

Psyllium seed forms a mucilaginous mass when mixed with water and has a bulk laxative effect. In people with diarrhea, the mucilage absorbs water, provides mass, and prolongs gastrointestinal transit (Newall et al. 1996; Blumenthal 1998). In individuals with constipation, the mucilage absorbs water, swells, and stimulates peristalsis, reducing gastrointestinal transit time (Newall et al. 1996; Blumenthal 1998).

7.6.3.3 Dosing and Preparation

As a laxative, the typical dose of psyllium seed is 10–30 grams per day (Blumenthal 1998; Gruenwald et al. 1998) in divided amounts. The FDA labeling recommends at least 8 ounces of water or other fluid with each dose. The ingestion of this product with insufficient liquid may result in choking.

7.6.3.4 Safety

Oral psyllium can cause transient flatulence and abdominal distention. When consumed without water, esophageal and bowel obstruction may occur (Agha et al. 1984; Newall et al. 1996). Psyllium should be avoided in people with fecal impaction, gastrointestinal obstructions, or narrowing. Allergic reactions to psyllium include allergic rhinitis, conjunctivitis, urticaria, and asthma (Gruenwald et al. 1998). Occupational exposure to psyllium can cause sensitization, of which symptoms include sneezing, watery eyes, chest congestion, and anaphylactoid reaction (Gruenwald et al. 1998). Psyllium may lower blood glucose levels in people with Type 2 diabetes and patients should monitor their levels carefully (Frati Munari et al. 1998).

7.6.3.5 Evidence

In a review of published studies, the use of psyllium in chronic constipation in older adults resulted in a high weekly stool frequency compared to docusate and placebo (Fleming and Wade 2010). The review stated that significant differences existed in the trial quality, methodology, and endpoints. An earlier systematic review rated the evidence supporting psyllium as moderate (Ramkumar and Rao 2005).

See Chapters 5 Cardiovascular Disease, 6 Endocrine Disorders, and 15 Obesity and Weight Loss for further discussion in other conditions.

7.6.3.6 Clinical Application

Psyllium has been commonly used as a bulk laxative to reduce constipation. It may also offer benefit for diarrhea and IBS as it is not absorbed and does not have systemic effects.

7.7 Inflammatory Bowel Disease

7.7.1 *Boswellia serrata*

7.7.1.1 Background

See Chapter 14 Musculoskeletal Conditions for discussion.

7.7.1.2 Pharmacognosy

See Chapter 14 Musculoskeletal Conditions for discussion.

7.7.1.3 Dosing and Preparation

The use of boswellia in inflammatory bowel disease (IBD) requires much higher doses than doses needed for osteoarthritis. In trials of ulcerative colitis and Crohn's disease, 300 mg three times daily appears to be the minimum dose needed for reduction in inflammation (Gupta et al. 1997).

7.7.1.4 Safety

See Chapter 14 Musculoskeletal Conditions for discussion.

7.7.1.5 Evidence

Data are mixed on whether boswellia presents an effective treatment for IBD. One study compared between *Boswellia serrata* and sulfasalazine for mild to moderate ulcerative colitis. Boswellia resin of 300 mg three times daily by mouth was given to 20 patients in the study, while 10 patients received 1 g of sulfasalazine three times daily. In 14 of the 20 patients given the botanical, remission was achieved, while 4 of the 10 achieved clinical remission using sulfasalazine (Gupta et al. 1997). For Crohn's disease, data are mixed. When the resin was compared to placebo over 12 months in 108 patients with Crohn's disease in remission, the rates of maintenance of remission, relapse time, and severity of symptoms were similar (Holtmeier et al. 2011).

7.7.1.6 Clinical Application

The evidence in ulcerative colitis and the mixed results in Crohn's disease have identified a potential role for boswellia in IBD if additional studies can confirm its benefits. Although promising, studies should always ensure the botanical is being compared to standard therapy for the specific phase of the disease such as induction versus maintenance of remission of disease flares.

7.7.2 Turmeric

7.7.2.1 Background

See Chapter 14 Musculoskeletal Conditions for discussion.

7.7.2.2 Pharmacognosy

See Chapter 14 Musculoskeletal Conditions for discussion.

7.7.2.3 Dosing and Preparation

Unlike turmeric products used in osteoarthritis, turmeric used in IBD is evaluated based on the quantity of curcumin rather than the overall extract. Turmeric doses used for IBD disease require approximately 1–2 grams orally daily of the active curcumin component to achieve symptom improvement (Hanai et al. 2006).

7.7.2.4 Safety

See Chapter 14 Musculoskeletal Conditions for discussion.

7.7.2.5 Evidence

One study of participants ages 13–65 years evaluated curcumin with sulfasalazine or mesalamine compared to sulfasalazine or mesalamine alone. In the 45 patients who received the additional 1 g twice daily of oral curcumin, researchers found significant decreases in clinical activity index and in levels of inflammation detected via endoscopic results at 6 months (Hanai et al. 2006). The rate of symptom recurrence was low with the addition of curcumin. A Cochrane review assessed this study to be of high quality with a low risk of bias (Garg et al. 2012).

Rectal therapy of mesalamine enemas or suppositories is a mainstay in the treatment of mild to moderate distal ulcerative colitis (Kornbluth and Sachar 2010). One study evaluated if rectal curcumin products could become an option for patients with ulcerative disease. Patients were randomized to receive either mesalamine with either a curcumin or placebo enema. Each curcumin enema contained 140 mg of curcumin product mixed with 20 milliliters of water. Patients in both the treatment and placebo arms of the study received 800 mg of oral mesalamine twice daily. The authors did not find statistical differences between the two sets of patients which may have been due to the small sample size. Serious adverse effects were not noted (Singla et al. 2014).

See Chapters 14 Musculoskeletal Conditions, 16 Cancer Prevention and Treatment, and 17 Supportive Care and Palliative Care for Cancer for further discussion in other conditions.

7.7.2.6 Clinical Application

With its favorable safety profile, turmeric and curcumin provide an option for inflammatory bowel disease if additional studies confirm these findings.

7.7.3 Wheatgrass

7.7.3.1 Background

Wheatgrass, *Triticum aestivum*, is produced from the seed leafs of the common wheat plant. Wheatgrass, specifically the young blades of the wheat plant, have been used in ancient Egyptian and Mesopotamian cultures. Consumption of wheatgrass in the western world is linked to the work of Dr. Charles F. Schnabel, who used dehydrated wheatgrass powder and fed it to family and friends.

7.7.3.2 Pharmacognosy

Wheatgrass is prepared by sprouting wheat berries until the leaf is able to produce chlorophyll, the compound in plants responsible for photosynthesis. Once sprouted, the leaf is cut and juiced or dried and powdered.

7.7.3.3 Dosing and Preparation

Wheatgrass is administered in several forms including enemas, however taking it in juice orally is the most common. Medicinal quantities of wheatgrass are up to 100 milliliters taken orally (Marawaha et al. 2004). When evaluating products, research has only been conducted on fresh wheatgrass (Ben-Arye et al. 2002).

7.7.3.4 Safety

Serious adverse effects have not been noted with the consumption of wheatgrass in medicinal quantitates for up to 18 months (Marawaha et al. 2004). The most common adverse effect of wheatgrass is nausea (Ben-Ayre et al. 2002).

7.7.3.5 Evidence

Recommendations for wheatgrass in inflammatory bowel disease are based on one randomized, double-blinded, placebo-controlled trial (Ben-Arye et al. 2002). A total of 23 patients who had ulcerative colitis disease limited to the distal portion of the colon were randomized to 100 mL of wheatgrass juice or placebo for one month. Nineteen patients completed the study and had full data. Investigators found a significant reduction in disease activity, abdominal pain, and severity of rectal bleeding. This trial had a short duration and follow-up was limited.

7.7.3.6 Clinical Application

Wheatgrass has been studied in ulcerative colitis, as well as beta-thalassemia. One small study has supported its benefit in ulcerative colitis and based on the available evidence, wheatgrass is a safe product.

7.7.4 Peppermint

7.7.4.1 Background

Peppermint (*Mentha piperta*) is an herb. The oil or volatile component of peppermint has been used in cooking, perfumery, candies, as well as for medicinal purposes for thousands of years (Balakrishnan 2015). Peppermint has a long history in both Eastern and Western medical traditions, including ancient Greek, Roman, and Egyptian cultures. Common medical uses for peppermint include digestive complaints such as diarrhea, indigestion, nausea, and vomiting, as well as many other conditions.

7.7.4.2 Pharmacognosy

Peppermint is native to Europe and Asia (Ramasubramania Raja 2012). Peppermint leaves, both fresh and dried, are distilled to extract the essential oil (McKay and Blumberg 2006). The chemical components of peppermint leaves and oil vary based on plant age, plant variety, growing conditions, and processing procedures (McKay and Blumberg 2006). The main volatile components are menthol and methone. The mechanism of peppermint may be related to its ability to inhibit muscular contractions in the gastrointestinal tract, antispasmodic properties, accelerated gastric emptying and action on the 5-HT(3) receptors (Rita and Animesh 2011; Hines et al. 2012; Balakrishnan 2015).

7.7.4.3 Dosing and Preparation

Peppermint oil is available in enteric-coated capsules, where each capsule contains about 0.2 mL of peppermint oil. Common dosing for irritable bowel syndrome is one capsule three times daily (Khanna et al. 2014).

7.7.4.4 Safety

Peppermint oil and tea are well tolerated with few adverse effects including heartburn and contact sensitivity in adults. In children and adults, caution should be taken as inhalation has cause apnea, laryngeal and bronchial spasms, acute respiratory distress, and respiratory arrest (Rita and Animesh 2011; Szema and Barnett 2011).

7.7.4.5 Evidence

Peppermint oil has been effective as an antispasmodic for irritable bowel syndrome. One meta-analysis evaluated nine trials using peppermint oil in 726 patients (Khanna et al. 2014). The use of peppermint oil showed superiority in global symptoms compared to placebo for the treatment of irritable bowel syndrome for up to 3 months. This was demonstrated with a risk ratio of 2.23, where 0–1 favors placebo and >1 favors peppermint (CI 1.78–2.81, $P < 0.00001$) (Khanna et al. 2014). In addition, the American College of Gastroenterology supports the use of peppermint oil for short-term relief of abdominal pain in irritable bowel syndrome (Brandt et al. 2009).

Peppermint aromatherapy has been evaluated in the treatment of postoperative nausea and vomiting. One study investigated the efficacy of peppermint aromatherapy as compared to isopropyl alcohol or placebo in 33 patients undergoing general surgery, orthopedic surgery, or gynecological surgery. Nausea was evaluated using a visual analogue scale with the groups similar in terms of the change in visual analogue scale (VAS) at 2 minutes or 5 minutes after receiving aromatherapy (Anderson and Gross 2004).

Three studies have evaluated the efficacy of peppermint aromatherapy in women undergoing surgical procedures (Tate 1997; Ferruggiari et al. 2012; Lane et al. 2012). These studies have had between 18 and 70 patients. Peppermint oil reduced the nausea rate after gynecologic surgeries when compared to placebo (Tate 1997). Similarly, peppermint aromatherapy reduced nausea based on an ordinal nausea scale when compared to placebo and standard antiemetics (Lane et al. 2012). However, a third study found no difference in nausea scores between the placebo, peppermint oil, and ondansetron groups (Ferruggiari et al. 2012).

One study investigated the use of peppermint aromatherapy in patients following cardiac surgery. Peppermint aromatherapy was administered via a nasal inhaler to a total of 34 patients without a comparator group. A five-point nausea scale was used to assess nausea pre- and post-use of the peppermint nasal inhaler. The average pre-nausea score was 3.29 (SD, 1.0) and 2 minutes after using the nasal inhaler the average score was 1.44 (SD, 1.3), demonstrating a significant reduction in the nausea score (Briggs et al. 2016).

7.7.4.6 Clinical Application

Peppermint oil offers a promising short-term option for IBS symptoms due to its success in treating abdominal pain and low rate of adverse effects. Future studies are needed to evaluate long-term use in IBS. Peppermint aromatherapy following surgery has yielded mixed results in the reduction in nausea.

7.8 Liver

7.8.1 Licorice

7.8.1.1 Background

See Section 7.2.1 under Upper GI.

7.8.1.2 Pharmacognosy

Glycyrrhizin may have beneficial effects on liver disease via multiple mechanisms. It has been found to have anti-inflammatory and antiapoptotic activities via its inhibitory action on the numerous cytokines including tumor necrosis factor-alfa (TNF-α), IL-10 and caspase-3 (Dhiman and Chawla 2005).

7.8.1.3 Dosing and Preparation

In Japan, cysteine and glycine are added to glycyrrhizin. This compound is known as Stronger Neominophagen C (SNMC) and is used in the treatment of acute and chronic hepatitis. The solution is administered intravenously and contains 0.2% glycyrrhizin, 0.1% cysteine and 2% glycine (Kaur et al. 2013). In the United States, glycyrrhizin is available as many nonstandardized oral formulations.

7.8.1.4 Safety

See Section 7.2.1 under Upper GI.

7.8.1.5 Evidence

7.8.1.5.1 Hepatitis C Virus Infection

Licorice root has been evaluated for the treatment of nonalcoholic fatty liver disease and chronic viral hepatitis C (HCV) (van Rossum et al. 1999). Most of the evidence is in the treatment of HCV. Studies have been conducted in Japan, as well as Europe, and have shown glycyrrhizin administered intravenously to decrease and normalize alanine aminotransferase (ALT) (van Rossum et al. 2001). This improvement was not maintained when the glycyrrhizin treatment was stopped.

One study has evaluated the potential for intermittent, long-term administration of 2 dosages of glycyrrhizin as SNMC to improve ALT values in patients with chronic HCV (Miyake et al. 2002). The ALT values were improved in both groups suggesting that glycyrrhizin may be effective at maintaining normal biochemical markers in this population.

Improvements in biochemical markers have yielded mixed results in terms of liver histology. A decreased rate of hepatocellular carcinoma was observed in patients with chronic HCV who received ALT suppressive therapy with glycyrrhizin (Ikeda et al. 2006; Orlent et al. 2006). Glycyrrhizin therapy does not appear to impact HCV directly as studies have shown HCV RNA values remain similar after receipt of intravenous glycyrrhizin. In a 52-week study, half of the patients experienced an improvement in HCV activity score or necroinflammation suggesting possible decrease in disease activity (Manns et al. 2012).

7.8.1.5.2 Nonalcoholic Fatty Liver Disease

A small Iranian study evaluated the use of glycyrrhizin in patients with nonalcoholic fatty liver disease (NAFLD). The use of glycyrrhizin resulted in statistically significant decreases in serum ALT and aspartate aminotransferase (AST) compared to placebo (Hajiaghamohammadi et al. 2012). The clinical significance is unclear as the ALT decreased from 64.09 to 51.27 IU/mL and AST from 58.18 to 49.45 IU/mL.

7.8.1.5.3 Autoimmune Hepatitis

Intravenous glycyrrhizin has also been investigated in the treatment of acute autoimmune hepatitis. In a Japanese study, 17 patients received treatment with SNMC and 14 received SNMC in addition to corticosteroids (Yasui et al. 2011). In the SNMC monotherapy group, ALT decreased in all patients and returned the ALT to normal, defined as less than 40 IU/L, in 14 patients.

7.8.1.6 Clinical Application

Licorice may be beneficial for decreasing disease progression associated with chronic hepatitis C in patients who are not eligible to receive treatment with direct acting antiviral agents. The intravenous form is not available in the United States.

7.8.2 Silymarin (Milk Thistle)

7.8.2.1 Background

Silybum marianum is native to Europe, southern Russia, Asia Minor, and northern Africa. Its use for liver disorders dates back to the Greco-Roman era (Kaur et al. 2013).

7.8.2.2 Pharmacognosy

Silymarin is an active compound extracted from the seeds and fruit of the *Silybum marianum* plant (Biba et al. 2003; Kaur et al. 2013). It is a flavonolignan composed of silibinin, silydianine, and silychristine. These flavonolignans have antioxidant, anti-inflammatory, antifibrotic, and membrane stabilizing properties, which may be the mechanism for its hepatoprotection and success in treatment of chronic inflammatory liver disorders. Silibinin, also known as silybin, is the most active of the components, makes up about 50%–70% of the silymarin extract and has also been separated into a pure substance (Abenavoli et al. 2010; Kaur et al. 2013).

7.8.2.3 Dosing and Preparation

In the clinical trials, daily doses of silymarin have ranged from 280 to 800 mg. The recommended dosage for active liver disease is 140 mg by mouth three times daily usually using a formulation with enhanced bioavailability (Dhiman and Chawla 2005). As silymarin is poorly water soluble, special formulations including Legalon®, Silipide, and Siliphos have been developed to enhance the bioavailability of silybin.

7.8.2.4 Safety

Silymarin has a good safety profile with no adverse effects observed in healthy volunteers who received a single 254 mg dose of silybin. Adverse effects have also not been observed in patients with liver disorders receiving 600–800 mg a day of oral silymarin (Dhiman and Chawla 2005; Li et al. 2014). Doses of silymarin above 1500 mg may cause a laxative effect (Del Prete et al. 2012). An intravenous formulation of silibinin is also available. Silymarin and silybin are not expected to have significant drug interactions based on an *in vivo* study (Kaur et al. 2013). *See Chapter 2 Pharmacokinetic and Pharmacogenomic Considerations for in-depth discussion of milk thistle's influence on drug metabolism.*

7.8.2.5 Evidence

7.8.2.5.1 Alcohol Induced Liver Disease

Silymarin and silibinin have been evaluated primarily for use in acute hepatitis, chronic hepatitis, and in the prevention of drug-induced liver injury (DILI). The available evidence is difficult to interpret due small sample sizes, the variable severity of liver disease, heterogeneous dosages, the inconsistent use of a control group, and poorly defined outcomes.

Three studies have evaluated the efficacy of milk thistle in patients with alcohol-induced liver disease. They have been primarily focused on the ability of silymarin to decrease elevations in biomarkers associated with hepatic damage, including AST, ALT, serum bilirubin, and gamma-glutamyl transferase (GGT) (Dhiman and Chawla 2005).

7.8.2.5.2 Viral Hepatitis

In a randomized, placebo-controlled trial, the efficacy of silymarin to normalize bilirubin, AST, and ALT was evaluated in 105 patients with acute hepatitis from a variety of etiologies (El-Kamary et al. 2009). The hepatitis was caused by acute hepatitis A (15.2%), acute B (33.3%) and chronic HCV infection with acute symptoms (17.1%) in most patients in the study. Patients treated with silymarin had a faster time to resolution of bilirubin (p = 0.042), however resolution of AST and ALT was similar between the groups.

Studies have also investigated oral silymarin for the treatment of chronic hepatitis C. While oral silymarin does not affect viral replication, it is theorized to decrease inflammatory and cytokine activity caused by the virus. The primary objective for most studies was normalization of AST and ALT. These studies have yielded mixed results with some showing improvements in liver enzymes, while others showing no benefit of silymarin over placebo (Loguercio and Festi 2011). These studies are difficult to interpret as they used different formulations and doses of silymarin.

While oral silymarin does not have antiviral properties, high dose intravenous silibinin was shown to have potent antiviral properties in patients with chronic viral hepatitis C whose disease did not respond to pegylated interferon and ribavirin (Kim et al. 2016).

Two dose ranging studies of intravenous silibinin have been conducted. Patients received 5, 10, 15, or 20 mg/kg/day. Both investigators found that HCV viral load decrease was dose dependent (Ferenci et al. 2008; Guedj et al. 2012). The speed of viral load decrease was noted to be four-fold higher than what is observed with pegylated interferon and ribavirin (Guedj et al. 2012). There were no differences noted between the dosing groups. Case reports have described the successful use of intravenous silibinin in an HIV-HCV co-infected patient and liver transplant patients with chronic HCV and limited treatment options (Dhiman & Chawla 2005; Loguercio & Festi 2011).

7.8.2.5.3 Drug Induced Liver Injury

Two studies have investigated the use of silymarin to prevent DILI in patients receiving standard treatment for pulmonary tuberculosis including isoniazid, rifampicin, pyrazinamide, and ethambutol. One trial did not show a benefit in the prevention of DILI (Zhang et al. 2015). The second trial was limited by small sample size and short follow-up with a study duration of only 4 weeks. Despite these limitations, the incidence of DILI at week 4 in the silymarin group was 3.7% compared to 32.1% in the placebo group (Luangchosiri et al. 2015).

See Chapters 8 Women's Health and 17 Supportive and Palliative Care for Cancer for additional discussion.

7.8.2.6 Clinical Application

The efficacy of silymarin have varied in the treatment of acute hepatitis, chronic hepatitis, alcoholic liver disease, and in the prevention of DILI. Data in support of its efficacy can be found for each disease state and the safety profile is excellent, although the botanical does not decrease the mortality rate from these diseases.

7.8.3 Phyllanthus (*P. amarus, P. urinaris*)

7.8.3.1 Background

Phyllanthus is a genus of shrubs, trees, and herbs of which more than 600 species exist. The species used most commonly for liver diseases are *P. amarus,* and *P. urinaris. P. amarus* is an annual plant indigenous to tropical and subtropical climates (Joseph and Raj 2011). *Phyllanthus* has been used as a treatment for kidney and urinary problems, intestinal infections, diabetes, and hepatitis B in many cultures including the Ayurvedic tradition (Calixto et al. 1998; Joseph and Raj 2011).

7.8.3.2 Pharmacognosy

Many species of the *Phyllanthus* genus have been studied phytochemically and pharmacologically. The lignans and tannins are considered the biologically active compounds of the genus (Calixto et al. 1998; Mao et al. 2016). The entire *P. amarus* plant is used to yield an extract, which can be dried and put in capsules. The extract contains lignans, geraniin, and five flavonaoids (Joseph and Raj 2011).

7.8.3.3 Dosing and Preparation

Clinical trials have used dosages of *P. amarus* ranging from 200 to 500 mg orally which are administered 3 or 4 times per day. The dosages of *P. urinaris* are higher at 1–3 grams three times daily.

7.8.3.4 Safety

Both *P. amarus* and *P. urinaris* have been well tolerated in clinical trials. A meta-analysis showed that *Phyllanthus* was well tolerated with studies reporting that no adverse effects were experienced by patients (Xia et al. 2011).

7.8.3.5 Evidence

7.8.3.5.1 Chronic Hepatitis B Infection

Both *P. amarus* and *P. urinaris* have evidence in the treatment of chronic viral hepatitis B (HBV). One study investigated the effects of *P. amarus* on chronic carriers of hepatitis B virus in Madras, India (Thyagarajan et al. 1988). A total of 60 patients ranging in age from under 10 to over 30 were randomized to receive 200 mg capsules orally three times daily of *P. amarus* or placebo for 30 days. Over half of the patients who received treatment with *P. amarus* lost hepatitis B surface antigen (HBsAg) compared to 1 (4%) in the placebo group. A subsequent study of adults showed no difference between patients treated with *P. amarus* and placebo in terms of HBsAg clearance (Doshi et al. 1994).

A phase 2 dose finding study was conducted on the efficacy of *P. urinaris* to decrease HBV DNA in patients with active HBV (Chan et al. 2003). A total of 42 Chinese patients were randomized to receive 1, 2, or 3 grams of *P. urinaris* or placebo three times daily for 6 months. At the end of treatment, a sustained virologic and biochemical response with *P. urinaris* was not statistically significant compared to placebo. *P. urinaris* was well tolerated with only abdominal pain, symptoms of upper respiratory tract infection, malaise, headache, myalgia, and dizziness identified.

Two systemic reviews have evaluated the efficacy and safety of the genus *Phyllanthus* for the treatment of chronic HBV. One study included a total of 17 trials and yielded positive results with respect to *Phyllanthus*' ability to clear serum HBsAg, although the studies had a wide range of methodologies and used different species (Liu et al. 2001). In a subsequent Cochrane review, 20 publications from 16 trials were included (Xia et al. 2011). *Phyllanthus* had a greater reduction of HBV DNA levels when used in combination with antiviral medications than when antivirals were used alone. Antivirals used included lamivudine, interferon alpha, adefovir dipivoxil, and thymosin. In chronic carriers of HBV, *Phyllanthus* was not effective in seroconversion from HBeAg to anti-HBe when compared to placebo (Xia et al. 2011).

7.8.3.5.2 Nonalcoholic Fatty Liver Disease

In addition, *P. urinaria* has been studied in the treatment of patients with NAFLD. In one study, 60 patients were randomized to receive *P. urinaria* 1 g three times daily or placebo. The primary outcome was the change in NAFLD activity score from baseline to week 24. The changes in the NAFLD score were small and not clinically significant between the two groups. ALT and AST, as well as glucose and lipids, were unchanged (Wong et al. 2012).

7.8.3.6 Clinical Application

Phyllanthus may be beneficial in the treatment of carriers of HBV, as well as those with active virus. *Phyllanthus* has been well tolerated with few adverse effects reported.

7.9 Summary

Gastrointestinal conditions are common globally. Multiple small studies have evaluated botanicals for the treatment of diverse gastrointestinal and hepatic diseases. Evidence has varied significantly for the use of botanicals in the treatment of upper gastrointestinal conditions, lower gastrointestinal conditions, and liver disorders.

REFERENCES

Abascal, K., and E. Yarnell. 2009. Clinical uses of Zingiber officinale (Ginger). *Alternative and Complementary Therapies*, 15(5): 231–237.

Abenavoli, L., R. Capasso, N. Milic, and F. Capasso. 2010. Milk thistle in liver diseases: Past, present, future. *Phytotherapy Research*, 24(10): 1423–1432.

Afzal, M., D. Al-Hadidi, M. Menon, J. Pesek, and M. S. Dhami. 2001. Ginger: An ethnomedical, chemical and pharmacological review. *Drug Metabolism and Drug Interactions*, 18(3–4): 159–190.

Agha, F. P., T. Nostrant, and R. G. Fiddian-Green. 1984. Giant colonic bezoar: A medication bezoar due to psyllium seed husks. *American Journal of Gastroenterology*, 79: 319–321.

Ahmad, B., M. U. Rehman, I. Amin et al. 2015. A review on pharmacological properties of zingerone (4-(4-hydroxy-3-methoxyphenyl)-2-butanone). *Scientific World Journal*: 816364.

Ahmad, I., M. Zahin, F. Aqil et al. 2008. Bioactive compounds from punica granatum, curcuma longa and zingiber officinale and their therapeutic potential. *Drugs of the Future*, 33(4): 329–346.

Al Habbal, M. J., Z. Al Habbal, and F. U. Huwez. 1984. A double-blind controlled clinical trial of mastic and placebo in the treatment of duodenal ulcer. *Clinical and Experimental Pharmacology and Physioliology*, 11(5): 541–544.

Alberts, D. S., M. E. Martinez, D. J. Roe et al. 2000. Lack of effect of a high-fiber cereal supplement on the recurrence of colorectal adenomas. Phoenix Colon Cancer Prevention Physicians' Network. *New England Journal of Medicine*, 342: 1156–1162.

Ali, B. H., G. Blunden, M. O. Tanira, and A. Nemmar. 2008. Some phytochemical, pharmacological and toxicological properties of ginger (zingiber officinale roscoe): A review of recent research. *Food and Chemical Toxicology: An International Journal Published for the British Industrial Biological Research Association*, 46(2): 409–420.

Anderson, L. A., and J. B. Gross. 2004. Aromatherapy with peppermint, isopropyl alcohol, or placebo is equally effective in relieving postoperative nausea. *J Perianesthesia Nurse*, 19(1): 29–35.

Armanini, D., S. Lewicka, C. Pratesi et al. 1996. Further studies on the mechanism of the mineralocorticoid action of licorice in humans. *Journal of Endocrinological Investigation*, 19: 624–629.

Balakrishnan, A. 2015. Therapeutic uses of peppermint—A review. *Journal of Pharmaceutical Sciences and Research*, 7(7): 474–476.

Ben-Arye, E., E. Goldin, D. D. Wengrower et al. 2002. Wheat grass juice in the treatment of active distal ulcerative colitis: A randomized double-blind placebo-controlled trial. *Scandinavian Journal of Gastroenterology*, 37(4): 444–449.

Berboucha, M., K. Ayouni, D. Atmani, and M. Benbouetra. 2010. Kinetic study on the inhibition of xanthine oxidase by extracts from two selected Algerian plants traditionally used for the treatment of inflammatory diseases. *Journal of Medical Food*, 13(4): 896–904.

Biba, B., R. Sevcik, M. Voldrich, and J. Kratka. 2003. Analysis of the active components of silymarin. *Journal of Chromatography A*, 990(1–2): 239–245.

Blumenthal, M. ed. 1998. *The Complete German Commission E Monographs: Therapeutic Guide to Herbal Medicines*. Trans. S. Klein. Boston, MA: American Botanical Council.

Brandt, L. J., W. D. Chey, A. E. Foxx-Orenstein et al. 2009. An evidence-based position statement on the management of irritable bowel syndrome. *American Journal of Gastroenterology*, 104(Suppl 1): S1–S35.

Briggs, P., H. Hawrylack, and R. Mooney. 2016. Inhaled peppermint oil for postop nausea in patients undergoing cardiac surgery. *Nursing*, 46(7): 61–67.

Calixto, J. B., A. R. Santos, V. Cechinel Filho, and R. A. Yunes. 1998. A review of the plants of the genus phyllanthus: Their chemistry, pharmacology, and therapeutic potential. *Medicinal Research Reviews*, 18(4): 225–258.

Chan, H. L., J. J. Sung, W. F. Fong et al. 2003. Double-blinded placebo-controlled study of Phyllanthus urinaris for the treatment of chronic hepatitis B. *Alimentary Pharmacology and Therapeutics*, 18(3): 339–345.

Clarke, T., L. I. Black, B. J. Stussman, P. M. Barnes, and R. L. Nahin. 2015. Trends in the use of complementary health approaches among adults: United States 2002–2012. *National Health Statistics Report*, 79: 1–16.

Cooke, C., I. Carr, K. Abrams, and J. Mayberry. 2000. Arrowroot as a treatment for diarrhoea in irritable bowel syndrome patients: A pilot study. *Arq Gastroenterology*, 37(1): 20–24.

Cosmetic Ingredient Review Expert Panel. 2007. Final report on the safety assessment of aloe andongensis extract, aloe andongensis leaf juice, aloe arborescens leaf extract, aloe arborescens leaf juice, aloe arborescens leaf protoplasts, aloe barbadensis flower extract, aloe barbadensis leaf, aloe barbadensis leaf extract, aloe barbadensis leaf juice, aloe barbadensis leaf polysaccharides, aloe barbadensis leaf water, aloe ferox leaf extract, aloe ferox leaf juice, and aloe ferox leaf juice extract. *International Journal of Toxicology*, 26(Suppl. 2): 1–50.

Dabos, K. J., E. Sfika, L. J. Vlatta, D. Frantzi, G. Amygdalos, and Giannikopoulos. 2010a. Is chios mastic gum effective in the treatment of functional dyspepsia? A prospective randomised double-blind placebo controlled trial. *Journal of Ethnopharmacology*, 127(2): 205–209.

Dabos, K. J., E. Sfika, L. J. Vlatta, and Giannikopoulos. 2010b. The effect of mastic gum on helicobacter pylori: A randomised pilot study. *Phytomedicine*, 17(3-4): 296–299.

Del Prete, A., A. Scalera, M. D. Iadevaia et al. 2012. Herbal products: Benefits, limits, and applications in chronic liver disease. *Evidence-Based Complementary and Alternative Medicine*, 2012: 837939.

Dhiman, R. K., and Y. K. Chawla. 2005. Herbal medicines for liver diseases. *Digestive Diseases and Sciences*, 50(10): 1807–1812.

Dorsch, W., D. Loew, E. Meyer-Buchtela, and H. Schilcher. 1998. Carvi fructus (Kummelfruchte). *Kopperation Phytopharmaka* 47–48.

Doshi, J. C., A. B. Vaidya, D. S. Antarkar, R. Deolalikar, and D. H. Antani. 1994. A two-stage clinical trial of phyllanthus amarus in hepatitis B carriers: Failure to eradicate the surface antigen. *Indian Journal of Gastroenterology*, 13(1): 7–8.

Dossett, M., R. B. Davis, A. J. Lembo, and G. Y. Yeh. 2014. Complementary and alternative medicine use by U.S. adults with gastrointestinal conditions: Results from the 2012 national health interview survey. *American Journal of Gastroenterology*, 109(11): 1705–1711.

El-Kamary, S. S., M. D. Shardell, M. Abdel-Hamid et al. 2009. A randomized controlled trial to assess the safety and efficacy of silymarin on symptoms, signs and biomarkers of acute hepatitis. *Phytomedicine*, 16(5): 391–400.

Ferenci, P., T. M. Scherzer, H. Kerschner et al. 2008. Silibinin is a potent antiviral agent in patients with chronic hepatitis C not responding to pegylated interferon/ribavirin therapy. *Gastroenterology*, 135(5): 1561–1567.

Ferruggiari, L., B. Ragione, E. R. Rich, and K. Lock. 2012. The effect of aromatherapy on postoperative nausea in women undergoing surgical procedures. *Journal of Perianesthesia Nurse*, 27(4): 246–251.

Fleming, V., and W. E. Wade. 2010. A review of laxative therapies for treatment of chronic constipation in older adults. *American Journal of Geriatric Pharmacotherapy*, 8(6): 514–550.

Foster, M., D. Hunter, and S. Samman. 2011. Chapter 3. Evaluation of the nutritional and metabolic effects of aloe vera. In: Benzie, I. F. F., and Wachtel-Galor, S. (eds). *Herbal Medicine: Biomolecular and Clinical Aspects*. 2nd edn. Boca Raton (FL): CRC Press/Taylor & Francis.

Frati Munari, A. C., W. Benitez Pinto, C. Raul Ariza Andraca, and M. Casarrubias. 1998. Lowering glycemic index of food by acarbose and plantago psyllium mucilage. *Archives of Medical Research*, 29: 137–141.

Freise, J., and S. Kohler. 1999. Peppermint oil-caraway oil fixed combination in non-ulcer dyspepsia—Comparison of the effects of enteric preparations. *Pharmazie*, 54(3): 210–215.

Fuchs, C. S., E. L. Giovannucci, G. A. Colditz et al. 1999. Dietary fiber and the risk of colorectal cancer and adenoma in women. *New England Journal of Medicine*, 340: 169–176.

Garg, S. K., V. Ahuja, M. J. Sankar, A. Kumar, and A. C. Moss. 2012. Curcumin for maintenance of remission in ulcerative colitis. *Cochrane Database of Systematic Reviews*, 10: CD008424.

Goerg, K. J., and T. Spilker. 2003. Effect of peppermint oil and caraway oil on gastrointestinal motility in healthy volunteers: A pharmacodynamic study using simultaneous determination of gastric and gall-bladder emptying and orocaecal transit time. *Alimentary Pharmacology and Therapeutics*, 17(3): 445–451.

Goulas, V., E. Stylos, M. V. Chatziathanasiadou et al. 2016. Functional components of carob fruit: Linking the chemical and biological space. *International Journal of Molecular Sciences*, 17(11): 1875.

Gruenwald, J., T. Brendler, and C. Jaenicke. 1998. *PDR for Herbal Medicines*. 1st edn. Montvale, NJ: Medical Economics Company, Inc.

Guedj, J., H. Dahari, R. T. Pohl et al. 2012. Understanding silibinin's modes of action against HCV using viral kinetic modeling. *Journal of Hepatology*, 56(5): 1019–1024.

Gupta, I., A. Parihar, H. Ammon et al. 1997. Effects of boswellia serrata gum resin in patients with ulcerative colitis. *European Journal Of Medical Research*, 2(1): 37–43.

Hajiaghamohammadi, A. A., A. Ziaee, and R. Samimi. 2012. The efficacy of licorice root extract in decreasing transaminase activities in non-alcoholic fatty liver disease: A randomized controlled clinical trial. *Phytotherapy Research*, 26(9): 1381–1384.

Hanai, H., T. Iida, K. Takeuchei et al. 2006. Curcumin maintenance therapy for ulcerative colitis: Randomized, multicenter, double-blind, placebo-controlled trial. *Clinical Gastroenterology and Hepatology*, 4(12): 1502–1506.

Hines, S., E. Steels, A. Chang, and K. Gibbons. 2012. Aromatherapy for treatment of postoperative nausea and vomiting. *Cochrane Database of Systematic Reviews*, (4): Cd007598.

Holtmeier, W., S. Zeuzem, W. Caspary et al. 2011. Randomized, placebo-controlled, double-blind trial of boswellia serrata in maintaining remission of crohn's disease: Good safety profile but lack of efficacy. *Inflammatory Bowel Diseases*, 17(2): 573–582.

Hostettler, M., R. Steffen, and A. Tschopp. 1995. Efficacy and tolerance of insoluble carob fraction in the treatment of travellers' diarrhoea. *Journal of Diarrhoeal Diseases Research*, 13(3): 155–158.

Huwez, F. U., and M. J. Al-Habbal. 1986. Mastic in treatment of benign gastric ulcers. *Gastroenterologia Japonica*, 21(3): 273–274.

Huwez, F. U., D. Thirlwell, A. Cockayne, and D. A. Ala'Aldeen. 1998. Mastic gum kills helicobacter pylori. *New England Journal of Medicine*, 339(26): 1946.

Ikeda, K., Y. Arase, M. Kobayashi et al. 2006. A long-term glycyrrhizin injection therapy reduces hepatocellular carcinogenesis rate in patients with interferon-resistant active chronic hepatitis C: A cohort study of 1249 patients. *Digestive Diseases and Sciences*, 51(3): 603–609.

Isbrucker, R. A., and G. A. Burdock. 2006. Risk and safety assessment on the consumption of licorice root (glycyrrhiza sp.), its extract and powder as a food ingredient, with emphasis on the pharmacology and toxicology of glycyrrhizin. *Regulatory Toxicology and Pharmacology*, 46(3): 167–192.

Joseph, B., and S. J. Raj. 2011. An overview: Pharmacognostic properties of phyllanthus atnarus linn. *International Journal of Pharmacology*, 7(1): 40–45.

Jung, W., S. Kwon, and J. Im. 2014. Influence of herbal complexes containing licorice on potassium levels: A retrospective study. *Evidence Based Complementary and Alternative Medicine*, 2014: 970385.

Kanauchi, O., T. Iwanaga, and K. Mitsuyama. 2001. Germinated barley foodstuff feeding. A novel neutraceutical therapeutic strategy for ulcerative colitis. *Digestion*, 63(Suppl. 1): 60–67.

Kanauchi, O., K. Mitsuyama, T. Saiki et al. 1998. Germinated barley foodstuff increases fecal volume and butyrate production at relatively low doses and relieves constipation in humans. *International Journal of Molecular Medicine*, 2(4): 445–450.

Kao, T. C., C. H. Wu, and G. C. Yen. 2014. Bioactivity and potential health benefits of licorice. *Journal of Agricultural and Food Chemistry*, 62(3): 542–553.

Kartalis, A., M. Didagelos, I. Georgiadis et al. 2016. Effects of chios mastic gum on cholesterol and glucosae levels of healthy volunteers: A prospective, placebo-controlled pilot study. *European Journal of Preventive Cardiology*, 23(7): 722–729.

Kaur, R., H. Kaur, and A. S. Dhindsa. 2013. Glycyrrhiza glabra: A phytopharmacological review. *International Journal of Pharmaceutical Sciences and Research*, 4(7): 2470–2477.

Khanna, R., J. K. MacDonald, and B. G. Levesque. 2014. Peppermint oil for the treatment of irritable bowel syndrome: A systematic review and meta-analysis. *Journal of Clinical Gastroenterology*, 6: 505–512.

Kim, M. S., M. Ong, and X. Qu. 2016. Optimal management for alcoholic liver disease: Conventional medications, natural therapy or combination? *World Journal of Gastroenterology*, 22(1): 8–23.

Kornbluth, A., and D. B. Sachar. 2010. Ulcerative colitis practice guidelines in adults: American college of gastroenterology, practice parameters committee. *American Journal Of Gastroenterology*, 105(3): 501–523.

Kottakis, F., K. Kouzi-Koliakou, S. Pendas et al. 2009. Effects of mastic gum pistacia lentiscus var. chia on innate cellular immune effectors. *European Journal of Gastroenterology and Hepatology*, 21(2): 143–149.

Lane, B., K. Cannella, C. Bowen et al. 2012. Examination of the effectiveness of peppermint aromatherapy on nausea in women post C-section. *Journal of Holistic Nursing*, 30(2): 90–96.

Langmead, L., R. M. Feakins, S. Goldthorpe et al. 2004. Randomized, double-blind, placebo-controlled trial of oral aloe vera gel for active ulcerative colitis. *Alimentary Pharmacology and Therapeutics*, 19: 739–747.

Li, J. Y., H. Y. Cao, P. Liu et al. 2014. Glycyrrhizic acid in the treatment of liver diseases: Literature review. *BioMed Research International*, 2014: 872139.

Liu, C., Y. Zheng, W. Xu, H. Wang, and N. Lin. 2014. Rhubarb tannins extract inhibits the expression of aquaporins 2 and 3 in magnesium sulphate-induced diarrhoea model. *BioMed Research International*, 2014: 619465.

Liu, J., H. Lin, and H. McIntosh. 2001. Genus Phyllanthus for chronic hepatitis B virus infection: A systematic review. *Journal of Viral Hepatitis*, 8(5): 358–366.

Loeb, H., Y. Vandenplas, P. Wursch, and P. Guesry. 1989. Tannin-rich carob pod for the treatment of acute-onset diarrhea. *Journal of Pediatric Gastroenterology and Nutrition*, 8(4): 480–485.

Loguercio, C., and D. Festi. 2011. Silybin and the liver: From basic research to clinical practice. *World Journal of Gastroenterology*, 17(18): 2288–2301.

Luangchosiri, C., A. Thakkinstian, S. Chitphuk et al. 2015. A double-blinded randomized controlled trial of silymarin for the prevention of antituberculosis drug-induced liver injury. *BMC Complementary and Alternative Medicine*, 15: 334.

Madisch, A., C. J. Heydenreich, V. Wieland et al. 1999. Treatment of functional dyspepsia with a fixed peppermint oil and caraway oil combination preparation as compared to cisapride. A multicenter, reference-controlled, double-blind equivalence study. *Arzneimittelforschung*, 49: 925–932.

Manns, M. P., H. Wedemeyer, A. Singer et al. 2012. Glycyrrhizin in patients who failed previous interferon alpha-based therapies: Biochemical and histological effects after 52 weeks. *Journal of Viral Hepatitis*, 19(8): 537–546.

Mao, X., L. F. Wu, H. L. Guo et al. 2016. The genus phyllanthus: An ethnopharmacological, phytochemical, and pharmacological review. *Evidence Based Complementary And Alternative Medicine*, 2016: 7584952.

Marawaha, R. K., D. Bansal, S. Kaur, and A. Trehan. 2004. Wheat grass juice reduces transfusion requirement in patients with thalassemia major: A pilot study. *Indian Pediatrics*, 41(7): 716–720.

Marx, W. M., L. Teleni, A. L. McCarthy et al. 2013. Ginger zZingiber officinale) and chemotherapy-induced nausea and vomiting: A systematic literature review. *Nutrition Reviews*, 71(4): 245–254. doi: 10.1111/nure.12016.

May, B., S. Kohler, and B. Schneider. 2000. Efficacy and tolerability of a fixed combination of peppermint oil and caraway oil in patients suffering from functional dyspepsia. *Alimentary Pharmacology and Therapeutics*, 14: 1671–1677.

McKay, D. L., and J. B. Blumberg. 2006. A review of the bioactivity and potential health benefits of peppermint tea (mentha piperita L.). *Phytotherapy Research*, 20(8): 619–633.

Melzer, J., W. Rosch, J. Reichling et al. 2004. Meta-analysis: Phytotherapy of functional dyspepsia with the herbal drug preparation STW 5 (Iberogast). *Alimentary Pharmacology and Therapeutics*, 20: 1279–1287.

Micklefield, G., O. Jung, I. Greving, and B. May. 2003. Effects of intraduodenal application of peppermint oil (WS(R) 1340) and caraway oil (WS(R) 1520) on gastroduodenal motility in healthy volunteers. *Phytotherapy Research*, 7(2): 135–140.

Micklefield, G. H., I. Greving, and B. May. 2000. Effects of peppermint oil and caraway oil on gastroduodenal motility. *Phytotherapy Research*, 14: 20–23.

Miyake, K., T. Tango, Y. Ota et al. 2002. Efficacy of Stronger Neo-Minophagen C compared between two doses administered three times a week on patients with chronic viral hepatitis. *Journal of Gastroenterology and Hepatology*, 17(11): 1198–1204.

Momeni, A., G. Rahimian, A. Kiasi, M. Amiri, and S. Kheiri. 2014. Effect of licorice versus bismuth on eradication of helicobacter pylori in patients with peptic ulcer disease. *Pharmacognosy Research*, 6(4): 341–344. doi: 10.4103/0974-8490.138289.

National Center for Complementary and Integrative Health. Access online: https://nccih.nih.gov. Accessed on June 6, 2018.

Newall, C.A., L. A. Anderson, and J. D. Philpson. 1996. *Herbal Medicine: A Guide for Healthcare Professionals*. London, UK: The Pharmaceutical Press.

Odes, H. S., and Z. Madar. 1991. A double-blind trial of a celandin, aloe vera and psyllium laxative preparation in adult patients with constipation. *Digestion*, 49: 65–71.

Orlent, H., B. E. Hansen, M. Willems et al. 2006. Biochemical and histological effects of 26 weeks of glycyrrhizin treatment in chronic hepatitis C: A randomized phase II trial. *Journal of Hepatology*, 45(4): 539–546.

Paraschos, S., P. Magiatis, S. Mitakou et al. 2007. *In vitro* and *in vivo* activities of chios mastic gum extracts and constituents against helicobacter pylori. *Antimicrobial Agents and Chemotherapy*, 551–559.

Quinkler, M., and P. M. Stewart. 2003. Hypertension and the cortisol-cortisone shuttle. *Journal of Clinical Endocrinology and Metabolism*, 88: 2384–2392.

Ramasubramania Raja, R. 2012. Medicinally potential plants of labiatae (lamiaceae) family: An overview. *Research Journal of Medicinal Plant*, 6(3): 203–213.

Ramkumar, D., and S. S. Rao. 2005. Efficacy and safety of traditional medical therapies for chronic constipation: Systematic review. *American Journal of Gastroenterology*, 00(4): 936–971.

Reynolds, T., and A. C. Dweck. 1999. Aloe vera leaf gel: A review update. *Journal of Ethnopharmacology*, 68: 3–37.

Rita, P., and D. K. Animesh. 2011. An updated overview on peppermint (Mentha piperita L.). *International Research Journal of Pharmacy*, 2(8): 1–10.

van Rossum, T. G., A. G. Vulto, W. C. Hop et al. 1999. Intravenous glycyrrhizin for the treatment of chronic hepatitis C: A double-blind, randomized, placebo-controlled phase I/II trial. *Journal of Gastroenterology and Hepatology*, 14(11): 1093–1099.

van Rossum, T. G., A. G. Vulto, W. C. Hop, and S. W. Schalm. 2001. Glycyrrhizin-induced reduction of ALT in European patients with chronic hepatitis C. *American Journal of Gastroenterology*, 96(8): 2432–2437.

Sabbadin, C., and D. Armanini. 2016. Syndromes that mimic an excess of mineralocorticoids. *High Blood Pressure & Cardiovascular Prevention*, 23(3): 231–235.

Saleem, M. N., and M. Idris. 2016. Formulation design and development of a unani transdermal patch for antiemetic therapy and its pharmaceutical evaluation. *Scientifica*, 2016: 7602347.

Saller, R., F. Iten, and J. Reichling. 2001. Dyspeptic pain and phytotherapy—A review of traditional and modern herbal drugs. *Forsch. Komplementarmed. Klass. Naturheilkd*, 8(5): 263–273.

Schatzkin, A., E. Lanza, D. Corle et al. 2000. Lack of effect of a low-fat, high-fiber diet on the recurrence of colorectal adenomas. Polyp Prevention Trial Study Group. *The New England Journal of Medicine*, 342: 1149–1155.

Schwertner, H. A., D. C. Rios, and J. E. Pascoe. 2006. Variation in concentration and labeling of ginger root dietary supplements. *Obstetrics and Gynecology*, 107(6): 1337–1343.

Shetty, P. S., and A. V. Kurpad. 1986. Increasing starch intake in the human diet increases fecal bulking. *American Journal of Clinical Nutrition*, 43(2): 210–212.

Singla, V., V. Pratap, S. K. Garg et al. 2014. Induction with NCB-02 (curcumin) enema for mild-to-moderate distal ulcerative colitis—A randomized, placebo-controlled, pilot study. *Journal of Crohn's Colitis*, 8(3): 208–214.

Szema, A. M., and T. Barnett. 2011. Allergic reaction to mint leads to asthma. *Allergy and Rhinology*, 2(1): 43–45.

Tate, S. 1997. Peppermint oil: A treatment for postoperative nausea. *Journal of Advanced Nursing*, 26(3): 543–549.

Thyagarajan, S. P., S. Subramanian, T. Thirunalasundari et al. 1988. Effect of Phyllanthus amarus on chronic carriers of hepatitis B virus. *Lancet*, 2(8614): 764–766.

Vaes, L. P., and P. A. Chyka. 2000. Interactions of warfarin with garlic, ginger, ginkgo, or ginseng: Nature of the evidence. *Annals of Pharmacotherapy*, 34: 1478–1482.

Vogler, B. K., and E. Ernst. 1999. Aloe vera: A systematic review of its clinical effectiveness. *British Journal of General Practice*, 49: 823–828.

Wong, V. W.-S., G. L.-H. Wong, A. W.-H. Chan et al. 2012. Treatment of non-alcoholic steatohepatitis with Phyllanthus urinaria: A randomized trial. *Journal of Gastroenterology and Hepatology*, 28(1): 57–62. https://doi.org/10.1111/j.1440-1746.2012.07286.x

Xia, Y., H. Luo, J. P. Liu, and C. Gluud. 2011. Phyllanthus species for chronic hepatitis B virus infection. *Cochrane Database of Systematic Reviews*, (4): Cd008960.

Yasui, S., K. Fujiwara, A. Tawada et al. 2011. Efficacy of intravenous glycyrrhizin in the early stage of acute onset autoimmune hepatitis. *Digestive Diseases and Sciences*, 56(12): 3638–3647.

Zhang , S., H. Pan, H. Lu et al. 2015. Preventive use of a hepatoprotectant against anti-tuberculosis drug-induced liver injury: A randomized controlled trial. *Journal of Gastroenteroogy Andl Hepatology*, 31(2): 409–416. doi: 10.1111/jgh/13070.

8

Women's Health

Renee A. Bellanger and Cheryl Horlen

CONTENTS

8.1 Introduction

Women have been using botanical products for millennia (Hardy 2000). According to the 2012 National Health Information Survey (NHIS) of U.S. households, over 22 million women (19.2%) had used a botanical supplement in the past year, which is more than 18 million men (16.4%) during the same period. Comparing this data with that of the 2002 survey, botanical supplement use was down from 21% of women, but still significantly higher than the use by men (16.7%) (Wu et al. 2014). Many women of childbearing potential use these supplements to alleviate symptoms of menstruation, fewer to aid in symptoms of pregnancy and to increase milk production during breastfeeding. Some use supplements as self-care, while others on the advice of midwives (Budzynska et al. 2016; Johnson et al. 2016). About half of women in Western countries ease symptoms of the menopausal transition with botanical products (Franco et al. 2016). Safety of botanical products used by women is a concern of all healthcare providers, especially during the time surrounding childbirth (Holst et al. 2011; Masullo et al. 2015). One survey has revealed that healthcare providers may recommend questionable products to pregnant women. Many items were traditionally used products that lacked substantial evidence of safety or efficacy in the literature (Holst et al. 2011; Kennedy et al. 2016).

8.2 Menstrual Problems

Women of childbearing potential may experience multiple menstrual-related problems during their reproductive years. Common menstrual-related conditions in which botanicals may offer relief include dysmenorrhea, premenstrual syndrome (PMS), and polycystic ovary syndrome (PCOS).

Dysmenorrhea is painful menstruation of uterine origin. The pain can vary in intensity and typically occurs with the onset of menstruation and lasts up to 72 hours. Primary dysmenorrhea, with an onset during adolescence, is due to an abnormally high release of prostaglandin F2α, which results in potent vasoconstriction and myometrial contraction. Secondary dysmenorrhea, with onset usually after the age of 25, is due to pelvic pathology. Examples of pathology that can cause secondary dysmenorrhea include endometriosis, uterine fibroids, and ovarian cysts (Dang et al. 2010).

Premenstrual syndrome is characterized by affective, physical, and behavioral symptoms that occur regularly in the luteal phase of the menstrual cycle and disappear shortly after the onset of menses (Ryu and Kim 2015). Severe PMS with functional or psychological impairment may be classified as premenstrual dysphoric disorder (PMDD) and is estimated to occur in 3%–8% of all reproductive age women (Bailey and Culhane 2010). Although the pathophysiology is not completely understood, women with PMS/PMDD may have an abnormal response to serotonin when ovarian steroid hormones decline in the luteal phase.

Polycystic ovary syndrome is a leading cause of anovulatory infertility among reproductive age women. Patients with PCOS often present with signs of hyperandrogenism, menstrual disturbances, and obesity. Inappropriate gonadotropic secretion, insulin resistance, and excessive androgen production all play a role in the pathophysiology of PCOS. Women with PCOS are at risk for the development of impaired glucose tolerance or diabetes, metabolic syndrome, obstructive sleep apnea, and endometrial hyperplasia, or cancer (Borgelt and Cheang 2010).

8.2.1 Bilberry (*Vaccinium myrtillus*)

8.2.1.1 Background

The bilberry plant is a small, deciduous, perennial shrub native to temperate regions of northern Europe, northern United States, and Canada. The plant flowers from April to June and produces purple-black berries, similar to American blueberries, from July through September. Historically, the twelfth century German herbalist Hildegard von Bingen recommended bilberry for the induction of menses. Today, bilberry is used for dysmenorrhea and fibrocystic breast disease (Freeman 2004; Foster and Johnson 2008; Ulbricht et al. 2009).

8.2.1.2 Pharmacognosy

The fruit of the bilberry plant is harvested for use in botanical medicine. The berries can be used fresh or dried, or their juice extracted and processed into a powder concentrate for use in capsules and pills (Foster and Johnson 2008). Bilberry contains tannins and flavonoid glycosides, but the key active compound are anthocyanosides, which scavenge free radicals, strengthen capillaries, and stimulate growth of healthy connective tissue. Anthocyanosides also decrease platelet aggregation through stimulating the formation of prostacyclin I2-like substances by vascular tissue (Freeman 2004; Ulbricht et al. 2009).

8.2.1.3 Dosing and Preparation

Dosing varies according to the intended use. An aqueous extract standardized to 25% anthocyanosides is often used. For dysmenorrhea, 160 mg of bilberry VMA extract twice daily for 8 days starting 3 days prior to menses has been used (Colombo and Vescovini 1985).

8.2.1.4 Safety

Since bilberry is also a food source, safety is often presumed, especially when consumed in amounts typically found in food or at recommended doses for short durations (Ulbricht et al. 2009). French postmarketing surveillance data revealed 4% of patients experienced adverse effects using one bilberry extract (Tegens®), with 1% of patients complaining of gastrointestinal discomfort (Ulbricht et al. 2009). Fresh bilberry may have a laxative effect, while dried bilberry may cause constipation. Although little human data is available, a theoretical risk of hypotension, hypoglycemia, and bleeding exists (Ulbricht et al. 2009). Due to bilberry reducing platelet aggregation, patients taking antithrombotic agents should be advised to avoid bilberry. Long-term safety has not been extensively studied (Ulbricht et al. 2009).

8.2.1.5 Evidence

The smooth muscle-relaxing activity of anthocyanosides may improve the symptoms of dysmenorrhea. Evidence of bilberry's role in the treatment of dysmenorrhea is limited to one randomized placebo-controlled double-blind study of 30 patients (Ulbricht et al. 2009). This study evaluated the effects of 160 mg twice daily of bilberry *V. myrtillus* anthocyanoside (Tegens®) given for 8 days, starting 3 days before menses, for two consecutive menstrual cycles. The authors found bilberry statistically significantly reduced pelvic pain, lumbosacral pain, breast pain, nausea, vomiting, and headache compared to placebo. Although the results were encouraging, study methods and baseline characteristics were not well described (Colombo and Vescovini 1985).

8.2.1.6 Clinical Application

Limited evidence of bilberry's effectiveness exists to reduce pain associated with menstruation. Bilberry may be associated with an increased risk of bleeding and lowered blood pressure and blood glucose.

8.2.2 Chasteberry (*Vitex angus-castus*)

8.2.2.1 Background

Native to the Mediterranean and Central Asia, the chaste tree is a deciduous shrub characterized by palmate leaves, blue-violet flowers, and dark red-black berries similar to peppercorns. Berries from the chaste tree have been used over 2500 years for gynecologic problems. In the historical record starting with Hippocrates, chasteberry has been used to promote normal menses without pain, to decrease bleeding after childbirth and promote lactation (Foster and Johnson 2008). In modern times, chasteberry is primarily used for menstrual irregularities due to intrauterine devices (Yavarikia et al. 2013). It is also used for symptoms of PMS and PMDD, including cyclic mastalgia (Atmaca et al. 2003; Berger et al. 2000; Carmichael 2008; Dinc and Coskun 2014; Halaska et al. 1999; Momoeda et al. 2014).

8.2.2.2 Pharmacognosy

The fruits of the chaste tree are used in botanical preparations. Ripe fruits are harvested in autumn and can be used fresh or dried or can be made into tinctures or teas. The berries contain essential oils, iridoid glycosides, flavonoids, and diterpenes (Brown 1994; Du Mee 1993; Upton 2001) Chasteberry preparations reduce follicle stimulating hormone (FSH) release while increasing luteinizing hormone (LH) and prolactin release from the anterior part of the pituitary gland. This leads to an increase in progesterone during the luteal phase of the menstrual cycle and may affect menstruation and alleviate symptoms of PMS (Foster and Johnson 2008). In women with hyperprolactinemia, chasteberry seems to suppress prolactin release. High doses of chasteberry may have agonistic effects at dopamine D2 receptors in the pituitary, resulting in an inhibition of prolactin release (Jarry et al. 1994; Wuttke 1996; Wuttke et al. 2003).

8.2.2.3 Dosing and Preparation

Dosing varies according to the intended use. Many preparations are standardized to contain 6% agnuside. An extract of 20–40 mg daily for 8 weeks has been used for the treatment of PMDD (Atmaca et al. 2003).

8.2.2.4 Safety

Chasteberry is generally well tolerated. Adverse effects include gastrointestinal symptoms, itching, rash, headache, and fatigue. Although human data is limited, patients with hormone sensitive cancers or conditions should avoid taking chasteberry. Due to the dopamine agonist effects of chasteberry, concerns exist about a potential interference with antipsychotic agents, metoclopramide, bromocriptine, and levodopa (Jarry et al. 1994; Meier et al. 2000; Wuttke 1996).

8.2.2.5 Evidence

Chasteberry has been studied in randomized controlled trials for the treatment of PMS/PMDD. Compared with placebo, the use of chasteberry has had mixed results. One study of 127 women receiving chasteberry or vitamin B6 for 3 months found both to be effective based on reductions in the premenstrual tension syndrome scale and improvements in clinical global impression (Whelan et al. 2009). A multicenter, double-blind, placebo-controlled prospective trial of varying doses of chasteberry was conducted in 142 women with stable PMS symptoms. Patients were randomized to placebo or *Vitex agnus castus* fruit extract (Ze 440) 8, 20, or 30 mg daily as a tablet during a meal for three full menstrual cycles. Patients assessed the intensity of six PMS-related symptoms by a five-point visual analogue scale (VAS) at baseline, for three consecutive days before the anticipated start of each menstruation, and end of therapy. Patients were allowed to continue current oral contraceptives and these patients were analyzed with their dosing group and separately. No effect of oral contraception was noted on any of the parameters studied.

There was no difference between study groups for any adverse events and no serious adverse events occurred. Overall, the group that received 20 mg of Ze 440 had the best reduction in PMS symptoms ($p < 0.001$). The higher dose, 30 mg Ze 440, did not have a significant effect on patients as compared to any of the other groups ($p = 0.599$ vs. 20 mg). The authors concluded that the 20 mg dose of the extract Ze 440 daily could be recommended to decrease PMS symptoms (Schellenberg et al. 2012).

Another study compared chasteberry to fluoxetine for 2 months in 38 women with PMDD. Both improved Hamilton Depression (HAM-D), Clinical Global Impressions (CGI), and Depression Symptom Rating (DSR) scores. Interestingly, chasteberry improved the physical symptoms of PMDD more than fluoxetine, including mastalgia. Fluoxetine improved psychological symptoms more than chasteberry. Adverse effects were mild in both groups, with nausea being the most common (Atmaca et al. 2003).

Chasteberry has also been used for the treatment of cyclic mastalgia. A double-blind, placebo controlled study found that a Vitex agnus castus extract-containing solution given for 3 months reduced pain 54% versus 40% with placebo as measured by a visual analog scale. Pain intensity also decreased faster with the use of chasteberry. Side effects were similar between groups (Halaska et al. 1999). Another study compared chasteberry to flurbiprofen in women less than 40 years old with cyclic mastalgia. After 3 months of treatment, both treatment groups had a similar amount of pain reduction. Side effects were limited to confusion and rash with chasteberry and dyspepsia and tinnitus with flurbiprofen (Dinc and Coskun 2014). Similarly, women with latent hyperprolactinemia or cyclic mastalgia were treated for 3 months with bromocriptine or chasteberry. Prolactin levels and breast pain both significantly decreased from pre-treatment levels; however, no significant differences between groups were observed (van Die et al. 2013).

Chasteberry has been evaluated for the treatment of primary dysmenorrhea in one study from Iran. Patients received either fennelin, vitagnus, mefenamic acid, or placebo starting one day before menses and continuing until the third day for two cycles. Both fennelin and vitagnus drops reduced pain during treatment better than mefenamic acid (Zeraati et al. 2014). While the results were positive, this study had inadequate descriptions of the products used, randomization, and statistical analysis.

8.2.2.6 Clinical Application

Chasteberry may be beneficial in reducing symptoms of PMS/PMDD. Patients receiving other dopaminergic agents should be cautioned not to use chasteberry products.

8.2.3 Cramp Bark (*Viburnum opulus*)

8.2.3.1 Background

Native to Europe, northern Africa, and northern Asia, cramp bark is an ornamental plant. The U.S. Pharmacopeia listed cramp bark in 1894. Historically used for treating a variety of cramps, the botanical is used now to relieve menstrual cramps, cramps during pregnancy, and muscle spasms (Hardy 2000).

8.2.3.2 Pharmacognosy

The bark of the plant contains scopoletin, proanthocyanidines and viopudial. Viopudial and scopoletin have antispasmodic effects on smooth muscle *in vitro* (Jarboe et al. 1966).

8.2.3.3 Dosing and Preparation

Cramp bark is usually dosed as an undiluted tincture at 3–5 mL (0.5–1 tsp) every 2 hours up to 3 days for acute dysmenorrhea. It can be started 1–2 days before the onset of menses to prevent dysmenorrhea (Yarnell 2015).

8.2.3.4 Safety

Adverse effects and its safety in pregnancy are unknown.

8.2.3.5 Evidence

Evidence for the use of cramp bark in patients with dysmenorrhea is limited to historical use.

8.2.3.6 Clinical Application

Cramp bark has been used to alleviate menstrual cramps, although clinical trials are not available to assess efficacy or safety.

8.2.4 Evening Primrose Oil (*Oenothera biennis*)

8.2.4.1 Background

Native to North America, the evening primrose plant grows in open areas with poor soil quality. The plant has lance-shaped leaves and yellow, lemon-scented flowers that open at dusk. Inside the flower, which only lasts for one night, are seed capsules (Foster and Johnson 2008). Oil made from the seeds is used for premenstrual syndrome, mastalgia, and menopausal symptoms (Cancelo Hidalgo et al. 2006; Ockerman et al. 1986; Pruthi et al. 2010; Puolakka et al. 1985; Wetzig 1994).

8.2.4.2 Pharmacognosy

Although the flowers and leaves of the evening primrose plant are edible, evening primrose oil is extracted from the seeds of the plant. The primary active ingredient is gamma-linolenic acid (GLA), an essential omega-6 fatty acid. GLA may suppress inflammation by increasing the production of prostaglandins (Belch and Hill 2000; Joe and Hart 1993; Morse et al. 1989).

8.2.4.3 Dosing and Preparation

Standardized capsules of evening primrose oil (EPO) 500–1300 mg contain linoleic acid (70%–73%), GLA (8%–10%), and some contain 10 IU of vitamin E to prevent oxidation. Efamol, a commercially available product used in several studies, is available as either 500 or 1000 mg EPO per capsule, which includes 115 mg of GLA and 10 mg of vitamin E per 1000 mg of EPO. Suggested daily dose is 3 g of EPO per day (Efamol Ltd.). Studies of evening primrose oil for premenstrual syndrome and mastalgia have used a wide range of doses (Bayles and Usatine 2009).

8.2.4.4 Safety

Evening primrose oil is generally well tolerated with reports of mild gastrointestinal discomfort. Theoretically, evening primrose oil may prolong bleeding time and increase the risk of bleeding especially in combination with other antithrombotic medications. Although reports are limited, and have confounding factors, a concern exists that evening primrose oil may lower the seizure threshold (Puri 2007).

8.2.4.5 Evidence

Although commonly used for mastalgia, premenstrual syndrome, and menopausal symptoms, evidence to support its use is limited. Studies evaluating evening primrose oil for mastalgia have produced conflicting results. Several studies with positive findings lacked a control group while more rigorous studies failed to show benefit (Parveen et al. 2007; Pashby et al. 1981; Sharma et al. 2012; Wetzig 1994). Randomized controlled trials evaluating evening primrose oil for premenstrual syndrome have not shown significant reductions in PMS symptoms (Whelan et al. 2009). One lesser quality study showed a reduction in depressive symptom with evening primrose oil compared to placebo (Whelan et al. 2009). In women with hot flushes and night sweats due to menopause, most studies have not shown a reduction in to these symptoms (Chenoy et al. 1994). A randomized, double-blinded trial in 56 symptomatic menopausal Iranian women who received 1 g per day of EPO extract or placebo for 6 weeks had a significant decrease in the severity of hot flushes, but not their duration or frequency. Some nausea was experienced by two women in the treatment group (Farzaneh et al. 2013).

8.2.4.6 Clinical Application

Evening primrose oil serves as a source of omega-6 fatty acids and GLA may exhibit anti-inflammatory effects. The benefit of evening primrose oil in premenstrual syndrome or menopause is not well established.

8.2.5 Blessed Thistle (*Cnicus benedictus*)

8.2.5.1 Background

Blessed thistle grows in southern Europe, western Asia and North Africa. It is considered a weed with hairy, leathery leaves and stems, and prickly pale yellow flower heads. It is a member of the *Asteraceae* family and has been used for cervical dysplasia, stimulation of lactation, and dysmenorrhea (Ulbricht et al. 2008a; Zapantis et al. 2012).

8.2.5.2 Pharmacognosy

Blessed thistle contains sesquiterpene lactone glycosides, cnicin, absinthin, and polyacetylene; triterpenoids; lignans; flavonoids; tannins and essential volatile oils. Cnicin and lignans may contribute to the bitter characteristics of the plant. Tannins may cause the gastrointestinal effects due to irritation of the mucous membranes and may be nephrotoxic over a period of time. The leaves and flowers of *Cnicus benedictus* are used in botanical extracts, teas, and flavorings (Al-Snafi 2016; Ulbricht et al. 2008a).

8.2.5.3 Dosing and Preparation

The usual daily dose in adult patients is 1.5–4 grams. It is often used as part of a combination of botanical ingredients. Traditionally, 2 tsp of dried leaves or 1.5–3 grams of dried flowering shoots are added to a cup of hot water as a tea and taken three times a day (Duke 2002; Blumenthal 2000; Ulbricht et al. 2008a).

8.2.5.4 Safety

Blessed thistle is likely safe when used as a flavoring agent. Allergy and hypersensitivity to blessed thistle is common. Patients with allergies to Asteraceae/Compositae family of plants may experience a cross sensitivity with blessed thistle. Patients with gastric ulcers or inflammatory bowel disease should not take blessed thistle. Acute doses over 5 g may cause stomach lining irritation and emesis. Blessed thistle has been used as an abortifacient and therefore use should be avoided in pregnancy (Ulbricht et al. 2008a). Information on the safety of blessed thistle during lactation is lacking (Zapantis et al. 2012). Drug interactions are based on anecdotal and traditional use of the plant. Clinical evidence is lacking for these safety concerns. Patients taking nonsteroidal anti-inflammatory drugs (NSAIDs) and antithrombotic agents should be cautioned about potential increased bleeding due to potential antagonism of platelet activating factor (Ulbricht et al. 2008a).

8.2.5.5 Evidence

No clinical data or trials are available.

8.2.5.6 Clinical Application

Traditionally, blessed thistle has been used to stimulate the start of menstruation. Due to its emmenagogue and abortifacient potential, women who are pregnant should not use blessed thistle. Blessed thistle should not be confused with milk thistle (*Silybum marianum*).

8.3 Pregnancy and Lactation

Women are sensitive to reports of the negative effects of prescription and over-the-counter (OTC) medications on their pregnancy and unborn child. Many women consider using "natural" alternatives to treat common ailments during pregnancy with the belief that these are safer, not realizing that these products may have similar safety concerns and may lack evidence to support efficacy (Dante et al. 2014; Kennedy et al. 2016). The efficacy and safety of botanical products used during the peripartum period and during lactation are not established (Dante et al. 2014; Holst et al. 2011; Kennedy et al. 2016). Published reports frequently do not indicate the specific trimester, quantity or quality of the product, or outcome of use (Hall and Jolly 2014). Prevalence of use of botanical medicines during pregnancy has been reported to be between 6% and 9% in North America and 58% in the United Kingdom (Holst et al. 2011; Kennedy et al. 2016).

Many women self-treat common complaints of pregnancy and chronic conditions with OTC medications and botanicals due to their own knowledge or sources of information other than from health care providers (Kennedy et al. 2013; Lupattelli et al. 2014). Women who use botanicals are generally married, over the age of 30, educated, urban, and employed outside the home (Kennedy et al. 2013; Frawley et al. 2015). Healthcare providers, including midwives, were involved in the recommendation to use botanicals about 22% of the time (Frawley et al. 2015; Kennedy et al. 2013).

The most common reasons for using botanicals during pregnancy include nausea, heartburn, constipation, upper respiratory symptoms, pain, sleeping concerns, relaxation, or preparation for labor (Hall and Jolly 2014; Holst et al. 2011; Kennedy et al. 2013). The most commonly used products were ginger, cranberry, valerian, raspberry, chamomile, peppermint, and echinacea (Frawley et al. 2015; Holst et al. 2011; Kennedy et al. 2013).

8.3.1 Nausea and Vomiting of Early Pregnancy (NVP, Morning Sickness)

8.3.1.1 Ginger (Zingiber officianale)

8.3.1.1.1 Background

From the tropical regions of Asia, ginger is used as a spice for food and as a botanical medicine in Chinese, Ayurvedic, and Arabic traditions to aid digestion. Ginger is used to treat nausea, painful menstrual periods, and pain. The oleoresin of ginger is also used as an ingredient in digestive, laxative, antitussive, antiflatulent, and antacid preparations (Ali et al. 2008; Mishra et al. 2012).

8.3.1.1.2 Pharmacognosy

The ginger plant can be harvested wild or cultivated in tropical locations, growing up to 90 cm in height. The perennial ginger plant's tuberous rhizome is used to prepare the spice and the medicinal products. The rhizome is aromatic, thick-lobed, pale yellowish and bears simple alternate narrow oblong lance-like leaves. Small yellowish green flowers may appear (Mishra et al. 2012).

Many constituent chemicals can be separated from the ginger rhizome and depend on the place of origin and the condition of the rhizome (fresh or dry). Gingerols are the major components in the fresh ginger rhizome, whereas shogaols, especially 6-shogaol, are the most abundant polyphenolic constituents of dried ginger (Ali et al. 2008; Mishra et al. 2012).

8.3.1.1.3 Dosing and Preparation

Th dosing has varied between 1 and 4 g per day in the published studies. In general, though the recommended dose is 250 mg orally four times a day, before meals and at bedtime. Ginger can be the fresh or dried rhizome prepared as a tea, candied, crystallized, or a cookie ingredient. Ginger extract can be used as a powder, syrup, or in a capsule or tablet. The concentrations of active ingredients, gingerols and shogaols, differ between the different preparations and the processing steps (Giacosa et al. 2015; Lete and Allue 2016).

8.3.1.1.4 Safety

Ginger in low to moderate doses is generally regarded as safe (GRAS) for humans by the FDA (National Center for Complementary and Integrative Health 2006). ACOG lists it as a non-pharmacologic agent to be used for nausea and vomiting of pregnancy in its treatment algorithm with an effective dose of less than 1500 mg in the reviewed studies (American Congress of Obstetricians and Gynecologists 2015). Minor gastrointestinal adverse effects are belching, heartburn, diarrhea, and mouth irritation (Viljoen et al. 2014). Ginger may have antiplatelet activity, so other antithrombotic agents should be avoided or monitored (National Center for Complementary and Integrative Health 2016).

A recent systemic review of ginger in the treatment of pregnancy-associated nausea and vomiting suggested that ginger reduces nausea with less adverse effects compared with pyridoxine and dimenhydrinate. When compared with metoclopramide, no differences in efficacy or adverse effects was observed (Viljoen et al. 2014).

8.3.1.1.5 Evidence

The use of ginger for NVP was explored using the Norwegian Mother and Child cohort data set (Heitmann et al. 2013). Ginger was reportedly used by 1020 women, (1.5%), of the entire study group of 68,522 women who gave birth in Norway between 1999 and 2008 and completed the questionnaire after being recruited near 17 weeks gestation. Of the women who reported taking ginger, 90% took it during their first trimester for NVP, dropping to almost 60% by the second half of the pregnancy. Of the women who took ginger, 15% also used other medications to reduce NVP, most often meclizine. Minor vaginal bleeding occurred more frequently in the group taking ginger after gestational week 17. No associations with serious adverse effects, such as fetal malformations, spontaneous abortion, premature birth, low birth weight, or diminished APGAR score were observed (Heitmann et al. 2013).

In a small single-blind study, women who were less than 20 weeks pregnant were assigned to ginger 250 mg capsules to be taken four times a day (n = 32) or a matched placebo capsule (n = 35) for symptoms of NVP. Symptom relief was assessed using a survey tool twice daily during the four-day study period and a personal interview at the end of the 4 days. More patients in the ginger group reported improvement in nausea symptoms compared with the placebo group (84% versus 56%). Also, the number of nausea events over the study period (185 versus 257) and reported intensity of nausea events was significantly reduced in the ginger group (p < 0.001). Vomiting was rare and not different between the two groups. No other adverse outcomes were reported (Ozgoli et al. 2009).

In Australia, women who were less than 16 weeks pregnant and had symptoms of nausea or vomiting were randomized in an equivalence trial to receive a capsule containing either ginger 350 mg (n = 146) or pyridoxine 25 mg (n = 145) three times a day for 3 weeks. At baseline, nausea and dry retching were experienced by almost all women and 60% of women reported vomiting. All symptoms were relieved at the same rate, between 53% and 55% improvement, by ginger and pyridoxine respectively, with nausea being relieved the most in both groups (p < 0.001). Women who continued taking other anti-emetic agents, including metoclopramide and prochlorperazine, had an additional reduction in nausea from 25% at baseline to 20% at 3 weeks. Belching was reported more frequently in the ginger group (9% vs 0%) (p < 0.05). More live births and fewer spontaneous abortions occurred in the ginger group. Overall the risk of pregnancy complications was similar between the groups. The authors concluded that ginger and pyridoxine were equivalent to improve pregnancy-induced nausea and vomiting (Smith et al. 2004).

Women less than 16 weeks pregnant with NVP were randomly allocated to take ginger 500 mg capsule (n = 85) or dimenhydrinate 50 mg (n = 85) twice daily for 1 week. Reduction in nausea and vomiting over the study period was assessed using a visual analog scale at baseline and twice daily for 7 days, along with the number of vomiting episodes daily. Nausea scores decreased similarly in both groups and the number of vomiting episodes were similar between groups by day three. Dimenhydrinate caused more sedation, while heartburn occurred in similar frequency in both groups (Pongrojpaw et al. 2007).

A group of pregnant women in their first trimester were randomly assigned to take capsules containing 500 mg ginger with 400 mcg of folic acid twice daily or metoclopramide 10 mg tablets three times a day for 21 days. Both groups had similar baseline characteristics. Ginger scores were better than baseline throughout, and had less vomiting at day 7, but not better than metoclopramide for nausea, vomiting at days 14 or 21, or overall symptom relief (Sharief and Shaker 2014).

A recent Cochrane review of treatments for NVP has suggested that ginger may be of benefit to relieve symptoms in early pregnancy, but conceded that evidence is limited except in comparison to placebo (Matthews et al. 2015).

See Chapters 7 Gastrointestinal Disease, 14 Musculoskeletal Conditions, and 17 Supportive and Palliative Care for Cancer for discussion of use in other conditions.

8.3.1.1.6 Clinical Application

Ginger may improve NVP symptoms in the first trimester in some patients. Due to reports of increased bleeding, ginger should not be used near the end of the third trimester or in those patients with a history of miscarriage, vaginal bleeding, or clotting disorders (Lindblad and Koppula 2016).

8.3.2 Cervical Ripening (Labor and Delivery)

8.3.2.1 Red Raspberry Leaf (Rubi idaei folium)

8.3.2.1.1 Background

Red raspberry leaf tea has been used as a women's tonic, as well as for diseases of the skin, respiratory tract, and gastrointestinal tract. Documentation exists of its use as a medicinal agent as early as the sixth century in texts from the Middle Ages in Europe (Hummer 2010; Simpson et al. 2001). The traditional uses of the leaf of the red raspberry shrub include treatment of diarrhea, to ease menstrual pain, or during late pregnancy to prevent miscarriage and facilitate childbirth (Holst et al. 2009; Simpson et al. 2001).

8.3.2.1.2 Pharmacognosy

The bioactive compounds of the leaves are hydrolysable tannins (2.6%–6.9% w/w), primarily ellagic acids. Flavanoids, quercetin, and kaemferol, are in higher concentration in the leaves (0.46%–1.05%) than the fruit (Ferlemi and Lamari 2016). The leaf also contains iron, calcium, manganese, magnesium, copper, zinc, vitamin C, vitamin E, and niacin (Gallaher et al. 2006). Red raspberry leaf extract alters uterine muscle tone and the strength and frequency of uterine contractions of the pregnant but not the non-pregnant uterine muscle in early animal and tissue models (Holst et al. 2009; Simpson et al. 2001).

8.3.2.1.3 Dosing and Preparation

Dosage recommendations are not standardized in the compendia. Doses are listed as 2 g dried leaf prepared in 4–8 ounces of water as a tea taken 2 to 4 times a day, 2.4 gm/day of tablet or capsule dried leaf preparations, and varying amounts of tincture due to concentration differences. Available capsule dosage forms contain 300–480 mg of dried red raspberry leaf. Multiple teas are available (Gallaher et al. 2006; Holst et al. 2009).

8.3.2.1.4 Safety

Red raspberry leaf is GRAS when used orally in amounts commonly found in foods. Its use should be limited to later pregnancy, after 32 weeks (Simpson et al. 2001). A review lists a disagreeable taste to the tea for some women, thus capsules and tablets may be preferred (Simpson et al. 2001). Adverse effects reported more commonly with raspberry leaf included constipation, strong uterine tightening, dizziness and bloating, but were not significant as compared to placebo (Simpson et al. 2001). Case reports of increased blood pressure should limit the use in specific populations of pregnant women (Holst et al. 2009). Reports of estrogenic effects are also limited but concerning in the pregnant woman (Eagon et al. 2000).

8.3.2.1.5 Evidence

A retrospective study of 108 women participating in a midwife program were asked by questionnaire if they had consumed raspberry leaf products during pregnancy at their postnatal hospital stay. The women that had taken raspberry products (n = 57) were the study group and the control group (n = 51) was randomly selected from women who had not. Raspberry leaf product of patient choice was started as early as 8 weeks up to 39 weeks gestation, with the majority of use between 30 and 34 weeks gestation. The majority of the women thought that the consumption of the raspberry leaf product had shortened their labor and positively affected the birth. Raspberry leaf did not affect gestation length, blood loss, use of medical augmentation of labor, or infant outcome. The authors felt that some clinical differences were in favor of the use of raspberry leaf during pregnancy, including a reduction in laboring time and reduced use of medical intervention of delivery (Parsons et al. 1999).

In a follow-up double-blind randomized controlled trial (Simpson et al. 2001) 240 pregnant women were recruited to receive red raspberry leaf 1.2 gram tablets containing 400 mg of 3:1 leaf extract twice daily with food or identical placebo regimen starting at 32 weeks gestation. Groups were asked to refrain from any other raspberry leaf forms during the study period. The results from 96 women in each group were able to be analyzed. The red raspberry leaf group had a higher diastolic blood pressure value before consumption of the product in early pregnancy and at 32 weeks gestation. No difference was found between groups comparing pre- and post-labor blood pressure values. Ten women in the raspberry leaf group and five women in the control group developed pregnancy-induced hypertension/pre-eclampsia. The authors felt that the red raspberry leaf group had a clinical advantage in the reduced length of the second stage of labor ($p = 0.28$), more unassisted vaginal deliveries (62.4% versus 50.6%; $p = 0.19$) and fewer forceps/vacuum extraction deliveries (19.3% versus 30.4%). The authors conceded that there is no significant relationship between raspberry leaf consumption and the outcomes between groups (Simpson et al. 2001).

A review of the safety and efficacy of red raspberry leaf use in pregnancy reveals a lack of clinical data, some of which is over 60 years old. In humans, a noncontrolled case report of three women taking raspberry leaf extract after delivery showed uterine relaxation measured by an intrauterine bag device. Other human trials reviewed are also described above. The authors conclude that evidence is insufficient to recommend red raspberry leaf products to pregnant women (Holst et al. 2009).

8.3.2.1.6 Clinical Application

Red raspberry leaf teas and other oral products have been used for women's health for centuries.

Some reports suggest a benefit in reduction of menstrual cramps. The use in pregnancy is regarded as safe under the care of a health professional. The use should be limited to later pregnancy, after 32 weeks' gestation. Women with increased blood pressure prior to pregnancy should avoid this product as it may be associated with hypertension of pregnancy and pre-eclampsia. Pregnant women who experience increased uterine contractions before approaching their due date while taking red raspberry leaf products should discontinue its use.

8.3.3 Galactagogue (Breastfeeding)

8.3.3.1 Fenugreek (Trigonella foenum-graecum)

8.3.3.1.1 Background

The fenugreek seed has been used for thousands of years, originating in the Middle East, North Africa, Egypt, and India. Fenugreek has been used for many women's health problems historically, for inducing childbirth and reducing menopausal symptoms. More recently, fenugreek is used for diabetes, hyperlipidemia, and as a galactagogue (Mandhare et al. 2016).

8.3.3.1.2 Pharmacognosy

Fenugreek seeds contain mucilage (galactomannan), fiber, fatty acids, amino acids (lysine, tryptophan, arginine, threonine, valine and methionine), alkaloids (trigonelline), flavonoids, saponins (coumarins), and vitamins A, C, D, B1, and minerals (calcium, iron, zinc). There are two proposed mechanisms of action for fenugreek to increase milk: an increase in production of sweat glands which leads to milk supply increases, or that fenugreek phytoestrogens and diosgenin, a steroid sapogenin, increases milk flow (Forinash et al. 2012; Turkyılmaz et al. 2011).

8.3.3.1.3 Dosing and Preparation

Fenugreek seed is taken as 3500–4000 mg/day (2 capsules of approximately 600 mg each with meals three times a day) until milk production is increased (Forinash et al. 2012; Zapantis et al. 2012). It can also be taken as a tea made from fenugreek seed powder (7.5 gm in 8 ounces of water) three times a day (Ghasemi et al. 2015; Zapantis et al. 2012).

8.3.3.1.4 Safety

Fenugreek is GRAS by the FDA in food products. It is possibly safe for women postpartum for up to 3 months, in doses as above, to enhance milk production (Zapantis et al. 2012). It is likely unsafe for women who are pregnant in doses greater than that found in a regular diet due to potential oxytocic effect and uterine stimulation (Zapantis et al. 2012). Persons with allergies to legume, chickpea, peanut or soy should avoid fenugreek because it is part of the Fabaceae "pea" family of plants (Zapantis et al. 2012). Adverse effects include minor gastrointestinal discomfort, headache, diarrhea and flatulence. After ingestion, the urine may smell of maple syrup. In infants, this can be mistaken for maple sugar urine disease, a metabolic disorder (Forinash et al. 2012). The mucilage component of fenugreek seed may decrease or delay absorption of other medications if taken concomitantly. There is a potential interaction with antithrombotics that may increase bleeding risk. Hypoglycemia may occur in some patients due to decreased absorption of carbohydrates. Blood glucose should be monitored when taking antidiabetic medications (Forinash et al. 2012; Zapantis et al. 2012).

8.3.3.1.5 Evidence

Fenugreek was given to 26 mothers of preterm infants, less than 31 weeks gestation, who were unable to breastfeed directly, in a randomized double blind, placebo controlled study. Three 575 mg capsules of either fenugreek or placebo were ingested three times a day for 21 days. The mothers were instructed in correct breast pump usage. Prolactin levels were drawn at baseline and then weekly during the study period. Study subjects kept a diary of pumping times, volume of breast milk expressed, kangaroo care (skin to skin) time, stress, sleep, and any side effects or illnesses experienced by the mother. Infants had their health, fluid status, gastrointestinal symptoms, respiratory symptoms, and weight changes documented by nursing staff at the hospital during the study duration. From the original 58 subjects recruited, 14 mothers that received fenugreek, and 12 taking placebo finished the study and were included. No differences in milk volume, prolactin level, emotion/stress levels, or infant data were found by the authors (Reeder et al. 2013).

A clinical report of 1200 women given fenugreek to stimulate lactation and seen in a breastfeeding clinic in California over a 6-year period, stated that both ease of breastfeeding and milk production were enhanced. Most women reported benefits within 72 hours of starting fenugreek capsules three times a day and then were able to discontinue fenugreek without loss of milk production (Huggins 1998).

Women with newborn infants were divided into three groups of 22 participants each. The intervention group received a tea containing fenugreek three cups a day, the placebo group received apple tea in the same volume, and the control group received no tea. All groups received routine postpartum advice. No differences in baseline data were found between groups. The volume of breast milk pumped over 15 minutes after 3 days was larger in the intervention group (73.2 ± 53.5 mL) than the placebo (38.8 ± 16.3 mL) or control groups (31.1 ± 12.9 mL). Infants in the intervention group had less weight loss after birth and regained birth weight sooner than the other groups. The tea containing fenugreek contained other herbs that may have contributed to the outcome (Turkyılmaz et al. 2011).

Another study of healthy breastfeeding term infant girls between birth and 4 months of age was conducted in Iran. Their mothers were randomized into two groups. The intervention group received black tea prepared with powdered fenugreek seeds and the placebo group received black tea with no other ingredients, one cup three times per day. None of the mothers had taken galactagogues previously. Baseline characteristics of mothers and infants in both groups were similar except for increased number of breastfeeding times per day in the placebo group. By week 4, the fenugreek infant group had gained more weight, had gained more in head circumference, had an increased number of wet and soiled diapers, and were feeding more frequently than the placebo group. Length of the infant was not significantly different. No adverse effects were noted in any group (Ghasemi et al. 2015).

See Chapters 6 Endocrine Disorders and 15 Obesity and Weight Loss for discussion of use in other conditions.

8.3.3.1.6 Clinical Application

Fenugreek is used to stimulate lactation in women with perceived low milk supply or other difficulty in breastfeeding an infant. The desired effect has been reported with both capsules and tea given three times a day (Sim et al. 2015). Evidence is limited on efficacy and safety.

8.3.3.2 Milk Thistle (Silybum marianum)

8.3.3.2.1 Background

Milk thistle is indigenous to India and southern Europe. Preparations of milk thistle seeds have been used medicinally from as early as fourth century B.C. Traditionally the seeds have been used in Europe as a galactogogue in nursing mothers. Milk thistle is also used for women's health issues including uterine complaints, menopausal symptoms, low breast milk supply, and infertility (Bhattacharya 2011).

8.3.3.2.2 Pharmacognosy

The active constituents of milk thistle seeds are silibinin (silybin), silychristin, and silidianin, collectively known as silymarin, extracted from the dried milk thistle seeds. Silibinin is the most biologically active component. The seeds also contain other flavonolignans, betaine, apigenin, silybonol, proteins, fixed oil and free fatty acids, which may contribute to the effects of milk thistle seeds (Bhattacharya 2011).

8.3.3.2.3 Dosing and Preparation

The average adult dose of powdered seed is 12–15 g/day; as dry standardized seed extract (silymarin): 200–400 mg/day; as liquid seed extract: 4–9 mL/day. Silymarin is poorly soluble in water, so milk thistle seed is not effective as a tea. Extracts from the seed are generally marketed as tablet and encapsulated form for oral use, usually containing an extract standardized to 70%–80% of silymarin (Bhattacharya 2011).

8.3.3.2.4 Safety

Women with allergies to the Asteraceae/Compositae family of plants may exhibit allergy to milk thistle. Most reported adverse reactions have been mild, including occasional gastrointestinal distress, pruritus, and headache. Silymarin has potential interactions including through inhibition of CYP2C9, CYP2D6 and CYP3A4, b-glucuronidase and P-glycoprotein (Zapantis et al. 2012). *See Chapter 2 Pharmacokinetic and Pharmacogenomic Considerations for more discussion.*

8.3.3.2.5 Evidence

Milk thistle micronized extract 420 mg (silymarin content 252 mg) (n = 25) or placebo (n = 25) was given twice daily to lactating women in Peru. At baseline, the women produced milk at about 15% of expected levels. The groups were similar for age, age of last child, quantity of breastmilk produced, or the macro constituents of their milk at baseline. Milk quantity increased in the treatment group over the placebo group at 30 days (990 mL vs. 650 mL) and 63 days (1119 mL vs 700 mL), but milk did not differ in water, protein, fat, or carbohydrate content. Silymarin or its components were not found in analysis of milk. The treatment group did not report adverse effects (Di Pierro et al. 2008).

A single blind randomized controlled study gave the micronized extract of milk thistle 420 mg (silymarin content 252 mg) twice daily or placebo for 28 days to women (N = 50) who gave birth to infants prematurely before 32 weeks' gestation. Milk production was quantified for 43 days. The women in the silymarin group had a higher production volume at baseline that continued through day 43. Milk production variation between groups was negligible during the period of product intake (day zero and days 26–28) (silymarin: 24.9 ± 38.1 g/day; placebo: 77.3 ± 24.9; difference silymarin-placebo: −52.4 ± 45.5 g/day, P = 0.872). The groups were asked about what product they believed that they were taking on the 28th day of the study. Women who believed they were taking silymarin had higher milk production at baseline and at days 26–28, even if they were in the placebo group. No important adverse events were reported for either mothers or infants. Silymarin concentration in human milk was not detectable (<0.3 mg/kg) at day 14 in any of the samples analyzed (Peila et al. 2015).

A double blind randomized controlled trial of mothers of preterm infants born between 27 and 33 weeks' gestation gave either 5 g of a product containing silymarin and galega (goat's rue) (n = 50) or lactose placebo (n = 50) for 25 days starting at 72 hours after birth. The primary outcome was milk volume 25% greater than historical norms for a similar group, or about 152 mL/day. Milk production was calculated from the volume of milk pumped at the hospital and that brought in from home by the mothers. The amount of milk was significantly higher in the galactagogue taking group at day 7 and 30 compared to the placebo group ($p < 0.05$). The volume of milk production from day 7 until 30 days after delivery was a mean amount of 200 mL in the galactagogue group (25% over historical mean) compared with 115 mL in the placebo group ($p < 0.0001$). Adverse reactions were not noted by the participants or their infants during the study period (Zecca et al. 2016).

8.3.3.2.6 Clinical Applications

The FDA does not list milk thistle as GRAS in food or supplements (Center for Food Safety and Applied Nutrition 2014). The evaluation of the benefit or safety of milk thistle as a galactagogue is limited. Adverse effects in the available studies are mild and reversible. Data on the outcomes of ingestion of milk thistle or its components by infants is limited to short-term use.

8.4 Perimenopause/Menopause

Perimenopause is a period of time prior to the last menstrual cycle and varies between women. Menopause is defined as the cessation of menses for a 12-month timeframe (Manson and Kaunitz 2016). The number of women over the age of 45 years that are likely to experience symptoms of menopause is increasing with the aging U.S. population (Gold et al. 2013). Most women report vasomotor symptoms, such as hot flushes and night sweats. Others may have mood changes, sleep disturbances, and memory loss, and some sexual dysfunction concerns. Many women are seeking non-hormonal remedies including botanicals for their menopausal symptoms (Manson and Kaunitz 2016).

8.4.1 Black Cohosh (*Actaea racemosa* or *Cimicifuga racemose*)

8.4.1.1 Background

Black cohosh was used by Native American for muscle aches and women's health concerns. It was adopted by early settlers to North America and termed "black snakeroot" in the nineteenth century USP. In Germany during the 1940s, black cohosh was introduced as a plant based estrogenic product to treat the hypophysis and "neurovegetative" symptoms including menstrual discomfort and menopausal symptoms (Lieberman 1998). In the United States, it is now found most frequently in dietary supplements and formulations taken for menopause, premenstrual syndrome, menstrual cramping, and preparation for childbirth.

8.4.1.2 Pharmacognosy

A herbaceous perennial plant from the family of *Ranunculaceae*, four American species of black cohosh exist (Betz et al. 2009). Black cohosh extracts are prepared from the roots and rhizomes. The plant is mostly gathered in the wild which brings concerns for proper identification by collectors. Recent attempts at cultivation have been successful, but may alter some of the plant's chemistry (Betz et al. 2009). The rhizome and attached roots of *Cimicifuga racemosa* are harvested in autumn and used fresh or in dried form. The rhizome of *Cimicifuga racemosa* contains triterpene glycosides including actein, cimicifugoside, cimiracemoside A, and 27-deoxyactein, as well as phenylpropanoids such as hydroxycinnamic acids. Further ingredients include alkaloids, N-methylserotonin, starch, fatty acids, resin, and tannins (Beer and Neff 2013).

8.4.1.3 Dosing and Preparation

To manage symptoms of menopause, the recommended dose of black cohosh is 40 mg of an alcoholic extract daily, standardized to contain 1 mg of the triterpene 27-deoxyactein per 20 mg, in 3 or 4 divided doses per day. Therapeutic effects generally begin after 2 weeks and maximum effects occur by week 8. The dried root product may be taken in quantities of 300–3000 mg per day in divided doses (Beer and Neff 2013; Low Dog et al. 2003).

8.4.1.4 Safety

Persons with liver disease should avoid black cohosh. Cases of hepatotoxicity have been associated with the use of black cohosh. The reported changes in liver function may be idiosyncratic, or due to patient specific factors or product adulteration (Betz et al. 2009). Black cohosh should not be used in women who are pregnant or may become pregnant. Drug interactions occur with estrogen containing products, docetaxel, and medications that are metabolized by the P450 CYP3A4 pathway such as midazolam (Low Dog et al. 2003). *See Chapter 2 Pharmacokinetic and Pharmacogenomic Considerations for more discussion.*

8.4.1.5 Evidence

In a double blind study, 304 symptomatic menopausal women from 24 centers were randomized to receive 2.5 mg of black cohosh 40% isopropanolic extract, equal to 20 mg of dry root (a single batch of commercial brand—Remifemin) or placebo tablets twice daily for 12 weeks. Baseline characteristics for all women were similar. No women were on hormone therapy, antiepileptics, psychiatric medications, or nutritional supplements such as soy and red clover for the duration of the study. The Menopause Rating Scale (MRS) was used to determine intensity of climacteric symptoms. After exclusions, 136 women were in each group that completed the study. The intervention group showed better scores on overall MRS scores ($p < 0.001$), Hot flushes markers ($p = 0.002$), Soma markers ($p < 0.48$) and Atrophy markers ($p < 0.001$) than the placebo group. A statistically relevant decline in the treatment difference occurred with increasing FSH level and women with over 3 years of menopausal symptoms. Adverse event reports were similar between groups (Osmers et al. 2005).

A multicenter RCT of 45- to 60-year-old postmenopausal women was conducted to determine the impact on hot flushes and vasomotor symptoms. These women were given black cohosh 6.5 mg dry root extract ($n = 42$) or matching placebo ($n = 42$) once daily with dinner for 8 weeks. Women with potential psychiatric, endocrine, or oncology concerns were excluded. The Greene vasomotor symptom scale and other internally validated diary type rubrics were used to determine the frequency and intensity of symptoms and any adverse effects. The intervention group had fewer vasomotor and hot flush symptoms at 4 and 8 weeks of the study ($p < 0.001$) (Shahnazi et al. 2013).

A retrospective chart review was conducted on 100 menopausal women who had been randomized to take a black cohosh containing supplement (84 mg black cohosh extract with St. John's wort) or placebo for hot flushes and vasomotor symptoms for 12 weeks. The women had PAP smears performed before and after the intervention. No differences were shown between groups' baseline characteristics. Maturation scores of vaginal cells were not different between groups. The authors conclude that there is no estrogenic effect of black cohosh on vaginal tissue (Hong et al. 2012).

In a recent review of the literature, the authors concluded that the extracts vary in their efficacy and safety. The isopranolic (iCR) extract 40 mg standardized dose per day was superior to placebo in relieving vasomotor symptoms especially in women in the first few years of menopause, reaching an average response rate of 70% to 80%. A combination of this extract iCR and St. John's wort have some efficacy in controlling anxiety, irritability, and depression. The ethanolic extract, BNO1055, has also shown benefit in menopausal symptom relief in uncontrolled studies. The authors state that studies performed in the United States with black cohosh products that are not certified have not shown efficacy for menopausal women. Adverse effects of black cohosh have not been different than those from placebo in controlled trials (Beer and Neff 2013).

A Cochrane review examined 16 RCTs with black cohosh as the intervention agent in over 2000 peri- and post-menopausal women. All studies administered oral preparations of black cohosh as monotherapy at a dose of 40 mg per day for a mean duration of 23.4 weeks. Hot flushes and night sweats did not differ between those taking black cohosh and placebo. The overall effect of black cohosh as compared to placebo did not change with use of any or a combination of menopausal symptom scoring systems (Kupperman index, Greene climacteric scale, Wiklund menopause symptom score). No study showed differences in adverse events in women taking black cohosh compared to placebo. Black cohosh was less effective against menopausal vasomotor symptoms compared to hormone therapy (HT). However,

HT had a much higher rate of adverse effects reported (1.46 events/subject versus 0.55 events/subject). Since the studies using any comparator were not similar enough in method or results, with some having missing methodology and/or data, conclusions about the efficacy or safety of black cohosh are not robust. The authors conclude that black cohosh is probably safe and may be useful for some women to reduce symptoms of menopause (Leach and Moore 2012).

8.4.1.6 Clinical Application

Black cohosh may relieve vasomotor symptoms for some women in early menopause. A trial of 40–80 mg per day of the isopranolic extract of black cohosh, or equivalent, may be warranted. Other dosing information depends on the extract/product utilized (Beer and Neff 2013; Hardy 2000; Osmers et al. 2005). Black cohosh should be discontinued at 12 weeks if no relief is experienced. It may continue for a year if relief or resolution of symptoms is experienced (Leach and Moore 2012).

8.4.2 Dong Quai (*Angelica sinensis*) (*Danggui, Tang-kuei*)

8.4.2.1 Background

A member of the plant family Apiaceae which also includes celery, parsley, carrots, and dill, dong quai originated in China. *Angelica sinensis* is used in Traditional Chinese Medicine (TCM) as a blood tonic and an anti-inflammatory agent, often in combination with other botanicals. It is used for gynecologic disorders, such as painful menstruation, anemia, premenstrual syndrome, menopause, fatigue and cardiovascular conditions. It is also called "female ginseng" (Hardy 2000; Wei et al. 2016).

8.4.2.2 Pharmacognosy

The active components of *Angelica sinensis* root are organic acids including folic acid, and ferulic acid, phthalides such asligustulide, and polysaccharides. The root also contains vitamins A, C, E, B12, niacin, and minerals which include iron, calcium, potassium, selenium, magnesium, zinc, manganese, and silicon. The dried root is used to prepare available encapsulated products and volatile oil. Dong quai is also used as a medicinal food. Fresh or dried root can be prepared into soup or wine. The mechanism of action in gynecologic disorders including menopause is unknown (Hook 2014; Ling et al. 2012; Wei et al. 2016).

8.4.2.3 Dosing and Preparation

A dose of 4.5 g per day (encapsulated dried root) can be taken as three 500 mg capsules three times a day. Powdered root in various forms is taken as 1–3 g three times a day. Other forms, including fluid extract tablets and tinctures, may have different doses. There is no proven dose for efficacy for relieving the symptoms of menopause. Products standardized to active component content are preferred, however this can vary between European, U.K. and Chinese markets. In general, *Angelica sinensis* is marked by its Z- ligustilide or trans-ferulic or ferulic acid content (Hook 2014).

8.4.2.4 Safety

Angelica sinensis is GRAS when taken orally in doses less than 15 gm per day by the FDA, although headache, hypotension and heart rhythm changes have been reported. Patients on antithrombotic agents may have an increased bleeding risk with the addition of *Angelica sinensis* (Heck et al. 2000; Stanger et al. 2012; Ulbricht et al. 2008b).

Dong quai should be avoided in women with a history of breast cancer as evidence exists of stimulation of breast cancer cell lines (MCF-7 and BT-20) (Lau et al. 2005). Women taking CYP2D6 or CYP3A4 substrates such as antidepressants, antipsychotics, beta-blockers, analgesics and anti-arrhythmic agents should avoid taking dong quai (Hook 2014).

Concerns regarding substitution of *Angelica acutiloba* or *Agylla gigas* for *Angelica sinensis* has led to more rigorous laboratory analysis for the preferred active constituents, ligustulide and ferulic acid, and for less preferred constituents of the substitutions, coumarins (Hook 2014; Ling et al. 2012; Wei et al. 2016).

8.4.2.5 Evidence

In a randomized double blind controlled trial, symptomatic menopausal women were given a dong quai supplement of dried root powder capsule standardized to 0.5 mg/kg of ferulic acid (n = 36) or placebo (n = 35). Three capsules were taken three times a day. Participants in the intervention arm received the equivalent of 4.5 grams of dong quai root daily for 24 weeks. Baseline characteristics for both groups were similar. Women were in clinic at baseline, 6, 12, and 24 weeks to evaluate blood pressure, weight, serum hormone levels, changes in endometrial and vaginal tissue, and menopausal symptoms. There were six drop outs in the placebo group and four in the intervention group for lack of efficacy, minor adverse effects, or change in health. No changes were noted in the number or quantity of hot flushes or other menopausal symptoms at any stage of evaluation. Kupperman scores were reduced by 30% from baseline but not significantly different between the groups. Endometrial thickness by ultrasound was increased by 2.3 mm from baseline in the placebo group and 0.8 mm the intervention group, not considered clinically significant. No hormonal or other changes were noted from baseline in either group. The authors concluded that dong quai did not benefit the menopausal women (Hirata et al. 1997).

In a Cochrane review of 22 randomized controlled studies of traditional Chinese botanical medicines that included *Angelica sinensis* used to alleviate menopausal vasomotor symptoms, there was insufficient evidence to show benefit over placebo. Minor adverse effects included gastrointestinal tract or breast tenderness (Zhu et al. 2016).

8.4.2.6 Clinical Application

Efficacy is based on traditional usage of dong quai when combined with other botanicals. Evidence does not support the use of *Angelica sinensis* products as monotherapy for the relief of menopausal symptoms. The use of dong quai in combination with other botanicals may be beneficial, but data is limited.

8.4.3 Asian Ginseng (*Panax ginseng*)

8.4.3.1 Background

The root of plants of the species Panax sp. (Family Araliaceae) is used medicinally. *Panax ginseng*, or Asian ginseng, is grown in Northeastern China and Korea. It is the oldest known botanical, considered powerful due to its root's physical form that looks like a human figure. *Panax* known as "all cure" and is a Greek root for word "panacea." Globally, the botanical is considered an adaptogen. The extract is used in TCM to restore "balance" and vital life force, and to enhance stamina. Ginseng is used to decrease fatigue, help improve concentration and cognitive function, improve female libido, and reduce menopausal symptoms (Geng et al. 2010; Kim et al. 2013a; Kim et al. 2012; Oh et al. 2010; Tode et al. 1999; Wiklund et al. 1999).

Ginseng is covered throughout this text for various conditions.

8.4.3.2 Pharmacognosy

White ginseng is unprocessed dried root and red ginseng is a steamed root. Dried root of *Panax ginseng* contains up to 200 components including ginsenosides, polysaccharides, polyacetylenes, peptides, and amino acids (Kim et al. 2013b). *See Chapter 10 Neurologic Conditions for more discussion.*

8.4.3.3 Dosing and Preparation

Red ginseng, a specific form of *Panax ginseng*, 36 grams daily in up to 3 divided doses for 4–12 weeks has been used (Kim et al. 2013b). *Panax ginseng* extract (G115, Ginsana®) 200–400 mg daily in the morning has also been used (Coon and Ernst 2002). *See Chapter 10 Neurologic Conditions for more discussion.*

8.4.3.4 Safety

Overall, adverse effects are mild in patients taking *Panax ginseng.* Controversy exists over the potential hormonal effects of *Panax ginseng.* There are reports of mastalgia and vaginal bleeding with use of topical or oral products in postmenopausal women. Phytoestrogenic effects on human breast cancer cells may be due to estrogen receptor binding. *Panax ginseng* has been associated with CNS stimulation in chronic users with psychiatric disorders. There is a potential increased bleeding risk with antithrombotic medications (Coon and Ernst 2002). *See Chapter 2 Pharmacokinetic and Pharmacogenomic Considerations for more discussion on potential drug interactions.*

8.4.3.5 Evidence

The effects of a standardized ginseng extract were compared at baseline and again at 16 weeks with those of a placebo in a randomized, multicenter, double-blind, parallel group study assessing quality of life and physiologic characteristics of 384 symptomatic menopausal women. Laboratory data on FSH and estradiol, as well as Pap smear samples, vaginal pH, and endometrial thickness by ultrasound, were obtained and three questionnaires gauging quality of life were completed by 193 women treated with ginseng standardized extract 200 mg daily and 191 women treated with placebo. Quality of life instruments were the Women's Health questionnaire, the psychological general well- being score, and the climacteric complaints by visual analog score. Results for patients receiving ginseng did not differ significantly from placebo for vasomotor symptoms, laboratory values, or cellular changes. Women did report reduced depression, better overall well-being, and health on one of the quality of life questionnaires (Psychological General Wellbeing index) in favor of ginseng compared with placebo ($p < 0.05$) (Wiklund et al. 1999).

A systematic review of randomized placebo controlled trials of ginseng for vasomotor and other symptoms in menopausal women was conducted. Of 87 trials screened, four trials met the inclusion criteria, with a total population of over 500 women. The largest trial was the one described above which used a standardized extract of ginseng in European women. The three smaller trials included used Korean red ginseng in Asian women. Differences in outcomes of these trials were considered due to dosing variations. Outcomes on relief of vasomotor symptoms and global health were considered favorable by the reviewers. No conclusions regarding efficacy or safety were stated due to variability of data and rigor of the trials (Kim et al. 2012).

8.4.3.6 Clinical Application

Ginseng does not have data to support its efficacy or safety in menopausal women.

8.4.4 Red Clover (*Trifolium pretense*)

8.4.4.1 Background

Red clover is a legume and part of the pea family Fabaceae/Leguminosae. It is cultivated in Europe and North America for nitrogen fixing of the soil. Cattle and sheep were found to have changes in fertility and increased risk of bloat and spontaneous abortion when grazed on it (Lethaby et al. 2013). Currently, red clover is used for menopausal symptoms (Beck et al. 2005; Lethaby et al. 2013).

8.4.4.2 Pharmacognosy

Red clover has a high content of isoflavones including genestein, daidzein, biochanin A and formononetin, as well as a smaller amount of coumestans. Pharmacologic effects are seen on estrogen, androgen, and progesterone receptors in yeast, animal, and human tissue models (Beck et al. 2005). The aboveground parts of the plant, including flower heads, leaves and stems are used to produce extracts (Booth et al. 2006).

8.4.4.3 Dosing and Preparation

The recommended dose is 40–80 mg daily of standardized isoflavone content (Beck et al. 2005; Lethaby et al. 2013). The isoflavone content differs in commercially available products (Wang et al. 2008).

8.4.4.4 Safety

Trials and reviews do not report differences between adverse effects of red clover supplements and placebo (Lethaby et al. 2013). Red clover extracts are safe when used for up to 3 years in medicinal amounts. No evidence of drug interactions is found with red clover. Patients with a high risk of bleeding, although unlikely, should avoid the botanical due to small amounts of coumarin compounds (Nelsen et al. 2002).

8.4.4.5 Evidence

A randomized multicenter double-blind placebo controlled study comparing the efficacy and safety of Promensil (41 mg of red clover isoflavones per tablet) or Remostil (28.6 mg of red clover isoflavones per tablet) was conducted in postmenopausal women 45–60 years of age with at least 35 hot flush episodes per week at baseline. Subjects had FSH serum concentrations of less than 30 mIU/mL. Vegetarians, subjects who consumed soy products regularly, or were taking medications that would decrease isoflavone absorption were excluded from study. Promensil has a higher concentration of biochanin A and genistein. Remostil has a greater concentration of mononetin and daidzein. The placebo tablets each contained less than 0.04 mg of total isoflavones. Subjects took two tablets once daily. Baseline data and physical exam were conducted before and at the end of a 2-week placebo period for all participants. Subjects that were 80% adherent to the 2-week regimen had a 24-hour urine samples taken and then took their randomized supplement treatment or placebo tablets for 12 weeks. Subjects were given a symptom and quality of life diary to complete and were contacted by phone throughout the study to encourage compliance and assess safety and efficacy. At the end of the study period, a pill count, another physical examination, laboratory analysis and 24-hour urine sample were collected. Of the 252 women who started, 98% (242) completed the study. Compliance was high with 98% of subjects taking at least 80% of the anticipated tablets. The number of hot flushes per week were reduced in all groups (41% in the Promensil group, 34% in the Rimostil group and 36% in the placebo group) by the end of the study ($p < 0.001$). Promensil reduced the frequency of hot flushes more rapidly than in the other groups. The supplements did not statistically differ from placebo at the end of the 12-week period. Women in all groups still experienced as many as five hot flush episodes per day at the end of the 12-week intervention. There was no correlation between urine isoflavone excretion in the urine and hot flush frequency ($p = 0.84$). Adverse effects were similar between groups (Tice et al. 2003).

The effects of a red clover extract on the vasomotor and general menopausal symptoms of symptomatic menopausal women over 40 years of age were analyzed. Subjects were randomized to received two capsules containing 80 mg of red clover isoflavones ($n = 50$) or a placebo ($n = 59$) for 90 days in a crossover design with a 7-day-washout period between the switch. Group A received the red clover supplement in the first phase and placebo in the second and Group B the reverse. Number of daily hot flushes/night sweats and menopausal symptom intensity, using the Kupperman index, were measured at baseline, 90, 97, and 187 days. No significant differences were found between groups in background of the subjects or characteristics, frequency, or intensity of menopausal symptoms at baseline. Both groups had decreased frequency of hot flushes in the red clover supplement time period. Night sweat frequency and Kupperman index scores, including that for anxiety and depression, decreased similarly in both groups during the ingestion of red clover supplementation. No adverse effects were reported in either group (Lipovac et al. 2012).

Nine trials, conducted from 1999 to 2010, which assessed the use of red clover extracts containing 40 to 120 mg of isoflavones on menopausal symptoms were analyzed within a Cochrane review of differing products containing isoflavones. The number and intensity of hot flushes and other vasomotor symptoms was reduced in many women in small studies, however, not in larger trials. The authors concluded that the variability of study design, size, and quality does not allow a strong conclusion as to the efficacy of red clover extract in reducing the number or intensity menopausal symptoms (Lethaby et al. 2013).

8.4.4.6 Clinical Application

Phytoestrogenic isoflavones derived from red clover can be considered for use in menopausal women to decrease frequency and intensity of vasomotor and other symptoms, although efficacy data is limited. Estrogenic effects on endometrial and breast tissue have not been demonstrated in human subjects at therapeutic doses. It may be prudent to avoid in women with a history of breast cancer.

8.4.5 Soy (*Glycine max*) Also Known as Daizu

8.4.5.1 Background

From the family Leguminosae, soy is cultivated in warm temperate zones from Asia to Australia. Soy beans have been used as a food staple with a high quality protein, oil and carbohydrate source in Asia and most recently used as a low glycemic index food for patients with diabetes. Medicinally, extracts have been used to protect bone density, heart health, and reduce menopausal symptoms in women (Aguiar and de Paula Barbosa 2014; Kalaiselvan et al. 2010).

8.4.5.2 Pharmacognosy

Soy contains daidzen, genistein, and glycitein, which is released from soy beans or powder during digestion. Equol is a digestive product of daidzen in humans who are genetically predisposed. Equol has weak estrogenic properties that mimics estradiol and can be active at hormonal receptors in the body. Soy isoflavones are secreted via enterohepatic circulation from bile. The beans are used as food and to produce multiple products, fermented and non-fermented foods, protein powders, and extracts (Kalaiselvan et al. 2010; Setchell et al. 2002).

8.4.5.3 Dosing and Preparation

Soy isolate or foods with combined isoflavone content of 40–120 mg/day may be used (Levis and Griebeler 2010). A meta-analysis showed that genistein dose should be a minimum of 19 mg/day (Taku et al. 2010).

8.4.5.4 Safety

Soy powder or beans used as a food stuff is GRAS. Women using soy powder as a supplement or extracts report bloating, nausea, weight gain, and bowel function changes. Some women in trials using soy powder prepared as a beverage disliked the taste of the supplement (Lethaby et al. 2013). A systematic review of 31 trials did not show an association of soy products with breast cancer in perimenopausal women from Western countries. There is inconsistent reports of the benefit of soy in prevention of breast cancer in pre- and post-menopausal Asian women (Chen et al. 2014). Soy has no well documented drug interactions and does not interact with tamoxifen. Soy does not generally cause symptoms in patients with known peanut allergy (Sicherer et al. 2000).

8.4.5.5 Evidence

A randomized crossover design comparing three soy protein supplements on plasma hormone concentrations was completed in 18 menopausal women with normal body mass index (BMI). Each subject consumed their usual diet but avoided foods with known phytoestrogens and alcoholic beverages. Soy protein powder supplements were added daily, contributing 348 calories, 63 grams protein, 21 grams carbohydrates, and 1.9 grams fat. Total isoflavone concentration varied in each of the three products, with the control contributing 0.11 mg, low content 1 mg and high content 2 mg per kg body weight of the subject daily. Dietary intake of calories did not differ between baseline and any of the intervention periods. Protein intake increased over baseline levels in all groups (p < 0.05). Carbohydrate, fat and fiber intake decreased from baseline in all groups (p < 0.05). Changes in FSH, estradiol, estrone, testosterone, DHEA-S, sex hormone binding globulin (SHBG) and thyroid binding globulin were demonstrated differing between the control and low from the high content supplements from baseline and at the end of study. Vaginal cytology and endometrial biopsy results did not vary from baseline or control product compared to either supplement. The authors state that soy components other than isoflavones may have complicated the results of the study (Duncan et al. 1999).

A randomized double blind placebo controlled study of soy isoflavone 100 mg per day was conducted in 80 menopausal women not taking any hormonal treatments in an effort to decrease menopausal symptoms, and cardiovascular risk, and to effect endogenous hormone levels. Subjects were excluded if they were on antidiabetic or lipid-lowering medications, ate soy or took other supplements, had uncontrolled hypertension or another cardiovascular risk. The Kupperman menopausal index, hormonal serum levels and physical data were assessed at baseline and at the end of the study. The baseline data were similar in both placebo and intervention arms. Patients on isoflavone therapy had a significantly lower Kupperman index and had fewer and less severe menopausal symptoms as compared to placebo at the end of the study period (p < 0.01). Cardiovascular risk markers, total cholesterol, and low density lipoprotein (LDL) cholesterol were significantly decreased in the treatment group as compared to baseline for both groups throughout and at the end of study for placebo (P < 0.001). High density lipoprotein (HDL) cholesterol (p < 0.005) and triglycerides (p < 0.05) increased from baseline in both groups. Blood pressure or plasma glucose were unchanged in both groups, as well as in hormonal or endometrial thickness by transvaginal sonography. The exception was an increase in 17 beta-estradiol at the end of study in the treatment group (p < 0.001), but this was not considered clinically significant (Han et al. 2002).

A systematic review and meta-analysis was conducted of double blind RCTs of soy to reduce menopausal hot flush frequency and severity published until the end of 2010. Inclusion criteria in the systematic review were met by 19 trials and 17 trials were included in the meta-analysis. The trials included in the systemic review were conducted in ten different countries on menopausal or perimenopausal women, sixteen trials were a crossover design and three were of parallel design. Soy isoflavone doses varied from 30 to 135 mg per day. Hot flush frequency was analyzed from data of 13 trials and 1,196 subjects and concluded that overall frequency decreased on both placebo and on soy. After eliminating the effect of placebo from the treatment data, hot flush frequency varied from a 3% to 57% decrease and 10 trials reported a benefit (p < 0.05). In the meta-analysis, daily ingestion of 30–80 mg of soy isoflavones for 6 weeks to 12 months significantly reduced overall hot flush frequency by 20% (p < 0.0001).

Severity of hot flushes was analyzed from nine trials including 988 women and resulted in a significant reduction in severity in response to soy intake as compared to placebo (p < 0.00001). Daily ingestion of a median dose of 54 mg of isoflavones for 12 weeks to 12 months significantly reduced hot flush severity as compared to placebo by 26% (p < 0.001) (Taku et al. 2012).

A model-based meta-analysis was developed to estimate the efficacy of soy on hot flushes in the English language literature from January 1990 to January 2014. The model was evaluated by graphic assessment using Monte Carlo simulations comparing placebo to soy effects. Effects of estradiol were compared to that of soy isoflavones using the same model. The authors conclude that the model indicates that soy isoflavones have an effect on menopausal hot flush frequency and severity of about 25% compared to placebo but only after 13.4 weeks. This is less than half of the effect of estradiol on menopausal symptoms and that estradiol only requires about 3 weeks to gain 80% of its maximal effect. The model suggests that to reach 80% of the maximal effect of soy 48 weeks of daily treatment would be required. No benefit of individual soy isoflavones was able to be identified (Li et al. 2015).

See Chapters 5 Cardiovascular Disease, 6 Endocrine Disorders, 14 Musculoskeletal Conditions, 16 Cancer Prevention and Treatment and 17 Supportive and Palliative Care for Cancer for discussion for other conditions.

8.4.5.6 Clinical Application

Soy products containing 40 mg or more of isoflavone given daily for 12–48 weeks may give some patients relief from hot flushes or other menopausal symptoms. Breast cancer patients may need to be aware of potential risks.

8.4.6 Wild Yam (*Dioscorea villosa*)

8.4.6.1 Background

D. villosa is a vine found in central southeastern U.S. Wild yam was popularized in the nineteenth century for antispasmodic effects when taken internally. Current topical use for menopausal symptoms is due to the belief that its diosgenin content can mimic progesterone (Dong et al. 2012).

8.4.6.2 Pharmacognosy

Extracts of Dioscorea root contain steroidal saponins, diosgenin, alkaloids, tannins, phytosterols, and starch (Borrelli and Ernst 2010; Dong et al. 2012). Diosgenin can be converted through chemical processing to norethindrone and cortisol (Dong et al. 2012). No evidence supports that diosgenin is converted by the human body into steroid hormones through the intermediate dehydroepiandrosterone to progesterone. *Dioscorea alata*, Chinese wild yam, may contain estrogenic compounds and may have weak effects on progesterone receptors in breast cancer cell cultures (Dietz et al. 2016).

8.4.6.3 Dosing and Preparation

Topical cream preparations of yam extracts can be administered as one teaspoonful of cream twice daily over intact skin in areas where fat deposits occur, such as abdomen, inner arms and thighs (Komesaroff et al. 2001).

8.4.6.4 Safety

Topical use of wild yam products, with an upper limit of 3.5% diosgen do not have documented adverse effects (Komesaroff et al. 2001).

8.4.6.5 Evidence

A small double-blind randomized crossover trial using wild yam or placebo in a topical cream delivery system to relieve menopausal symptoms in 23 women was conducted over a 6-month period. Women kept a diary during a one-month baseline observation period and then for a week each month during the treatment phases. No differences were observed in blood levels collected to measure FSH, estradiol, triglyceride, HDL cholesterol, glucose, and LDL cholesterol levels or salivary progesterone levels during the baseline period and at 3 months for each arm. The number and severity of diurnal flushing, nocturnal sweating, or other menopausal symptoms reported by the subjects showed similar minor positive effects in both active and placebo periods. No changes were reported on weight or blood pressure. No adverse effects were reported by the subjects (Komesaroff et al. 2001).

8.4.6.6 Clinical Application

Clinical data is limited on the use of wild yam or its extracts on the relief of menopausal symptoms.

8.4.7 Fennel (*Foeniculum vulgare*)

8.4.7.1 Background

Foeniculum vulgare, fennel, originated in the southern Mediterranean region and has been used as an aromatic agent, in culinary efforts and for medicinal purposes since early southern European and Middle Eastern cultures. Fennel has been cultivated throughout Asia, Europe, and North America. This aromatic perennial herb belongs to the plant family *Apiaceae* (Kooti et al. 2015; Rather et al. 2012). The seeds have been used to alleviate gastrointestinal complaints, as a diuretic, and has demonstrated estrogenic effects (Kooti et al. 2015).

8.4.7.2 Pharmacognosy

The dried fruit/seed can be manufactured into a powder or an essential oil product. The essential oil derived from the fruit of the fennel plant contains palmitic, oleic, linoleic, and petrocylic acids and an aromatic essence is used in medicinal products. The estrogenic effects of fennel are from anethole or its derivatives (Rather et al. 2012).

8.4.7.3 Dosing and Preparation

Fennel seeds, one teaspoonful per cup, can be made into a tea. Fennel alcoholic extract is available in a concentration of 1 g per 1 mL.

8.4.7.4 Safety

Fennel seeds are GRAS (Rather et al. 2012) Estragole, found in the essential oil and in extracts of fennel seed, may cause mutagenic changes in a DNA repair test in cell culture. No specific tumor formation or teratogenicity has been reported in humans (Rather et al. 2012; Kooti et al. 2015). As reported in a case series of four girls under the age of five premature thelarche, breast tissue enlargement, was associated with ingestion of fennel tea multiple times a day. The children had elevated serum estradiol levels to 15 times normal levels. After discontinuing fennel tea administration, serum estradiol reduced to normal levels and tissue changes resolved. The authors state that a menopausal woman resumed menses with similar use (Türkyılmaz et al. 2008).

8.4.7.5 Evidence

A 5% fennel seed extract in an emulsion cream base or placebo was randomly assigned to 60 postmenopausal women who were not taking any hormonal supplements or other phytoestrogen products. The women applied 5 g of the assigned cream vaginally once daily for 8 weeks. Symptoms were assessed by questionnaire and physical examination at baseline and every 2 weeks during the study period. After 8 weeks of intervention, every participant in the fennel cream group showed symptom relief including itching ($p < 0.017$), dryness ($p < 0.001$), pallor ($p < 0.0.001$), and dyspareunia ($p < 0.001$). Vaginal burning was relieved in the fennel group but did not show a significant difference from placebo cream. On vaginal swab examination at 8 weeks, vaginal pH decreased in the fennel group ($p < 0.001$). Also, superficial cells increased ($p < 0.001$) and intermediate and parabasal cells decreased in the fennel group which determined an increased maturation vaginal index of 65–100 versus 50–64 in the placebo group ($p < 0.001$). No reports of adverse reactions occurred from either group (Yaralizadeh et al. 2016).

Fennel essential oil obtained by steam distillation (30%) in sunflower oil and sunflower oil placebo were manufactured into 100 mg soft capsules. There were no differences in demographic data between the intervention (n = 40) and the placebo (n = 39) groups. Participants, investigators and data analysts were all blinded to group. Each participant received two capsules daily for 8 weeks. Menopausal symptoms were assessed and scored using the MRS questionnaire at baseline and at weeks 4, 8, and 10 after start of study. Participants were contacted each week of the study period to assess compliance and adverse effects. In the intervention group, MRS scoring was different at 4, 8, and 10 weeks from baseline ($p < 0.001$), but not in the placebo group ($p = 0.402$). When the groups were compared, the MRS scores differed at weeks 4, 8, and 10 ($p < 0.001$) but not at baseline ($p = 0.77$). Minor adverse effects were noted in both groups, including one allergic skin reaction and a description of hot flashes in the intervention group and one digestive complaint in the control group. Overall, the participants who received active fennel capsules, each containing 71–90 mg anethole content, had reduction of somatic, psychologic, and urogenital menopausal symptoms as compared to placebo (Rahimikian et al. 2017).

8.4.7.6 Clinical Application

Clinical data is sparse for the use of fennel to relieve menopausal symptoms. Safety is demonstrated with a long history of culinary use. The essential oil of fennel and fennel tea may have minor adverse effects but data is limited.

8.5 Conclusion

Women's health has been area of medicine where botanical supplement use traditionally has been very common. Throughout history women have used botanical products to ease pain, aid pregnancy, childbirth and lactation, and facilitate the hormonal changes through and after the menopause.

REFERENCES

Aguiar, P. M., and A. de Paula Barbosa. 2014. "Use of soy isoflavones on hormone replacement therapy during climacteric." *African Journal of Pharmacy and Pharmacology* 8 (42): 1071–1078.

Al-Snafi, A. E. 2016. "The constituents and pharmacology of cnicus benedictus: A review." *The Pharmaceutical and Chemical Journal* 3 (2): 129–135.

Ali, B. H., G. Blunden, M. O. Tanira, and A. Nemmar. 2008. "Some phytochemical, pharmacological and toxicological properties of ginger (zingiber officinale roscoe): A review of recent research." *Food and Chemical Toxicology* 46 (2): 409–420.

American Congress of Obstetricians and Gynecologists. 2015. "Practice bulletin summary no. 153: Nausea and vomiting of pregnancy." *Obstetrics and Gynecology* 126 (3): 687–688. doi: 10.1097/01. AOG.0000471177.80067.19

Atmaca, M., S. Kumru, and E. Tezcan. 2003. "Fluoxetine versus vitex agnus castus extract in the treatment of premenstrual dysphoric disorder." *Human Psychopharmacology* 18 (3): 191–195.

Bailey, T. M. and N. S. Culhane. 2010. "Premenstrual Syndrome and Premenstrual Dysphoric Disorder." In *Women's Health Across the Lifespan: A Pharmacotherapeutic Approach*, edited by L. M. Borgelt, M. B. O'Connell, J. A. Smith, and K. A. Calis, 195–206. Bethesda, MD: ASHP.

Bayles, B., and R. Usatine. 2009. "Evening primrose oil." *American Family Physician* 80 (12): 1405–1408.

Beck, V., U. Rohr, and A. Jungbauer. 2005. "Phytoestrogens derived from red clover: An alternative to estrogen replacement therapy?" *The Journal of Steroid Biochemistry and Molecular Biology* 94 (5): 499–518.

Beer, A. M., and A. Neff. 2013. "Differentiated evaluation of extract-specific evidence on cimicifuga racemosa's efficacy and safety for climacteric complaints." *Evidence-Based Complementary and Alternative Medicine: eCAM* 2013: 860602.

Belch, J. J., and A. Hill. 2000. "Evening primrose oil and borage oil in rheumatologic conditions." *The American Journal of Clinical Nutrition* 71 (1 Suppl.): 6S.

Berger, D., W. Schaffner, E. Schrader, B. Meier, and A. Brattstrom. 2000. "Efficacy of vitex agnus castus L. extract Ze 440 in patients with pre-menstrual syndrome (PMS)." *Archives of Gynecology and Obstetrics* 264 (3): 150–153.

Betz, J. M., L. Anderson, M. I. Avigan, J. Barnes, N. R. Farnsworth, B. Gerdn, L. Henderson, E. J. Kennelly, U. Koetter, and S. Lessard. 2009. "Black cohosh: Considerations of safety and benefit." *Nutrition Today* 44 (4): 155–162.

Bhattacharya, S. 2011. "Phytotherapeutic properties of milk thistle seeds: An overview." *J Adv Pharm Educ Res* 1: 69–79.

Blumenthal, M. 2000. *Herbal Medicine: Expanded Commission E Monographs*. Vol. 534. Boston, MA: Integrative Medicine Communications.

Booth, N. L., C. R. Overk, P. Yao, S. Totura, Y. Deng, A. S. Hedayat, J. L. Bolton, G. F. Pauli, and N. R. Farnsworth. 2006. "Seasonal variation of red clover (trifolium pratense L., fabaceae) isoflavones and estrogenic activity." *Journal of Agricultural and Food Chemistry* 54 (4): 1277–1282.

Borgelt, L. M., and K. I. Cheang. 2010. "Polycystic Ovary Syndrome." In *Women's Health Across the Lifespan: A Pharmacotherapeutic Approach*, edited by L. M. Borgelt, M. B. O'Connell, J. A. Smith, and K. A. Calis, 235–248. Bethesda, MD: ASHP.

Borrelli, F., and E. Ernst. 2010. "Alternative and complementary therapies for the menopause." *Maturitas* 66 (4): 333–343.

Brown, D. J. 1994. "Vitex agnus castus clinical monograph." *Qtrly Rev Natural Med* 2: 111–121.

Budzynska, K., A. C. Filippelli, E. Sadikova, T. Low Dog, and P. Gardiner. 2016. "Use and factors associated with herbal/botanical and nonvitamin/nonmineral dietary supplements among women of reproductive age: An analysis of the infant feeding practices study II." *Journal of Midwifery & Women's Health* 61 (4): 419–426.

Cancelo Hidalgo, M. J., C. Castelo-Branco, J. E. Blumel, J. L. Lanchares Perez, J. I. Alvarez De Los Heros, and Isona Study Group. 2006. "Effect of a compound containing isoflavones, primrose oil and vitamin E in two different doses on climacteric symptoms." *Journal of Obstetrics and Gynaecology: The Journal of the Institute of Obstetrics and Gynaecology* 26 (4): 344–347.

Carmichael, A. R. 2008. "Can vitex agnus castus be used for the treatment of mastalgia? What is the current evidence?" *Evidence-Based Complementary and Alternative Medicine* 5 (3): 247–250.

Center for Food Safety and Applied Nutrition, Food and Drug Administration. "GRAS Notice Inventory— Agency Response Letter GRAS Notice no. GRN 000066." Center for Food Safety and Applied Nutrition, last modified Oct 15, accessed Nov 8, 2016, http://www.fda.gov/Food/IngredientsPackagingLabeling/GRAS/NoticeInventory/ucm153979.htm

Chen, M., Y. Rao, Y. Zheng, S. Wei, Y. Li, T. Guo, and P. Yin. 2014. "Association between soy isoflavone intake and breast cancer risk for pre-and post-menopausal women: A meta-analysis of epidemiological studies." *PloS One* 9 (2): e89288.

Chenoy, R., S. Hussain, Y. Tayob, P. M. O'Brien, M. Y. Moss, and P. F. Morse. 1994. "Effect of oral gamolenic acid from evening primrose oil on menopausal flushing." *BMJ (Clinical Research Ed.)* 308 (6927): 501–503.

Colombo, D., and R. Vescovini. 1985. "Controlled clinical trial of anthocyanosides from vaccinium myrtillus in primary dysmenorrhea." *G Ital Obstet Ginecol* 7: 1033–1038.

Coon, J. T., and E. Ernst. 2002. "Panax ginseng: A systematic review of adverse effects and drug interactions." *Drug Safety* 25 (5): 323–344.

Dang, D. K., F. Wang, and K. A. Calis. 2010. "Dysmenorrhea." In *Women's Health Across the Lifespan: A Pharmacotherapeutic Approach*, edited by L. M. Borgelt, M. B. O'Connell, J. A. Smith, and K. A. Calis, 181–193. Bethesda, MD: ASHP.

Dante, G., G. Bellei, I. Neri, and F. Facchinetti. 2014. "Herbal therapies in pregnancy: What works?" *Current Opinion in Obstetrics & Gynecology* 26 (2): 83–91.

Di Pierro, F., A. Callegari, D. Carotenuto, and M. M. Tapia. 2008. "Clinical efficacy, safety and tolerability of BIO-C (micronized silymarin) as a galactagogue." *Acta Bio-Medica: Atenei Parmensis* 79 (3): 205–210.

van Die, M. D., H. G. Burger, H. J. Teede, and K. M. Bone. 2013. "Vitex agnus-castus extracts for female reproductive disorders: A systematic review of clinical trials." *Planta Medica* 79 (07): 562–575.

Dietz, B. M., A. Hajirahimkhan, T. L. Dunlap, and J. L. Bolton. 2016. "Botanicals and their bioactive phytochemicals for women's health." *Pharmacological Reviews* 68 (4): 1026–1073.

Dinc, T., and F. Coskun. 2014. "Comparison of fructus agni casti and flurbiprofen in the treatment of cyclic mastalgia in premenopausal women." *Ulusal Cerrahi Dergisi* 30 (1): 34–38.

Dog, L. T., K. L. Powell, and S. M. Weisman. 2003. "Critical evaluation of the safety of cimicifuga racemosa in menopause symptom relief." *Menopause (New York, N.Y.)* 10 (4): 299–313.

Dong, S. H., D. Nikolic, C. Simmler, F. Qiu, R. B. van Breemen, D. D. Soejarto, G. F. Pauli, and S. N. Chen. 2012. "Diarylheptanoids from dioscorea villosa (wild yam)." *Journal of Natural Products* 75 (12): 2168–2177.

Du Mee, C. 1993. "Vitex agnus castus." *Aust Journal of Medical Herbalism* 5 (3): 63–65.

Duke, J. A. 2002. *Handbook of Medicinal Herbs*. CRC press.

Duncan, A. M., K. E. Underhill, X. Xu, J. Lavalleur, W. R. Phipps, and M. S. Kurzer. 1999. "Modest hormonal effects of soy isoflavones in postmenopausal women." *The Journal of Clinical Endocrinology and Metabolism* 84 (10): 3479–3484.

Eagon, P. K., M. S. Elm, and D. S. Hunter. 2000. *Medicinal Herbs: Modulation of Estrogen Action. Era of Hope Mtg, Dept Defense*. Atlanta, GA: Breast Cancer Res Prog, 8–11.

Efamol Ltd. "Efamol Evening Primrose Oil Product Information." Product Information: Efamol Evening Primrose Oil, accessed Dec 8, 2016, http://www.efamol.com/products/efamol-woman-pure-evening-primrose-oil/information.php

Farzaneh, F., S. Fatehi, M.-R. Sohrabi, and K. Alizadeh. 2013. "The effect of oral evening primrose oil on menopausal hot flashes: A randomized clinical trial." *Archives of Gynecology and Obstetrics* 288 (5): 1075–1079.

Ferlemi, A. V., and F. N. Lamari. 2016. "Berry leaves: An alternative source of bioactive natural products of nutritional and medicinal value." *Antioxidants (Basel, Switzerland)* 5 (2).

Forinash, A. B., A. M. Yancey, K. N. Barnes, and T. D. Myles. 2012. "The use of galactogogues in the breastfeeding mother." *The Annals of Pharmacotherapy* 46 (10): 1392–1404.

Foster, S., and R. L. Johnson. 2008. *National Geographic Desk Reference to Nature's Medicine.* National Geographic Books.

Franco, O. H., R. Chowdhury, J. Troup, T. Voortman, S. Kunutsor, M. Kavousi, C. Oliver-Williams, and T. Muka. 2016. "Use of plant-based therapies and menopausal symptoms: A systematic review and meta-analysis." *Jama* 315 (23): 2554–2563. doi: 10.1001/jama.2016.8012.

Frawley, J., J. Adams, A. Steel, A. Broom, C. Gallois, and D. Sibbritt. 2015. "Women's use and self-prescription of herbal medicine during pregnancy: An examination of 1,835 pregnant women." *Women's Health Issues Official Publication of the Jacobs Institute of Women's Health* 25 (4): 396–402.

Freeman, L. W. 2004. *Mosby's Complementary & Alternative Medicine: A Research-Based Approach.* St. Louis, Mo.: Mosby.

Gallaher, R. N., K. Gallaher, A. J. Marshall, and A. C. Marshall. 2006. "Mineral analysis of ten types of commercially available tea." *Journal of Food Composition and Analysis* 19: 53–57.

Geng, J., J. Dong, H. Ni, M. S. Lee, T. Wu, K. Jiang, G. Wang, A. L. Zhou, and R. Malouf. 2010. "Ginseng for cognition." *The Cochrane Database of Systematic Reviews* (12): CD007769.

Ghasemi, V., M. Kheirkhah, and M. Vahedi. 2015. "The effect of herbal tea containing fenugreek seed on the signs of breast milk sufficiency in iranian girl infants." *Iranian Red Crescent Medical Journal* 17 (8): e21848.

Giacosa, A., P. Morazzoni, E. Bombardelli, A. Riva, G. Bianchi Porro, and M. Rondanelli. 2015. "Can nausea and vomiting be treated with ginger extract? *"European Review for Medical and Pharmacological Sciences* 19 (7): 1291–1296.

Gold, E. B., S. L. Crawford, N. E. Avis, C. J. Crandall, K. A. Matthews, L. E. Waetjen, J. S. Lee, R. Thurston, M. Vuga, and S. D. Harlow. 2013. "Factors related to age at natural menopause: Longitudinal analyses from SWAN." *American Journal of Epidemiology* 178 (1): 70–83.

Halaska, M., P. Beles, C. Gorkow, and C. Sieder. 1999. "Treatment of cyclical mastalgia with a solution containing a vitex agnus castus extract: Results of a placebo-controlled double-blind study." *Breast (Edinburgh, Scotland)* 8 (4): 175–181.

Hall, H. R., and K. Jolly. 2014. "Women's use of complementary and alternative medicines during pregnancy: A cross-sectional study." *Midwifery* 30 (5): 499–505.

Han, K. K., J. M. Soares Jr, M. A. Haidar, G. R. de Lima, and E. C. Baracat. 2002. "Benefits of soy isoflavone therapeutic regimen on menopausal symptoms." *Obstetrics and Gynecology* 99 (3): 389–394.

Hardy, M. L. 2000. "Herbs of special interest to women." *Journal of the American Pharmaceutical Association (Washington, D.C.: 1996)* 40 (2): 234–242.

Heck, A. M., B. A. DeWitt, and A. L. Lukes. 2000. "Potential interactions between alternative therapies and warfarin." *American Journal of Health-System Pharmacy: AJHP: Official Journal of the American Society of Health-System Pharmacists* 57 (13): 30.

Heitmann, K., H. Nordeng, and L. Holst. 2013. "Safety of ginger use in pregnancy: Results from a large population-based cohort study." *European Journal of Clinical Pharmacology* 69 (2): 269–277.

Hirata, J. D., L. M. Swiersz, B. Zell, R. Small, and B. Ettinger. 1997. "Does dong quai have estrogenic effects in postmenopausal women? A double-blind, placebo-controlled trial." *Fertility and Sterility* 68 (6): 981–986.

Holst, L., S. Haavik, and H. Nordeng. 2009. "Raspberry leaf—Should it be recommended to pregnant women? *"Complementary Therapies in Clinical Practice* 15 (4): 204–208.

Holst, L., D. Wright, S. Haavik, and H. Nordeng. 2011. "Safety and efficacy of herbal remedies in obstetrics: Review and clinical implications." *Midwifery* 27 (1): 80–86.

Hong, S. N., J. H. Kim, H. Y. Kim, and A. Kim. 2012. "Effect of black cohosh on genital atrophy and its adverse effect in postmenopausal women." *The Journal of Korean Society of Menopause* 18 (2): 106–112.

Hook, I. L. 2014. "Danggui to angelica sinensis root: Are potential benefits to european women lost in translation? A review." *Journal of Ethnopharmacology* 152 (1): 1–13.

Huggins, K. E. 1998. "Fenugreek: One remedy for low milk production." *Rental Roundup* 15 (1): 16–17.

Hummer, K. E. 2010. "Rubus pharmacology: Antiquity to the present." *HortScience* 45 (11): 1587–1591.

Jarboe, C. H., C. M. Schmidt, J. A. Nicholson, and K. A. Zirvi. 1966. "Uterine relaxant properties of viburnum." *Nature* 212 (5064): 837.

Jarry, H., S. Leonhardt, C. Gorkow, and W. Wuttke. 1994. "In vitro prolactin but not LH and FSH release is inhibited by compounds in extracts of agnus castus: Direct evidence for a dopaminergic principle by the dopamine receptor assay." *Experimental and Clinical Endocrinology* 102 (6): 448–454.

Joe, L. A., and L. L. Hart. 1993. "Evening primrose oil in rheumatoid arthritis." *The Annals of Pharmacotherapy* 27 (12): 1475–1477.

Johnson, P. J., K. B. Kozhimannil, J. Jou, N. Ghildayal, and T. H. Rockwood. 2016. "Complementary and alternative medicine use among women of reproductive age in the united states." *Women's Health Issues: Official Publication of the Jacobs Institute of Women's Health* 26 (1): 40–47.

Kalaiselvan, V., M. Kalaivani, A. Vijayakumar, K. Sureshkumar, and K. Venkateskumar. 2010. "Current knowledge and future direction of research on soy isoflavones as a therapeutic agents." *Pharmacognosy Reviews* 4 (8): 111–117.

Kennedy, D. A., A. Lupattelli, G. Koren, and H. Nordeng. 2013. "Herbal medicine use in pregnancy: Results of a multinational study." *BMC Complementary and Alternative Medicine* 13: 355. doi: 10.1186/1472-6882-13-355

Kennedy, D. A., A. Lupattelli, G. Koren, and H. Nordeng. 2016. "Safety classification of herbal medicines used in pregnancy in a multinational study." *BMC Complementary and Alternative Medicine* 16.101.

Kim, H. G., J. H. Cho, S. R. Yoo, J. S. Lee, J. M. Han, N. H. Lee, Y. C. Ahn, and C. G. Son. 2013a. "Antifatigue effects of panax ginseng C.A. Meyer: A randomised, double-blind, placebo-controlled trial." *PloS One* 8 (4): e61271.

Kim, M. S., H. J. Lim, H. J. Yang, M. S. Lee, B. C. Shin, and E. Ernst. 2013b. "Ginseng for managing menopause symptoms: A systematic review of randomized clinical trials." *Journal of Ginseng Research* 37 (1): 30–36.

Kim, S. Y., S. K. Seo, Y. M. Choi, Y. E. Jeon, K. J. Lim, S. Cho, Y. S. Choi, and B. S. Lee. 2012. "Effects of red ginseng supplementation on menopausal symptoms and cardiovascular risk factors in postmenopausal women: A double-blind randomized controlled trial." *Menopause (New York, N.Y.)* 19 (4): 461–466.

Komesaroff, P. A., C. V. Black, V. Cable, and K. Sudhir. 2001. "Effects of wild yam extract on menopausal symptoms, lipids and sex hormones in healthy menopausal women." *Climacteric: The Journal of the International Menopause Society* 4 (2): 144–150.

Kooti, W., M. Moradi, S. A. Akbari, N. Sharafi-Ahvazi, M. Asadi-Samani, and D. Ashtary-Larky. 2015. "Therapeutic and pharmacological potential of foeniculum vulgare mill: A review." *Journal of HerbMed Pharmacology* 4 (1).

Lau, C. B., T. C. Ho, T. W. Chan, and S. C. Kim. 2005. "Use of dong quai (angelica sinensis) to treat peri- or postmenopausal symptoms in women with breast cancer: Is it appropriate?" *Menopause (New York, N.Y.)* 12 (6): 734–740.

Leach, M. J., and V. Moore. 2012. "Black cohosh (cimicifuga spp.) for menopausal symptoms." *The Cochrane Database of Systematic Reviews* (9): CD007244.

Lete, I., and J. Allue. 2016. "The effectiveness of ginger in the prevention of nausea and vomiting during pregnancy and chemotherapy." *Integrative Medicine Insights* 11: 11–17.

Lethaby, A., J. Marjoribanks, F. Kronenberg, H. Roberts, J. Eden, and J. Brown. 2013. "Phytoestrogens for menopausal vasomotor symptoms." *The Cochrane Database of Systematic Reviews* (12): CD001395.

Levis, S., and M. L. Griebeler. 2010. "The role of soy foods in the treatment of menopausal symptoms." *The Journal of Nutrition* 140 (12): 2321S.

Li, L., Y. Lv, L. Xu, and Q. Zheng. 2015. "Quantitative efficacy of soy isoflavones on menopausal hot flashes." *British Journal of Clinical Pharmacology* 79 (4): 593–604.

Lieberman, S. 1998. "A review of the effectiveness of cimicifuga racemosa (black cohosh) for the symptoms of menopause." *Journal of Women's Health* 7 (5): 525–529.

Lindblad, A. J., and S. Koppula. 2016. "Ginger for nausea and vomiting of pregnancy." *Canadian Family Physician Medecin De Famille Canadien* 62 (2): 145.

Ling, F., X.-f. Xiao, C.-x. Liu, and H. E. Xin. 2012. "Recent advance in studies on angelica sinensis." *Chinese Herbal Medicines* 4 (1): 12–25.

Lipovac, M., P. Chedraui, C. Gruenhut, A. Gocan, C. Kurz, B. Neuber, and M. Imhof. 2012. "The effect of red clover isoflavone supplementation over vasomotor and menopausal symptoms in postmenopausal women." *Gynecological Endocrinology: The Official Journal of the International Society of Gynecological Endocrinology* 28 (3): 203–207.

Lupattelli, A., O. Spigset, M. J. Twigg et al. 2014. "Medication use in pregnancy: A cross-sectional, multinational web-based study." *BMJ Open* 4 (2): 004365.

Mandhare, T. A., S. B. Udugade, P. S. Gaikwad, and S. S. Mahamuni. 2016. "A review on astonishing benefits of fenugreek (trigonella foenum-graecum)." *International Journal of Pharmaceutical and Chemical Sciences* 5 (4): 213–217.

Manson, J. E., and A. M. Kaunitz. 2016. "Menopause management: Getting clinical care back on track." *The New England Journal of Medicine* 374 (9): 803–806.

Masullo, M., P. Montoro, A. Mari, C. Pizza, and S. Piacente. 2015. "Medicinal plants in the treatment of women's disorders: Analytical strategies to assure quality, safety and efficacy." *Journal of Pharmaceutical and Biomedical Analysis* 113: 189–211.

Matthews, A., D. M. Haas, D. P. O'Mathuna, and T. Dowswell. 2015. "Interventions for nausea and vomiting in early pregnancy." *The Cochrane Database of Systematic Reviews* (9): CD007575.

Meier, B., D. Berger, E. Hoberg, O. Sticher, and W. Schaffner. 2000. "Pharmacological activities of vitex agnus-castus extracts in vitro." *Phytomedicine : International Journal of Phytotherapy and Phytopharmacology* 7 (5): 373–381.

Mishra, R. K., A. Kumar, and A. Kumar. 2012. "Pharmacological activity of zingiber officinale." *International Journal of Pharmaceutical and Chemical Sciences* 1 (3): 1073–1078.

Momoeda, M., H. Sasaki, E. Tagashira, M. Ogishima, Y. Takano, and K. Ochiai. 2014. "Efficacy and safety of vitex agnus-castus extract for treatment of premenstrual syndrome in japanese patients: A prospective, open-label study." *Advances in Therapy* 31 (3): 362–373.

Morse, P. F., D. F. Horrobin, M. S. Manku, J. C. Stewart, R. Allen, S. Littlewood, S. Wright, J. Burton, D. J. Gould, and P. J. Holt. 1989. "Meta-analysis of placebo-controlled studies of the efficacy of epogam in the treatment of atopic eczema. Relationship between plasma essential fatty acid changes and clinical response." *The British Journal of Dermatology* 121 (1): 75–90.

National Center for Complementary and Integrative Health. 2016. "Ginger." NCCIH, last modified -05-01T13:33:03-04:00, accessed Oct 18, 2016, https://nccih.nih.gov/health/ginger.

Nelsen, J., C. Ulbricht, E. P. Barrette, D. Sollars, C. Tsourounis, A. Rogers, S. Basch, S. Hashmi, S. Bent, and E. Basch. 2002. "Red clover (trifolium pratense) monograph: A clinical decision support tool." *Journal of Herbal Pharmacotherapy* 2 (3): 49–72.

Ockerman, P. A., I. Bachrack, S. Glans, and S. Rassner. 1986. "Evening primrose oil as a treatment of the premenstrual syndrome." *Recent Advanced Clinical Nutrition* 2: 404.

Oh, K. J., M. J. Chae, H. S. Lee, H. D. Hong, and K. Park. 2010. "Effects of korean red ginseng on sexual arousal in menopausal women: Placebo-controlled, double-blind crossover clinical study." *The Journal of Sexual Medicine* 7 (4 Pt 1): 1469–1477.

Osmers, R., M. Friede, E. Liske, J. Schnitker, J. Freudenstein, and H. H. Henneicke-von Zepelin. 2005. "Efficacy and safety of isopropanolic black cohosh extract for climacteric symptoms." *Obstetrics and Gynecology* 105 (5 Pt 1): 1074–1083.

Ozgoli, G., M. Goli, and M. Simbar. 2009. "Effects of ginger capsules on pregnancy, nausea, and vomiting." *Journal of Alternative and Complementary Medicine (New York, N.Y.)* 15 (3): 243–246.

Parsons, M., M. Simpson, and T. Ponton. 1999. "Raspberry leaf and its effect on labour: Safety and efficacy." *Australian College of Midwives Incorporated Journal* 12 (3): 20–25.

Parveen, S., G. Sarwar, M. Ali, and G. A. Channa. 2007. "Danazol versus oil of evening primrose in the treatment of mastalgia." *Pakistan Journal of Surgery* 23 (1): 10–13.

Pashby, N. L., R. E. Mansel, L. E. Hughes, J. Hanslip, and P. E. Preece. 1981. *A Clinical Trial of Evening Primrose Oil in Mastalgia.* Blackwell Science, 801.

Peila, C., A. Coscia, P. Tonetto et al. 2015. "Evaluation of the Galactogogue effect of silymarin on mothers of preterm newborns (32 weeks)." *La Pediatria Medica E Chirurgica : Medical and Surgical Pediatrics* 37 (3): 2015105. doi: 10.4081/pmc.2015.105

Pongrojpaw, D., C. Somprasit, and A. Chanthasenanont. 2007. "A randomized comparison of ginger and dimenhydrinate in the treatment of nausea and vomiting in pregnancy." *Journal of the Medical Association of Thailand = Chotmaihet Thangphaet* 90 (9): 1703–1709.

Pruthi, S., D. L. Wahner-Roedler, C. J. Torkelson, S. S. Cha, L. S. Thicke, J. H. Hazelton, and B. A. Bauer. 2010. "Vitamin e and evening primrose oil for management of cyclical mastalgia: A randomized pilot study." *Alternative Medicine Review: A Journal of Clinical Therapeutic* 15 (1): 59–67.

Puolakka, J., L. Makarainen, L. Viinikka, and O. Ylikorkala. 1985. "Biochemical and clinical effects of treating the premenstrual syndrome with prostaglandin synthesis precursors." *The Journal of Reproductive Medicine* 30 (3): 149–153.

Puri, B. K. 2007. "The safety of evening primrose oil in epilepsy." *Prostaglandins, Leukotrienes, and Essential Fatty Acids* 77 (2): 101–103.

Rahimikian, F., R. Rahimi, P. Golzareh, R. Bekhradi, and A. Mehran. 2017. "Effect of foeniculum vulgare mill. (fennel) on menopausal symptoms in postmenopausal women: A randomized, triple-blind, placebo-controlled trial." *Menopause* 24 (9): 1017–1021.

Rather, M. A., B. A. Dar, S. N. Sofi, B. A. Bhat, and M. A. Qurishi. 2012. "Foeniculum vulgare: A comprehensive review of its traditional use, phytochemistry, pharmacology, and safety." *Arabian Journal of Chemistry* 9https://doi.org/10.1016/j.arabjc.2012.04.011

Reeder, C., A. Legrand, and S. K. O'Connor-Von. 2013. "The effect of fenugreek on milk production and prolactin levels in mothers of preterm infants." *Clinical Lactation* 4 (4): 159–165.

Ryu, A., and T. H. Kim. 2015. "Premenstrual syndrome: A mini review." *Maturitas* 82 (4): 436–440.

Schellenberg, R., C. Zimmermann, J. Drewe, G. Hoexter, and C. Zahner. 2012. "Dose-dependent efficacy of the vitex agnus castus extract Ze 440 in patients suffering from premenstrual syndrome." *Phytomedicine* 19 (14): 1325–1331.

Setchell, K. D., N. M. Brown, and E. Lydeking-Olsen. 2002. "The clinical importance of the metabolite equol-a clue to the effectiveness of soy and its isoflavones." *The Journal of Nutrition* 132 (12): 3577–3584.

Shahnazi, M., J. Nahaee, S. Mohammad-Alizadeh-Charandabi, and S. Bayatipayan. 2013. "Effect of black cohosh (cimicifuga racemosa) on vasomotor symptoms in postmenopausal women: A randomized clinical Ttrial." *Journal of Caring Sciences* 2 (2): 105–113.

Sharief, M., and S. A. Shaker. 2014. "Comparison of effectiveness of ginger and metoclopramide on the treatment of nausea and vomiting in pregnancy." *Scientific Journal of Medical Science* 3 (8): 357–364.

Sharma, N., A. Gupta, P. K. Jha, and P. Rajput. 2012. "Mastalgia cured! Randomized trial comparing centchroman to evening primrose oil." *The Breast Journal* 18 (5): 509–510.

Sicherer, S. H., H. A. Sampson, and A. W. Burks. 2000. "Peanut and soy allergy: A clinical and therapeutic dilemma." *Allergy* 55 (6): 515–521.

Sim, T. F., H. L. Hattingh, J. Sherriff, and L. B. Tee. 2015. "The use, perceived effectiveness and safety of herbal galactagogues during breastfeeding: A qualitative study." *International Journal of Environmental Research and Public Health* 12 (9): 11050–11071.

Simpson, M., M. Parsons, J. Greenwood, and K. Wade. 2001. "Raspberry leaf in pregnancy: Its safety and efficacy in labor." *Journal of Midwifery & Women's Health* 46 (2): 51–59.

Smith, C., C. Crowther, K. Willson, N. Hotham, and V. McMillian. 2004. "A randomized controlled trial of ginger to treat nausea and vomiting in pregnancy." *Obstetrics and Gynecology* 103 (4): 639–645.

Stanger, M. J., L. A. Thompson, A. J. Young, and H. R. Lieberman. 2012. "Anticoagulant activity of select dietary supplements." *Nutrition Reviews* 70 (2): 107–117.

Taku, K., M. K. Melby, F. Kronenberg, M. S. Kurzer, and M. Messina. 2012. "Extracted or synthesized soybean isoflavones reduce menopausal hot flash frequency and severity: Systematic review and meta-analysis of randomized controlled trials." *Menopause (New York, N.Y.)* 19 (7): 776–790.

Taku, K., M. K. Melby, J. Takebayashi, S. Mizuno, Y. Ishimi, T. Omori, and S. Watanabe. 2010. "Effect of soy isoflavone extract supplements on bone mineral density in menopausal women: Meta-analysis of randomized controlled trials." *Asia Pacific Journal of Clinical Nutrition* 19 (1): 33–42.

Tice, J. A., B. Ettinger, K. Ensrud, R. Wallace, T. Blackwell, and S. R. Cummings. 2003. "Phytoestrogen supplements for the treatment of hot flashes: The isoflavone clover extract (ICE) study: A randomized controlled trial." *Jama* 290 (2): 207–214.

Tode, T., Y. Kikuchi, J. Hirata, T. Kita, H. Nakata, and I. Nagata. 1999. "Effect of korean red ginseng on psychological functions in patients with severe climacteric syndromes." *International Journal of Gynaecology and Obstetrics: The Official Organ of the International Federation of Gynaecology and Obstetrics* 67 (3): 169–174.

Turkyılmaz, C., E. Onal, I. M. Hirfanoglu, O. Turan, E. Koç, E. Ergenekon, and Y. Atalay. 2011 Feb 1. "The effect of galactagogue herbal tea on breast milk production and short-term catch-up of birth weight in the first week of life." *The Journal of Alternative and Complementary Medicine* 17 (2): 139–142.

Türkyılmaz, Z., R. Karabulut, K. Sönmez, and A. Can Başaklar. 2008. "A striking and frequent cause of premature thelarche in children: Foeniculum vulgare." *Journal of Pediatric Surgery* 43 (11): 2109–2111.

Ulbricht, C., E. Basch, S. Basch et al. 2009. "An evidence-based systematic review of bilberry (vaccinium myrtillus) by the natural standard research collaboration." *Journal of Dietary Supplements* 6 (2): 162–200.

Ulbricht, C., E. Basch, C. Dacey, S. Dith, P. Hammerness, S. Hashmi, E. Seamon, M. Vora, and W. Weissner. 2008a. "An evidence-based systematic review of blessed thistle (cnicus benedictus) by the natural standard research collaboration." *Journal of Dietary Supplements* 5 (4): 422–437.

Ulbricht, C., W. Chao, D. Costa, E. Rusie-Seamon, W. Weissner, and J. Woods. 2008b. "Clinical evidence of herb-drug interactions: A systematic review by the natural standard research collaboration." *Current Drug Metabolism* 9 (10): 1063–1120.

Upton, R. 2001. "Chaste tree fruit, vitex agnus-castus: Standards of analysis, quality control, and therapeutics." *American Herbal Pharmacopoeia and Therapeutic Compendium*: 1–37.

Viljoen, E., J. Visser, N. Koen, and A. Musekiwa. 2014. "A systematic review and meta-analysis of the effect and safety of ginger in the treatment of pregnancy-associated nausea and vomiting." *Nutrition Journal* 13: 20.

Wang, S. W., Y. Chen, T. Joseph, and M. Hu. 2008. "Variable isoflavone content of red clover products affects intestinal disposition of biochanin A, formononetin, genistein, and daidzein." *Journal of Alternative and Complementary Medicine (New York, N.Y.)* 14 (3): 287–297.

Wei, W. L., R. Zeng, C. M. Gu, Y. Qu, and L. F. Huang. 2016. "Angelica sinensis in china-A review of botanical profile, ethnopharmacology, phytochemistry and chemical analysis." *Journal of Ethnopharmacology* 190: 116–141.

Wetzig, N. R. 1994. "Mastalgia: A three-year australian study." *The Australian and New Zealand Journal of Surgery* 64 (5): 329–331.

Whelan, A. M., T. M. Jurgens, and H. Naylor. 2009. "Herbs, vitamins and minerals in the treatment of premenstrual syndrome: A systematic review." *Canadian Journal of Clinical Pharmacology* 16 (3): 407–429.

Wiklund, I. K., L. A. Mattsson, R. Lindgren, and C. Limoni. 1999. "Effects of a standardized ginseng extract on quality of life and physiological parameters in symptomatic postmenopausal women: A double-blind, placebo-controlled trial. Swedish Alternative Medicine Group." *International Journal of Clinical Pharmacology Research* 19 (3): 89–99.

Wu, C. H., C. C. Wang, M. T. Tsai, W. T. Huang, and J. Kennedy. 2014. "Trend and pattern of herb and supplement use in the united states: Results from the 2002, 2007, and 2012 National Health Interview Surveys." *Evidence-Based Complementary and Alternative Medicine : eCAM* 2014: 872320.

Wuttke, W. 1996. "Dopaminergic action of extracts of agnus castus." *Forschende Komplementarmedizen* 3: 329–330.

Wuttke, W., H. Jarry, V. Christoffel, B. Spengler, and D. Seidlova-Wuttke. 2003. "Chaste tree (vitex agnus-castus)--Pharmacology and clinical indications." *Phytomedicine : International Journal of Phytotherapy and Phytopharmacology* 10 (4): 348–357.

Yaralizadeh, M., P. Abedi, S. Najar, F. Namjoyan, and A. Saki. 2016. "Effect of foeniculum vulgare (fennel) vaginal cream on vaginal atrophy in postmenopausal women: A double-blind randomized placebo-controlled trial." *Maturitas* 84: 75–80. doi: 10.1016/j.maturitas.2015.11.005, http://www.ncbi.nlm.nih.gov/pubmed/26617271

Yarnell, E. 2015. "Herbal medicine for dysmenorrhea." *Alternative and Complementary Therapies* 21 (5): 224–228.

Yavarikia, P., M. Shahnazi, S. Hadavand Mirzaie, Y. Javadzadeh, and R. Lutfi. 2013. "Comparing the effect of mefenamic acid and vitex agnus on intrauterine device induced bleeding." *Journal of Caring Sciences* 2 (3): 245–254.

Zapantis, A., J. G. Steinberg, and L. Schilit. 2012. "Use of herbals as galactagogues." *Journal of Pharmacy Practice* 25 (2): 222–231.

Zecca, E., A. A. Zuppa, A. D'Antuono, E. Tiberi, L. Giordano, T. Pianini, and C. Romagnoli. 2016. "Efficacy of a galactogogue containing silymarin-phosphatidylserine and galega in mothers of preterm infants: A randomized controlled trial." *European Journal of Clinical Nutrition* 70 (10): 1151–1154.

Zeraati, F., F. Shobeiri, M. Nazari, M. Araghchian, and R. Bekhradi. 2014. "Comparative evaluation of the efficacy of herbal drugs (fennelin and vitagnus) and mefenamic acid in the treatment of primary dysmenorrhea." *Iranian Journal of Nursing and Midwifery Research* 19 (6): 581–584.

Zhu, X., Y. Liew, and Z. L. Liu. 2016. "Chinese herbal medicine for menopausal symptoms." *The Cochrane Database of Systematic Reviews* 3: CD009023.

9

Men's Health

Kelly M. Shields

CONTENTS

9.1 Introduction

Men's health encompasses multiple conditions involved with physical, mental, and psychological wellness. This chapter focuses on benign prostatic hyperplasia and erectile dysfunction, two of the most common conditions for which botanical products have been used.

9.2 Benign Prostatic Hyperplasia

Benign prostatic hyperplasia (BPH) is common, progressive condition in men whereby the prostate is enlarged and presses against the urethra. This pressure can result in a variety of symptoms impacting quality of life. Symptoms can be classified as irritative (urgency, nocturia) or obstructive (dribbling, hesitancy, retention). Symptoms do not correlate well with objective measures such as prostate size, or the post void residual volume. Although its etiology is not fully understood, BPH is associated with age-related hormone changes. One theory focuses on the potential role of dihydrotestosterone (DHT). Research indicates that even with decreases in serum testosterone concentrations, patients may continue to accumulate high levels of DHT as testosterone is converted to DHT via 5 alpha reductase (Lawrentschuk and Perara 2016).

Common treatment options for BPH include selective alpha-1 blockers such as tamsulosin or 5-alpha reductase inhibitors such as finasteride or surgery. In addition, the first-line treatment is often simply watchful waiting. Men may prefer using a botanical product initially as well, as some prescription agents are associated with adverse effects such as erectile dysfunction which are especially impactful in terms of quality of life.

9.2.1 Saw Palmetto

9.2.1.1 Background

Saw palmetto (*Serenoa repens*, *Serenoa serrulata*), or the dwarf palm, is used popularly in Europe for the management of BPH symptoms.

9.2.1.2 Pharmacognosy

Saw palmetto is comprised of sterols and fatty acids. It has several proposed mechanisms of action, the one most likely related to BPH symptom improvement is inhibition of 5-alpha-reductase activity similar to finasteride. In human tissue cultures, saw palmetto has also demonstrated inhibition of androgen activity by competition with dihydrotestosterone.

9.2.1.3 Dosing and Preparation

Patients should take a daily dose of 320 mg with 80%–90% liposterolic content.

9.2.1.4 Safety

Clinical trials have noted minimal safety issues with short term use of saw palmetto. The most common adverse effects included abdominal pain, diarrhea, nausea, and decreased libido all of which had rates similar to those with placebo.

9.2.1.5 Evidence

A 2012 Cochrane systematic review extracted information from 32 randomized, controlled trials providing results from 5,666 men (MacDonald et al. 2012). The duration of the trials ranged from 4 to 72 weeks with a mean follow-up period of 29 weeks. The interventions included brand name product Permixon®, combination product Prostagutt® containing saw palmetto and stinging nettle, as well as non-branded saw palmetto products. Overall, symptoms did not improve compared to placebo. The American Urological Association (AUA) total scores showed no significant changes compared to placebo. The number of AUA clinical responders was 442 per 1,000 in the placebo group compared to 424 per 1,000 in the saw palmetto group. Nocturia, peak urine flow, and prostate size also did not have statistically significant improvement compared to placebo. The review concluded that the use of saw palmetto had minimal benefits on the objective and subjective measures of BPH.

A 2009 Cochrane review published similar findings from 30 randomized, controlled trials (Tacklind et al. 2009). This earlier report did identify that nocturia showed a greater benefit (−0.78 nocturnal visits, $p < 0.05$) with saw palmetto than placebo in nine trials. However, this observation was more commonly reported in the smaller, lower quality trials. When considering only higher quality, larger trials, the results showed −0.31 nocturnal visits, $p < 0.05$).

9.2.1.6 Clinical Application

Saw palmetto's clinical benefits are modest at best. The best candidate for use of this product would be a man with mild BPH, as trials involving participants with moderate to severe symptoms show no significant benefit. If a man chooses to use saw palmetto, any potential symptomatic relief will not be seen for several weeks. Unlike finasteride, saw palmetto does not reduce the actual size of the prostate. In addition, levels of prostate specific antigen (PSA) are unchanged. Although saw palmetto has not been associated with significant adverse effects, the botanical is not an effective first-line therapy for most men.

9.2.2 Pygeum

9.2.2.1 Background

The African plum tree (*Pygeum africanum*), also commonly referred to as pygeum, is native to central and southern Africa. Its lipid-soluble bark has been used medicinally for thousands of years and traditional African healers have used pygeum to treat BPH symptoms.

9.2.2.2 Pharmacognosy

The effects of pygeum are related to multiple potential mechanisms of action including anti-inflammatory properties and 5-alpha reductase inhibition. Pygeum contains triterpenes, fatty acids and phytosterols.

9.2.2.3 Dosing and Preparation

Men who are interested in pygeum should be advised to take 75–200 mg of the standardized extract daily. Products are often standardized to 14% triterpenes.

9.2.2.4 Safety

The adverse effects from pygeum reported in clinical trials have been generally mild and gastrointestinal (GI) in nature such as nausea, constipation, diarrhea, and abdominal discomfort.

9.2.2.5 Evidence

A 2011 Cochrane review of pygeum for BPH evaluated 18 randomized controlled trials involving 1,562 patients (Wilt and Ishani 2011). Doses of pygeum ranged from 75 to 200 mg daily. The duration of the trials ranged from 30 to 122 days, with a mean treatment length of 64 days. Twelve of the 13 placebo-controlled trials reported beneficial effects of pygeum. Compared to placebo, pygeum reduced symptoms of nocturia by 19%, increased peak urine flow by 23%, and reduced residual urine volume by 24%. Patients were also twice as likely to be rated by their physician as having improved overall symptoms compared to those in the placebo arms (Wilt and Ishani 2011).

9.2.2.6 Clinical Application

Although direct comparisons of pygeum to standard prescription drugs are not available, the standardized extract may offer symptomatic benefit to men.

9.2.3 Stinging Nettle

9.2.3.1 Background

The root of the stinging nettle (*Urtica dioca*) has been historically used for many conditions, and most commonly studied for BPH.

9.2.3.2 Pharmacognosy

Multiple mechanisms of action have been proposed for stinging nettle. Among the potential mechanisms are that the polysaccharides contribute to its anti-inflammatory effects or possibly beta-sitosterols. *See Section 9.2.5 for beta-sitosterol discussion.*

9.2.3.3 Dosing and Preparation

Dosages have varied, but generally 300 mg twice daily is an appropriate dose. Some combination products may contain lower doses of stinging nettle.

9.2.3.4 Safety

Stinging nettle is generally safe with its adverse effects primarily GI-related complaints. This product should be avoided in patients with allergy to nettles. Stinging nettle leaves contain vitamin K, leading to potential concern about its use by individuals who are also taking warfarin.

9.2.3.5 Evidence

A comprehensive review of 34 published studies with stinging nettle demonstrated the wide variations in their results (Chrubasik et al. 2007). Most trials were not placebo controlled studies. The controlled studies which showed benefits on symptoms were conducted using a specific formulation Bazoton®. The International Prostate Symptom Score (IPSS) was used as the outcome measure in many studies and statistically significant improvements occurred between 12 weeks and 12 months. The dosages of stinging nettle has ranged between 350 and 459 mg daily in clinical trials.

Stinging nettle has also been studied in combination with saw palmetto. The product PRO® 160/120 (extracts from saw palmetto fruits and stinging nettle roots) has been evaluated in multiple trials. A summary of four controlled clinical studies showed that the use of this product twice daily for 24–48 weeks improved symptoms, notably nocturnal voiding compared to placebo (Oelke et al. 2014). The analysis included the results of 922 patients with the benefit present at the end of 24 weeks of treatment. It is unclear whether the saw palmetto or the stinging nettle component was primarily responsible for the reported benefits.

9.2.3.6 Clinical Application

Stinging nettle may provide some benefit as a single ingredient product but the data is mixed. Based on the available evidence, stinging nettle has limited safety concerns.

9.2.4 Rye Grass Extract

9.2.4.1 Background

Rye grass pollen (*Secale cereal*) has also been studied for impact on BPH symptoms.

9.2.4.2 Pharmacognosy

The rye grass extract contains beta-sterols, and one appears to be similar to stigmasterol (Buck et al. 1990). These compounds may relax urethral smooth muscle tone and increase bladder muscle contraction. Some evidence suggests that alpha-adrenergic receptors may be affected and relax the internal and external bladder sphincter muscles (MacDonald et al. 2000).

9.2.4.3 Dosing and Preparation

Studies have focused primarily on the use of Cernilton®. This branded product has one standard formulation which is registered as a pharmaceutical agent and is used throughout western Europe. The standard dose of Cernilton® contains 60 mg of Cernitin T60, a water-soluble pollen extract fraction, and 3 mg of Cernitin GBX, an acetone-soluble pollen extract fraction (Cernelle AB). The acetone-soluble fraction contains β-sterols (MacDonald et al. 2000).

9.2.4.4 Safety

The trials with Cernilton® have reported no significant safety issues or adverse effects with the product. Since this product is derived from rye grass, it is expected that patients with grass allergies, especially to rye grass, may experience symptoms of allergic rhinitis.

9.2.4.5 Evidence

A systematic review of four controlled trials presented the results from 444 patients (MacDonald et al. 2000). The trials ranged in length from 12 to 24 weeks. Although the trials had significant limitations including no active controls, short durations, and small populations, participants did report improved clinical symptoms. These benefits were noted in nocturia and overall symptom scores.

9.2.4.6 Clinical Application

Although data are limited, Cernilton® is a potential agent that could be tried for patients seeking a botanical therapy.

9.2.5 Beta-Sitosterol

9.2.5.1 Background

Beta-sitosterol has been used for hypercholesterolemia, as well as the treatment of BPH. Beta-sitosterol can be found in foods like flax seed, pumpkin seeds, and wheat germ. It is also found in the African wild potato which has been promoted for the management of BPH symptoms.

9.2.5.2 Pharmacognosy

This plant-based sterol product is thought to decrease prostate proliferation, possibly through the inhibition of growth factors, and to improve the symptoms of BPH. Animal research has indicated that inhibition of 5-alpha-reductase activity may also occur, although data in humans is not available.

9.2.5.3 Dosing and Preparation

The daily dosage ranges between 60 and 130 mg of β-sitosterol orally in 2–3 divided doses.

9.2.5.4 Safety

Beta-sitosterol has had few adverse effects noted, with the most common being GI intolerance. Theoretically, beta-sitosterol supplements could have an additive effect with lipid-lowering medications such as statins. For that reason, increased cholesterol monitoring is recommended for patients on these medications.

9.2.5.5 Evidence

One of the earlier BPH studies of this supplement evaluated 200 patients who were treated with either 20 mg of beta-sitosterol (Harzol®) three times daily or placebo for 6 months (Berges et al. 1995). This primary outcome measure for this trial was change in Boyarsky score with a decrease of −6.7 (SD 4) points in the beta-sitosterol group compared to −2.1 (SD 3.2) in the placebo group, $p < 0.01$. The beta-sitosterol group noted improvement in patient symptoms as measured by the IPSS questionnaire −7.4 points in the treatment group versus −2.1 points in the placebo group. An open label follow-up to this trial was conducted (Berges et al. 2000). Researchers noted that for the group continuing on beta-sitosterol results from the first 6 months were maintained throughout the 18-month time period; however, no further benefits were noted.

Another trial evaluated the effects of 130 mg beta-sitosterol (Azuprostat®) daily in 177 men with BPH over a 6-month time period (Klippel et al. 1997). Patients were assessed using the changes in IPSS scores as a primary outcome measure. Researchers found a statistically significant greater improvement in IPSS scores for patients using the beta-sitosterol product (51%) than those in the placebo group (19%).

9.2.5.6 Clinical Application

The use of beta-sitosterol 60–130 mg orally in 2–3 divided doses daily appears to significantly improve urinary symptoms, specifically maximum urinary flow. Adverse effects are limited primary to GI disturbances.

9.2.6 Pumpkin Seed

9.2.6.1 Background

Pumpkin seed (*Cucurbita pepo*) has been used historically for micturition disorders and has some trial data evaluating its role in management of BPH symptoms.

9.2.6.2 Pharmacognosy

Pumpkin seed contains glutamic acid, aspartic acid, leucine, phytosterols (beta-sitosterol), and potassium (Caili et al. 2006). Its mechanism of action is not well understood and may be related to improvement in bladder and urethral function.

9.2.6.3 Dosing and Preparation

Studies have used from 60 to 130 mg in divided doses daily.

9.2.6.4 Safety

In the available trials, no significant adverse events have been reported.

9.2.6.5 Evidence

One recent study compared pumpkin seed (GRANU FINK®), pumpkin seed extract (GRANU FINK Prosta forte®), and placebo (Vahlensieck et al. 2015). This trial included 1,431 patients and evaluated a portion of patients noting "response," which was defined as a reduction of at least five points on the IPSS. Investigators noted over the 12-month trial period most patients reported a response; these included 46.3% of the pumpkin seed extract, 58.5% of the pumpkin seed, 47.8% of the placebo group.

An additional trial compared pumpkin seed extract to prazosin, an alpha-1 blocker; the study did not specify the dosages used (Shirvan et al. 2014). In this 6-month trial, patients in both groups reported a statistically significant reduction in the IPSS from 14.50 ± 3.49 to 9.24 ± 3.60 in the pumpkin seed group and from 14.54 ± 5.36 to 8.08 ± 2.93 in the prazosin group.

9.2.6.6 Clinical Application

Overall, the efficacy data for pumpkin seed extract is limited, however the supplement is safe and so it may be an option for men interested in a botanical for BPH.

9.2.7 Lycopene

9.2.7.1 Background

Lycopene is a carotenoid that provides yellow, red, and orange coloring to vegetables and fruits. One important dietary source of lycopene is tomato and tomato-based products.

9.2.7.2 Pharmacognosy

Lycopene is a carotenoid, but not a precursor to vitamin A. It does possess antioxidant properties. Lycopene is relatively heat resistant, and heat helps release lycopene, increasing bioavailability in processed tomato products.

9.2.7.3 Dosing and Preparation

Lycopene is most often found in commercial products with other ingredients. Depending on the product used, the dosage can range from 5 to 15 mg daily.

9.2.7.4 Safety

Lycopene is well tolerated with minimal adverse effects and drug interactions have not been documented.

9.2.7.5 Evidence

Evidence from clinical trials on the potential benefits of lycopene on BPH symptoms is limited. One study of 40 patients compared lycopene 15 mg daily to placebo for 6 months (Schwarz et al. 2008). Patients experienced a statistically significant reduction in serum PSA levels (−0.74 mcg/L in treatment versus −0.04 mcg/L in the placebo group). In addition, both groups noted similar improvements in patient-reported symptoms as measured by the IPSS tool, with a reduction of about two points in each group. A noncontrolled study of 43 men evaluated effect of adding 50 g of tomato paste, which is about 13 mg of lycopene, daily for 10 weeks on PSA levels (Edinger and Koff 2006). A statistically significant reduction in PSA levels was noted (baseline 6.51 ng/mL compared to 5.81 ng/mL at 10th week), but patient symptoms were not recorded.

9.2.7.6 Clinical Application

Due to the limited information about lycopene for BPH, it should not be routinely recommended, but certainly should be a component of a healthy diet. If a man is interested in lycopene, there are no significant safety concerns with the supplement.

9.3 Erectile Dysfunction

Erectile dysfunction (ED) is frequently considered a symptom of the aging process in men. However, multiple factors contribute to ED including medications and concurrent conditions such as hypertension, diabetes, and hyperlipidemia. Erectile dysfunction can be classified as psychogenic, organic, or of mixed etiology. First-line treatment involves identifying and resolving the underlying cause if possible. When medications are warranted, the phosphodiesterase inhibitors such as sildenafil are often utilized first. However, some men may desire to treat erectile dysfunction without seeking medical treatment and may try any of the variety of over the counter sexual enhancement products available.

9.3.1 Yohimbe

9.3.1.1 Background

Yohimbe is the common name for the *Pausinystalia yohimbine* tree, which is native to areas of central and western Africa.

9.3.1.2 Pharmacognosy

The bark of this tree contains the alkaloid yohimbine, although levels are low and vary greatly. Yohimbine is the principal alkaloid from the plant yohimbe. Yohimbine hydrochloride, available as a prescription product Yocon® has been prescribed for the treatment of erectile dysfunction, although this is not an FDA approved use and its evidence is limited. Yohimbine may block alpha-2 adrenergic receptors in the corpus cavernosum.

9.3.1.3 Dosing and Preparation

Most trials have used a dose of 5–100 mg in divided doses, representing about 6 mg of yohimbine per dose.

9.3.1.4 Safety

Unlike other botanical supplements for men's health, the use of yohimbine has been associated with serious adverse cardiovascular effects due to increased norepinephrine including hypertension, hypertensive crisis, atrial fibrillation, and myocardial infarction (Kearney et al. 2010).

9.3.1.5 Evidence

Clinical trials of yohimbe itself are not available, although studies of its constituent yohimbine have been published. A meta-analysis of seven trials of yohimbine showed a benefit over placebo in the treatment of erectile dysfunction (Ernst and Pittler 1998). The trials included 419 men total, with mixed etiology of their ED. The studies ranged from 2–10 weeks in length. Most trials used a dosage of 5.4 mg three times daily. The results from the yohimbine trials cannot be extrapolated to products provided in other dosage forms.

9.3.1.6 Clinical Application

Yohimbe lacks published evidence of its efficacy and significant potential safety concerns exist. In addition, an important issue is that many men considering its use would likely be older and could have cardiovascular risk factors. This product should not be recommended to most men.

9.3.2 Pycnogenol

9.3.2.1 Background

Pycnogenol is a patented water extract of the French maritime pine (*Pinus pinaster*). The product has been used for many conditions including chronic venous insufficiency, allergies, attention deficit hyperactivity disorder, osteoarthritis, and ED.

9.3.2.2 Pharmacognosy

Multiple bioflavonoids, including oligomeric proanthocyanidins (OPCs), are present in the extract. Among its proposed mechanisms of action, pycnogenol is known to decrease inflammation through a reduction in C-reactive protein, provide antioxidant effects, impact erythrocyte membrane fluidity, and reduce platelet aggregation. In the treatment of ED, pycgnogenol may work by activating endothelial nitric oxide synthase therefore increasing nitrous oxide production and promoting vasodilation (Therapeutic Research Center 2017).

9.3.2.3 Dosing and Preparation

Different brands of pycnogenol have been used in studies with Prelox®, a combination of pycnogenol and L-arginine, being the most common. An additional consideration is that confusion may exist regarding products containing grape seed oil as they also contain OPCs, however the data on the two products are not interchangeable as OPCs are just one element of each plant product.

9.3.2.4 Safety

Pycnogenol, either as a single ingredient or in combination with L-arginine, is generally safe. Reports of mild GI symptoms did not lead to treatment discontinuation by participants in the published studies.

9.3.2.5 Evidence

As a single ingredient product, a double-blind trial compared pycnogenol 120 mg daily to placebo in 21 patients over a 3-month time period (Ďuračková et al. 2003). Patients were assessed using the International Index of Erectile Function (IIEF) to determine the treatment benefit. Based on questionnaire responses at the end of the study, a statistically significant improvement in symptoms was present, moving the participants' ED classification from moderate to mild. This benefit was not maintained after stopping the pycnogenol treatment.

   More trials of ED have been completed using pycnogenol in conjunction with L-arginine. The largest of these trials compared two Prelox®, each tablet contained pycnogenol 20 mg plus L-arginine 700 mg, twice daily versus placebo (Ledda et al. 2010). The trial evaluated IIEF results in 124 men after 3 and then after 6 months of therapy. At 3 months, the IIEF score was statistically significantly improved, and at 6 months, all domains and the overall IIEF score showed statistically significant improvement over placebo.

9.3.2.6 Clinical Application

Pycnogenol combined with L-arginine provides benefit in management of erectile dysfunction, although at least several weeks will be needed in order to observe a response. The combination is generally safe with only reports of mild GI symptoms.

9.3.3 Panax Ginseng

9.3.3.1 Background

Panax ginseng is considered an adaptogen and has been used for many diseases including ED.

9.3.3.2 Pharmacognosy

See Chapter 10 Neurological Conditions for discussion.

9.3.3.3 Dosing and Preparation

In clinical trials, the most common dosage has been 600 mg three times daily; other studies used 900 mg three times daily or 1,000 three times daily. *See Chapter 10 Neurological Conditions for discussion.*

9.3.3.4 Safety

Adverse events with Panax ginseng in ED studies were rare and consisted primarily of headache and mild gastrointestinal upset. *See Chapter 2 Pharmacokinetic and Pharmacogenomic Considerations and 10 Neurological Conditions for further discussion.*

9.3.3.5 Evidence

A systematic review of seven randomized, controlled trials evaluated the potential effects of *Panax ginseng* on treatment of ED (Jang et al. 2008). The trials varied widely in their design, and most were of low quality. Six trials had a placebo control and all six reported therapeutic efficacy which was defined as improvement of erectile function with ginseng compared to placebo. Four used a validated questionnaire and those trials reported positive effects.

One subsequent double-blind, placebo-controlled study focused on the role of ginseng berry extract in the management of mild to moderate ED (Choi et al. 2013). This trial followed 119 men taking two tablets each with 350 mg of standardized ginseng berry extract, two times daily. Patients noted a statistically significant improvement in IIEF erectile function score after 8 weeks of treatment, specifically improvement in subscores of intercourse satisfaction, sexual desire, and overall satisfaction were noted at 4 weeks for the treatment group. This trial was unique in that it used the berry extract and not products derived from ginseng root.

9.3.3.6 Clinical Application

Panax ginseng products may provide some patients with a perceived benefit in sexual functioning in ED. The adverse effects have been minimal in published studies.

9.4 Summary

Benign prostatic hyperplasia and erectile dysfunction are common conditions in many men, especially as they age. For both conditions, botanical supplements may provide modest benefits and are safe, with the potential exception of yohimbe in individuals with underlying cardiovascular conditions. While none of the botanicals have demonstrated superiority to the available prescription drugs, they may offer alternatives to patients seeking options.

REFERENCES

Berges, R. R., A. Kassen, and T. Senge. 2000. Treatment of symptomatic benign prostatic hyperplasia with b-sitosterol: An 18-month follow-up. *British Journal of Urology International* 85, no. 7 (May): 842–846.

Berges, R. R., J. Windeler, H. J. Trampisch, and T. Senge. 1995. Randomised, placebo-controlled, double-blind clinical trial of beta-sitosterol in patients with benign prostatic hyperplasia. *Lancet* 345, no. 8964: 1529–1532.

Buck, A. C., R. Cox, R. W. Rees, L. Ebeling, and A. John. 1990. Treatment of outflow tract obstruction due to benign prostatic hyperplasia with the pollen extract, cernilton. A double blind placebo controlled study. *British Journal of Urology* 66, no. 4 (Oct): 398–404.

Caili, F., S. Huan, and L. Quanhon. 2006. A review on pharmacological activities and utilization technologies of pumpkin. *Plant Food for Human Nutrition* 6, no. 12 (Jun): 73–80. doi:10.1007/s11130-006-0016-6

Choi, Y. D., C. W. Park, J. Jang, S. H. Kim, H. Y. Jeon, W. G. Kim, S. J. Lee, and W. S. Chung. 2013. Effects of Korean ginseng berry extract on sexual function in men with erectile dysfunction: A multicenter, placebo-controlled, double-blind clinical study. *International Journal of Impotence Research* 25, no. 2 (Mar): 45. doi:10.1038/ijir.2012.45

Chrubasik, J. E., S. Chrubasik, B. D. Roufogalis, and H. Wagner. 2007. A comprehensive review on the stinging nettle effect and efficacy profiles. Part II: Urticae radix. *Phytomedicine* 14, no. 7: 568–579.

Ďuračková, Z., B. Trebatický, V. Novotný, I. Žitňanová, and J. Breza. 2003. Lipid metabolism and erectile function improvement by Pycnogenol®, extract from the bark of pinus pinaster in patients suffering from erectile dysfunction-a pilot study. *Nutrition Research* 23, no. 9: 1189–1198.

Edinger, M. S. and W. J. Koff. 2006. Effect of the consumption of tomato paste on plasma prostate-specific antigen levels in patients with benign prostate hyperplasia. *Brazilian Journal of Medical and Biological Research* 39, no. 8 (Aug): 1115–1119.

Ernst, E. and M. H. Pittler. 1998. Yohimbine for erectile dysfunction: A systematic review and meta-analysis of randomized clinical trials. *The Journal of Urology* 159, no. 2: 433–436. doi:10.1016/S0022-5347(01)63942-9.

Jang, D-J., M. S. Lee, B-C. Shin, Y-C. Lee, and E. Ernst. 2008. Red ginseng for treating erectile dysfunction: A systematic review. *British Journal of Clinical Pharmacology* 66, no. 4 (Oct): 444–450.

Kearney, T., N. Tu, and C. Haller. 2010. Adverse drug events association with yohimbine-containing products: A retrospective review of the california poison control system reported cases. *Annals of Pharmacology* 44: 1022–1029.

Klippel, K. F., D. M. Hiltl, and B. Schipp. 1997. A multicentric, placebo-controlled, double-blind clinical trial of b-sitosterol (phytosterol) for the treatment of benign prostatic hyperplasia. *British Journal of Urology International* 80, no. 3 (Sep): 427–432.

Lawrentschuk, N. and M. Perara. *"Benign Prostate Disorders" in Endotext.* South Dartmouth: MDText.com, 2016.

Ledda, A., G. Belcaro, M. R. Cesarone, M. Dugall, and F. Schönlau. 2010. Investigation of a complex plant extract for mild to moderate erectile dysfunction in a randomized, double-blind, placebo-controlled, parallel-arm study. *British Journal of Urology International* 106, no. 7 (Oct): 1030.

MacDonald, R., A. Ishani, I. Rutks, and T. J. Wilt. 2000. A systematic review of cernilton for the treatment of benign prostatic hyperplasia. *British Journal of Urology International* 85, no. 7 (May): 836–841.

MacDonald, R., J. W. Tacklind, I. Rutks, and T. J. Wilt. 2012. Serenoa repens monotherapy for benign prostatic hyperplasia (BPH): An updated cochrane systematic review. *British Journal of Urology International* 109, no. 12 (Jun): 1756–1761.

Oelke, M., R. Berges, S. Schläfke, and M. Burkart. 2014. Fixed-dose combination PRO 160/120 of sabal and urtica extracts improves nocturia in men with LUTS suggestive of BPH: Re-evaluation of 4 controlled clinical studies. *World Journal of Urology* 32, no. 5 (Oct): 1149–1154.

Schwarz, S., U. C. Obermüller-Jevic, E. Hellmis, W. Koch, G. Jacobi, and H-K. Biesalski. 2008. Lycopene inhibits disease progression in patients with benign prostate hyperplasia 1,2. *The Journal of Nutrition* 138, no. 1 (Jan): 49.

Shirvan, M. K., M. Reza, D. Mahboob, M. Masuminia, and S. Mohammadi. 2014. Pumpkin seed oil (prostafit) or prazosin? Which one is better in the treatment of symptomatic benign prostatic hyperplasia. *JPMA. Journal of the Pakistan Medical Association* 64, no. 6 (Jun): 683.

Tacklind, J., R. MacDonald, I. Rutks, and T. J. Wilt. 2009. Serenoa repens for benign prostatic hyperplasia. *The Cochrane Database of Systematic Reviews* no. 2: CD001423.

Therapeutic Research Center. Pycnogenol. Natural Medicines [database online]. Available at: http://naturalmedicines.therapeuticresearch.com. Accessed: May, 1, 2017.

Vahlensieck, W., C. Theurer, E. Pfitzer, B. Patz, N. Banik, and U. Engelmann. 2015. Effects of pumpkin seed in men with lower urinary tract symptoms due to benign prostatic hyperplasia in the one-year, randomized, placebo-controlled GRANU study. *Urologia Internationalis* 94, no. 3: 286–295.

Wilt, T. J. and A. Ishani. 2011. Cochrane database of systematic reviews: Pygeum africanum for benign prostatic hyperplasia. *Progress in Neurology and Psychiatry* 15, no. 4 (Jul): 29–31.

10

Neurological Conditions

Jacintha S. Cauffield and Jack J. Chen

CONTENTS

10.1 Introduction

Neurological conditions are often chronic and conventional treatments are not fully effective. Adults with common neurological conditions use complementary and alternative medicine (CAM) more frequently than those without these conditions (44.1% versus 32.6%, $p < 0.0001$) (Wells et al. 2010). For example, nearly half of adults with memory loss or migraines have reported the use of CAM (Wells et al. 2010). Patients may also use CAM because conventional treatments are perceived as too costly, inconvenient to access, or associated with undesirable adverse effects. As a result, these patients seek CAM therapies, such as botanical products, even though their efficacy may not be well characterized. Understanding the evidence of botanical products for neurologic conditions is important and can help clinicians better facilitate patient care and outcomes.

10.2 Dementia

The global market for supplements targeting cognitive function reached U.S. $1.39 billion in 2012 and is projected to continue to grow (Benedict 2015). This includes nootropics, which are supplements, drugs, or other substances designed to enhance cognitive function, including memory, creativity, motivation, and executive function. Many supplements including Bacopa monnieri, Ginkgo biloba, Panax ginseng and related species, and huperzine A from Huperzia serrata are used in patients with dementia, as well as to help prevent memory loss.

10.2.1 Bacopa (*Bacopa monnieri*)

10.2.1.1 Background

Bacopa monnieri (synonyms *Bacopa monniera, Graticola monnieri, Herpestis monniera, Lysimachia monnieri,* and *Moniera cuneifolia*) is a small, creeping perennial aquatic herb from the family Scrophulariaceae. It is native to the wetlands of southern India, Australia, and South America. It is a popular aquarium plant. Bacopa is also known as "water hyssop" or "Brahmi" and has been used for centuries in Ayurvedic medicine as a "medhyarasayana" to improve memory and intellect (Russo and Borrelli 2005).

10.2.1.2 Pharmacognosy

The plant stem and leaves are used. The principal active components are triterpene saponins of the dammarane class called bacosides and bacopasaponins. The main chemical constituent thought to contribute to the memory-enhancing properties is bacoside A, which usually occurs with its optically-rotated component bacoside B, the latter of which is thought to be an artifact of the isolation of bacoside A. Bacoside A is derived from two triterpenoid saponins: pseudojujubogenin and jujubogenin on acid hydrolysis. This in turn yields the bacogenins A1, A2, A3, and A4 present in bacoside A (Rajan et al. 2015).

10.2.1.3 Dosing and Preparation

Two different standardized extracts have been used in clinical trials. The first, available in capsule form (Keenmind®, CDRI 08, from Soho Flordis International [SFI]), is a standardized ethanolic extract standardized for a minimum of 55% combined bacosides A and B. Each capsule contains 150 mg *B. monnieri* extract (20:1) equivalent to 3 g dried herb (Stough et al. 2001). The second, available in tablet form (BacoMind® from Suanfarma, Inc.), is an alcoholic 20:1 herb to extract ratio standardized to contain a total bacosides content of 40%–50%. It is standardized to nine active constituents: bacoside A3, bacopaside I, bacopaside II, jujubogenin isomer of bacopasaponin C, bacopasaponin C, bacosine, luteolin, apigenin, and b–sitosterol-d-glucoside. Each 300 mg tablet contains an equivalent of 6,000 mg of dried herb (Morgan and Stevens 2010).

10.2.1.4 Safety

Bacopa monnieri extracts are well tolerated. The most common adverse effects with BacoMind® tablets included increased stool frequency, nausea, abdominal cramping, and diarrhea (Morgan and Stevens 2010). Additional adverse effects that occurred with KeenMind® capsules included a decrease in felt stress, dry mouth, increased thirst, increased or decreased appetite, palpitations, and headaches (Stough et al. 2001).

10.2.1.5 Evidence

Although interest exists in using *B. monnieri* to treat dementia, clinical studies are not available in this population. All trials to date have focused on some aspect of cognitive performance. One systematic review identified six trials that examined effects of Bacopa extracts on validated cognitive outcomes. All studies were conducted over 12 weeks and were randomized, double-blind, parallel group, and placebo controlled. Subjects were healthy, without chronic medical conditions. The majority of the assessment measures focused on the domain of free recall memory, with the most frequently used test being the auditory verbal learning test (AVLT). Of six tests in the AVLT, the results on only one was found to be significantly improved by Bacopa extracts. The ability to recall short stories or passages was not improved (Pase et al. 2012). In a second meta-analysis, nine trials were identified. Of these, seven were conducted in healthy individuals, and two were conducted in patients with cognitive impairment. There was no association between Bacopa and memory improvement with the exception of a 17.9 msec decrease in the time to complete a task in subjects taking Bacopa (Kongkeaw et al. 2014).

10.2.1.6 Clinical Application

Bacopa is used in Ayurvedic medicine to treat memory and intellect. Despite the availability of standardized extracts (Bacomind® and KeenMind®), data regarding in benefits in patients with dementia is lacking. The extracts are well tolerated, with mild gastrointestinal (GI) adverse effects being the most common.

10.2.2 Ginkgo Biloba (*Ginkgo biloba*)

10.2.2.1 Background

Ginkgo is derived from the leaf of ginkgo biloba, one of the oldest living tree species and the sole surviving species of the large plant division Ginkgophyta, once widespread throughout the world 180 million years ago. Ginkgo has a long history of medicinal use in Asia and Europe and ginkgo biloba extracts have been widely used in the treatment of dementia for decades (Birks and Grimley Evans 2009). One of the largest medicinal *Ginkgo biloba* plantations is located in South Carolina.

10.2.2.2 Pharmacognosy

The most widely studied ginkgo formulation is the extract of ginkgo biloba 761 (EGb 761). Utilizing *Ginkgo biloba* leaves, this 27-step extraction process was patented by the pharmaceutical firm of Willmar Schwabe, Karlsruhe, Germany. The process produces a standard product containing 24% flavone glycosides primarily quercetin, kaempferol, and isorhamnetin, 6% terpene lactones consisting of 2.8%–3.4% ginkgolides A, B, and C, and 2.6%–3.2% bilobalide, and <5 ppm ginkgolic acid which is a known allergen naturally found in *Ginkgo biloba* (Nash and Shah 2015). Another extraction process produces LI-1370, a standardized extract of 25% ginkgo glycosides and 6% lactones.

The physiologic effects of EGb 761 are likely due to the combined activities of several constituents. *Ginkgo biloba* extracts have demonstrated antioxidative effects and attenuation of hypoxia-induced cellular damage. Additionally, pharmacologic mechanisms include improved blood rheology, enhanced microcirculation, alterations in neurotransmitter levels, enhanced neuroplasticity, prevention of brain edema, and neuroprotection (Nash and Shah 2015). The half-life of ginkgo flavonoids range from 2–4 hours and that of the terpenoids ranges from 3–10 hours. The constituents of *Ginkgo biloba* extract readily cross the blood brain barrier.

10.2.2.3 Dosing and Preparation

The recommended dosages of EGb 761 are 120–240 mg per day administered in two divided doses. A period of at least 8 weeks may be required for the onset of benefits. The standardized EGb 761 product, Tebonin is manufactured by the German-based pharmaceutical manufacturer of Murdock, Madaus, and Schwabe. In the United States, Nature's Way, a division of the German-based manufacturer, also manufactures Egb 761 as Ginkgold. Another standardized *Ginkgo biloba* formulation, LI-1370, has also been extensively studied in Europe and is available in the United States as Ginkai, Lichtwer Pharma, Berlin, Germany.

10.2.2.4 Safety

Ginkgo biloba extract (i.e., EGb 761) is well tolerated. The most common adverse effects are nausea and diarrhea, occurring in up to 5% of patients. The use of nonstandardized products may be associated with a greater risk of adverse effects, such as rash and seizures. Potent contact allergens including ginkgolic acids and other alkyphenols are present in significant amounts in *Ginkgo biloba* nuts and to a lesser extent in *Ginkgo biloba* leaves. For safety purposes, the extraction process for EGb 761 removes these allergens to 5 ppm or less (Baron-Ruppert and Luepke 2001).

Excessive consumption of *Ginkgo biloba* nuts, a delicacy in Asian cultures, can result in severe neurotoxicity. The responsible toxin is believed to be ginkgotoxin (4-O-methylpyridoxine), an inhibitor of gamma-aminobutyric acid (GABA) synthesis. Rarely, seizures have been associated with *Ginkgo biloba* administration and it is possible that nonstandardized products containing *Ginkgo biloba* nuts may have been responsible (Granger 2001; Gregory 2001). Based on case reports, non-EGb 761 *Ginkgo biloba* products may lower the seizure threshold and may increase the risk of seizures in patients. Caution should be exercised when recommending non-EGb 761 *Ginkgo biloba* products to patients with a history of seizures. Vitamin B6 50 mg daily has been shown to provide protection against ginkgotoxin-induced neurotoxicity (Jang et al. 2015).

Insulin activity may also be affected by EGb 761. In one study, EGb 761 administration reduced insulin secretion in patients with non-insulin dependent diabetes and concurrent hyperinsulinemia (Kudolo 2001). However, in the absence of hyperinsulinemia, insulin secretion was enhanced. Therefore, patients with diabetes should have blood glucose monitored regularly when EGb 761 is initiated.

Ginkgolides may act as platelet-activating factor antagonists, inhibiting platelet aggregation and case reports have associated *Ginkgo biloba* ingestion with an increased risk of bleeding when used with or without concurrent antithrombotic drugs (Rosenblatt and Mindel 1997; Matthews 1998; Beckert et al. 2007; Pedroso et al. 2011). However, in one study involving healthy subjects, EGb 761 reduced platelet aggregation but had no effect on coagulation assays or bleeding time (Guinot et al. 1989). In a randomized controlled study of healthy men, administration of EGb 761 240 mg per day for 7 days was not associated with abnormal platelet and coagulation parameters (Kohler et al. 2004). A meta-analysis of 18 randomized controlled trials on the effect of *Ginkgo biloba* extract on coagulation found only small and clinically insignificant changes (Kellerman and Kloft 2011). Regarding a potential drug interaction with warfarin, analysis of data from a large clinical repository demonstrated that concurrent administration of ginkgo with warfarin is associated with a significantly increased risk of bleeding (hazard ratio = 1.38, 95% CI: 1.20 to 1.58, p < 0.001) (Stoddard et al. 2015). Overall, as a precaution, since the half-life of ginkgolides ranges from 3–10 hours, *Ginkgo biloba* should be held at least 48 hours prior to surgery to reduce the risk for excessive bleeding. *See Chapter 2 Pharmacokinetic and Pharmacogenomic Considerations for further discussion.*

10.2.2.5 Evidence

10.2.2.5.1 Treatment of Cognitive Impairment/Dementia

A 2009 Cochrane review included 36 clinical studies (Birks and Grimley Evans 2009). Most studies had a small sample size and short duration, typically 3 months. Nine studies (n = 2016) had an adequate sample size and duration of 6 months. In these studies, most patients were diagnosed with either Alzheimer or vascular type dementia. Most studies tested the standardized EGb 761 extract at different dosages and demonstrated inconsistent results on cognition, activities of daily living, mood, depression, and carer burden outcomes. The *Ginkgo biloba* extract and placebo groups were similar in the proportion of subjects experiencing adverse events. A subgroup analysis of patients with Alzheimer-type dementia showed no consistent pattern of benefit associated with *Ginkgo biloba* extract. Overall, the Cochrane review concluded the evidence that *Ginkgo biloba* extract has a predictable and clinically significant benefit in dementia or cognitive impairment was inconsistent and unreliable.

In a subsequent meta-analysis which included three new studies, EGb 761 in a dosage of at 120–240 mg per day was efficacious and well tolerated in patients with Alzheimer, vascular, and mixed types of dementia (Gauthier and Schlaefke 2014). The meta-analysis data set consisted of 2,625 outpatients (1,396 for EGb 761 and 1,229 for placebo) randomized to receive treatment for 22 to 26 weeks. Statistically significant benefits of EGb 761 over placebo was confirmed by responder analyses as well as for standardized mean differences for change in cognition (−0.52; 95% confidence interval [CI] −0.98, −0.05; P = 0.03), activities of daily living (−0.44; 95% CI −0.68, −0.19; P < 0.001), and global rating (−0.52; 95% CI −0.92, −0.12; P = 0.01). The risk of adverse events was similar in the EGb 761 and placebo groups.

In a 2016, meta-analysis which included studies comparing *Ginkgo biloba* products to conventional drug therapy such as cholinesterase inhibitors, the botanical in combination with these therapies was associated with a statistically significant improvement on Mini-Mental State Examination (MMSE) scores at 24 weeks for patients with Alzheimer type dementia [mean difference (MD) 2.39, 95% CI 1.28 to 3.50, P < 0.0001] and mild cognitive impairment (MD 1.90, 95% CI 1.41 to 2.39, P < 0.00001). Activities of Daily Living (ADL) scores also improved at 24 weeks for patients with Alzheimer type dementia (MD −3.72, 95% CI −5.68 to −1.76, P = 0.0002) (Yang et al. 2016). This meta-analysis differed from other published studies in that the authors included trials from four major Chinese literature databases. A total of 21 randomized controlled trials involving 2,608 patients met the inclusion criteria. However, the authors found that the general methodological quality of included trials was moderate to poor.

In a systematic review of 10 systematic reviews [Alzheimer type dementia (n = 3), vascular dementia (n = 1), mixed dementia (n = 5), mild cognitive impairment (n = 1)], treatment with *Ginkgo biloba* extracts was associated with improvement in cognition, neuropsychiatric symptoms, and ADL scores (Zhang et al. 2016). The effect of EGB 761 was dose-dependent with efficacy demonstrated with 240 mg per day. Overall adverse events were similar to placebo. The authors concluded that the evidence supports the efficacy and safety of *Ginkgo biloba* extracts in the treatment of mild cognitive impairment and dementia.

10.2.2.5.2 *Prevention of Cognitive Impairment/Dementia*

In a primary prevention study of 118 normal adults aged over 85 years for over 42 months, *Ginkgo biloba* extract containing at least 6% terpene lactones and 24% flavone glycosides 80 mg three times daily did not prevent the development of dementia or cognitive decline, but was associated with an increase in stroke and transient ischemic attack (Dodge et al. 2008). However, a secondary analysis taking into account medication adherence showed a protective effect of *Ginkgo biloba* extract on progression of memory impairment.

In the Ginkgo Evaluation of Memory (GEM) study, elderly individuals with normal cognition and those with mild cognitive impairment were randomized to receive placebo or EGb 761 120 mg twice daily (DeKosky et al. 2008). Over a median follow-up of 6.1 years, EGb 761 had no effect on reducing incident Alzheimer type dementia or all-cause dementia but was associated with a insignificant doubling in the risk of hemorrhagic stroke.

In a third prevention study, known as GuidAge, 2,854 patients were randomized to EGb 761 120 mg twice daily or placebo. The study population included individuals aged 70 years and older and who had spontaneously reported memory problems to a primary care practitioner. After 5 years, use of EGb 761 did not reduce the risk of progression to Alzheimer type dementia compared with placebo (Vellas et al. 2012)

See Chapter 5 Cardiovascular Disease for use in other conditions.

10.2.2.6 Clinical Application

Ginkgo biloba extracts used as monotherapy or adjunctive to conventional therapies in patients with Alzheimer and mixed types of dementia is safe and associated with some improvements in cognition, neuropsychiatric symptoms, and ADL scores. The standardized EGb 761 extract was specifically used in most studies. Because nonstandardized products may be associated with a greater risk of adverse effects, EGb 761 should be the preferred product. *Ginkgo biloba* does not appear to prevent cognitive impairment in healthy adults.

10.2.3 Ginseng (*Panax ginseng*)

10.2.3.1 Background

Panax ginseng (synonym *Panax schinseng*, "true ginseng," Asian or Korean ginseng) is a slow-growing perennial member of the family Araliaceae. It has been used medicinally for thousands of years, and is the most consumed medicinal botanical in the world. It is highly valued in Asia, where a piece of a 115-year-old root was sold for U.S. $157 million (Smith et al. 2014). It was native to the forests of China and Korea, but demand for wild ginseng has made it all but extinct in those areas. It is widely cultivated in cooler climates in Asia and North America. The genus name "Panax" is Greek for "all-heal" and comes from the same root as "panacea." The species name "ginseng" is derived from the Chinese words "jen shen" or "ren shen," meaning roughly "man root" because the rhizome is thought to look like a miniature person. According to the Doctrine of Signatures, which states that a plant that resembles a part of the human body is good for treating ailments of that body part, ginseng was believed to be good for treating a wide range of ailments. Ginseng has been used as a general tonic for well-being, to promote longevity, and as an "adaptogen" to increase resistance to a wide range of stressors, including environmental, chemical, and biological. Additional uses include stimulation of immune function, increasing physical and athletic stamina, treating fatigue, and as an aphrodisiac. Ginseng is used to improve a number of neurological and psychiatric conditions, including cognitive function, memory, concentration, dementia, depression, and anxiety (TRC 2017).

10.2.3.2 Pharmacognosy

The plant root or rhizome is used medicinally. The major active components of *Panax ginseng* are the dammarane or triterpenoid glycosides, which are also known as ginsengosides or panaxosides. Over 100 different types have been identified and isolated from different parts of ginseng. The method of ginseng preparation changes the composition of ginsengosides. Several ginsengosides and ginsengoside metabolites have beneficial effects on the central nervous system, including ginsingosides Rb1, Rd, Re and Rg1 have demonstrated neuroprotective benefits in animal models. Rb1 protects hippocampal neurons against ischemic damage and delays death of neurons from damage induced by transient forebrain ischemia. In rats with cerebral injury, Rg1 has a protective effect against transient focal ischemic injury. Ginsengoside Rb1 increases the uptake of choline in cerebral cholinergic nerve endings, as well as modulating acetylcholine release and uptake. Both Rb1 and Rg1 improve scopolamine-induced amnesia in rats, and Rg3 improves learning in animal models. GInsengoside Re, Rg1, Rg3, Rh2, and gintonin reduce the accumulation of beta-amyloid protein in cultured neurons and transgenic AD mice, and improve learning (Geng et al. 2010; Rokot et al. 2016). Total ginsenosides, Rb1, Rd, and Rg1 appear to decrease hyperphosphorylated tau protein (Rokot et al. 2016). Compound K, a major metabolite of *Panax*, also may play an important role in the neuroprotection properties of *Panax ginseng* (Smith et al. 2014).

10.2.3.3 Dosing and Preparation

A number of plants go by the common name of "ginseng," but *Panax ginseng* is considered to be the species of interest. Other species include *Panax quinquefolius* (American ginseng), *Panax notoginseng* (Chinese ginseng), and are of medicinal interest, but the chemical constituents vary. For this reason, clinical trials should identify the exact species of "ginseng" used in the study. Because *Panax ginseng* products are frequently adulterated, a product should be from a company that uses Good Manufacturing Practices (GMP) and standardization. In addition, *Panax ginseng* is used in many different forms. Drying the fresh root in the sun yields white ginseng, whereas red ginseng is produced by steaming fresh ginseng at 95–100°C for 2–3 hours prior to drying. Red ginseng is the form most frequently used in Traditional Chinese Medicine (TCM). Ginseng can also be fermented (Smith et al. 2014). A new formulation called Sun ginseng (SG-135) is produced by heat treatment of raw ginseng at 120°C for 3 hours, which results in a different chemical composition than the other forms (Heo et al. 2012).

Trials have used multiple *Panax ginseng* formulations. In the treatment of Alzheimer type dementia, 4.5–9 gm/day of red Korean ginseng or 4.5 gm/day of either white ginseng or SG-135 has been used (Lee et al. 2009; Heo et al. 2012; Heo et al. 2016). For cognitive performance, 200–400 mg daily of G115 (Pharmaton SA, Lugano, Switzerland) has been used (Geng et al. 2010). *Panax ginseng* extract (Gerimax Ginseng Extract; Dansk Droge A/S Ishoj, Denmark) 400 mg/day has also been used for enhancing cognitive performance (Geng et al. 2010).

10.2.3.4 Safety

Panax ginseng has been well-tolerated in trials with few or no adverse effects reported. Adverse effects have included fever, nausea, vomiting, diarrhea, constipation, gastric complaints, headache, anorexia, dizziness, and dermatitis or eczema (Lee et al. 2009; Geng et al. 2010). Data suggest that ginseng is safe for use for up to 6 months, but longer term data is lacking (TRC 2017). Most concerns about drug or disease interactions are theoretical. Given the wide range of ginseng species and formulations used, identifying interactions may be difficult at present. *See Chapter 2 Pharmacokinetic and Pharmacogenomic Considerations for further discussion.*

10.2.3.5 Evidence

A Cochrane review examined the effects of ginseng on cognitive performance (Geng et al. 2010). The review included all *Panax* species. Nine randomized, double-blind, placebo-controlled trials met inclusion criteria. Eight trials included healthy subjects, and one enrolled patients with age-associated memory impairment. Only five of these trials in healthy subjects had results that were extractable for review. All were performed at hospitals at university centers. Four were conducted in European countries, and one in South Korea. Three trials were conducted in patients in their 20s and 30s, and two were conducted in middle-aged patients. One trial used a *Panax quinquefolius* extract, two used G115, one used the Korean ginseng extract Cheong Kwan Jang and one used Gerimax Ginseng Extract. The results suggested improvements in specific tests of working memory (Speed of Carrying out 3-Back task), speed of processing (Mental Arithmetic), two aspects of psychomotor performance (Choice Reaction Time and Tapping Test and in one aspect of learning and memory (Selective Reminding). However, the results are not generalizable to the larger population, nor do they suggest how *Panax ginseng* might help patients with neurocognitive impairment.

Clinical trials that have examined the effects of *Panax ginseng* on Alzheimer type dementia have been of low quality. A systematic review identified two open label trials (Lee et al. 2009) that used ginseng as an adjunct to conventional treatment versus conventional treatment alone (control). One trial used Korean red ginseng (KRG) at doses of 4.5 and 9 gm/day versus control. The high dosage, but not the low one, showed significant improvements in MMSE, but not in the Alzheimer's Disease Assessment Scale-cognitive subscale (ADAs-cog) at 12 weeks. The other trial used 4.5 gm/day of white ginseng powder versus control and also showed significant improvements on both the MMSE and ADAs-cog. Combined, the two trials enrolled 158 patients and showed significant benefits on both MMSE and ADAS-cog. However, given the low quality of the trials, firm conclusions cannot be drawn.

In a 24-week, open-label trial, 40 patients with MMSE of 20 or less were randomized to receive a daily dose of 1.5, 3 or 4.5 gm of SG-135 versus a control, only the high dosage group showed significant improvement in MMSE, ADAs-cog and ADAS-noncog (Heo et al. 2012). Treatment with 4.5 gm/day KRG in 14 patients for 12 weeks had no significant impact on MMSE (Heo et al. 2016). Of note, all of the studies that examined *Panax ginseng* in patients with Alzheimer type dementia were performed in Asian populations, and may not be generalizable to other populations.

10.2.3.6 Clinical Application

Panax ginseng is relatively safe when used short term to treat dementia, but the data for its use are not strong. Studies have used variable preparations and frequently have not identified the specific species used which limit the application of the available evidence to date.

10.2.4 Huperzia (*Huperzia serrata*)

10.2.4.1 Background

Huperzia serrata (synonym *Lycopodium serrata*), is commonly known as Chinese club moss. Native to India and Southeast Asia, traditionally it was used to relieve pain, as an antidote for poison and to relieve swelling. Today it is known as the source of the alkaloid huperzine A. Huperzine A has been approved for the treatment of Alzheimer type dementia by the State Food and Drug Administration of China since 1994. It is also used to treat vascular dementia, schizophrenia, and insomnia (Zhang 2012).

10.2.4.2 Pharmacognosy

Chinese club moss is not itself used medicinally. The alkaloid huperzine A is isolated from the whole Chinese club moss plant. Huperzine A has a number of enantiomers that have variable stereoselectivity. Levorotatory huperzine A [(-)-huperzine A] is the enantiomer with the highest biological activity (TRC 2015). It acts as a potent and reversible acetylcholinesterase inhibitor (AChEI) (Zhang 2012).

10.2.4.3 Dosing and Preparation

Huperzine A was given in dosages ranging from 0.1 to 0.5 mg/day, in one to three divided doses. Huperzine A is not sold as an extract of *Huperzia serrata*, but as a single chemical entity.

10.2.4.4 Safety

The most common adverse effects are cholinergic in nature, and include dizziness, anorexia, diarrhea, nausea, insomnia and somnolence. Constipation was also listed as a side effect (Li et al. 2008). One case of withdrawal secondary to anorexia and nausea occurred in one trial, and two cases of withdrawal occurred in another trial due to nausea, anorexia and mild abdominal pain. In both studies, the numbers of withdrawals were similar between treatment and placebo groups (Li et al. 2008). Because huperzine A has AChEI activity, it should not be combined with other AChEIs and not administered with anticholinergic agents.

10.2.4.5 Evidence

10.2.4.5.1 Treatment of Cognitive Impairment/Dementia

A Cochrane review identified 17 potential trials, all of which were from China (Li et al. 2008). Of these, six trials of 454 patients met the criteria for inclusion. The dosage of huperzine A ranged from 0.2 to 0.4 mg daily. The average duration of Alzheimer type dementia ranged from 3 months to 10 years in one trial, 2.7–3.4 years in four trials, and was not specified in one trial. The length of treatment ranged from 8 to 36 weeks. Compared with placebo, huperzine A improved cognitive function as measured by the MMSE and the ADAs-cog. These findings were based on a small number of the included trials, and the trials were of low methodological quality. The review concluded that evidence was insufficient for the effects of huperzine A on the symptoms of Alzheimer type dementia. A Cochrane review also did not find evidence to support the use of huperzine A to treat mild cognitive impairment (Yue et al. 2012). A Cochrane review identified one study that used huperzine A to treat vascular dementia (Hao et al. 2009). Huperzine A had no significant effect on cognitive function over placebo as measured by the MMSE.

A more recent meta-analysis (Xing et al. 2014) identified eight trials that met inclusion criteria for the use of huperzine A to treat Alzheimer's disease and two trials that used huperzine A to treat vascular dementia. The median Jadad score for the Alzheimer's disease trials was 3.75, with four trials scoring greater than four, and the median Jadad score for the vascular dementia trials at 3.5. Huperzine had a significant positive effect on the MMSE and ADLs, and the effect appeared to increase with the duration of treatment from 6–16 weeks. Heterogeneity was apparent in the Alzheimer type dementia results, with strong suggestion of publication bias, which confounds the results. Findings were similar for vascular dementia with positive effects on MMSE and ADLs, as well as high heterogeneity and high risk of publication bias.

10.2.4.6 Clinical Application

Huperzine A possesses AChEI activity and is approved for use to treat dementia associated with Alzheimer's disease in China. Although clinical trials have shown positive effects of huperzine A on cognitive function in patients with Alzheimer's disease and vascular dementia, the trials are of lower quality, have a high degree of heterogeneity and a strong publication bias. More rigorous trials need to be performed in order to clarify the role of huperzine A in the treatment of dementia.

10.3 Headaches

In the 2007 National Health Interview Survey, 49.5% of adults with migraines or severe headaches in the US adults used some form of CAM in the past 12 months, compared with 33.9% of those who did not have headaches (Wells et al. 2011). Mind-body techniques, including deep breathing exercises, meditation, yoga, progressive relaxation, and guided imagery were most common (30.2% versus 17.2%) of those without headaches. Compared with 18.4% of patients without headaches, 26.7% of patients with migraines or severe headaches used some form of botanical or other supplement for treatment, most commonly feverfew.

10.3.1 Butterbur (*Petasites hybridus*)

10.3.1.1 Background

Butterbur (*Petasites hybridus;* synonyms *Petasites officinalis, Tussilago hybrida*) is a member of the Asteraceae/Compositae family. The botanical genus name, *Petasites*, derives from the Greek word petastos, referring to a broad brimmed sun hat worn by ancient Greek farmers or travelers. It refers to the plant's large leaves, which can reach 3 feet in diameter, and were used to wrap butter on warm days thus, the common name of butterbur (Giles et al. 2005). The perennial shrub grows in wet, marshy ground, and can be found in damp forests and adjacent to rivers or streams. It is native to central Europe, ranging from the British Isles to the Europe-Asia border, and from southern Scandinavia to southern Italy (GBIF 2016). Other common names include blatterdock, bog rhubarb, bogshorns, butterdock, and pestwurz (Sutherland and Sweet 2010). Butterbur has been used medicinally for over 2,000 years to treat fever, bubonic plague in the Middle Ages, urogenital tract spasms, gastrointestinal conditions, aches and pains, and lung conditions. It is used to treat allergic rhinitis, asthma, allergic skin conditions, and for migraine prophylaxis.

10.3.1.2 Pharmacognosy

Butterbur extracts are prepared from the rhizomes, roots, and leaves. Pharmacological activity, including antispasmotic and anti-inflammatory properties, comes from the eremophilane sesquiterpenoids petasin, isopetasin, S-petasin, and iso-S-petasin. These compounds are collectively referred to as petasins. Butterbur has anti-inflammatory activity from the isopetasin component. Antispasmotic activity is secondary to petasin causing smooth muscle and vascular wall relaxation. Petasins block calcium influx into the smooth muscle cells via voltage-dependent channels. Petasins appear to have high affinity for cerebral blood vessels (Sutherland and Sweet 2010). In addition, petasin has anti-inflammatory activity through inhibition of lipoxygenase activity and down-regulation of leukotriene synthesis. Isopetasin also inhibits the synthesis of leukotrienes (Giles et al. 2005).

10.3.1.3 Dosing and Preparation

The formulation used in clinical trials for migraine prophylaxis is a supercritical CO_2 extract of the *Petasites hybridus* rhizome standardized to contain a minimum of 15% petasins (Petadolex®, Weber and Weber GmbH & Co, KG, Germany). The drug:extract ratio is 28:44, and each 50 mg capsule contains is 7.5 mg of petasin and isopetasin. Dosing in adults is 50–75 mg twice daily. In clinical trials, children aged 6–9 received 25 mg twice daily for 2 months, with the option to increase to 25 mg three times daily if needed to achieve response. Dosing in children aged 10–17 is 50 mg twice daily, with the option to increase to 50 mg three times daily after two months if needed (Pothmann and Danesch 2005).

10.3.1.4 Safety

Warnings have been issued in the United States not to consume unprocessed butterbur plant or raw extracts because the plant contains pyrrolizidine alkaloids (PAs). These compounds cause hepatotoxicity in humans, including veno-occlusive disease and have been shown to be carcinogenic in animal studies (Sutherland and Sweet 2010). Petadolex® is specially prepared to remove PAs to less than 0.088 ppm, the lowest detectable level set for PAs. Because PAs are metabolized to toxic compounds by cytochrome P450 3A4, inducers of 3A4 such as St. John's Wort and carbamazepine should be avoided.

Petadolex® was well tolerated in clinical trials and most adverse effects did not differ significantly from placebo. Most adverse effects were mild to moderate in intensity and included burping, nausea, and abdominal pain (Grossmann and Schmidramsl 2000; Diener et al. 2004; Lipton et al. 2004). Adverse effects in children also included mild burping, nausea, regurgitation, diarrhea, and bitter taste sensation, as well as dermatologic/allergic symptoms of itching, rash, and allergic rhinitis. Other symptoms included arthralgia, dizziness, fatigue, and asthmatic symptoms (Pothmann and Danesch 2005; Oelkers-Ax et al. 2008). Mild elevations in liver enzymes were observed in some studies, but they were transient and not clinically relevant (Pothmann and Danesch 2005; Oelkers-Ax et al. 2008).

Few drug-drug or drug-disease interactions have been documented with butterbur. Patients with allergies to other members of the Asteracae/Compositae family such as ragweed, daisies, and chrysanthemums may have cross-sensitivity to Petadolex®. Caution is urged when combining Petadolex® with anticholinergic agents due to theoretical additive effects (Giles et al. 2005).

10.3.1.5 Evidence

Evidence for the efficacy of the butterbur extract, Petadolex®, for migraine prevention comes from two trials in adults (Grossmann and Schmidramsl 2000; Diener et al. 2004), one of which went through a second round of analysis (detailed below, Lipton et al. 2004) and two trials in children (Pothmann and Danesch 2005; Oelkers-Ax et al. 2008). Both trials in adults involved a 4-week run-in period in which patients had to be off all preventive migraine medication and have at least two migraine headaches, followed by 12 weeks' treatment with either Petadolex® or placebo. In the first trial (Grossman and Schmidramsl 2000), patients were randomized to either 50 mg twice daily (n = 33) or placebo (n = 27). In the original analysis, the primary endpoint was frequency of headaches per 4-week period. Compared with placebo, the frequency of migraine attacks decreased significantly from baseline for patients on Petadolex® when compared with placebo at all time points. The intensity and duration of migraines also decreased, but were statistically significant only at the 8-week time point. Pain intensity decreased by 1.5 points on a 10-point scale (4.3–2.8) by week 8 in the treatment group, and was significantly less than placebo (4.1 and 3.8, respectively) but increased back to 3.2 by the end of 12 weeks versus 3.8 in placebo.

The re-analysis of the Grossman trial (Lipton et al. 2004) employed an intention-to-treat (ITT) rather than per-protocol analysis. Of patients receiving the extract, 45% were responders defined by at least a 50% reduction in migraine frequency versus 15% in the placebo group. The number of migraines in the treatment group declined from 3.4 at baseline to 1.9, 1.4, and 1.6 at weeks 4, 8, and 12, respectively versus 2.9 at baseline, and 2.2, 2.4, and 2.6, respectively in the placebo group. All changes were in favor of butterbur, including changes in pain intensity. Patients receiving the butterbur extract also had a significant decrease in use of medications to treat acute headaches from 44% at baseline to 18% at 12 weeks versus 27% and 26%, respectively in the placebo group.

The second trial in adults (Diener et al. 2004) randomized patients to Petadolex® 50 mg twice daily (n = 71), 75 mg twice daily (n = 68), or placebo (n = 63) for 12 weeks. The primary endpoint, a reduction in the mean number of migraine attacks was measured as the percentage reduction from baseline in migraine attacks per month across the 4-month treatment period. The outcome was significant only in the 75 mg group (45% versus 32% for 50 mg and 28% for placebo, p < 0.05). By month 4, 68% of subjects taking 75 mg were responders versus 56% on 50 mg and 49% on placebo; p < 0.05 for 75 mg only). Based on these two trials, the American Academy of Neurology (AAN) Evidence-based Guidelines states that Petadolex®, the petasites purified extract, is established as effective and should be considered for migraine prevention (Holland et al. 2012).

A 4-month, open-label trial examined the effects of Petadolex® in 29 children aged 6–9 years and 79 adolescents aged 10–17 years (Pothmann and Danesch 2005). Headache attacks were reduced by a mean of 63.2% after 4 months, 67% and 61.9%, respectively, in children and adolescents. Most of the study population, 85.7% and 74.1%, respectively, were defined as responders to therapy. The results were limited by the lack of a placebo group.

In another study, the efficacy of Petadolex® (n = 19) was compared to music therapy (n = 20) and placebo (n = 19) in school aged children in a 28-week trial (Oelkers-Ax et al. 2008). Double-blinding occurred for butterbur treatment (with either Petadolex® or placebo), but not for music therapy. There was an 8-week run-in period, followed by a 12-week treatment phase, an 8-week post-treatment phase, and another 8-week follow-up period. Baseline headache frequency was significantly reduced during the after treatment, but only music therapy was significantly reduced when compared with placebo. Headache frequency was similar among the three groups during the follow-up period.

10.3.1.6 Clinical Application

A specific extract of *Petsites hybridus*, standardized to petasin and isopetasin content and free of pyrrolizidine alkaloids (Petadolex®) used as monotherapy for migraine prophylaxis in adults is safe and is associated with significant reductions in migraine frequency. Data for the use of the same extract in children is promising. Butterbur should not be ingested, either whole or in part, or as unprocessed extracts, due to the presence of hepatotoxic pyrrolizidine alkaloids.

10.3.2 Feverfew (*Tanacetum parthenium*)

10.3.2.1 Background

Feverfew (*Tanacetum parthenium*) is a daisy-like perennial plant whose name is derived from the Latin word febrifugia or "fever reducer" and was used by ancient Greeks and early Europeans as an antipyretic. The origins of *Tanacetum parthenium* can be traced to Southeastern Europe, but the plant is now found throughout Asia, Australia, Europe, North and South America, and North Africa. It is also known as "featherfew," because of its feathery leaves. Its yellow flowers resemble those of chamomile (*Matricaria chamomilla*), for which they are sometimes confused and its yellow-green leaves are pinnate–bipinnate (chrysanthemum-like). Common names for feverfew include *Chrysanthemum parthenium*, featherfew, bachelor's button, and wild chamomile.

10.3.2.2 Pharmacognosy

A principal bioactive ingredient of feverfew is parthenolide, a sesquiterpene lactone (Bohlmann and Zdero 1982). Parthenolide is found in the leaves, but not in the stems, and comprises up to 85% of the total sesquiterpene content (Heptinstall et al. 1992). Overall, its antimigraine properties are attributed to antiplatelet, vasoactive, and anti-inflammatory mechanisms (Pareek et al. 2011). Parthenolides have been shown to inhibit prostaglandin biosynthesis, but unlike salicylates, does not inhibit cyclo-oxygenation by prostaglandin synthase (Collier et al. 1980). Parthenolides inhibit the secretion of serotonin (5-HT) and parthenolides derived from fresh leaf extracts inhibit both contraction and relaxation of vascular smooth muscles (Barsby et al. 1993; Mittra et al. 2000). Parthenolide inhibits the transcription factor nuclear factor kappa B (NF-kβ) and attenuates inducible nitric oxide synthase (iNOS) expression (Hehner et al. 1999; Tassorelli et al. 2005). This activity is relevant to migraine pathophysiology because in patients with migraine, NF-k B activity peaks after attack onset and is accompanied by up-regulation of iNOS (Sarchielli et al. 2006). The proinflammatory transcription factor, NF-kβ, increases transcription of endothelial cell nitric oxide synthase (eNOS). Both eNOS and iNOS synthesizes nitric oxide, a known inducer of headaches.

10.3.2.3 Dosing and Preparation

In the United States, feverfew is commercially available as a dried-leaf extract preparation, with variable concentrations of parthenolides and sesquiterpene lactones. Feverfew supplements should be standardized to contain at least 0.2% parthenolide. For the prophylaxis of migraine headaches, the Drugs Directorate of Health Canada has cleared a feverfew product that contains 125 mg of standardized authenticated feverfew leaf powder providing a minimum of 0.2% parthenolide, or 0.25 mg parthenolide per tablet (Tanacet 125®) (Carty 1996). A supercritical carbon dioxide extracted feverfew formulation, MIG-99 (Schaper & Bruemmer GmbH & Co) has been effective at doses providing an equivalent of 0.5 mg parthenolide once daily for migraine prevention in randomized controlled trials, but it is not available commercially.

10.3.2.4 Safety

Feverfew is reasonably well tolerated. Abrupt discontinuation of long-term feverfew ingestion has been reported to result in the development of a transient "post feverfew syndrome" characterized by disturbed sleep, increased headache frequency, joint aches, and nervousness (Johnson 1985). Mouth ulcers and inflammation of the oral mucosa and tongue has been reported with ingestion of raw feverfew leaves or powdered feverfew leaf preparations (Johnson 1985). Pregnant women should not take feverfew, as it may cause uterine contractions (Sun-Edelstein and Mauskop 2011). Patients with allergies to other members of the Asteracae/Compositae family such as ragweed, daisies, and chrysanthemums may have cross-sensitivity to feverfew and anecdotal reports describe contact dermatitis (e.g., Burry 1980; Hausen and Osmundsen 1983).

Extracts of the feverfew have been shown to inhibit human blood platelet aggregation *in vitro* and isofraxidin, a coumarin derivative, has been isolated from the roots of *T. parthenium* (Losche et al. 1987; Kisiel and Stojakowska 1997). In a human study, feverfew did not have a clinically significant effect on platelet function (Biggs et al. 1982).

10.3.2.5 Evidence

In an early double-blind, placebo-controlled study of chronic feverfew users, 17 subjects were randomized to receive two capsules containing 50 mg powdered freeze-dried feverfew leaves, equivalent of two small leaves, every morning or placebo (i.e., feverfew withdrawal) (Johnson 1985) for 6 months. The withdrawal of feverfew led to a statistically significant increase in headache frequency. Subjects randomized to feverfew capsules experienced a mean 1.69 headaches per month, which was identical with the frequency of headache attacks when they were taking raw feverfew leaves. Subjects randomized to placebo capsules experienced 3.13 headaches per month, which was significantly higher than the frequency when they were taking raw feverfew leaves (p < 0.02). In another early double-blind, placebo-controlled study, 72 patients wcrc randomized to receive one capsule daily containing powdered dried feverfew leaves or placebo for 4 months and then crossed over to the other treatment arm for an additional 4 months (Murphy et al. 1988). Each feverfew capsule contained on average 82 mg feverfew powder, equivalent to approximately 2.2 μmol (0.5 mg) of parthenolide which corresponded to about two medium-sized leaves. Feverfew treatment was associated with a statistically significant reduction in migraine frequency. There was a 24% reduction (95% CI, 14%–34%) in the number of attacks during feverfew treatment.

Studies using a stable formula of *T. parthenium*, MIG-99, have been conducted. In the first study, 147 migraine patients, with or without aura, were divided into four dosing groups: MIG-99 2.08 mg (corresponding to 0.17 mg parthenolide), 6.25 mg (0.5 mg parthenolide), 18.75 mg (1.5 mg parthenolide), and placebo administered three times a day. The study found no significant beneficial results at any dose, although a subset of high-frequency migraineurs appeared to benefit from treatment (Pfaffenrath et al. 2002). The finding that patients who had at least four migraine attacks within 4 weeks at baseline showed a significant benefit with MIG-99 compared to placebo is a positive finding. In a follow-up study, 170 patients with four to six monthly migraine attacks were randomized to MIG-99 6.25 mg three times daily or placebo. The MIG-99 treated group experienced a significant reduction in the number of attacks per month from 4.76 to 1.9 compared to placebo and the 50% responder rate for feverfew as 30.3% compared to 17.3% for placebo (Diener et al. 2005). Based on these and other studies, the AAN Evidence-based Guidelines states that MIG-99 is probably effective and should be considered for migraine prevention (Holland et al. 2012). Likewise, a 2015 Cochrane evidence-based review concluded that feverfew is effective in migraine prevention although the quality of evidence is low (Wider 2015).

10.3.2.6 Clinical Application

Feverfew (*Tanacetum parthenium*) extracts appear to be safe and effective for reducing the frequency of migraine headaches, especially in patients with four or more headaches per month. Studies show that *T. parthenium* at dosages providing an equivalent of 0.5 mg parthenolide per day are required.

10.4 Cannabis/Medical Marijuana Use in Clinical Neurology

For background information, please refer to Chapter 18 Therapeutic Potential of Cannabis.

10.4.1 Efficacy

10.4.1.1 Multiple Sclerosis

Use of dietary supplements is common among patients with multiple sclerosis (MS). Between 33% and 80% of patients report use, as well as the use of cannabinoids (Yadav et al. 2014). A systematic review conducted by the AAN (Koppel et al. 2014) examined the effects of various cannabinoids on the symptoms of multiple sclerosis. Cannabinoids in all forms were ineffective in improving objective measures of spasticity such as the Ashworth Spasticity Scale over 12–15 weeks, but might improve scores over 1 year.

Several forms of cannabinoids were found to significantly improve patient-reported spasticity and pain. Oral cannabinoid extract (OCE) was scored as effective for reducing patient reported scores, whereas THC and nabiximols were rated as probably effective, and smoked cannabis was rated as having uncertain efficacy due to insufficient evidence. With regard to central pain or painful spasms, OCE was rated as effective for reducing central pain, whereas THC and nabiximols were rated as probably effective for MS-related pain and painful spasms. Smoked marijuana was found to impair posture and balance in patients with spasticity (Koppel et al. 2014).

Of the 1,619 patients included in the systematic review, 6.9% stopped cannabinoid products due to adverse effects versus 2.2% of patients receiving placebo. Data on adverse reactions was not always complete, but nausea, fatigue, increased weakness, behavioral and/or mood changes, suicidal ideation and/or hallucinations, dizziness and/or vasovagal symptoms, and feelings of intoxication were reported most frequently. As a result, the AAN recommended that OCE might be recommended to patients with MS in order to reduce patient reported symptoms of spasticity and pain, that THC might be offered to patients with MS to reduce patient-reported symptoms of spasticity and pain (excluding central neuropathic pain), and nabiximols might be offered to patients with MS to reduce symptoms of pain and spasticity. In all cases, the recommendations cautioned that cannabinoids might not improve objectives measures. The organization also suggested that effects with OCE and THC might persist for 1 year (Yadav et al. 2014).

10.4.1.2 Seizure Disorders

In a Cochrane review of cannabinoids for epilepsy, four trials were identified for inclusion (Gloss and Vickrey 2014). The sample sizes were small including only 9–15 patients per trial, of short duration between 3 weeks to 12 months, and blinding methods were unclear for most. Cannabidiol (CBD) was used in dosages ranging from 200 to 300 mg daily. The seizure frequency was similar in two of the trials, and several patients on cannabidiol were seizure free in the other two trials. The sample sizes were small so a statistical analysis was not practical. No adverse effects were observed in three of the four trials, mild drowsiness only reported in the fourth. The authors noted that the formal search process for the Cochrane review failed to identify more than half of the trials they considered for inclusion and thus may have missed additional trials. An AAN systematic review concluded that data were insufficient to either confirm or refute the efficacy of cannabinoids to decrease seizure frequency (Koppel et al. 2014).

In a systematic review of cannabinoids as adjunctive treatments for treatment-resistant epilepsy, 36 trials were identified: 6 randomized controlled trials (RCTs) and 30 observational studies (non-RCTs). The RCTs included a total of 555 patients, whereas the non-RCTs included 2,865 patients. The mean age in the RCTs was 16.3 years (range 2.3–49 years), whereas the mean age range in the non-RCTs was 15 years (range 0.5–50 years). All RCTs studied CBD. The more recent trials used weight based dosing (2.5–20 mg/kg/day) over a mean treatment length of 14 weeks. The earlier RCTs used CBD 100 mg administered two to three times daily. The non-RCTs used a variety of cannabinoids, but CBD was the most common. The primary outcome of the systematic review was 50% reduction in seizure frequency, which was reported in nineteen total studies (two RCTs and 17 non-RCTs). CBD was more likely than placebo to produce a >50 reduction in seizures in the two RCTs (RR 1.74, 95% CI 1.24 to 2.43, low GRADE rating) with a NNT of 8. An estimated 48.5% of patients in the non-RCTs achieved a >50% reduction in seizures, but the evidence was deemed to be of mixed quality. Complete seizure freedom was also assessed, with a RR of 6.17 for CBD (95% CI 1.50 to 25.32, low GRADE rating) and a NNT of 171.

There was mixed quality of evidence suggesting CBD improved quality of life. There was no difference in likelihood of study withdrawal between CBD and placebo in the RCTs. Evidence was more mixed for the non-RCT trials. The most common AEs noted for CBD in the RCTs were drowsiness, diarrhea, fatigue and changes in appetite. Ataxia was also noted in the non-RCTs (Stockings et al. 2018).

In April 2018, the FDA voted unanimously to approve cannabidiol oral solution (Epidiolex®) for the adjunctive treatment of seizures associated with Dravet Syndrome and Lennox-Gastaut syndrome (LGS) in children ≥2 years old.

10.5 Conclusion

Use of botanical preparations for neurological conditions is common, particularly for headaches and dementia. *Bacopa monnieri*, *Ginkgo biloba*, *Panax ginseng*, and huperzine A from *Huperzia serrata* have been used to treat dementia. While specific extracts from all have been relatively safe for short term use, only the *Ginkgo biloba* extract Egb 761 and huperzine A have any data suggesting possible efficacy. Feverfew (*Tanacetum parthenium*) and butterbur (*Petasites hybridus*) have been used to treat headaches. A specific butterbur extract (Petadolex®) that is free of pyrrolizidine alkaloids has been shown to be safe and have some efficacy in the prevention of migraines. Specific formulations of feverfew are likewise safe and have some efficacy in preventing migraines. Medical marijuana and cannabis preparations have been used to treat spasticity in multiple sclerosis with improvement in subjective, but not objective measures. Data on the use of cannabinoids in the treatment of epilepsy are strongest for cannabidiol as an adjunct for treatment-resistant epilepsy. Data on the use of other forms of cannabinoids are insufficient to determine the effects on epilepsy.

REFERENCES

Baron-Ruppert, G., and N. P. Luepke. 2001. "Evidence for toxic effects of alkylphenols from ginkgo biloba in the hen's egg test (HET)." *Phytomedicine* 8 (2):133–8. doi: 10.1078/0944-7113-00022.

Barsby, R. W., U. Salan, D. W. Knight, and J. R. Hoult. 1993. "Feverfew and vascular smooth muscle: Extracts from fresh and dried plants show opposing pharmacological profiles, dependent upon sesquiterpene lactone content." *Planta Med* 59 (1):20–5. doi: 10.1055/s-2006-959596.

Beckert, B. W., M. J. Concannon, S. L. Henry, D. S. Smith, and C. L. Puckett. 2007. "The effect of herbal medicines on platelet function: An *in vivo* experiment and review of the literature." *Plast Reconstr Surg* 120 (7):2044–50. doi: 10.1097/01.prs.0000295972.18570.0b.

Benedict, S. 2015. "Food for thought: marketing supplements for improved cognition." *Natural Products Insider.* https://www.naturalproductsinsider.com/healthy-living/food-thought-marketing-supplements-improved-cognition.

Biggs, M. J., E. S. Johnson, N. P. Persaud, and D. M. Ratcliffe. 1982. "Platelet aggregation in patients using feverfew for migraine." *Lancet* 2 (8301):776.

Birks, J., and J. Grimley Evans. 2009. "Ginkgo biloba for cognitive impairment and dementia." *Cochrane Database of Systematic Reviews* (1):Cd003120. doi: 10.1002/14651858.CD003120.pub3.

Bohlmann, F., and C. Zdero. 1982. "Sesquiterpene lactones and other constituents from Tanacetum parthenium." *Phytochemistry* 21 (10):2543–2549. https://doi.org/10.1016/0031-9422(82)85253-9.

Burry, J. N. 1980. Compositae dermatitis in South Australia: Contact dermatitis from *Chrysanthemum parthenium. Contact Dermatitis* 6(6):445.

Carty, H. C. 1996. "Herbal preparations under scientific scrutiny." *Cmaj* 155 (9):1236.

Collier, H. O., N. M. Butt, W. J. McDonald-Gibson, and S. A. Saeed. 1980. "Extract of feverfew inhibits prostaglandin biosynthesis." *Lancet* 2 (8200):922–3.

DeKosky, S. T., J. D. Williamson, A. L. Fitzpatrick, R. A. Kronmal, D. G. Ives, J. A. Saxton, O. L. Lopez et al. 2008. "Ginkgo biloba for prevention of dementia: A randomized controlled trial." *Jama* 300 (19):2253–62. doi: 10.1001/jama.2008.683.

Diener, H. C., V. Pfaffenrath, J. Schnitker, M. Friede, and H. H. Henneicke-von Zepelin. 2005. "Efficacy and safety of 6.25 mg t.i.d. feverfew CO2-extract (MIG-99) in migraine prevention--a randomized, double-blind, multicentre, placebo-controlled study." *Cephalalgia* 25 (11):1031–41. doi: 10.1111/j.1468-2982.2005.00950.x.

Diener, H. C., V. W. Rahlfs, and U. Danesch. 2004. "The first placebo-controlled trial of a special butterbur root extract for the prevention of migraine: Reanalysis of efficacy criteria." *European Neurology* 51 (2):89–97. doi: 10.1159/000076535.

Dodge, H. H., T. Zitzelberger, B. S. Oken, D. Howieson, and J. Kaye. 2008. "A randomized placebo-controlled trial of Ginkgo biloba for the prevention of cognitive decline." *Neurology* 70 (19 Pt 2):1809–17. doi: 10.1212/01.wnl.0000303814.13509.db.

Gauthier, S., and S. Schlaefke. 2014. "Efficacy and tolerability of Ginkgo biloba extract EGb 761(R) in dementia: A systematic review and meta-analysis of randomized placebo-controlled trials." *Clinical Intervention Aging* 9:2065–77. doi: 10.2147/cia.s72728.

Geng, J., J. Dong, H. Ni, M. S. Lee, T. Wu, K. Jiang, G. Wang, A. L. Zhou, and R. Malouf. 2010. "Ginseng for cognition." *Cochrane Database System Review* (12):Cd007769. doi: 10.1002/14651858.CD007769.pub2.

Giles, M., C. Ulbricht, K. P. Khalsa, C. D. Kirkwood, C. Park, and E. Basch. 2005. "Butterbur: An evidence-based systematic review by the natural standard research collaboration." *Journal of Herb Pharmacother* 5 (3):119–43.

Global Biodiversity Information Facility (GBIP) Secretariat. 2016. "Petasites hybridus." In *GBIF Backbone Taxonomy*.

Gloss, D., and B. Vickrey. 2014. "Cannabinoids for epilepsy." *Cochrane Database System Review* (3):Cd009270. doi: 10.1002/14651858.CD009270.pub3.

Granger, A. S.. 2001. "Ginkgo biloba precipitating epileptic seizures." *Age Aging* 30 (6):523–5.

Gregory, P. J. 2001. "Seizure associated with ginkgo biloba?" *Annals of Internal Medicine* 134 (4):344.

Grossmann, M., and H. Schmidramsl. 2000. "An extract of petasites hybridus is effective in the prophylaxis of migraine." *International Journal of Clinica Pharmacology Therapy* 38 (9):430–5.

Guinot, P., E. Caffrey, R. Lambe, and A. Darragh. 1989. "Tanakan inhibits platelet-activating-factor-induced platelet aggregation in healthy male volunteers." *Haemostasis* 19 (4):219–23.

Hao, Z., M. Liu, Z. Liu, and D. Lv. 2009. "Huperzine A for vascular dementia." *Cochrane Database System Review* (2):Cd007365. doi: 10.1002/14651858.CD007365.pub2.

Hausen, B. M., P. E. Osmundsen. 1983. Contact allergy to parthenolide in *Tanacetum parthenium* (L.) Schulz-Bip. (feverfew, Asteraceae) and cross-reactions to related sesquiterpene lactone containing Compositae species. *Acta Derm Venereol.* 63(4): 308–14.

Hehner, S. P., T. G. Hofmann, W. Droge, and M. L. Schmitz. 1999. "The antiinflammatory sesquiterpene lactone parthenolide inhibits NF-kappa B by targeting the I kappa B kinase complex." *Journal of Immunology* 163 (10):5617–23.

Heo, J. H., S. T. Lee, K. Chu, M. J. Oh, H. J. Park, J. Y. Shim, and M. Kim. 2012. "Heat-processed ginseng enhances the cognitive function in patients with moderately severe alzheimer's disease." *Nutritional Neuroscience* 15 (6):278–82. doi: 10.1179/1476830512y.0000000027.

Heo, J. H., M. H. Park, and J. H. Lee. 2016. "Effect of Korean Red Ginseng on cognitive function and quantitative EEG in patients with Alzheimer's disease: A preliminary study." *Journal of Alternative Complementary Medicine* 22 (4):280–5. doi: 10.1089/acm.2015.0265.

Heptinstall, S., D. V. Awang, B. A. Dawson, D. Kindack, D. W. Knight, and J. May. 1992. "Parthenolide content and bioactivity of feverfew (tanacetum parthenium (L.) Schultz-Bip.). Estimation of commercial and authenticated feverfew products." *Journal of Pharm Pharmacology* 44 (5):391–5.

Holland, S., S. D. Silberstein, F. Freitag, D. W. Dodick, C. Argoff, and E. Ashman. 2012. "Evidence-based guideline update: NSAIDs and other complementary treatments for episodic migraine prevention in adults: Report of the quality standards subcommittee of the american academy of neurology and the american headache society." *Neurology* 78 (17):1346–53. doi: 10.1212/WNL.0b013e3182535d0c.

Jang, H. S., S. Y. Roh, E. H. Jeong, B. S. Kim, and M. K. Sunwoo. 2015. "Ginkgotoxin induced seizure caused by vitamin B6 deficiency." *Journal of Epilepsy Residents* 5 (2):104–6. doi: 10.14581/jer.15018.

Johnson, E. S., N. P. Kadam, D. M. Hylands, P. J. Hylands. 1985. Efficacy of feverfew as prophylactic treatment of migraine. *Br Med J.* 291:569–73.

Kellermann, A. J., and C. Kloft. 2011. "Is there a risk of bleeding associated with standardized ginkgo biloba extract therapy? A systematic review and meta-analysis." *Pharmacotherapy* 31 (5):490–502. doi: 10.1592/phco.31.5.490.

Kisiel, W., and A. Stojakowska. 1997. "A sesquiterpene coumarin ether from transformed roots of Tanacetum parthenium." *Phytochemistry* 46 (3):515–6. https://doi.org/10.1016/S0031-9422(97)87091-4.

Kohler, S., P. Funk, and M. Kieser. 2004. "Influence of a 7-day treatment with ginkgo biloba special extract EGb 761 on bleeding time and coagulation: A randomized, placebo-controlled, double-blind study in healthy volunteers." *Blood Coagul Fibrinolysis* 15 (4):303–9.

Kongkeaw, C., P. Dilokthornsakul, P. Thanarangsarit, N. Limpeanchob, and C. Norman Scholfield. 2014. "Meta-analysis of randomized controlled trials on cognitive effects of Bacopa monnieri extract." *Journal of Ethnopharmacology* 151 (1):528–35. doi: 10.1016/j.jep.2013.11.008.

Koppel, B. S., J. C. Brust, T. Fife, J. Bronstein, S. Youssof, G. Gronseth, and D. Gloss. 2014. "Systematic review: Efficacy and safety of medical marijuana in selected neurologic disorders: Report of the guideline development subcommittee of the american academy of neurology." *Neurology* 82 (17):1556–63. doi: 10.1212/wnl.0000000000000363.

Kudolo, G. B. 2001. "The effect of 3-month ingestion of Ginkgo biloba extract (EGb 761) on pancreatic beta-cell function in response to glucose loading in individuals with non-insulin-dependent diabetes mellitus." *Journal of Clinical Pharmacology* 41 (6):600–11.

Lee, M. S., E. J. Yang, J. I. Kim, and E. Ernst. 2009. "Ginseng for cognitive function in alzheimer's disease: A systematic review." *Journal of Alzheimers Disease* 18 (2):339–44. doi: 10.3233/jad-2009-1149.

Li, J., H. M. Wu, R. L. Zhou, G. J. Liu, and B. R. Dong. 2008. "Huperzine A for alzheimer's disease." *Cochrane Database System Review* (2):Cd005592. doi: 10.1002/14651858.CD005592.pub2.

Lipton, R. B., H. Gobel, K. M. Einhaupl, K. Wilks, and A. Mauskop. 2004. "Petasites hybridus root (butterbur) is an effective preventive treatment for migraine." *Neurology* 63 (12):2240–4.

Losche, W., A. V. Mazurov, S. Heptinstall, W. A. Groenewegen, V. S. Repin, and U. Till. 1987. "An extract of feverfew inhibits interactions of human platelets with collagen substrates." *Thromb Res* 48 (5):511–8.

Matthews, M. K., Jr. 1998. "Association of ginkgo biloba with intracerebral hemorrhage." *Neurology* 50 (6):1933–4.

Mittra, S., A. Datta, S. K. Singh, and A. Singh. 2000. "5-Hydroxytryptamine-inhibiting property of feverfew: Role of parthenolide content." *Acta Pharmacology Sin* 21 (12):1106–14.

Morgan, A., and J. Stevens. 2010. "Does bacopa monnieri improve memory performance in older persons? Results of a randomized, placebo-controlled, double-blind trial." *Journal of Alternative Complementary Medicine* 16 (7):753p9. doi: 10.1089/acm.2009.0342.

Murphy, J. J., S. Heptinstall, and J. R. Mitchell. 1988. "Randomised double-blind placebo-controlled trial of feverfew in migraine prevention." *Lancet* 2 (8604):189–92.

Nash, K. M., and Z. A. Shah. 2015. "Current Perspectives on the Beneficial Role of Ginkgo biloba in Neurological and Cerebrovascular Disorders." *Integr Med Insights* 10:1–9. doi: 10.4137/imi.s25054.

Oelkers-Ax, R., A. Leins, P. Parzer, T. Hillecke, H. V. Bolay, J. Fischer, S. Bender, U. Hermanns, and F. Resch. 2008. "Butterbur root extract and music therapy in the prevention of childhood migraine: An explorative study." *Eur J Pain* 12 (3):301–13. doi: 10.1016/j.ejpain.2007.06.003.

Pareek, A., M. Suthar, G. S. Rathore, and V. Bansal. 2011. "Feverfew (Tanacetum parthenium L.): A systematic review." *Pharmacogn Rev* 5 (9):103–10. doi: 10.4103/0973-7847.79105.

Pase, M. P., J. Kean, J. Sarris, C. Neale, A. B. Scholey, and C. Stough. 2012. "The cognitive-enhancing effects of Bacopa monnieri: A systematic review of randomized, controlled human clinical trials." *J Altern Complement Med* 18 (7):647–52. doi: 10.1089/acm.2011.0367.

Pedroso, J. L., C. C. Henriques Aquino, M. L. Escorcio Bezerra, R. F. Baiense, M. M. Suarez, L. A. Dutra, P. Braga-Neto, and O. G. Povoas Barsottini. 2011. "Ginkgo biloba and cerebral bleeding: A case report and critical review." *Neurologist* 17 (2):89–90. doi: 10.1097/NRL.0b013e3181f097b4.

Pfaffenrath, V., H. C. Diener, M. Fischer, M. Friede, and H. H. Henneicke-von Zepelin. 2002. "The efficacy and safety of Tanacetum parthenium (feverfew) in migraine prophylaxis--a double-blind, multicentre, randomized placebo-controlled dose-response study." *Cephalalgia* 22 (7):523–32. doi: 10.1046/j.1468-2982.2002.00396.x.

Pothmann, R., and U. Danesch. 2005. "Migraine prevention in children and adolescents: Results of an open study with a special butterbur root extract." *Headache* 45 (3):196–203. doi: 10.1111/j.1526-4610.2005.05044.x.

Rajan, K. E., J. Preethi, and H. K. Singh. 2015. "Molecular and Functional Characterization of Bacopa monniera: A Retrospective Review." *Evid Based Complement Alternat Med* 2015:945217. doi: 10.1155/2015/945217.

Rokot, N. T., T. S. Kairupan, K. C. Cheng, J. Runtuwene, N. H. Kapantow, M. Amitani, A. Morinaga, H. Amitani, A. Asakawa, and A. Inui. 2016. "A role of ginseng and its constituents in the treatment of central nervous system disorders." *Evid Based Complement Alternat Med* 2016:2614742. doi: 10.1155/2016/2614742.

Rosenblatt, M., and J. Mindel. 1997. "Spontaneous hyphema associated with ingestion of Ginkgo biloba extract." *N Engl J Med* 336 (15):1108. doi: 10.1056/nejm199704103361518.

Russo, A., and F. Borrelli. 2005. "Bacopa monniera, a reputed nootropic plant: An overview." *Phytomedicine* 12 (4):305–17. doi: 10.1016/j.phymed.2003.12.008.

Sarchielli, P., A. Floridi, M. L. Mancini, C. Rossi, F. Coppola, A. Baldi, L. A. Pini, and P. Calabresi. 2006. "NF-kappaB activity and iNOS expression in monocytes from internal jugular blood of migraine without aura patients during attacks." *Cephalalgia* 26 (9):1071–9. doi: 10.1111/j.1468-2982.2006.01164.x.

Smith, I., E. M. Williamson, S. Putnam, J. Farrimond, and B. J. Whalley. 2014. "Effects and mechanisms of ginseng and ginsenosides on cognition." *Nutr Rev* 72 (5):319–33. doi: 10.1111/nure.12099.

Stockings, E., D. Zagic, G. Campbell, M. Weier, W.D. Hall, S. Nielsen, G.K. Herkes, M. Farrell, and L. Degenhardt. "Evidence for cannabis and cannabinoids for epilepsy: A systematic review of controlled and observational evidence." *J Neurol Neurosurg Psychiatry* 2018; 0:1–13. doi: 10.1136/jnnp-2017-317168.

Stoddard, G. J., M. Archer, L. Shane-McWhorter, B. E. Bray, D. F. Redd, J. Proulx, and Q. Zeng-Treitler. 2015. "Ginkgo and Warfarin Interaction in a Large Veterans Administration Population." *AMIA Annu Symp Proc* 2015:1174–83.

Stough, C., J. Lloyd, J. Clarke, L. A. Downey, C. W. Hutchison, T. Rodgers, and P. J. Nathan. 2001. "The chronic effects of an extract of Bacopa monniera (Brahmi) on cognitive function in healthy human subjects." *Psychopharmacology (Berl)* 156 (4):481–4.

Sun-Edelstein, C., and A. Mauskop. 2011. "Alternative headache treatments: Nutraceuticals, behavioral and physical treatments." *Headache* 51 (3):469–83. doi: 10.1111/j.1526-4610.2011.01846.x.

Sutherland, A., and B. V. Sweet. 2010. "Butterbur: An alternative therapy for migraine prevention." *Am J Health Syst Pharm* 67 (9):705–11. doi: 10.2146/ajhp090136.

Tassorelli, C., R. Greco, P. Morazzoni, A. Riva, G. Sandrini, and G. Nappi. 2005. "Parthenolide is the component of tanacetum parthenium that inhibits nitroglycerin-induced Fos activation: Studies in an animal model of migraine." *Cephalalgia* 25 (8):612–21. doi: 10.1111/j.1468-2982.2005.00915.x.

Therapeutic Research Center (TRC). 2015. "Huperzine A." In *Natural Medicines*.

Therapeutic Research Center (TRC). 2017. "Panax Ginseng." In *Natural Medicines*.

Vellas, B., N. Coley, P. J. Ousset, G. Berrut, J. F. Dartigues, B. Dubois, H. Grandjean et al. 2012. "Long-term use of standardised Ginkgo biloba extract for the prevention of Alzheimer's disease (GuidAge): A randomised placebo-controlled trial." *Lancet Neurol* 11 (10):851–9. doi: 10.1016/s1474-4422(12)70206-5.

Wells, R. E., S. M. Bertisch, C. Buettner, R. S. Phillips, and E. P. McCarthy. 2011. "Complementary and alternative medicine use among adults with migraines/severe headaches." *Headache* 51 (7):1087–97. doi: 10.1111/j.1526-4610.2011.01917.x.

Wells, R. E., R. S. Phillips, S. C. Schachter, and E. P. McCarthy. 2010. "Complementary and alternative medicine use among US adults with common neurological conditions." *J Neurol* 257 (11):1822–31. doi: 10.1007/s00415-010-5616-2.

Wider, B., M. H. Pittler, E. Ernst. 2015. Feverfew for preventing migraine. *Cochrane Database of Systematic Reviews* 4. Art. No.: CD002286.

Xing, S. H., C. X. Zhu, R. Zhang, and L. An. 2014. "Huperzine a in the treatment of Alzheimer's disease and vascular dementia: A meta-analysis." *Evid Based Complement Alternat Med* 2014:363985. doi: 10.1155/2014/363985.

Yadav, V., C. Bever, Jr., J. Bowen, A. Bowling, B. Weinstock-Guttman, M. Cameron, D. Bourdette, G. S. Gronseth, and P. Narayanaswami. 2014. "Summary of evidence-based guideline: Complementary and alternative medicine in multiple sclerosis: Report of the guideline development subcommittee of the American Academy of Neurology." *Neurology* 82 (12):1083–92. doi: 10.1212/wnl.0000000000000250.

Yang, G., Y. Wang, J. Sun, K. Zhang, and J. Liu. 2016. "Ginkgo Biloba for mild cognitive impairment and Alzheimer's disease: A systematic review and meta-analysis of randomized controlled trials." *Curr Top Med Chem* 16 (5):520–8.

Yue, J., B. R. Dong, X. Lin, M. Yang, H. M. Wu, and T. Wu. 2012. "Huperzine A for mild cognitive impairment." *Cochrane Database Syst Rev* 12:Cd008827. doi: 10.1002/14651858.CD008827.pub2.

Zhang, H. F., L. B. Huang, Y. B. Zhong, Q. H. Zhou, H. L. Wang, G. Q. Zheng, and Y. Lin. 2016. "An overview of systematic reviews of Ginkgo biloba extracts for mild cognitive impairment and dementia." *Front Aging Neurosci* 8:276. doi: 10.3389/fnagi.2016.00276.

Zhang, H. Y. 2012. "New insights into huperzine A for the treatment of Alzheimer's disease." *Acta Pharmacol Sin* 33 (9):1170–5. doi: 10.1038/aps.2012.128.

11

Psychiatric Disorders

Jessica L. Gören and Sara E. Dugan

CONTENTS

11.1 Introduction

Depression and anxiety are two of the most common mental health disorders (Kessler et al. 1994, Baxter et al. 2013, Kessler and Bromel 2013). In addition, 1/3 of adults report at least one symptom of insomnia (Roth 2007). The use of complementary therapies is particularly high among these patients. Reports indicate persons using complementary therapy are more likely to have psychiatric symptoms than those who do not. Community surveys demonstrate depression, anxiety, and insomnia are among the most common reasons cited for complementary and alternative medicine (CAM) use (Kessler et al. 2001). Use of botanicals was reported in 18.6% of adult survey respondents with depression (Tindle et al. 2005). Complementary and alternative medicine use is also common in pediatric patients with up to 2/3 of parents reporting use or interest in CAM for their children with attention deficit hyperactivity disorder (ADHD) (Chan et al. 2003, Sinha and Efron 2005). Therefore, knowledge of botanicals is of particular importance when working with patients with psychiatric disorders (Wong et al. 1998, Knaudt et al. 1999, Yager et al. 1999, Kessler et al. 2001, Barnes et al. 2008).

11.2 Anxiety

Although prevalence varies across cultures, anxiety disorders are among the most common psychiatric disorders in adults across Europe and the United States (U.S.) (Kessler et al. 2001, Wittchen et al. 2011). Studies indicate anxiety is associated with dysfunction of the noradrenergic, serotonergic, and gamma-aminobutyric acid (GABA) systems. Other research indicates chronically elevated cortisol levels from activation of the hypothalamic-pituitary-adrenal axis may play a role in the manifestation of anxiety disorders. Pharmacotherapy for anxiety disorders involves enhancement of GABA effects via interaction with voltage-gated ion channels and benzodiazepine receptors or manipulation of serotonergic function (Sarris et al. 2011a, 2013b,c).

11.2.1 Chamomile (*Matricaria recutita*)

11.2.1.1 Background

See Chapter 13 Dermatologic Conditions for discussion.

11.2.1.2 Pharmacognosy

Historically, chamomile's mechanism of action for anxiety was thought to be through interactions with the GABAergic system (Sarris et al. 2011a, 2013b,c). However, several preclinical studies have concluded this is unlikely. An alternate anxiolytic mechanism may be through modulation of the neuroendocrine system.

11.2.1.3 Dosing and Preparation

The most effective dose of chamomile for anxiety has not been established. Doses used in clinical trials for anxiety ranged from 220 to 1,100 mg. Studies differed in frequency of administration, although the most rigorous study used thrice daily dosing. A tea made from the flowers has been used as a nonspecific calming agent. Chamomile tea can be prepared from commercially available tea bags of dried chamomile or by pouring boiling water over chamomile flowers and steeping for 5 minutes. For insomnia, the dose is 270 mg (given twice daily) or 540 mg nightly of the dried extract.

11.2.1.4 Safety

See Chapter 13 Dermatologic Conditions for discussion.

11.2.1.5 Evidence

One 8-week randomized, double blind placebo-controlled trial assessed the efficacy of chamomile extract in 57 patients with generalized anxiety disorder (Amsterdam et al. 2009). Doses of 220–1,100 mg were found to be effective in decreasing symptoms in those with mild to moderate anxiety. Participants were instructed to take chamomile at their convenience, either as once daily or in divided doses. Chamomile use did not result in significant adverse events, but one patient reported abdominal discomfort. The authors noted a greater decrease in resting heart rate with chamomile, but the difference was not clinically or statistically significant. Adverse effects did not increase with higher doses of chamomile.

The single randomized placebo-controlled trial of 34 patients with insomnia for 6 months or more failed to find any benefit with 270 mg of chamomile twice daily. There were some modest improvements in daytime functioning by self-report, although these did not reach statistical significance. Given the small number of participants and trends towards some benefits, particularly in improvement in daytime functioning, larger studies may demonstrate significant improvements (Zick et al. 2011). *See Chapter 13 Dermatologic Conditions for further discussion.*

11.2.1.6 Clinical Application

Chamomile has limited evidence to support its use in mild to moderate anxiety disorders. The dose of chamomile for the treatment of generalized anxiety disorder is still unknown, although doses up to 1,100 mg daily did not result in adverse effects. It is likely safe to use in doses of 220–1,100 mg with other psychotropic medications, but data is lacking to support its efficacy. Chamomile does not appear to be effective for chronic insomnia, although data are limited.

11.2.2 Kava (*Piper methysticum*)

11.2.2.1 Background

Kava is a member of the pepper family from the South Pacific. It is a slow growing perennial whose root has been used for religious ceremonies and to treat anxiety and social phobia for many years. In Western countries, kava has been used for the treatment of anxiety disorders.

11.2.2.2 Pharmacognosy

The anxiolytic effects of kava are due to kavalactones extracted from the peeled root. While numerous kavalactones have been identified, the anxiolytic effects appear to be mediated by kavain, dihyrkavain, methsticin, dihydromethysticum, demethoxyyangonin, and yangonin (Sarris et al. 2013a,b,c). Kavalactones' pharmacologic activity in the central nervous system (CNS) may be due to effects on voltage-gated sodium ion channels, neurotransmitter function and release, $GABA_A$ receptors, monoamine oxidase B function, and cyclooxygenase (Sarris et al. 2013a,b,c).

11.2.2.3 Dosing and Preparation

Kava is available in many formulations. No standard dose for kava has been identified. Clinical trials used doses of 60–300 mg of kavalactones with doses of 105–210 mg being most common. While the mechanism of kava-induced hepatotoxicity has not been established, it may be due to ingestion of aerial parts or root peelings of the plant, contaminants from growing or processing conditions, or ingestion of acetonic and ethanolic extracts (Pittler and Ernst 2010, Teschke et al. 2012, Sarris et al. 2013a,b,c). Therefore, only aqueous extracts of the peeled root should be used (Sarris et al. 2011a,b, Teschke et al. 2011, 2012, Sarris et al. 2013a,b,c). While aqueous extracts are preferred, they have also been associated with rare cases of hepatotoxicity (Teschke et al. 2012).

11.2.2.4 Safety

Medicinal kava was withdrawn from the European Union markets due to concerns regarding hepatotoxicity (Kutcha et al. 2005, Sarris et al. 2011b, Schmidt 2014). However, the decision to withdraw marketing authorization for kava was overturned in a German court in 2014. The regulatory agency has since filed an appeal. In May 2015, the European Medicines Agency's Committee on Herbal Medicinal Products issued a request for scientific data on kava indicating the availability of medicinal kava in Europe may change (Schmidt 2014). Kava remains available as a dietary supplement in Europe and the U.S.

Hepatic failure can be severe, but appears to be rare with kava use. In Germany, it was estimated that 450 million daily doses of medicinal kava had been sold between 1999 and 2001. During that time, there were 26 cases of hepatic failure reported with kava. Of these reports, only three were believed to have been caused by kava (Schmidt 2014, Kutcha et al. 2015).

A Cochrane review of placebo controlled trials identified 12 randomized double blind placebo trials of kava (60–280 mg of kavalactones) for anxiety (Pittler and Ernst 2010). Six trials reported adverse events including stomach complaints, restlessness, drowsiness, tremor, headache and tiredness. There were no reports of hepatotoxicity, even in the seven studies that monitored liver function tests. Similar adverse effects were reported in a subsequent randomized controlled trial published after the Cochrane review was completed (Sarris et al. 2013a). While poorly described in the literature, a kava-induced dermopathy has been reported that is more common and severe with chronic, heavy kava use (Norton and Ruze 1994).

Concomitant use of kava with other CNS depressants or alcohol may lead to significant sedation and should be avoided. Kava is a potent inhibitor of cytochrome P450 enzymes including 1A2, 2C9, 2C19, 2D6, and 3A4 (Anke and Ramzan 2004). There are case reports of kava worsening parkinsonian symptoms and inducing parkinsonism in patients without Parkinson's disease (Meseguer et al. 2002, Izzo and Ernst 2009). Therefore, careful review for drug interactions and comorbid disease states should be conducted prior to initiation of kava.

11.2.2.5 Evidence

Data from seven trials (n = 380) were included in a Cochrane meta-analysis which concluded kava in a dose of 60–280 mg kavalactones is effective for the treatment of anxiety although the effect size is small (Pittler and Ernst 2010). In a randomized controlled trial (n = 75) not included in the meta-analysis, kava decreased symptoms of anxiety and increased the number of patients in remission compared with placebo. The effect size was large (d = 0.8) in patients with higher symptom burden (Sarris et al. 2013a).

11.2.2.6 Clinical Application

Kava appears to have modest benefits in generalized anxiety disorder in doses of 60–280 mg of kavalactones daily. Kava was administered as once daily and multiple daily doses in the studies with thrice daily administration being most commonly studied. Overall, it is well tolerated with headache and stomach complaints being the most common adverse effects reported in clinical trials. Although rare, reports of hepatotoxicity are worrisome. This specific adverse event and the limited data supporting kava's efficacy should be weighed against the adverse effects of drug classes such as benzodiazepines and antidepressants. Patients should be advised to ingest only aqueous extracts of the peeled root. Kava should be avoided when the process by which kava was prepared is not known. Special care should be taken to assess for potential drug interactions with kava use and in patients with hepatic dysfunction or Parkinson's disease.

11.2.3 Lavender (*Lavandula angustifolia* or *officianilis*)

11.2.3.1 Background

Lavender, from the mint family lamiaceae, is an aromatic evergreen plant with small blue and purple flowers native to the Mediterranean, Arabian peninsula, Russia, and Africa. It has been used for centuries as a medicine and culinary herb. It is available as aromatherapy and for oral ingestion.

11.2.3.2 Pharmacognosy

When distilled from the dried plant as an oil, lavender has been shown to contain more than 160 different constituents (Kasper 2013). The therapeutic properties of orally ingested lavender are most likely due to multiple substances including linalool and linalyl. *In vitro* studies indicate inhibition of calcium channels and GABA effects may contribute to lavender's anxiolytic effect.

11.2.3.3 Dosing and Preparation

Lavender is available in many forms including as an oil and spray for aromatherapy and oral formulations. In Germany, a standardized oral formulation is available, while in other countries lavender is sold as a supplement.

To prepare lavender tea, 1–2 tsp of dried lavender flowers are steeped in one cup of hot water. Lavender oil for oral ingestion is derived from distillation of the entire plant and is typically dosed at 80–100 mg daily.

11.2.3.4 Safety

Lavender appears safe for oral ingestion. In clinical trials, eructation and dyspepsia were the most common adverse effects reported. Lavender has significantly fewer adverse effects than lorazepam and was not associated with sedation in one clinical trial (Woelk and Schlafke 2010). In another study, adverse effects were equal to those of the placebo group and less than with paroxetine (Kasper et al. 2014). Discontinuation of lavender after 10 weeks does not lead to any appreciable withdrawal symptoms. Topical application may result in dermatitis.

Pharmacokinetic studies found no interaction of lavender with CYP450 enzymes (Kasper 2013). There are no known drug interactions when ingested orally.

11.2.3.5 Evidence: Aromatherapy

Several studies have demonstrated that lavender aromatherapy effectively decreases anxiety in stressful situations. In one study (n = 200), ambient lavender and orange odors' effects on anxiety were compared with music and neither music nor aromatherapy controls for patients in a dentist's waiting room. Anxiety and mood were improved with ambient lavender scent when compared with music (Lehrner et al. 2015). Another study (n = 340) demonstrated patients in dental waiting rooms with ambient lavender scent had less anxiety than patients in a similar setting with no odor (Kristsidima et al. 2010). In a third study, (n = 597) patients had lower anxiety levels when there was ambient lavender scent in a dental waiting area (Zabirunnisa et al. 2014). A study of graduate student nurses taking an exam reported lavender decreased stress and heart rate (McCaffrey et al. 2009).

A study of lavender aromatherapy for pain and anxiety when undergoing peripheral venous cannulation reported patients (n = 106) had less pain, lower anxiety and higher satisfaction with care when in the lavender scented rooms (Karaman et al. 2016). However, in another trial (n = 60) lavender aromatherapy on days 2 and 3 after coronary bypass surgery did not decrease anxiety (Seifi et al. 2014). A randomized placebo controlled study of 106 women tested lavender inhalation for the pain and anxiety with intrauterine device insertion. Lavender inhalation 30 minutes prior to procedure was associated with significant reduction in anxiety, although the overall effect was small (Shahnazi et al. 2012). A trial of 140 women demonstrated lavender aromatherapy decreased anxiety and depression during the 4 weeks postpartum (Klanpour et al. 2016).

11.2.3.6 Evidence: Oral Administration

Results with oral administration of lavender are mixed. In one study (n = 97), prior administration with oral lavender (100, 200 micromol) did not prevent anxiety when watching anxiety-provoking film clips (Bradley et al. 2009). A randomized, double-blind, placebo- and paroxetine-controlled study (n = 539) reported lavender in doses of 80 mg and 160 mg daily significantly reduced anxiety scores in patients with generalized anxiety disorder. Of the patients in the 160 mg dose group, 60% showed a reduction of anxiety score greater than or equal to 50% and 46% had a Hamilton Anxiety Rating Scale (HAM-A) score of less than 10, indicating minimal residual anxiety symptoms. This was numerically, but not statistically, superior to the 80 mg dose (Kapser et al. 2014). A 6-week study comparing 80 mg of lavender to 0.5 mg of lorazepam found lavender was equivalent to lorazepam in the treatment of generalized anxiety disorder (Woelk and Schlafke 2010).

In one randomized, single-blind crossover trial of lavender aromatherapy for insomnia, ten patients reported improvements in sleep but the difference did not reach statistical significance (Lewith et al. 2005). In a 12-week trial of 67 women, aged 45–55 years old, inhalation of lavender for 20 minutes twice weekly improved subjective sleep quality.

11.2.3.7 Clinical Application

Lavender aromatherapy appears to be safe and effective for reducing mild anxiety in stressful situations, although the effect size is small. Most studies involved exposure 30 minutes prior to the experience. Ambient lavender scent in dental waiting rooms or other stressful environments is reasonable given its relative safety but may not be acceptable to all patients in the waiting area. Some studies indicate benefits with lavender aromatherapy prior to minor medical procedures. Lavender aromatherapy after more invasive medical interventions was ineffective. Oral lavender in doses of 80–160 mg was effective for generalized anxiety disorder in some well-designed trials. Lavender has no drug known interactions and is a reasonable option for those with mild anxiety.

Lavender aromatherapy does not appear to be effective for insomnia but data are limited. Patients have reported some improvements in sleep quality. Given the safety of aromatherapy, lavender would be a reasonable adjunct to behavioral therapy.

11.2.4 Lemon Balm (*Melissa officinalis*)

11.2.4.1 Background

Lemon balm is a perennial herb from the mint family. Lemon balm has been widely grown in parts of the Middle East and southern Europe (Shakeri et al. 2016). It has been reported to have a calming effect and has been used for anxiety and insomnia. Topically, lemon balm has been used to treat cold sores. *See Chapters 6 Endocrine Disorders and 12 Botanicals for Common Infections for further discussion.*

11.2.4.2 Pharmacognosy

The active constituents of lemon balm are derived from the leaves and flowers of the plant. The active constituents include polyphenolics, flavonoids, and triterpenes which appear to inhibit GABA transaminase, increase GABA levels, reduce serum and brain corticosterone levels, and inhibit monoamine oxidase (Sarris et al. 2013b,c, Shakeri et al. 2016).

11.2.4.3 Dosing and Preparation

As a tea, 1.5–4.5 grams of lemon balm leaves are steeped in one cup of hot water and administered as needed. Capsules of 300 mg of standardized extract made from distillation of leaves and flowers is available in the U.S. and Europe. Doses of 300–900 mg daily were found to be effective for anxiety symptoms with most studies reporting 300 mg twice daily.

11.2.4.4 Safety

The long history of use and lack of reported adverse effects indicates lemon balm is relatively safe (European Medicine Agency 2013). No adverse effects were reported in the clinical trials of anxiety (Kennedy et al. 2002, 2004, Cases et al. 2011). Lemon balm can cause sedation and should be used cautiously with other CNS depressants including alcohol. It has also been reported to decrease serum glucose and use should be avoided in those on antihyperglycemic medications (Chung et al. 2010). It has been associated *in vitro* and in animal models with decreased thyroid stimulating hormone and thyroid secretion (Auf'mkolk et al. 1984, Santini et al. 2003). Therefore, care should be used in patients treated for hypothyroidism. In one trial, lemon balm inhibited CYP450 2D6; thus, it should not be administered with CYP450 2D6 substrates or medications requiring this isoenzyme system for conversion to active metabolites, such as tamoxifen (Grappe et al. 2014).

11.2.4.5 Evidence

One open label study of 20 patients with anxiety and insomnia reported a decrease in anxiety and associated symptoms (18% and 15%, respectively) at doses of 300–900 mg daily (Cases et al. 2011). Fourteen patients achieved full remission of anxiety and 70% achieved remission of both their anxiety and insomnia. A 42% decrease in insomnia symptoms in 20 patients (Cases et al. 2011). A total of 85% of patients achieved full remission for insomnia.

In a randomized, placebo-controlled, double-blind, crossover study (n = 20) of mood and cognitive performance, doses of 300–900 mg daily have been shown to increase self-rated calmness, a secondary outcome, after cognitive testing (Kennedy et al. 2002). A second randomized controlled trial of 18 patients reported dosing of 600 mg significantly increased self-ratings of calmness (Kennedy et al. 2004). *See Chapters 6 Endocrine Disorders and 12 Botanicals for Common Infections for further discussion.*

11.2.4.6 Clinical Application

Lemon balm is relatively effective for mild anxiety and to promote self-reported calmness. The studies are quite small and further research is needed to assess the efficacy of lemon balm in anxiety disorders. Data are insufficient to draw conclusions regarding the use of lemon balm in insomnia. It does have the risk for drug interactions and care should be taken when used with other medications. Adverse effects were rare in the clinical trials with sedation being the most common one (Kennedy et al. 2002, 2004, Cases et al. 2011).

11.2.5 Passionflower (*Passiflora incarnate*)

11.2.5.1 Background

Passiflora incarnate is a perennial evergreen climbing vine (Miroddi et al. 2013). It has been grown for thousands of years by indigenous people of South America and the U.S. Its fruit has been used in jams and jellies, while the leaves have been used for medicinal purposes.

11.2.5.2 Pharmacognosy

Passionflower has numerous active constituents including amino acids, chrysin, cyanogenic glycosides, indole alkaloids, and flavanoids (Miroddi et al. 2013, Sarris et al. 2013b,c). The indole alkaloids inhibit monoamine oxidase, but they are present only in small quantities; it is unlikely that this serves as the pharmacologic basis for anxiolytic effects (Miroddi et al. 2013). While chrysin binds with the benzodiazepine receptor, it has a low binding affinity making this an unlikely source of anxiolytic properties (Sarris et al. 2013b,c). Other studies indicate leaf extracts may inhibit GABA-transaminase, while extracts from the whole plant appear to inhibit GABA uptake (Sarris et al. 2013a,b,c). Extracts of passionflower contain some GABA and pretreatment with flumazenil, a benzodiazepine receptor antagonist, lessens the effects of passionflower, but the exact mechanism is unknown. It is likely that GABA-ergic effects account for some of passionflower's anxiolytic effects (Miroddi et al. 2013, Sarris et al. 2013b,c).

11.2.5.3 Dosing and Preparation

Forty-five drops of passionflower extract and 90 mg capsules have both been used for the treatment of anxiety. Administration of the dried herb, an infusion of 2 g in 150 mL, 2 mL of a 1:1 fluid extract and 10 mL of a 1:5 tincture 3–4 times daily have been used in clinical trials of anxiety. A passionflower tea for insomnia can be made with 2 g of dried leaves, stems, seeds, and flowers infused in one cup of boiling water for 10 minutes.

11.2.5.4 Safety

Passionflower is calming and may enhance the effects of other sedating medications and alcohol. Adverse events in one study consisted of dizziness, drowsiness and confusion. It may cause uterine contraction and be an abortifacient in high doses, so passionflower should be avoided in women trying to conceive or who are pregnant (De Smet 2002).

11.2.5.5 Evidence

Two randomized, placebo-controlled trials reported passionflower was more effective than placebo in treating anxiety before surgery. In one trial of 60 patients undergoing ambulatory surgery, pretreatment with 500 mg of passionflower 90 minutes before surgery led to improvement in anxiety before and up to 90 minutes afterwards compared with placebo (Movafegh et al. 2008). In another study of 60 participants, administration of passionflower 30 minutes before surgery resulted in decreased anxiety immediately preceding spinal anesthesia compared with placebo (Aslanargun et al. 2012). One trial directly compared passionflower with oxazepam in 36 patients with generalized anxiety disorder. Both interventions were equally effective, although oxazepam had a faster onset of action. The oxazepam group experienced greater impairment in their job performance compared with the passionflower group. (Akhondzadeh et al. 2001). In a double-blind, randomized controlled trial of 162 subjects with neurosis/anxiety, passionflower was compared with mexazolam in a dose of 90 mg daily (Mori et al. 1993). Those taking passionflower were less likely to be sedated, although this finding was not statistically significant. In a Cochrane review of two trials including 198 patients, passionflower was as effective as benzodiazepines for anxiety (Miyasaka et al. 2007).

In one pre-post study of 41 patients, the consumption of passionflower tea yielded improvements in subjective sleep quality (Ngan and Conduit 2011). However, in the 10 patients who underwent polysomnography, objective measures of sleep were not altered.

11.2.5.6 Clinical Application

Preliminary studies indicate passionflower is effective for generalized anxiety disorder and as pretreatment for anxiety associated with surgery based on several small studies. Its use should be avoided women who are pregnant. In healthy, nonpregnant patients who are not on any interacting medications, passionflower would be a reasonable treatment for anxiety.

Data are insufficient to draw conclusions regarding the efficacy of passionflower in insomnia. Given its potential for adverse effects, drug interactions and lack of safety in pregnancy, passionflower should not be routinely used for the treatment of insomnia.

11.2.6 Saffron (*Crocus sativus*)

See Section 11.3.1 in Depression for discussion of use for anxiety.

11.3 Depression

Depression affects 350 million people globally and is the leading cause of disability worldwide (WHO 2016). The pathophysiology of depression is related to a complex interplay of genetics, hormones, and life experiences. It has long been purported that alterations in monoamine function in the brain cause depression. However, given the limitations of drug therapy targeting these mechanisms it seems likely the cause of depression is much more complex.

11.3.1 Saffron (*Crocus sativus*)

11.3.1.1 Background

Saffron is a perennial herb used as a spice, perfume and medicine for many years (Sarris et al. 2011a). Saffron's progenitor may be *Crocus cartwrightianus* which is native to Greece and Southwest Africa, but it has been propagated throughout much of the world. Saffron comes from the dried styles and stigma (i.e., threads) of *Crocus sativus* (Pitsikas 2016). It has been used for many ailments including stomach ache, teething pain, depression, anxiety, and insomnia.

11.3.1.2 Pharmacognosy

Saffron consists of at least 150 compounds with 40 to 50 believed to be active. Four constituents, crocins, crocetin, picrocrocin, and safranaol are believed to be pharmacologically active (Loprest and Drummond 2014, Sarris et al. 2011, 2013b,c, Pitikis et al 2016). Most of the other constituents have not been extensively studied (Sarris et al. 2013a,b,c, Pitikis et al 2016).

Saffron is an N-methyl-D-aspartate (NMDA) receptor antagonist and a GABA agonist which may account for its anxiolytic effects (Sarris et al. 2011a, 2013b,c). Crocins appear to regulate the release of corticosterone from the adrenal cortex in rats which may account for saffron's efficacy in animal models of anxiety (Pitikis et al. 2008). Flavonoids may decrease anxiety through interaction with the $GABA_A$ receptor. Other potential mechanisms underlying saffron's effects for psychiatric disorders include antioxidant and anti-inflammatory properties, and dopaminergic, noradrenergic, and serotonergic effects (Loprest and Drummond 2014). Although this last effect is less well supported in the literature, animal models demonstrate saffron has antidepressant effects (Pitsikas et al. 2008).

11.3.1.3 Dosing and Preparation

Saffron extract is prepared from the stigma and flowers of the plant. Studies have found extracts from both sources to be effective. Saffron products typically contain 30% crocins, 5%–15% picrocrocin, and 5% volatile compounds including safranal (Sarris et al. 2011a). The stigma has been used in four studies while the petals were used in two studies of depression. Outcomes were similar for products derived from either part (Loprest and Drummond 2014). Standardized (n = 3) and non-standardized extracts had similar outcomes in studies. The most commonly used dose was 15 mg twice daily.

11.3.1.4 Safety

In most studies, there was a non-significant trend towards increased adverse effects with saffron when compared to placebo (Sarris et al. 2011a, 2013b,c). Adverse effects included anxiety, tachycardia, nausea, dyspepsia, and appetite changes. In clinical trials, sedation/drowsiness, headache, dry mouth, constipation, and sexual dysfunction occurred more frequently with antidepressants while anxiety/nervousness, increased appetite, nausea, and headache occurred more frequently with saffron when compared with placebo (Loprest and Drummond 2014). In one study of safety and tolerability, doses of 400 mg of saffron were associated with decreased red blood cell counts, hemoglobin, hematocrit and platelets, and increased sodium, blood urea nitrogen, and creatinine. While blood pressure was significantly lowered, vital signs and laboratory indices remained within normal limits (Modeghegh et al. 2008).

Doses of saffron of 10 grams daily or greater can lead to serious adverse effects including kidney injury, miscarriage, and death. High doses of saffron lead to uterine contractions and saffron is considered unsafe for use in pregnancy. There is no information available on saffron drug interactions.

11.3.1.5 Evidence

Two 6-week, placebo-controlled studies of 40 patients with mild to moderate depression reported significant improvement with saffron 30–90 mg daily (Akhondzadeh et al. 2005, Moshiri et al. 2006). In a 6-week randomized, controlled trial, saffron 30 mg daily was as effective as imipramine 100 mg daily for the treatment of mild to moderate depression (Akhondzadeh et al. 2004). In two randomized, controlled trials, 15 mg twice daily of saffron was as effective as fluoxetine in patients with mild to moderate depression. In each study, both groups achieved a 25% remission rate (Noorbala et al. 2005, Akhondzadeh et al. 2007). Improvements began within one week of treatment and continued over the duration of the studies.

In a 4-week randomized, placebo-controlled trial of 40 patients with major depressive disorder, crocin 15 mg twice daily or placebo were added to ongoing selective serotonin reuptake inhibitor treatment. The crocin group had significant improvements on anxiety ratings compared with placebo (Talaei et al. 2015). However, interpretation of the results is limited by a high dropout rate. In a 12-week, placebo-controlled trial of 60 adults, 50 mg of saffron led to significant improvements in anxiety and depression (Mazidi et al. 2016).

11.3.1.6 Clinical Application

In standard doses of 30 mg daily, saffron appears to be safe and may have some benefit for mild depression and mild anxiety. Given its potential adverse effects and limited number of study participants, saffron should not be routinely used for depression, especially by pregnant women or those trying to conceive. The use of higher doses is dangerous and should be avoided due to the risk of blood dyscrasias.

11.3.2 St. John's Wort (*Hypericum perforatum*)

11.3.2.1 Background

St. John's wort is a shrubby flowering perennial herb originating from Europe, western Asia and North Africa. It has been introduced broadly throughout the world (Muszynska et al. 2015). It has been used for centuries for psychiatric disorders and is a commonly purchased botanical in the US (Linde et al. 2008, Muszynska et al. 2015).

11.3.2.2 Pharmacognosy

The buds, leaves, and flowers from the plant are used for medicinal purposes (Linde et al. 2008). More than 150 constituents have been identified, with hypericin, pseudohypericin, hyperforin and pseudohyperforin generally considered to be the pharmacologically active components (Linde et al. 2008, Muszynska et al. 2015). While St. John's wort does inhibit monoamine oxidase, this effect is minimal at normal doses and is not considered the primary source of its efficacy in depression (Lind 2009, Muszynska et al. 2015). Inhibition of the reuptake of monoamines such as dopamine, norepinephrine, and serotonin most likely accounts for antidepressant properties (Linde et al. 2008, Muszynska et al. 2015).

11.3.2.3 Dosing and Preparation

While extracts can be made by pressing the plant, most supplements are dried extracts (Lind 2009). In Europe, St. John's wort is available as a medicinal product but in other parts of the world, including the U.S. it is a dietary supplement. Doses most commonly used for depression are between 500 and 1,200 mg daily (Linde et al. 2008).

11.3.2.4 Safety

One open-label 52-week study of 440 patients with mild to moderate depression treated with 500 mg of St. John's wort demonstrated its safety when administered over a long period of time (Brattstron 2009). In the study, 217 patients reported 504 adverse effects of which 30 (6%) were thought to be related to active treatment. Gastrointestinal and skin complaints were the most commonly reported. Skin complaints consisted of rash, urticaria, discoloration, and photosensitivity. No changes in body mass index were noted over the course of the study.

In a randomized, double-blind, 52-week trial, adverse effects from a standardized extract of 900 mg daily were similar to placebo (Kasper et al. 2008). A 2008 systematic review reported St. John's wort had fewer adverse effects than standard antidepressant treatments (Linde et al. 2008). Dropout rates due to adverse effects were similar between St. John's wort and placebo. However, in the one study that systematically assessed adverse effects at baseline and changes over the course of treatment, St. John's wort had significantly more diarrhea, constipation, dry mouth, nausea, and vomiting compared with placebo (Rapaport et al. 2011). The rate of complaints with St. John's wort was similar to citalopram, although only 40% of St. John's wort patients reported them as distressing compared with 60% of citalopram. Although not reaching statistical significance, the patients receiving St. John's wort had more sleep problems than the placebo group (Rapaport et al. 2011).

Adverse events with St. John's wort were comparable to placebo and less frequent than with antidepressants in a meta-analysis of 34 trials randomized controlled trials which reported safety outcomes. The analysis reported the dropout rate and incidence of significant adverse events with St. John's wort was comparable to placebo. The authors note that the quality and heterogeneity across studies limited the assessment of rare adverse events with St. John's wort (Apaydin et al. 2016). *See Chapter 2 Pharmacokinetic and Pharmacogenomic Considerations for detailed discussion related to drug interactions.*

11.3.2.5 Evidence

A 2008 systematic review of 29 studies that included 5,489 patients reported that St. John's wort was more efficacious than placebo and equally efficacious with active comparators for mild to moderate depression. Eighteen of the trials were placebo-controlled and 17 trials used an antidepressant as an active comparator. While doses of 240 mg to 1,800 mg daily of St. John's wort were studied, most trials used 500–1,200 mg daily (Linde et al. 2008). The largest improvements were in German studies, where standardized extracts are prescribed by medical professionals. One open-label study reported that the benefits with St. John's wort were sustained for 52 weeks (Brattstron 2009). In another 8-week randomized, controlled trial for mild (n = 100) to moderate (n = 100) atypical depression, St. John's wort was not effective on the primary outcome measure of percent reduction of HAMD score. However, the absolute reduction in symptoms, as well as the results for both primary and secondary outcomes, were significant when the analysis was restricted to those with moderate depression (Mannel et al. 2010). In a 26-week continuation study of 124 patients with major depressive disorder, no significant difference for St. John's wort 900–2,500 mg or sertraline 50–100 mg were reported when compared with placebo. However, symptoms were significantly improved from baseline. The authors speculated that a large placebo response obscured the benefits of active treatment (Sarris et al. 2012). In a meta-analysis of 35 randomized controlled trials of 6,993 patients, St. John's wort was more effective than placebo and equally effective with antidepressants for mild to moderate depression. The authors note that the data supporting altered response by depression symptom severity was weak (Apaydin et al. 2016). *See Chapters 13 Dermatological Conditions and 15 Obesity and Weight Loss for further discussion.*

11.3.2.6 Clinical Application

St. John's wort in doses of 500–1,200 mg daily is a reasonable option for the treatment of depression under medical supervision. Working with a provider may increase the likelihood of positive outcomes and would allow for close monitoring of adverse effects and drug interactions. While adverse effects are fewer than with traditional antidepressants, gastrointestinal effects and sleep disturbances have been noted.

11.4 Insomnia

Insomnia is a persistent problem in falling asleep, staying asleep, or both. People with insomnia wake feeling unrefreshed which can impact their daytime functioning. There are numerous causes of insomnia and it is often a symptom of other diseases. Historically drug therapy for insomnia has focused on enhancing GABAergic effects or nonspecific sedation associated with a myriad of medications. The American College of Physicians recommends the use of cognitive behavioral therapy before drug therapy for chronic insomnia (Qaseem et al. 2016). Therefore, botanicals should be reserved for use after behavioral treatments for chronic insomnia have failed. In addition, a recent meta-analysis failed to find any evidence that botanicals are effective for insomnia (Leach and Page 2015). The use of botanicals as hypnotics for short-term or chronic insomnia is unlikely to provide significant benefits. However, reports also did not find increased adverse effects with botanicals compared with placebo.

11.4.1 Chamomile

See Section 11.2.1 in Anxiety for discussion of use for insomnia.

11.4.2 Lavender

See Section 11.2.3 in Anxiety section for discussion of use for insomnia.

11.4.3 Lemon Balm

See Section 11.2.4 in Anxiety section for discussion of use for insomnia.

11.4.4 Passionflower

See Section 11.2.5 in Anxiety section for discussion of use for insomnia.

11.4.5 Valerian (*Valeriana officinalis*)

11.4.5.1 Background

Valerian is a perennial plant originally native to Europe and Asia, but has since been widely introduced to other parts of the world. It has been used for centuries as a perfume and treatment of insomnia.

11.4.5.2 Pharmacognosy

Valepotriates and the esquiterpenoid, valerenic acid, are thought to be the primary active constituents of valerian (Sarris et al. 2011a). Extracts of valerian may modulate GABA, serve as a GABA-A receptor agonist, and a partial serotonin$_{5A}$ partial agonist (Sarris et al. 2011a).

11.4.5.3 Dosing and Preparation

Valerian extracts and teas are made from the roots and rhizomes of the plant. It is available in multiple oral dosage forms, liquid extracts, and teas. Doses used in studies ranged from 250 to 3,000 mg daily, typically standardized to 0.8% valerenic acids.

11.4.5.4 Safety

Most studies report no adverse effects with valerian including a lack of hangover effect. One study that did identify adverse effects reported an increased risk of diarrhea with valerian (Bent et al. 2006). In a systematic review and meta-analysis, patients treated with valerian did report increased adverse effects compared with placebo (Leach and Page 2015).

Seven cases of valerian-associated hepatitis have been reported. In all but one case, discontinuation of valerian led to full resolution of the symptoms. In the final case, treatment with a corticosteroid resulted in improvement (Kia et al. 2016). Data are not available on any clinically significant drug interactions with valerian (Kelber et al. 2014).

11.4.5.5 Evidence

A systematic review and meta-analysis reported valerian was effective for insomnia. However, of the 16 studies, only six reported a dichotomous outcome (i.e., improved or not improved) and could be included in the meta-analysis (Bent et al. 2006). The studies had methodological issues and evidence of publication bias was present, limiting reliability of the data. Another review reported that in well-designed trials, valerian was ineffective for the treatment of insomnia (Taibi et al. 2007). A large randomized web-based study of 400 individuals with self-reported insomnia reported valerian decreased self-reported awakenings and improvements in overall sleep, although neither were the primary outcome measure (Culpepper and Wingertzahn 2015).

11.4.5.6 Clinical Application

Data are insufficient to draw conclusions regarding the use of valerian in insomnia, although patient self-report supports the botanical as a hypnotic. Given its long history of use, relative safety and trends toward improvements in self-rated sleep quality, valerian would be a reasonable option with behavioral therapy. Valerian lacks the hangover effect seen with many prescription hypnotics making it an appealing alternative. However, traditional hypnotics have more data supporting their efficacy in the treatment of insomnia. Valerian should be avoided in people with liver disease, as there may be a small risk of hepatitis.

11.5 Attention Deficit Hyperactivity Disorder (ADHD)

Attention deficit hyperactivity disorder (ADHD) is among the most common of the neuropsychiatric disorders diagnosed in children and adolescents, with a worldwide prevalence estimated at 5.3% (Polanczyk et al. 2007). Clinical treatment guidelines recommend use of stimulants such as methylphenidate and non-stimulant medications such as atomoxetine as first-line treatment for ADHD (Wolraich et al. 2011). A survey of 117 parents or caregivers of children or adolescent patients at five community mental health centers found that 23 participants (19.6%) reported current or recent botanical use, and ADHD was the disorder most frequently reported as having benefited from the botanical therapy (Cala et al. 2003). The products considered for use in patients with ADHD may act by increasing neurotransmitter levels, specifically dopamine, serotonin, or norepinephrine, or to be directly stimulating within the brain (Shakibaei et al. 2015).

11.5.1 Ginkgo (*Ginkgo biloba*)

11.5.1.1 Background

Ginkgo biloba is a unique tree species native to Asia, the extract has been utilized for treatment of a number of different conditions including ADHD (Ahn et al. 2016). *See Chapter 10 Neurologic Conditions for more discussion.*

11.5.1.2 Pharmacognosy

The exact mechanism of action for *ginkgo biloba* is unknown. The extract of *ginkgo biloba* most often used contains terpenoids, flavonol glycosides, and proanthocyanidins (Brondino et al. 2013, Shakibaei et al. 2015). Results from animal studies suggest that *ginkgo biloba* extract inhibits platelet-activating factor and enhances nitric oxide production in vessels, with subsequent effects on both peripheral and cerebral blood flow (Heck et al. 2000, Brondino et al. 2013, Ahn et al. 2016). Additional studies suggest that *ginkgo biloba* extract can reversibly inhibit monoamine oxidase (MAO) A and B activity, and prevent the synaptosomal uptake of dopamine, serotonin, and norepinephrine, both of these actions contribute to increasing concentrations of neurotransmitters (Brondino et al. 2013). Improvement of cerebrovascular blood flow and increased activity of neurotransmitters may contribute to alleviation of ADHD symptoms such as hyperactivity (Brondino et al. 2013, Ahn et al. 2016).

11.5.1.3 Dosage and Preparation

See Chapter 10 Neurologic Conditions for discussion.

11.5.1.4 Safety

Adverse effects were reported as being mild in most cases and included abdominal pain, constipation, diarrhea, headache, insomnia, loss of appetite, and stomach ache (Niederhofer 2010, Salehi et al. 2010). *See Chapters 2 Pharmacokinetic and Pharmacogenomic Considerations and 10 Neurologic Conditions for further discussion.*

11.5.1.5 Evidence

An open-label study of six subjects ages 17–19 years with attention deficit disorder (ADD) were given *ginkgo biloba* extract 200 mg daily for 4 weeks with no other medications. Using the 60-item Wender Utah Questionnaire, the subjects had significantly fewer ADD symptoms during treatment (baseline mean 1.16 and 4-week mean of 0.84, $p < 0.013$) (Niederhofer 2010). This was a small sample size, studied over a short period of time, but an improvement in symptoms was suggested with *ginkgo biloba* extract use (Niederhofer 2010).

A larger open-label pilot trial was conducted in 20 children ages 6–13 years with ADHD who were given 240 mg of *ginkgo biloba* extract tablets daily for 3–5 weeks. Participants were evaluated on changes in parents' assessment of their children's attentiveness between the start and end of therapy using the German ADHD rating scale questionnaire. The authors reported significant improvements in parents' assessment of attentiveness ($p < 0.01$), and decreases in the total score, hyperactivity and impulsivity items ($p < 0.01$) (Ubel-von Sandersleben et al. 2014). This was also a small sample size, studied over a short period of time, and while there were trends related to improvement on other cognitive tests and imaging trials, the significance is difficult to interpret.

Two randomized, controlled trials of *ginkgo biloba* in ADHD have been conducted. In one study, 50 children ages 6–14 years with ADHD were randomized to receive either methylphenidate 20–30 mg per day or *ginkgo biloba* extract in tablet form 80–120 mg per day for 6 weeks (Salehi et al. 2010). The primary endpoint was change from baseline in ADHD Rating Scale (ADHD-RS-IV), which is an instrument that uses a four-point Likert scale to assess the 18 ADHD symptoms from the Diagnostic and Statistical Manual (DSM-IV). There was a statistically significant difference between the *ginkgo biloba* extract and methylphenidate groups at 6 weeks on both the parent rating scales for inattention ($p = 0.02$) and for hyperactive/impulsive symptoms ($p = 0.003$) (Salehi et al. 2010). Analysis of the teacher ADHD rating scales also showed improvement at 6 weeks for inattention ($p = 0.0001$) and hyperactive/impulsive symptoms ($p = 0.03$) (Salehi et al. 2010). Since this was a stronger trial methodologically it suggests use of *ginkgo biloba* extract may improve ADHD symptoms (Salehi et al. 2010).

A second randomized, double-blind, placebo-controlled trial of 66 children ages 6–12 years with ADHD was conducted in Iran (Shakibaei et al. 2015) After 2 weeks without medications, participants were all given methylphenidate 20–30 mg per day based on weight and then randomized to receive placebo or *ginkgo biloba* extract 80–120 mg per day based on weight for 6 weeks. Outcomes were measured using the ADHD RS-IV and Children's Global Assessment Scale (CGAS), which measures general functioning in ten areas, each scored from 1–10. Both groups demonstrated similar improvement in ADHD symptoms from baseline (Shakibaei et al. 2015). Clinical treatment response rate defined as a 27% or greater improvement from baseline was significantly higher with *ginkgo biloba* extract versus placebo on the parent rating scale (93.5% (*ginkgo biloba* extract) versus 58.6% (placebo), $p = 0.002$). No difference in treatment response rate was seen with the teachers' ratings (83.9% (*ginkgo biloba* extract) versus 79.3% (placebo), $p = 0.451$) (Shakibaei et al. 2015). All participants improved on their CGAS scores from baseline but no significant difference was seen between the groups (Shakibaei et al. 2015). *See Chapters 5 Cardiovascular Disease and 10 Neurologic Conditions for further discussion.*

11.5.1.6 Clinical Application

Ginkgo biloba extract appears to have modest improvement in ADHD symptoms at doses 80–240 mg, although the degree of improvement is less than that with methylphenidate. Tolerability information has not been rigorously collected, but no major adverse effects have been reported. Additional studies especially comparing *ginkgo biloba* extract to options such as atomoxetine and longer-term trials evaluating safety information are needed to determine its place in therapy.

11.5.2 Ginseng (*Panax ginseng*)

11.5.2.1 Background

Ginseng contains ginsenosides, a class of phytochemicals with antioxidant and neuroprotective effects (Ahn et al. 2016). *See Chapter 10 Neurologic Conditions for more discussion.*

11.5.2.2 Pharmacognosy

The exact mechanism of action for ginseng is unknown. Ginsenosides have been reported to increase levels of neurotransmitters dopamine and norepinephrine in animal models, these neurotransmitters are targeted by existing treatments for ADHD (Ahn et al. 2016). Ginsenosides have been shown to increase brain glucose utilization indicating more efficient metabolism, as well as increasing factors that influence nerve growth factor, suggesting a potential role long-term to promote growth in underdeveloped areas of the brain (Lyon et al. 2001).

11.5.2.3 Dosage and Preparation

See Chapter 10 Neurologic Conditions for discussion.

11.5.2.4 Safety

The adverse effects of ginseng include headache, fatigue, perspiration and taste aversion (Niederhofer 2009, Lee et al. 2011, Ko et al. 2014). In a combination trial of *ginkgo biloba* and *Panax quinquefolium*, increased ADHD symptoms and aggressiveness were reported along with sweating, headache, and tiredness (Lyon et al. 2001). This suggests that additional larger trials are necessary to establish a better picture of the safety of ginseng in these patients, both for monotherapy or in combination with other medications. *See Chapters 2 Pharmacokinetic and Pharmacogenomic Considerations and 10 Neurologic Conditions for further discussion.*

11.5.2.5 Evidence

A case report of two patients 14 years and 17 years old with ADHD previously treated with methylphenidate, were given *Panax ginseng* extract 250 mg for 4 weeks followed by placebo for 4 weeks to evaluate symptoms. The total ADHD RS IV score, inattention and hyperactive/impulsive scores all decreased (total 24 to 20; inattention 22 to 18; hyperactive/impulsive 46 to 38) during the study period. Scores during the placebo period were similar to baseline scores, with a total score of 42, inattention 20 and hyperactive/impulsive 22 (Niederhofer 2010). The continuous performance test which uses computerized scores to identify inattention or concentration difficulties found an improvement with methylphenidate but no change with the use of *Panax ginseng* (Niederhofer 2010).

In an observational study of 18 children ages 6–14 years with ADHD, participants received either Korean red ginseng 1,000 mg or placebo both administered twice daily for 8 weeks (Lee et al. 2011). Efficacy outcomes were changes in omission errors scores as measured by the computerized ADHD diagnostic system (ADS) and the Conners ADHD rating scale. The ADS measures inattentiveness, and significant decreases in the omission errors scores has been associated with restoration of impaired cognitive function in children with ADHD. Omission errors scores significantly improved in the ginseng group compared to the placebo group at 8 weeks (p < 0.023) (Lee et al. 2011). The Conners ADHD rating scale also showed significant improvement over 8 weeks (p < 0.024) (Lee et al. 2011). Korean red ginseng did demonstrate benefit in computer analyzed programs that measure inattentiveness, but with only 18 children in the study, larger trials are needed that include other clinical outcomes including academic performance.

In a randomized, double-blind, placebo-controlled trial of 72 children ages 6–15 years, with ADHD received either Korean red ginseng extract 1 gm (KRG) (n = 35) twice daily or placebo (n = 37) for 8 weeks (Ko et al. 2014). Primary outcome was an 18-item questionnaire evaluating the DSM-IV symptoms with nine questions for inattention and nine questions for hyperactivity/impulsivity. Both groups demonstrated an improvement in total and inattention scores from baseline to week eight (KRG p < 0.001; placebo p = 0.002) (Ko et al. 2014). The KRG group had a statistically significant difference on the hyperactivity score compared to placebo at week 8 (p = 0.019) (Ko et al. 2014). This trial included a larger number of children over 8 weeks and provides support that *Panax ginseng* may have some benefit for treatment of hyperactivity symptoms of ADHD.

An open-label, pilot study evaluated the use of a combination product including *Ginkgo biloba* 50 mg and *Panax quinquefolium* 200 mg. Thirty-six children between the ages of 3–17 years with ADHD were given the combination product twice daily for 4 weeks. The primary outcome was the Conners Parent Rating Scale. At week two, improvements were present on the hyperactive/impulsive, cognitive problems, and oppositional categories in more than half of the participants. These improvements persisted through week 4 with 22/34 (65%) showing improvement in hyperactivity/impulsivity, 18/34 (53%) improving on cognitive problems, and 21/34 (62%) improving in the oppositional category (Lyon et al. 2001). While this is a slightly different product than the Korean red ginseng, ginkgo and ginseng combination products appear to have some potential benefit for the treatment of ADHD. *See Chapters 5 Cardiovascular Disease, 6 Endocrine Disorders, and 10 Neurologic Conditions for further discussion in different disease states.*

11.5.2.6 Clinical Application

Data on *Panax ginseng* or *Korean red ginseng*, demonstrated modest benefits in the treatment of ADHD symptoms with doses from 250 to 1,000 mg. Although symptom improvement was inconsistent with some trials demonstrating markers of inattention improved while others demonstrated improvement in hyperactivity/impulsivity measurements. The American ginseng was only studied in combination with ginkgo; therefore, it is not clear if the benefit was due to the combination or to one of the ingredients alone. At this time, the use of American ginseng as monotherapy is not justified for the treatment of ADHD (Table 11.1).

TABLE 11.1

Hyperprolactinemia – Licorice

Hyperprolactinemia is an adverse effect reported with the use of antipsychotic medications. Symptoms of hyperprolactinemia include oligomenorrhea, amenorrhea, gynecomastia, and sexual dysfunction; which may be barriers to sustained adherence to antipsychotic therapy. Conventional treatment of hyperprolactinemia with dopamine agonists such as bromocriptine is challenging as this may impact the efficacy of the antipsychotic medication. A botanical preparation of licorice also known as peony-glycyrrhiza decoction (PGD) has been evaluated for the treatment hyperprolactinemia (defined as a serum prolactin concentration over 50 mcg/L) in 20 Chinese women who were taking risperidone and experiencing symptoms of hyperprolactinemia. This was a crossover study where participants received either PGD 45 gm per day or bromocriptine 5 mg daily for 4 weeks. This was followed by a 4-week washout period and an additional 4 weeks of the other treatment. PGD produced significant decreases in serum prolactin levels by 24% from baseline which was similar to the decrease seen with bromocriptine that ranged from 21% to 38%. A greater proportion of patients on PGD demonstrated an improvement in symptoms of hyperprolactinemia compared to bromocriptine treatment (56% PGD vs. 17% bromocriptine, p = 0.037). Participants did not show an increase in psychotic symptoms or changes in other hormone levels while on PGD therapy (Yuan et al. 2008). This is a short-term trial, but it does provide some evidence that the PGD compounds may have a role in the treatment of symptomatic hyperprolactinemia in patients on antipsychotic therapy.

11.6 Conclusion

Patients may use botanicals to treat psychiatric disorders. The evidence suggests that mild anxiety may be treated with chamomile, kava, lavender, lemon balm, and passion flower. Depression may be treated successfully with St. John's Wort or saffron and ADHD symptoms may improve with gingko or Korean red ginseng. Although the safety profiles are not complete, most appear to be well tolerated. Botanicals may have a role in the treatment of mild psychiatric disorders, and future trials comparing these options to prescription medications will help clarify their place in therapy.

REFERENCES

Ahn, J., H.S. Ahn, J.H. Cheong et al. 2016. Natural product-derived treatments for attention-deficit/hyperactivity disorder: Safety, efficacy, and therapeutic potential of combination therapy. *Neural Plast* article ID 1320423.

Akhondzadeh, S., E. Moshiri, A. Noorbala et al. 2007. Comparison of petal of crocus sativus L. and fluoxetine in the treatment of depressed outpatients: A pilot double-blind randomized trial. *Progressive Neuropsychopharmacolology and Biololigical Psychiatry* 30:439–443.

Akhondzadeh, S., H. Fallah-Pour, K. Afkham et al. 2004. Comparison of crocus sativus L. and imipramine in the treatment of mild to moderate depression: A pilot double-blind randomized trial. [ISRCTN45683816]. *BMC Complementary Alternative Medicine* 4:12.

Akhondzadeh, S., H.R. Naghavi, M. Vazirian et al. 2001. Passionflower in the treatment of generalized anxiety disorder: A pilot double-blind randomized controlled trial with oxazepam. *Journal of Clinical Pharmacology Therapy* 26(5):363–367.

Akhondzadeh, S., N. Tahmacebi-Pour, A.A. Noorbala et al. 2005. Crocus sativus L. in the treatment of mild to moderate depression a double-blind, randomized, placebo-controlled trial. *Phytotherapy Res* 19:148–151.

Amsterdam, J.D., Y. Li, I. Soeller et al. 2009. A randomized, double blind, placebo-controlled trial of oral Matricaria recutita (chamomile) extract therapy for generalized anxiety disorde *Journal of Clinical Psychopharmacolology* 29(4):378–382.

Anke, J., I. Ramzan. 2004. Pharmacokinetic and pharmacodynamic drug interactions with kava (piper methysticum forst). *Journal of Ethnopharmacolology* 93(2–3):153–160.

Apaydin, E.A., A.R. Maher, R. Shanmam et al. 2016. A systematic review of St. John's wort for major depressive disorder. *System Review* 5(1):148.

Aslanargun, P., O. Cuvas, B. Dikmen, E. Aslan, and M.U. Yuksel. 2012. Passiflora incarnate Linneaus as an anxiolytic before spinal anesthesia. *J Anesth* 2(1):39–44.

Auf'mkolk, M., J.A. Ingbar, S.M. Amir et al. 1984. Inhibition by certain plant extracts of the binding of adenylate cyclase stimulatory effect of bovine thyrotropin in human thyroid membranes. *Endocrinology* 115:527–534.

Barnes, P.K., B. Bloom, and R. Nahin. 2008. Complementary and alternative medicine use among adults and children, United States, 2007. National Health Statistics report; no. 12. National Center for Health Statistics, MD, USA.

Baxter, A.J., K.M. Scott, T. Vos, and H.A. Whiteford. 2013. Global prevalence of anxiety disorders: A systematic review and meta-regression. *Psychological Medicine* 43(5):897–910.

Bent. S., A. Padula, D. Moore, M. Patterson, and W. Mehling. 2006. Valerian for sleep: A systematic review and meta-analysis. *American Journal of Medicine* 119(12):1005–1012.

Bradley, B.F., S.L. Brown, S. Chu, and R.W. Lea. 2009. Effects of orally administered lavender essential oil on response to anxiety-provoking film clips. *Human Psychopharmacology* 24(4):319–330.

Brattstron, A. 2009. Long-term effects of St. John's wort (hypericum perforatum) treatment: A 1-year safety study in mild to moderate depression. *Phytomedicine* 16(4):277–283.

Brondino, N., A. De Silvestri, S. Re et al. 2013. A systematic review and meta-analysis of ginkgo biloba in neuropsychiatric disorders: From ancient tradition to modern-day medicine. *Evidence-Based Complementary and Alternative Medicine* 2013:1–11.

Cala, S., M.L. Crismon, J. Baumgartner. 2003. A survey of herbal use in children with attention-deficit-hyperactivity disorder or depression. *Pharmacotherapy* 23(2):222–230.

Cases, J., A. Ibarra, N. Feuillere et al. 2011. Pilot trial of Melissa officinalis L. leaf extract in the treatment of volunteers suffering from mild-to-moderate anxiety disorders and sleep disturbances. *Medical Journal of Nutrition Metabolism* 4(3):211–218.

Chan, E., L.A. Rappaport, K.L. Kemper. 2003. Complementary and alternative therapies in childhood attention deficit and hyperactivity disorder. *J Dev Behav Pediatr* 24:4–8.

Chung, M.J., S.Y. Cho, M.J. Bhuiyan, L.H. Kim, S.J. Lee. 2010. Anti-diabetic effects of lemon balm (Melissa officinalis) essential oil on glucose- and lipid-regulating enzymes in type 2 diabetic mice. *British Journal of Nutrition* 104(2):180–188.

Culpepper, L., M.A. Wingertzahn. 2015. Over-the-counter agents for the treatment of occasional disturbed sleep or transient insomnia: A systematic review of the efficacy and safety. *Prim Care Companion CNS Disord* 17(6):10.4088.

De Smet PA. 2002. Herbal remidies *N Engl J Med* 19;347(25):2045–2056.

European Medicines Agency Science Medicines Health. Committee on herbal medicines products. Assessment report on Melissa officinalis L., folium. EMA/HMPC/196746/2012. May 2013. Accessed 7/21/2016 at http://www.ema.europa.eu/docs/en_GB/document_library/Herbal_-_HMPC_assessment_report/2013/08/WC500147187.pdf

Grappe, F., G. Nance, L. Coward, G. Gorman. 2014. In vitro inhibitory effects of herbal supplements on tamoxifen and irinotecan metabolism. *Drug Metabol Drug Interact* 29(4):269–279.

Heck, A.M., B.A. DeWitt, A.L. Lukes. 2000. Potential interactions between alternative therapies and warfarin. *Am J Health Syst Pharm* 57(13):1221–1227.

Izzo, A.A., E. Ernst. 2009. Interactions between herbal medicines and prescribed drugs: An updated systematic review. *Drugs* 69(13):1777–1798.

Karaman, T., S. Karaman, S. Dogru et al. 2016. Evaluating the efficacy of lavender aromatherapy on peripheral venous cannulation pain and anxiety: A prospective, randomized study. *Complement Ther Pract* 23:64–68.

Kasper, S. 2013. An orally administered lavandula oil preparation for anxiety disorder and related conditions: An evidence based review. *International J of Psychiatry in Clinical Practice* 17:15–22.

Kasper, S., H.P. Volz, H.J. Moller, A. Dienel, M. Kieser. 2008. Continuation and long-term maintenance treatment with Hypericum extract WS 5570 after recovery from an acute episode of moderate depression – a double-blind, randomized, placebo controlled long-term trial. *Eur Neuropsychopharmacol* 18(11):803–813.

Kasper, S., M. Gastpar, W.E. Muller et al. 2014. Lavender oil preparation Silexan is effective in generalized anxiety disorder – a randomized, double-blind comparison to placebo and paroxetine. *Int J Neuropsychopharmacol* 17(6):859–869.

Kelber, O., K. Nieber, K. Kraft. 2014. Valerian: No evidence for clinically relevant interactions. *Evid Based Complement Alternat Med* article ID 879396.

Kennedy, D.O., A.B. Scholey, N.T.J. Tildesley et al. 2002. Modulation of mood and cognitive performance following acute administration of Melissa officinalis (lemon balm). *Pharmacol Biochem Behav* 72(4):953–964.

Kennedy, D.O., W. Little, A.B. Scholey. 2004. Attenuation of laboratory induced stress in humans after acute administration of Melissa officinalis (lemon balm). *Psychosom Med* 72(4):953–964.

Kessler, R.C., E.J. Bromel. 2013. The epidemiology of depression across cultures. *Annu Rev Public Health* 34:119–138.

Kessler, R.C., J. Soukup, R.B. Davis et al. 2001. The use of complementary and alternative therapies to treat anxiety and depression in the United States. *Am J Psychiatry* 158(2):289–294.

Kessler, R.C., K.A. McGonagle, S. Zhao et al. 1994. Lifetime and 12 month prevalence of DSM III-R psychiatric disorders in the United States. *Arch Gen Psychiatry* 51:8–19.

Kia, Y.H., S. Alexander, D. Dowling, R. Standish. 2016. A case of steroid-responsive valerian-associated hepatitis. *Intern Med J* 46(1):118–119.

Klanpour, M., A. Mansouri, T. Mehrabi, G. Asghari. 2016. Effects of lavender scent inhalation on prevention of stress, anxiety and depression in the post partum period. *Iran J Nur Midwifery Res* 21(2):197–201.

Knaudt, P.R., K.M. Connor, R.H. Weisler, L.E. Churchill, J.R. Davidson. 1999. Alternative therapy use by psychiatric outpatients. *J Ner Ment Dis* 187:7692–7695.

Ko, H.J., I. Kim, J.B. Kim et al. 2014. Effects of Korean red ginseng extract on behavior in children with symptoms of inattention and hyperactivity/impulsivity: A double-blind randomized placebo-controlled trial. *J Child Adolesc Psychopharmacol* 24(9):501–508.

Kristsidima, M., T. Newton, K. Asimakopoulu. 2010. The effects of lavender scent on dental patient anxiety levels: A cluster randomized-controlled trial. *Community Dent Oral Epidemiol* 38(1):83–87.

Kutcha, K., M. Schmidt, A. Nahrstedt. 2015. German Kava ban lifted by court: The alleged hepatotoxicity of Kava (Piper methysticum) as a case of ill-defined herbal drug identity, lacking quality control, and misguided regulatory politics. *Planta Med* 18:1647–1653.

Leach, M.J., A.T. Page. 2015. Herbal medicines for insomnia: A systematic review and meta-analysis. *Sleep Med Rev* 24:1–12.

Lee, S.H., W.S. Park, M.H. Lim. 2011. Clinical effects of Korean red ginseng on attention deficit hyperactivity disorder in children: An observational study. *J Ginseng Res* 35(2):226–234.

Lehrner, J., G. Marwinski, S. Leh, P. Johren, L. Deecke. 2015. Ambient odors of orange and lavender reduce anxiety and improve mood in a dental office. *Physiology Behavior* 86(1–2):92–95.

Lewith, G.T., A.D. Godfrey, P. Prescott. 2005. A single-blind, randomized pilot study evaluating the aroma of Lavandula augustifolia as a treatment for mild insomnia. *J Altern Complement Med* 11(4):631–637.

Lind, K. 2009. St. John's wort – an overview. *Frosch Komplementmed* 26:146–155.

Linde, K., M.M. Berner, L. Kriston. 2008. St. John's wort for major depression (review). *Cochrane Database of Systematic Reviews* 4:Art No. CD000448.

Loprest, A.L., P.D. Drummond. 2014. Saffron (crocus sativus) for depression: A systematic review of clinical studies and examination of underlying antidepressant mechanisms of action. *Hum Psychopharmacol* 29:517–527.

Lyon, M.R., J.C. Cline, J.T. De Zepetnek et al. 2001. Effect of the herbal extract combination panax quinquefolium and ginkgo biloba on attention-deficit hyperactivity disorder: A pilot study. *J Psychiatry Neurosci* 26(3):221–228.

Mannel, M., U. Kuhn, U. Schmidt, M. Plich, H. Murck. 2010. St. John's wort extract LI160 for the treatment of depression with atypical features – a double-blind, randomized, and placebo-controlled trial. *J Psychiatr Res* 44(12):760–767.

Mazidi, M., M. Shemshian, S.H. Mousavi et al. 2016. A double-blind, randomized and placebo-controlled trial of saffron (crocus sativus L.) in the treatment of anxiety and depression. *J Comlement Integr Med* 13(2):195–199.

McCaffrey, R., D.J. Thomas, A.O. Kinzelman. 2009. The effects of lavender and rosemary essential oils on test-taking anxiety among graduate nursing students. *Holist Nurs Pract* 23(2):88–93.

Meseguer, E., R. Taboada, V. Sanchez et al. 2002. Life-threatening parkinsonism induced by kava-kava. *Mov Disorder* 17(1):195–196.

Miroddi, M., G. Calapai, M. Navarra, P.L. Mincuillo, S. Gangemi. 2013. Passiflora incarnate L.: Ethnopharmacology, clinical application, safety and evaluation of clinical trials. *J Ethnopharmacol* 150(3):791–804.

Miyasaka, L.S., A.N. Atallah, B.G.O. Soares. 2007. Passiflora for anxiety disorders. *Cochrane Database Systematic Review* (1) Article ID CD004518-2007. doi: 10.1002/14651858.CD004518.pub2.

Modeghegh, M.H., M. Shahabian, H.A. Esmaeli, O. Rajbai, H. Hosseinzadeh. 2008. Safety evaluation of saffron (Crocus sativus) tablets in healthy volunteers. *Phytomedicine* 15(12):1031–1037.

Mori, A., K. Hasegawa, M. Murasaki et al. 1993. Clinical evaluation of passiflamin (passiflora extract) on neurosis – multicentered double blind study in comparison with mexazolam. *Clinical Evaluation* 21:383–440.

Moshiri, E., A.A. Basti, A.A. Noorbala et al. 2006. Crocus sativus L. (petal) in the treatment of mild to moderate depression: A double-blind, randomized and placebo-controlled trial. *Phytomedicine* 13(9–10):607–611.

Movafegh, A., R. Alizadeh, F. Hajimohamadi, F. Esfehani, M. Nejatfar. 2008. Preoperative oral passiflora incarnate reduces anxiety in ambulatory surgery patients: A double-blind, placebo-controlled study. *Anesth Analg* 106(6):1728–1732.

Muszynska, B., M. Lojewski, J. Rojowski, W. Opoka, K. Sulkowaska-Ziaja. 2015. Natural products of relevance in the prevention and supportive treatment of depression. *Psychiatr Pol* 49(3):435–453.

Niederhofer, H. 2009. Panax ginseng may improve some symptoms of attention-deficit hyperactivity disorder. *J Diet Suppl* 6(1):22–27.

Niederhofer, H. 2010. Ginkgo biloba treating patients with attention-deficit disorder. *Phytotherapy Research* 24:26–27.

Ngan, A., R. Conduit. 2011. A double-blind, placebo-controlled investigation of the effects of Passiflora incarnata (passionflower) herbal tea on subjective sleep quality. *Phytother Res* 25(8):1153–1159.

Noorbala, A.A., S. Akhondzadeh, N. Tahmacebi-Pour, A.H. Jamshidi. 2005. Hydro-alcoholic extract of rocus sativus L. versus fluoxetine in the treatment of mild to moderate depression: A double-blind randomized pilot trial. *J Ethnopharmacol* 97:281–281.

Norton, S.A., P. Ruze. 1994. Kava dermopathy. *J American Academy Dermatology* 31(1):89–97.

Pitsikas, N. 2016. Constituents of saffron (crocus Sativus L.) as a potential candidate for the treatment of anxiety disorders and schizophrenia. *Molecules* 21:303–314.

Pitsikas, N., A. Boultadakis, F. Georgiadou, P.A. Tarantilis, N. Sakellaridis. 2008. Effects of the active constituents of Crocus sativus L., crocins, in an animal model of anxiety. *Phytomedicine* 15(12): 1135–1139.

Pittler, M.H., E. Ernst. 2010. Kava extract versus placebo for treating anxiety. *Cochrane Database of Systematic Reviews [Serial Online]* May 10, 2010:6. Article No.: CD003383. doi: 10.1002/14651858.CD003383

Polanczyk, G., M. Silva de Lima, B.L. Horta, J. Biederman, L.A. Rohde. 2007. The worldwide prevalence of ADHD: A systematic review and metaregression analysis. *Am J Psychiatry* 104(6):942–948.

Qaseem, A., D. Kansagara, M.A. Forciea et al. 2016. Management of chronic insomnia disorder in adults: A clinical practice guideline from the American College of Physicians. *Ann Intern Med* 165:125–133.

Rapaport, M.H., A.A. Nierenberg, R. Howland, C. Dording, P.J. Schettler, D. Mischoulon. 2011. The treatment of minor depression with St. John's wort or Citalopram: Failure to show benefit over placebo. *J Psychiatr Res* 45(7):931–941.

Roth, T. 2007. Insomnia: Definition, prevalence, etiology and consequences. *J Clin Sleep Med* 3(Suppl 5):s7–s10.

Salehi, B., R. Imani, M.R. Mohammadi et al. 2010. Ginkgo biloba for attention-deficit/hyperactivity disorder in children and adolescents: A double blind, randomized controlled trial. *Progress in Neuro-Psychopharmacology & Biol Psychiatry* 34:76–80.

Santini, F., P. Vitti, G. Ceccarini et al. 2003. In vitro assay of thyroid disruptors affecting TSH-stimulating adenylate cyclase activity. *Endocrinology* 26:950–955.

Sarris, J., A. Panossian, I. Schweitzer, C. Stough, A. Scholey. 2011a. Herbal medicine for depression, anxiety and insomnia: A review of psychopharmacology and clinical evidence. *European Neuropsychopharmacol* 21:841–860.

Sarris, J., C.A. Bousman, Z.T. Wahid et al. 2013a. Kava in the treatment of generalized anxiety disorder. A double blind, randomized, placebo-controlled trial. *J Clin Psychopharmacol* 33:643–648.

Sarris, J., E. McIntyre, D.A. Camfield. 2013b. Plant-based medicines for anxiety disorders, part 2: A review of clinical studies with supporting preclinical evidence. *CNS Drugs* 27:301–319.

Sarris, J., E. McIntyre, D.A. Camfield. 2013c. Plant-based medicines for anxiety disorders, part 1: A review of preclinical studies. *CNS Drugs* 27:207–219.

Sarris, J., M. Fava, I. Schweitzer, D. Mischoulon. 2012. St. John's wort (hypericum perforatum) versus sertraline and placebo in major depressive disorder: Continuation data from a 26-week RCT. *Pharmacopsychiatry* 45(7):275–278.

Sarris, J., R. Teschke, C. Stough et al. 2011b. Re-introduction of kava (piper methysticum) to the EU: Is there a way forward? *Planta Med* 77(2):107–110.

Schmidt, M. 2014. German court ruling reverses kava ban; German regulatory authority appeals decisions. *HerbalEGram* 11(7). Accessed 7/20/2016 at: http://cms.herbalgram.org/heg/volume11/07July/GermanKavaBanReversal.html?ts=1469198341&signature=d13fe3958c81ef0bb101177196fd4e91

Seifi, Z., A. Beikmoradi, K. Oshvandi, J. Poorolajal, M. Araghchian, R. Safiaryan. 2014. The effect of lavender essential oil on anxiety level in patients undergoing coronary artery bypass graft surgery: A double-blind randomized clinical trial. *Iran J Nurs Midwifery Res* 19(6):574–580.

Shahnazi, M., R. Nikjoo, P. Yavarika, S. Mohammad-Alizadeh-Charandabi. 2012. Inhaled lavender effect on anxiety and pain caused from intrauterine device insertion. *J Caring Sci* 1(4):255–261.

Shakeri, A., A. Sahebkar, B. Javadi. 2016. Melissa officinalis L. – A review of traditional uses, phytochemistry and pharmacology. *J Ethnopharmacol* 188:204–228.

Shakibaei, F., M. Radmanesh, B. Salari Em Mahaki. 2015. Ginkgo biloba in the treatment of attention-deficit/hyperactivity disorder in children and adolescents. A randomized, placebo-controlled, trial. *Complementary Therapies in Clinical Practice* 21:61–67.

Sinha, D., D. Efron. 2005. Complementary and alternative medicine use in children with attention deficit hyperactivity disorder. *J Pediatr Child Health* 41:23–26.

Taibi, D.M., C.A. Landis, H. Petry, M.V. Vitiello. 2007. A systematic review of valerian as a sleep aid: Safe bit note effective. *Sleep Med Rev* 11:209–230.

Talaei, A., M. Hassanpour Moghadam, S.A. Sajadi Tabassi, S.A. Mohajeri. 2015. Crocin, the main active saffron constituent, as an adjunctive treatment in major depressive disorder: A randomized, double-blind, placebo-controlled, pilot clinical trial. *J Affect Disord* 174:51–56.

Teschke, R., J. Sarris, I. Schweitzer. 2012. Kava hepatoxicity in traditional and modern use: The presumed Pacific kava paradox hypothesis revisted. *J Clin Pharmacol* 73(2):170–174.

Teschke, R., J. Sarris, X. Glass et al. 2011. Kava, the anxiolytic herb: Back to basics to prevent liver injury? *Br J Clin Pharm* 71(3):445–448.

Tindle, H.A., R.B. Davis, R.S. Phillips, D.M. Eisenberg. 2005. Trends in the use of complementary and alternative medicine by US adults, 1997-2002. *Altern Ther Health Med* 11:42–49.

Ubel-von Sandersleben, H., A. Rothenberger, B. Albrecht, L.G. Rothenberger, S. Klement, N. Bock. 2014. Ginkgo biloba extract EGb 761 in children with ADHD preliminary findings in an open multilevel dose finding study. *Zeitschrift fur Kinder- und Jugendpsychiatri und Psychotherapie* 42:337–347.

Wittchen, H.U., F. Jacobi, J. Rehm et al. 2011. The size and burden of mental disorders and other disorders of the brain in Europe 2010. *Eur Neuropsychopharmacol* 21(9):655–679.

Wolraich, M., L. Brown, R.T. Brown et al. 2011. ADHD: Clinical practice guideline for diagnosis, evaluation, and treatment of attention-deficit/hyperactivity disorder in children and adolescents. *Pediatrics* 128(5):1007–1022.

Woelk, H., S. Schlafke. 2010. A multi-center, double-blind, randomized study of lavender oil preparation Silexan in comparison to lorazepam for generalized anxiety disorder. *Phytomedicine* 17(2):94–99.

Wong, A.H., A.H. Smith, H.S. Boon. 1998. Herbal remedies in psychiatric practice. *Arch Gen Psychiatry* 55:1032–1044.

World Health Organization. Depression fact sheet, April 2016. Accessed 8/2/2016 at: http://www.who.int/mediacentre/factsheets/fs369/en/

Yager, J., S.L. Siegfreid, T.L. DiMatteo. 1999. Use of alternative remedies by psychiatric patients: Illustrative vignettes and a discussion of the issues. *Am J Psychiatry* 156:1432–1438.

Yuan, H.N., C.Y. Wang, C.W. Sze et al. 2008. A randomized, crossover comparison of herbal medicine and bromocriptine against riperidone-induced hyperprolactinemia in patients with schizophrenia. *J Clin Psychopharm* 28(3):264–270.

Zabirunnisa, M., J. Gadagi, P. Gadde, N. Myla, J. Koneru, C. Thatimatla. 2014. Dental patient anxiety: Possible deal with lavender fragrance. *J Res Pharm Pract* 3(3):100–103.

Zick, S.M., B.D. Wright, A. Sen, J.T. Arnedt. 2011. Preliminary examination of the efficacy and safety of a standardized chamomile extract for chronic primary insomnia: A randomized placebo-controlled pilot study. *BMC Complement Altern Med* 22(11):78.

12

Botanicals for Common Infections

Thamer Almangour, Gary N. Asher, and Amanda Corbett

CONTENTS

12.1 Introduction

The discovery of penicillin by Alexander Fleming was one of the greatest inventions of the 20th century, after which, several antimicrobial agents were discovered and saved millions of lives from infection-related deaths. However, accelerated antimicrobial resistance, which is immerging globally, in conjunction with the decline in the number of newly developed antibiotics, has become a major public health threat. In 2013, the Centers for Disease Control and Prevention (CDC) reported that resistant bacteria infects 2 million people annually in the United States and results in 23,000 deaths (CDC 2013). In February of 2017, the World Health Organization (WHO) declared its first list of antibiotic-resistant priority pathogens to guide and promote research and development of new antimicrobials (WHO 2017b).

In addition to the antimicrobial resistance threat, the cost burden due to increased antimicrobial use and antimicrobial adverse reactions are major concerns. One example includes *Clostridium difficile* infections secondary to antimicrobial use, which caused half a million infections among patients in the United States in a single year according to a recent CDC study, with an estimated 15,000 deaths (CDC 2015). These concerns highlight the importance of having alternative and effective strategies to treat and prevent microbial infections. Botanicals can serve as options to treat such infections. For example, an extract of the plant *Berberis lyceum* demonstrated antimicrobial activity against multiple microorganisms, as well as, the inability for *E. coli* to develop resistance following continuous exposure to the *Berberis lyceum* methanolic extract (Malik et al. 2017). This information, considering the recent increase in multidrug-resistant strains of *E. coli* and other pathogens, shows promise for botanicals serving as antimicrobials. Some examples are described in the following chapter.

12.2 Urinary Tract Infections

Urinary tract infection (UTI) is one of the most commonly acquired bacterial infections. An estimated 60% of women age 18 and over will have at least one episode of lower UTI at some point in their lives (Foxman et al. 2015). In a prospective study of nearly 180 women age 17–82 years with an initial diagnosis of lower UTI, 44% experienced at least one recurrent episode of UTI over 12 months necessitating additional antibiotic treatment courses (Ikaheimo et al. 1996). In a U.S. national survey from 1997, UTIs led to an estimated 7 million health provider office visits plus 1 million emergency department visits and 100,000 hospitalizations (Schappert 1999).

12.2.1 Cranberry

12.2.1.1 Background

Cranberry is an evergreen shrub that is a member of the Ericaceae family. Two species are commonly found, *Vaccinium macrocarpon*, the North American cranberry and *V. oxycoccos*, the European cranberry. The North American cranberry was used for medicinal purposes by Native Americans and has the most clinical data on prevention and treatment of UTIs. In 1914, Blatherwick first reported that individuals ingesting cranberry had acidic urine, which was secondary to the presence of benzoic acid. It was believed for several years that cranberry exerts its beneficial effect through urinary acidification (Blatherwick 1914). The applicable part of the plant is the fruit.

12.2.1.2 Pharmacognosy

Escherichia coli is the most common pathogen causing UTIs. *E. coli* has a cell protein structure called fimbriae, which are responsible for bacterial adhesion to the carbohydrates or lipid components of the host urothelium. Several theories have been proposed on the mechanism of cranberry on prevention of UTIs. The most supported theories are that cranberry inhibits uropathogen (specifically *E. coli*) P-fimbriae binding to mannose-like residues on mucosal cells via mannose-specific, lectin-like structures and that cranberry inhibits binding of *E. coli* type I pili to bladder epithelial cells. Data is insufficient to show acidification of the urine via cranberry ingestion prevents UTIs (Guay 2009). The proanthocyanidins (PACs) in cranberry inhibit the adhesion of both antibiotic susceptible and resistant *E. coli* (Guay 2009, Howell 2007).

12.2.1.3 Dosing and Preparation

Dosing, strength, formulations, frequency, and duration vary widely across different trials. Cranberry juice, tablets, capsules, and syrup have been used in clinical trials (Jepson and Craig 2007). Most trials do not fully describe any standardization of the studied product such as amount of proanthocyanidins. In women ages 18–40 years for prevention of recurrent UTIs, 250–500 mg twice daily of 1.5% proanthocyanidin standardized whole cranberry powder was used (Sengupta et al. 2011). Many studies have used cranberry juice for prevention of recurrent UTIs in otherwise healthy women, pregnant women, elderly women, and children. For the few studies in adults that did provide specific information used doses of 240 mL juice twice daily with an average of 112 mg of proanthocyanidin per 240 mL and 240 mL juice three times daily with an average of 80 mg of proanthocyanidin per 240 mL (Barbosa-Cesnik et al. 2011, Wing et al. 2008).

12.2.1.4 Safety

Cranberry capsules or tablets are generally well tolerated. In trials using cranberry juice, the dropout rate is often high due to the taste of the juice (Jepson et al. 2012). Other adverse effects are generally similar between the active cranberry arm and placebo or control arm. Most adverse effects were gastrointestinal in nature such as nausea, vomiting, diarrhea, and gastroenteritis (Jepson et al. 2012). Cranberry may increase the risk of urinary calcium oxalate and uric acid stone formation (Gettman et al. 2005). Caution should be taken with sugar-sweetened cranberry juice cocktail in patients with diabetes.

Cranberry does not appear to inhibit or induce drug-metabolizing enzymes CYP1A2, CYP2C9, and CYP3A4 and therefore, interactions with medications metabolized by these enzymes are unlikely (Lilja et al. 2007). In addition, ingestion of 240 mL twice daily of cranberry juice for 7 days did not affect the prothrombin time in subjects taking warfarin (Mellen et al. 2010).

12.2.1.5 Evidence

Many clinical studies have evaluated the effects of cranberry for the prevention of recurrent UTI. A 2012 Cochrane review evaluated 24 studies using cranberry juice/concentration, tablets, or capsules compared to placebo or active comparators such as methenamine hippurate, antibiotics, or lactobacillus (Jepson et al. 2012). Overall, cranberry did not reduce the occurrence of symptomatic UTI (RR 0.86, 95% CI 0.71 to 1.04). This review included studies in pregnant and nonpregnant women, older individuals, cancer patients, children, and individuals with neuropathic bladder or spinal injury. Of note, UTI recurrence did not differ in trials comparing cranberry to antibiotics (RR 1.31, 95% CI 0.85 to 2.02) (Jepson et al. 2012). This is promising as use of antibiotics may be reduced in these populations.

Two studies are specifically worth noting. One trial of 60 women with a history of recurrent UTI and a culture positive, mildly symptomatic UTI, used a 1.5% standardized proanthocyanidin product dosed as 250 mg encapsulated powder twice daily (low dose) or 500 mg encapsulated powder twice daily (high dose) compared to placebo (Sengupta et al. 2011). After 90 days, there was no difference in the presence of *E. coli* in the urine in the placebo group compared to baseline (p = 0.72). A significant *E. coli* reduction occurred in both the low dose (p < 0.01) and high dose groups (p < 0.0001). In addition, symptomatic relief was present in both cranberry groups, but not in the control arm. A second trial evaluated 319 college women with an acute UTI who were randomized to 27% cranberry juice standardized to an average of 112 mg of proanthocyanidin per 240 mL of juice given twice daily for 6 months or placebo juice (Barbosa-Cesnik et al. 2011). They were followed for the recurrence of a second UTI. Based on an intent to treat analysis, the recurrence rate was similar between the cranberry group (19.3%) and placebo (14.6%) (p = 0.21).

A recent meta-analysis of nonpregnant, otherwise healthy, women found a 26% reduction in risk of UTI recurrence in those taking cranberry vs those not (RR 0.74, 95% CI 0.55 to 0.98, $I^2 = 54\%$) (Fu et al. 2017). Seven RCTs were included in this analysis with four of those being published after the Jepson, 2012 analysis. Both cranberry juice, tablets, and encapsulated powders were used. Six of the trials included a placebo arm.

12.2.1.6 Clinical Application

Cranberry juice, tablets, and encapsulated powders have been studied in diverse populations. Overall, it may be reasonable to use cranberry products for the prevention of recurrent UTI. Trials of healthy women have the strongest data, and importantly, used products that standardize the proanthocyanidin content. Use of cranberry in lieu of antibiotics for UTI prevention may be advantageous in that antibiotic use will be decreased and the risk of antibiotic resistance may be lessened.

12.2.2 Uva Ursi

12.2.2.1 Background

Uva ursi, *Arctostaphylos uva-ursi*, also known as bearberry, is an evergreen shrub that has been used in Europe for treating UTI since the thirteenth century. The glycoside, arbutin, is the main active constituent and accounts for 4%–12% of the dried leaves (EMA 2012, ESCOP 2012, WHO 2004). However, the whole extract of bearberry leaves is responsible for its pharmacological action (EMA 2012, ESCOP 2012, WHO 2004).

12.2.2.2 Pharmacognosy

In vitro, aqueous extract of bearberry enhances the cell surface hydrophobicity of gram-negative bacteria including *E. coli and Acinetobacter baumannii*, although the extract does not demonstrate bactericidal activity. This suggests that bearberry affects the cell surface of microbes by increasing aggregation of microorganisms enhancing bacterial excretion from the urinary tract rather than disrupting bacterial cell membranes causing bacterial death (Turi et al. 1997). Arbutin is a hydroquinone glycoside that is absorbed in the small intestine, deglycosylated in the liver, and immediately metabolized to glucuronide and sulfate conjugates (de Arriba et al. 2013, Schindler et al. 2002). Arbutin is renally eliminated primarily in the form of hydroquinone conjugates with only small proportion as free hydroquinone. (de Arriba et al. 2013, Schindler et al. 2002, Siegers et al. 2003).

12.2.2.3 Dosing and Preparation

The recommended daily dose is 3 g of dried leaf to 150 mL water as an infusion or cold maceration up to four times a day or 400–840 mg hydroquinone derivatives calculated as water-free arbutin (Blumenthal and Busse 2016).

12.2.2.4 Safety

Clinical evidence to evaluate the safety of uva ursi is limited. UVA-E™ (Medic Herb AB, Goteborg, Sweden), which contains bearberry leaves extract with a standardized content of arbutin and methylarbutin, plus the hydroalcoholic extract of dandelion root (*Taraxacum officinale),* when given as three tablets three times daily was well tolerated when used for up to one month (Larsson et al. 1993). Due to the known carcinogenicity and mutagenicity of hydroquinone, as well as the lack of long-term safety data, the use of uva ursi should be limited to no longer than one month. In a case report, a 56-year old woman who complained of decreased visual acuity was found to have bull's-eye maculopathy, diffused retinal thinning, and paracentral scotomas, which were suspected to be due to the ingestion of uva ursi prepared as tea for 3 years to prevent recurrent UTIs. This adverse effect was proposed to be due to the ability of hydroquinone to inhibit tyrosine kinase and consequently melanin synthesis in retinal epithelium and choroidal layers (Wang and Del Priore 2004).

Drug interactions have not been fully evaluated with uva ursi; therefore, caution should be used when combined with prescription and nonprescription medications. Theoretically, interactions may occur with lithium based on uva ursi's potential diuretic properties. In addition, as uva ursi seems to be most effective in alkaline urine, substances that acidify the urine may reduce its effectiveness.

12.2.2.5 Evidence

The clinical evidence supporting the use of uva ursi is limited. In a prospective, randomized, double-blind, placebo-controlled trial, 57 women ages 32–63 years who had three or more UTIs during the preceding year and at least one episode in the past 6 months, were randomly assigned to receive either UVA-E™ (Medic Herb AB, Goteborg, Sweden) (n = 30) or placebo (n = 27) three tablets three times daily for 1 month. All participants were followed for up to one year. At the end of the study, the rate of recurrent UTIs in the uva ursi/dandelion group was lower compared to placebo, with none of the patients who received uva ursi/dandelion experiencing a recurrent UTI compared to five (23%) patients in placebo group (p < 0.05) (Larsson et al. 1993). A randomized controlled factorial design trial in adult women with suspected UTIs is currently comparing ibuprofen, uva-ursi, a combination of both, or placebo to relieve urinary symptoms and reduce antibiotic use (ATAFUTI trial) (Trill et al. 2017).

12.2.2.6 Clinical Application

Based on the limited data on efficacy and drug interactions, uva ursi is not recommended as a first line therapy for UTI. However, there may be a role for use in individuals with uncomplicated UTIs who want to avoid antimicrobial drugs. The results of the ATAFUTI trial may provide additional information on the use of uva ursi in symptom relief and delay of antibiotics in treatment of UTI.

12.3 Influenza

Each year, approximately 3–5 million people worldwide become severely ill due to influenza, and up to a half-million influenza-associated deaths occur according to the WHO (WHO 2016). Although prevention through vaccination is the most effective approach to reduce influenza-related morbidty and mortality, antivirals such as neuraminidase inhibitors, for example, are a mainstay when antimicrobial treatment is indicated (WHO 2016, Ghebrehewet et al. 2016). However, a recent meta-analysis has questioned the risk to benefit of these drugs (Jefferson et al. 2014). One botanical, elderberry, has been shown to be effective in the treatment of influenza.

12.3.1 Elderberry

12.3.1.1 Background

Elderberry, *Sambucus nigra*, also known as black elder, was used in German medicine to treat upper respiratory tract infections, back pain, neuropathic pain, headache, constipation, and was also used as a diuretic (Vlachojannis et al. 2010). The applicable plant part for medicinal use is the ripened fruit.

12.3.1.2 Pharmacognosy

Elderberries contain anthocyanins which are thought to be responsible for its biological activities with the primary ones being cyanidin-3-glucoside and cyanidin-3-sambubioside. (Zakay-Rones et al. 2004, Wu et al. 2002). Sambucol® (SAM), a trade formulation of elderberry contains a high amount of three flavonoids that have shown antiviral activity against herpes virus, respiratory syncytial virus, parainfluenza, and influenza (Amoros et al. 1992, Mahmood et al. 1993, Nagai et al. 1990, Zakay-Rones et al. 1995). Elderberry can inhibit the viral cell surface protein, hemagglutinin, inhibiting the adhesion of the virus to the host cell and consequently viral replication. For its immunostimulatory effect, elderberry stimulates the production of inflammatory cytokines such as interleukins and tumor necrosis factor (Barak et al. 2001, Zakay-Rones et al. 2004).

12.3.1.3 Dosing and Preparation

Sambucol® (SAM) is dosed as 15 ml of the syrup formulation containing 38% of the standardized elderberry extract plus small amounts of raspberry extract, glucose, citric acid and honey given four times daily for 5 days to start within 48 hours of onset of symptoms has been used for treatment of influenza (Zakay-Rones et al. 2004). In addition, 175 mg elderberry extract formulated as a slow-dissolve lozenge for 2 days to start within 24 hours of onset symptoms has also been used (Kong 2009).

12.3.1.4 Safety

Elderberry fruit extract is generally safe when used orally in the amounts and duration that were tested in clinical studies. In the well-designed clinical trials described below, no adverse effects were reported for the use of elderberry (Kong 2009, Zakay-Rones et al. 1995, 2004). Plant parts other than ripe fruit should be avoided; seeds, bark, leaves, flowers, and unripened fruit of elderberries contain cyanide, which may cause nausea, vomiting, and severe diarrhea (Sambucus nigra, 2014).

In terms of drug interactions, elderberry stimulates immune function by enhancing the production of the inflammatory cytokines (Barak et al. 2001). Therefore, a theoretical concern exists that elderberry may interfere with immunosuppressants such as corticosteroids, calcineurin inhibitors, target of rapamycin inhibitors, and antimetabolites. Relatedly, a concern exists that elderberry might worsen autoimmune diseases such as rheumatoid arthritis, multiple sclerosis, and systemic lupus erythematosus. Although no human studies on elderberry's effect on CYP450 enzymes are available, two *in vitro* studies demonstrated no inhibitory effect of elderberry on five UGT enzymes, CYP1A2, CYP2D6, or CYP3A4 (Choi et al. 2014, Langhammer and Nilsen 2014).

12.3.1.5 Evidence

Several small clinical trials have demonstrated the effectiveness of elderberry in reducing influenza-like symptoms. In a multicenter, placebo-controlled study, 60 participants, aged 18–54 years who presented with influenza-like symptoms for less than 48 hours and subsequently had confirmed influenza virus antigen, were randomized to 15 ml of the standardized elderberry extract syrup formulation contained 38% of the standardized extract plus small amounts of raspberry extract, glucose, citric acid, and honey or to placebo four times daily for 5 days. All participants were otherwise healthy and did not belong to high-risk groups. Baseline symptom severity and symptom improvement was assessed using a 10-point visual analogue scale. In the elderberry group, symptom relief occurred in 3–4 days compared to 7–8 days in the placebo (p < 0.001) (Zakay-Rones et al. 2004). These findings were comparable to the results of an earlier double-blind study of individuals living in an agricultural community during an influenza outbreak. Symptoms resolved within 2–3 days in the elderberry-treated group compared with 6 or more days in the placebo group (p < 0.001) (Zakay-Rones et al. 1995). In another double-blind study, 64 patients aged 16–60 years with influenza-like symptoms for less than 24 hours were randomly assigned to receive 175 mg elderberry extract lozenges four times daily or placebo for 2 days. The severity of symptoms was assessed using a visual analogue scale. After 48 hours of treatment, 88% in the elderberry group were void of all symptoms or showed relief from some symptoms whereas only 16% of patients in the placebo group showed symptomatic improvement while no one achieved complete recovery (Kong 2009).

12.3.1.6 Clinical Application

Based on the available safety and efficacy data, it is reasonable to consider elderberry for the treatment of influenza. Its use does not override recommendations for influenza vaccination and use of standard treatment for influenza in high risk populations such as the elderly, young children, pregnant women, and those with underlying lung disease. Populations in which stimulation of the immune system could be detrimental should avoid the use of elderberry.

12.4 Herpes Simplex Virus Infection

Herpes simplex virus (HSV) is categorized as HSV-1, which mostly causes oral-facial herpes or cold sores, and HSV-2, which mostly causes genital herpes. Worldwide, an estimated 3.7 billion people under age 50 have HSV-1 infection. The highest reported prevalence was in Africa and the lowest in the Americas. HSV-1 is associated with tingling, itching or burning sensation around the mouth followed by ulcers or blisters. Highly contagious, the virus can be transmitted by oral-oral contact or to the genitalia through oral-genital or genital-genital contact (WHO 2017a).

12.4.1 Lemon Balm

12.4.1.1 Background

Lemon balm, also known as *Melissa officinalis*, belongs to the *Lamiaceae/Labiatae* family. It is a perennial lemon-scented herb, native to southern Europe, Asia, and North Africa. The applicable part of the plant is the leaf. Its medicinal use dates back over 2,000 years with a recommendation by Paracelsus (1493–1541) that lemon balm would completely revive a man and should be used for "all complaints supposed to proceed from a disordered state of the nervous system" (Grieve 1980, Kennedy et al. 2002). Traditional uses have included anxiety, stress, sleep disturbances, pain, headache, and gastrointestinal problems. *See Chapters 6 Endocrine Disorders and 11 Pyschiatric Disorders for further discussion.*

12.4.1.2 Pharmacognosy

Lemon balm possesses antiviral activity against HSV through a direct botanical-virus interaction (Allahverdiyev et al. 2004, Kucera et al. 1965, Schnitzler et al. 2008). In an *in vitro* study, the volatile oil and its components were responsible for inhibiting the protein synthesis of HSV-2 (Allahverdiyev et al. 2004). Virucidal and antiviral effects of lemon balm aqueous extract against HSV-1 has also been demonstrated (Astani et al. 2014, Dimitrova et al. 1993).

12.4.1.3 Dosing and Preparation

A 1% dried extract from *Melissa officinalis* leaves (drug/extract 70:1) in a cream base to be applied on the affected sites up to five times daily for up to 14 days has been used in trials (Koytchev et al. 1999, Wolbling and Leonhardt 1994)

12.4.1.4 Safety

Lemon balm is generally well tolerated when applied topically with the dosages and duration used in clinical trials. In one clinical trial using topical cream, 3 of 115 subjects reported a burning sensation and paresthesia; however, this was not conclusively related to the cream since these are also common symptoms of genital HSV (Wolbling and Leonhardt 1994). One case of skin irritation and one withdrawal from the study due to exacerbation of herpes symptoms were reported (Wolbling and Leonhardt 1994).

In vitro, lemon balm was shown to inhibit the activation of both tamoxifen and irinotecan (Grappe et al. 2014). Clinical data is needed to confirm this potential interaction. Oral and potentially absorbable topical lemon balm should potentially be avoided in patients taking these medications. Human studies assessing the drug interaction potential of lemon balm have not been conducted; therefore, caution should be used with oral lemon balm products in patients with concomitant medications.

12.4.1.5 Evidence

Evidence supporting the topical use of lemon balm to treat HSV infection of the skin or transitional mucosa is limited. In a double-blind, placebo-controlled trial, 66 patients with a history of recurrent herpes labialis, with at least four episodes per year, were randomized to either 1% dried extract of *Melissa officinalis* leaves (drug/extract 70:1) in a cream base (Lomaherphan®) (n = 34) or placebo (n = 32). It was applied to the affected skin four times daily for 5 days and was started no later than 4 hours after the onset of symptoms of itching, tingling, burning, and tautness. The primary endpoint was the combined symptoms score for complaints, number of blisters, and size of the lesion in cm² on day 2 of treatment, based on a 4-point scale where zero indicates no symptoms and 3 indicates pronounced symptoms. The two groups differed in the combined symptoms score with mean ± SEM value of 4.03 ± 0.33 in the lemon balm group and 4.94 ± 0.40 in the placebo group, p = 0.04 (Koytchev et al. 1999). A significantly faster healing of the herpetic infection of the skin or transitional mucosa when Lomaherphan®, 1% dried extract from *Melissa officinalis* leaves (drug/extract 70:1) in a cream base, was applied in early stage of the infection compared to placebo for up to 14 days (Wolbling and Leonhardt 1994). *See Chapters 6 Endocrine Disorders and 11 Pyschiatric Disorders for further discussion.*

12.4.1.6 Clinical Application

Despite multiple *in vitro* studies demonstrating the antiviral activity of lemon balm on herpes simplex virus, limited clinical data exist. However, due to its safety profile and low potential for drug interactions, it is reasonable to suggest the use of topical lemon balm for treatment of oral herpes labialis.

12.5 Immune Support

12.5.1 Echinacea

12.5.1.1 Background

Echinacea extract has been used by Native Americans since the 1600s as a general medicine for various conditions including sore gums, coughs, bowel issues, and snakebites (Blumenthal and Busse 2016). It was included on the U.S. national formulary in the early 1900s but became less popular after the 1930s with the introduction of sulfa antibiotics. The use of echinacea has come back in the past several decades as many studies have focused on its use in upper respiratory tract infections (Gunning 1999, Shah et al. 2007).

The German Commission E states that Echinacea "supports and promotes the natural powers of resistance of the body, especially in infectious conditions of the nose and throat" (Blumenthal and Busse 2016).

Commonly known as purple coneflower, echinacea belongs to the *Asteraceae* or *Compositae* family. It is cultivated for medicinal purposes in the U.S., Canada, and Europe, especially Germany. *Echinacea angustifolia, Echinacea purpurea,* and *Echinacea pallida* are the three species used for medicinal purposes including the root and aerial components (Barrett 2003). The most common use of echinacea is the treatment and prevention of common cold and upper respiratory tract infections. Based on data from the 2012 National Health Interview Survey, despite a decline in its use from 2007 to 2012, echinacea remains the most frequently used botanical in the United States (Clarke et al. 2015).

12.5.1.2 Pharmacognosy

Echinacea likely has immunomodulating effects. The proposed immunomodulating mechanism is based on the aklamide, glycoprotein, polysaccharide, and caffeic acid derivative components of the plant activating macrophages, stimulating neutrophil phagocytosis, increasing the number of natural killer cells, and upregulation of tumour necrosis factor (Bauer et al. 1989, Gertsch et al. 2004). Echinacea also has antiviral activity (Bodinet et al. 2002).

12.5.1.3 Dosage and Preparation

Over 800 echinacea products are commercially available worldwide (Ernst 2002). The dosages and preparation for the treatment and prevention of the common cold vary widely across studies. Pressed juice, alcohol tinctures, and tablets from dried extract were the most common preparations used in clinical trials (Linde et al. 2006, Shah et al. 2007). Two products, Echinaguard® and Echinacin® have demonstrated benefit in prevention and treatment of the common cold in multiple clinical trials. For the treatment of the common cold, 4–5 mL of a 40% ethanol extraction diluted with a half glass of water of a standardized echinacea formulation containing concentrated extract of alkamides/cichoric acid/polysaccharides at concentrations of 0.25/2.5/25.5 mg/mL, respectively, eight to ten times the first day of cold then three to four times daily the following 6 days has been studied (Goel et al. 2004, 2005). A 6-day protocol giving 5–6 cups of a tea preparation containing 1275 mg of dried botanical and root of echinacea per bag the first day of symptoms, then 1 cup per day for the subsequent days has been used (Lindenmuth and Lindenmuth 2000). For the prevention of the common cold, 0.9 mL of echinacea extract given three times daily (equivalent to 2,400 mg echinacea extract daily) titrated up to 0.9 mL five times daily (equivalent to 4,000 mg echinacea extract daily) at first onset of symptoms has been studied (Jawad et al. 2012).

12.5.1.4 Safety

Echinacea is generally safe when used orally in the dosages and durations evaluated in clinical trials. Mild adverse effects such as nausea, heart burn, constipation, abdominal pain, mouth irritation, dry mouth, bad taste, numbness of the tongue, headache, dizziness, and skin rash have been reported (Barrett et al. 2011, Goel et al. 2004, Parnham 1996, Schapowal et al. 2009, Turner et al. 2005, Yale and Liu 2004). Some individuals may have an allergic reaction to echinacea, which may be severe.

Due to its immunostimulatory effect, a theoretical concern exists that echinacea may interfere with immunosuppressants such as corticosteroids or worsen autoimmune diseases (Lindenmuth and Lindenmuth 2000, Goel et al. 2004, Taylor et al. 2003, Woelkart et al. 2005). Based on clinical studies, echinacea does not appear to induce or inhibit the activity of CYP2D6, CYP2C9, or P-gp. (Asher et al. 2017, Gorski et al. 2004, Gurley et al. 2004, Gurley et al. 2008a,b). Echinacea inhibits intestinal CYP3A activity but induces hepatic CYP3A (Gorski et al. 2004). *See Chapter 2: Pharmacokinetic and Pharmacogenomic Considerations for additional information.*

12.5.1.5 Evidence

Many clinical studies with varied dosing, duration, preparation, echinacea species, and plant parts have been published with conflicting results. A well designed 2007 meta-analysis evaluated clinical trials of echinacea in either prevention or treatment of the common cold (Shah et al. 2007). After extensive screening, 14 trials were evaluated which concluded 58% decreased risk (OR 0.42, 95%CI 0.25 to 0.71, Q statistic $p < 0.001$) of developing the common cold and a decrease in duration of illness by 1.4 days (weighted mean difference −1.44, 95% CI −2.24 to −0.64; $p = 0.01$). The majority of these trials were using single *Echinacea purpurea* products, although two trials included a combination product [(*Echinacea purpurea*, *Echinacea angustifolia*, vitamin C, Propolis) and (*Echinacea purpurea*, vitamin C, rosemary leaf, eucalyptus, fennel seed)].

A Cochrane systematic review evaluated the effectiveness and safety of echinacea preparations in the prevention and treatment of the common cold. Twenty-four randomized controlled trials were included in qualitative synthesis only, due to the heterogeneity of the preparations studied (Karsch-Volk et al. 2014). Ten trials evaluated treatment, while 15 trials evaluated prevention of colds (one trial addressed both treatment and prevention). Study authors concluded the evidence was weak supporting echinacea for prevention and treatment of cold, and the treatment effects were likely small and of questionable clinical significance. In comparing their results to the Shah meta-analysis, authors noted that the Shah study used different inclusion criteria, combined trials of different echinacea preparations, and included treatment and prevention trials together in their meta-analyses.

12.5.1.6 Clinical Application

The data on the efficacy of echinacea for prevention and treatment of the common cold is extensive and conflicting. Minimal adverse effects have been noted. A risk of rash and potentially severe allergic reaction indicates that caution should be used as with any other medication. Individuals taking medications metabolized by CYP 450 1A2 or 3A4 should be cautious when taking concomitant echinacea. Based on these data, individuals with the common cold may benefit from taking echinacea, although again the evidence is inconclusive. It is recommended that either *Echinacea purpurea* or a combination with *Echinacea angustifolia* be used. Daily use for prevention of the common cold is not recommended.

12.5.2 Astragalus

12.5.2.1 Background

Astragalus, also known as *Astragalus membranaceus, Astragalus mongholicus* or *Astragalus complanatus*, belongs to the *Fabaceae/Leguminosae* family. It is a perennial botanical found in temperate and arid regions. It has been used in traditional Chinese medicine for centuries to treat various diseases and has been shown *in vitro* to stimulate cell-mediated immunity (Block and Mead 2003). *See Chapter 16 Supportive and Palliative Care for Cancer for further discussion.*

12.5.2.2 Pharmacognosy

Flavonoids, saponins, and polysaccharides are the active constituents of astragalus with the root being the applicable part used for medicinal purposes (Ibrahim et al. 2013, Li et al. 2014). The polysaccharide component of *Astragalus membranaceus* has immunostimulating activities through different mechanisms. For instance, astragalus polysaccharides activate B cells and macrophages, but not T cells (Shao et al. 2004). Astragalus can also stimulate interferon induction in mice and human (Hou et al. 1981). An *in vitro* study showed that astragalus stimulates mononuclear cells and increases lymphocyte production (Sun et al. 1983). In another *in vitro* study, astragalus stimulates the proliferation of peripheral blood mononuclear cells, cytokine production of peripheral blood mononuclear cells, and promotes the IgG production of peripheral blood B cells (Wang et al. 2002). It may also increase the phagocytosis of the macrophages (Zhang et al. 2012).

12.5.2.3 Dosing and Preparation

Eighty mg of *Astragalus membranaceus* root extract per capsule containing standardized 40% polysaccharide in a dose of two capsules twice daily for up to 6 weeks has been used in patients with seasonal allergic rhinitis (Matkovic et al. 2010).

12.5.2.4 Safety

Astragalus is generally well tolerated when used orally. In a clinical trial, 10 of 41 patients had mild to moderate adverse effects including rhinosinusitis, pharyngitis, enterocolitis, nausea, lacunar angina, and vulvitis. Most of these effects were due to the studied condition and may not have been directly related the astragalus (Matkovic et al. 2010). Kidney and liver cysts were shown in a CT scan in a patient who consumed astragalus tea every day for one month. The report concluded that this case strongly suggested that repeated oral administration of *Astragalus membranaceus* may lead to the formation of liver and kidney cysts (Tong et al. 2014).

Since astragalus enhances immune function, a concern exists that the botanical may interfere with immunosuppressants (Hou et al. 1981, Shao et al. 2004, Sun et al. 1983, Wang et al. 2002, Zhang et al. 2012). In addition, astragalus has a diuretic effect which may affect serum lithium concentrations and necessitate monitoring serum lithium levels (Ma et al. 1998). Due to the effect on immune function, a theoretical concern exists that astragalus may also worsen autoimmune diseases (Hou et al. 1981, Shao et al. 2004, Sun et al. 1983, Wang et al. 2002, Zhang et al. 2012). A study in human liver microsomes and one in rats suggests *Astragalus membranaceus* may inhibit CYP 450 3A4 enzymes (Pao et al. 2012).

12.5.2.5 Evidence

Although astragalus has immunostimulating activity, clinical studies in reducing the symptoms of common cold and upper respiratory tract infections are lacking. The available data is limited on the effectiveness of astragalus to improve the symptoms of allergic rhinitis. In a double-blind, placebo-controlled trial, 48 patients with seasonal allergic rhinitis were randomized to receive two capsules (80 mg each) of *Astragalus membranaceus* root extract as an active ingredient standardized to contain 40% of polysaccharides (n = 32) or placebo (n = 16). The primary endpoints were mean change in the total symptom score (total score of individual symptoms based on a 4-point scale: rhinorrhea, nasal congestion, sneezing, itching or burning eyes), quality of life (using a questionnaire with total score of individual symptoms based on a 4-point scale), and specific serum IgE and IgG. Secondary endpoints included investigator and patient global evaluation of treatment efficacy using a 5-point scale and change in nasal eosinophils. Compared to baseline, total symptom score improved after 3 and 6 weeks of treatment (p = 0.002 and 0.001, respectively) and quality of life also improved after 6 weeks of treatment (p < 0.001). Compared to placebo after 3 weeks, there was a reduction in the individual symptom of rhinorrhea in the *Astragalus membranaceus* group (p = 0.048), but no difference in other symptoms, serum IgE and IgG, or nasal eosinophils. Investigators' and patients' global evaluation showed that *Astragalus membranaceus* is more efficacious than placebo (p = 0.003 and 0.026, respectively) (Matkovic et al. 2010). *See Chapter 16 Supportive and Palliative Care for Cancer for further discussion.*

12.5.2.6 Clinical Application

Data is limited on the efficacy of astragalus as an immune modulator. One study suggests it may be effective for use in seasonal allergic rhinitis. A potential exists for drug interactions via effects on immune modulation, diuretic effects, and as an inhibitor of CYP450 3A4. This botanical has been used in Chinese medicine for centuries, so if astragalus is to be used, individuals should not be taking other medications and should be in the care of a Chinese medicine specialist.

12.5.3 Andrographis

12.5.3.1 Background

Andrographis, also known as *Andrographis paniculate*, belongs to the *Acanthaceae* family, and has been used in the Ayurvedic and Chinese systems of medicine for the treatment of digestive problems, diarrhea, malaria, and hepatitis (Burgos et al. 2009, Coon and Ernst 2004, Poolsup et al. 2004). Inflammatory and infectious diseases such as upper respiratory tract infections have also been treated with this botanical.

12.5.3.2 Pharmacognosy

The diterpene lactone, andrographolide, is the main constituent which is believed to provide the biological activity and is found mostly in the leaves of the plant (Jayakumar et al. 2013). Andrographolide has an immunomodulating effect and particularly, immunostimulatory activity. This constituent enhances production of the antibody and the delayed-type hypersensitivity response to foreign antigens, macrophages phagocytosis, and proliferation of splenic lymphocytes (Puri et al. 1993). *In vitro*, a fixed combination of andrographolide and Kan Jang™ (a standardized combination of *Andrographis paniculata* extract and *Eleutherococcus senticosus extract*) enhances the formation of interferon-gamma, neopterin, and β2 microglobulin (Panossian et al. 2002)

12.5.3.3 Dosing and Preparation

Four 100 mg tablets of *Andrographis paniculata* dried extract administered three times daily for 5 days has been used (Caceres et al. 1999). In addition, 200 mg daily (100 mg capsule twice daily) of an extract of *Andrographis paniculata* for 5 days has been used (Saxena et al. 2010). Three to six grams of *Andrographis paniculata* for 7 days has been used for pharyngotonsillitis (Thamlikitkul et al. 1991). For prevention of common cold symptoms, a dose of 200 mg of *Andrographis paniculata* dried extract daily for 3 months has been used (Caceres et al. 1997). Eighty-five mg of a standardized extract of *Andrographis paniculata* and 10 mg of *Eleutherococcus senticosus* extract four tablets three times daily for 5 days has been used (Gabrielian et al. 2002).

12.5.3.4 Safety

Andrographis is well tolerated when consumed in the amounts and durations that were used in clinical trials. Adverse effects are mild, reversible, and infrequent. The adverse effects include vomiting, epistaxis, urticaria, diarrhea, headache, dizziness, fatigue, pruritus, and rash (Coon and Ernst 2004, Saxena et al. 2010).

Andrographis has antithrombotic effects (Amroyan et al. 1999, Zhao and Fang 1991). It might potentially increase the risk of bleeding in patients receiving antithrombotic agents and caution should be used in patients with bleeding disorders or those undergoing surgery. In addition, andrographis has caused a significant fall in blood pressure in an animal study (Zhang et al. 1998). A theoretical concern exists that its concomitant use with antihypertensives may potentiate the hypotensive effect. In addition, andrographis theoretically might interfere with immunosuppressants or worsen autoimmune disorders (Panossian et al. 2002, Puri et al. 1993). In rat and human hepatocytes, andrographis decreased the activity of CYP 450 1A2, 2C9, 2D6, 3A4 suggesting potential inhibition (Tan and Lim 2015).

12.5.3.5 Evidence

In a 2017 systematic review and meta-analysis of 33 randomized controlled trials enrolling 7175 patients with acute respiratory tract infections, *Andrographis paniculata*, alone or with usual care significantly improved the overall symptoms of acute respiratory tract infections compared with placebo, usual care, and other herbal therapies as well as shortened the duration to symptom resolution. It improved cough (n = 596, standardized mean difference: −0.39, 95% confidence interval [−0.67, −0.10]) and sore throat (n = 314, SMD: −1.13, 95% CI [−1.37, −0.89]) compared with placebo (Hu et al. 2017). This data should be interpreted cautiously, however, due to between-study heterogeneity and the poor quality of included studies.

12.5.3.6 Clinical Application

Limited data exist for the use of andrographis in treating symptoms of upper respiratory infections. Based on the systematic review, andrographis may potentially decrease cough and sore throat. Although only *in vitro* data on drug interactions exists, concomitant use of andrographis with medications should likely be avoided.

12.6 Symptom Management

12.6.1 Thyme

12.6.1.1 Background

Thyme is a perennial plant also known as *Thymus vulgaris* belonging to the *Lamiaceae/Labiatae* family and is cultivated in several European countries, the United States, and the Mediterranean region. It is widely used as traditional medicine in the western Mediterranean region (Nagoor Meeran et al. 2017). In the early 20th century with the early use of hemodialysis, thymol was used as sterilizer to allow multiple reuse of hemodialyzers. Thymol containing plants have been used in traditional medicine to treat cough, headache, diarrhea, and warts (Marchese et al. 2016). Flowers, leaves, and the plant essential oil are used for medicinal purposes.

12.6.1.2 Pharmacognosy

Flavonoids from thyme have demonstrated spasmolytic activity of smooth muscle in the trachea and ileum in animal models. This occurs by inhibiting the activity of acetylcholine, histamine, and L-noradrenaline or by calcium channel antagonism (Reiter and Brandt 1985, Van Den Broucke and Lemli 1983). The phenolic monoterpene thymol is the major compound of thyme (Jukic et al. 2007).

12.6.1.3 Dosing and Preparation

Several standardized thyme extracts in syrup or tablet formulations in cough preparations are available and different dosages have been used. For example, 1–2 g of dried botanical in boiling water to be ingested multiple times daily as needed has been used to relieve upper respiratory tract symptoms (Blumenthal and Busse 2016, Jellin 2017).

12.6.1.4 Safety

Thyme is generally safe and has Generally Recognized as Safe (GRAS) status in the U.S. When taken orally, it should be used in the dosage and duration in clinical trials (Marzian 2007). Mild gastrointestinal adverse effects have been reported with extracts from thyme and ivy leaves (Ernst et al. 1997).

In vitro data suggests that thyme demonstrates antithrombotic activity (Tognolini et al. 2006, Yamamoto et al. 2005). It might theoretically increase the risk of bleeding in patients receiving antithrombotic agents, in patients with bleeding disorders or patients undergoing surgery (Tognolini et al. 2006, Yamamoto et al. 2005). *In vitro* data also showed that thyme has the affinity to bind to estrogen receptors and therefore, may interfere with the activity of estrogen replacement therapy (Zava et al. 1998). In addition, *in vitro* data showed that thymol has an acetylcholine esterase inhibitory effect and might theoretically antagonize the effect of anticholinergics and potentiate the effect of cholinomimetics (Jukic et al. 2007).

In vitro data shows thyme inhibits CYP 450 1A2, 2C9, 2C19, and 3A4 (Brahmi et al. 2011, Foster et al. 2003). It is unclear whether CYP 450 2D6 is inhibited as the results of the two studies were not in agreement.

12.6.1.5 Evidence

Several studies have evaluated the effectiveness of thyme in improving symptoms associated with bronchitis. In a controlled multicenter study including 7783 adults and children with acute bronchitis, the use of a product containing 60 mg of dried extract of *Primulae radix* and 160 mg of dried extract of thyme was, on average, more effective than synthetic secretolytic drugs in symptomatic treatment. However, this benefit was less pronounced in children compared to adults (Ernst et al. 1997). In a double-blind, placebo-controlled, multicenter trial, 150 patients with acute bronchitis for less than 48 hours were randomly assigned to receive 30 drops (1 mL) of Bronchicum Tropfen™, a fixed combination of thyme extract and primose root tincture (n = 75) five times daily or placebo (n = 75) for 7–9 days. The primary endpoint was the bronchitis severity score at the end of the study compared to baseline. A 5.8-point reduction in the bronchitis severity score was apparent in the treatment group compared to placebo (p ≤ 0.001). More patients were symptom free in the treatment group (58.7%) compared to placebo (5.3%) (Gruenwald et al. 2005).

In a single-blind, non-inferiority trial, 189 individuals with acute bronchitis for less than 48 hours were randomly assigned to receive either thyme fluid extract and primrose root fluid extract as 5 mL six times daily (Bronchicum Elixir S™, fluid test medication, n = 94) or a fixed combination of thyme fluid extract and primrose root tincture 1 mL 5 times daily (Bronchcium Tropfen™, drops test medication, n = 95) for 7–9 days. The primary endpoint was the bronchitis severity score at the end of the study compared to baseline. The bronchitis severity score was significantly reduced at the end of the study compared to the baseline in both groups but no difference between groups. Noteworthy, 52.1% of patients in the fluid test medication group and 53.7% of the patients in drops test medication group were symptom free at the end of the study (Gruenwald et al. 2006).

In another double-blind, placebo-controlled, multicenter study, 361 patients with acute bronchitis and over 10 coughing fits per day were randomized to either Bronchipret Saft™, a thyme-ivy combination syrup 16.2 mL daily in three divided doses (n = 182) or placebo (n = 179). The primary endpoint was the frequency of coughing fits on days 7–9. Compared to baseline, the treatment group had a mean 68.7% reduction in coughing fits on days 7–9 compared to 47.6% in placebo (p < 0.0001) (Kemmerich et al. 2006).

12.6.1.6 Clinical Application

Based on the available safety and efficacy data, it is reasonable to recommend thyme for reducing symptoms of acute bronchitis. In the efficacy trials, combination products including Bronchcium Tropfen™, Bronchicum Elixir S™, or Bronchipret Saft™ were used and could be recommended. Although data on drug interactions is limited, a potential for inhibition of CYP 450 enzymes exists.

12.6.2 Propolis

12.6.2.1 Background

Propolis, also known as bee glue, is a resin mixture, made by honeybees using juices and residue from trees, bees wax, and its saliva to produce a product to seal bee hives. It is known to have antibacterial, antifungal, antiviral, and anti-inflammatory effects and commonly used to treat upper respiratory infections. Propolis has been used in folk medicine for centuries. Egyptians used it for embalming and Aristotle in 350 BC first reported its use as a medicine. Centuries later the Greeks reported its use as a medicine and in the 12th century it was documented for treating mouth and throat infections as well as dental caries (de Groot 2013).

12.6.2.2 Pharmacognosy

Due to the various plant sources used to make propolis, it has a variable composition. The Poplar-type propolis is the most widely available in the world and has more than 400 identified components. These components include long-chain fatty acids from the bees wax component as well as flavonoids, aromatic acids, esters, glycerol, amino acids, sugars, etc. (de Groot 2013). *In vitro* data reveals that propolis has antibacterial activity against many bacteria including *Streptococcus pneumoniae, Haemophilus influenzae, Haemophilus parainfluenzae, Moraxella catarrhalis*, and *Streptococcus pyogenes* (Speciale et al. 2006). Propolis has also demonstrated antiviral and antifungal properties. Although the exact mechanism is not known, its antimicrobial properties may be due to the high flavonoid content (Grange and Davey 1990).

12.6.2.3 Dosing and Preparation

A preparation containing 50 mg/mL of echinacea extract, 50 mg/mL of propolis, and 10 mg/mL of vitamin C with a dose of 5 mL in children ages 1–3 years and 7.5 mL in children aged 4–7 years twice daily for 12 weeks has been tested for the prevention of respiratory tract infections (Cohen et al. 2004).

12.6.2.4 Safety

The most common adverse effects are allergic contact dermatitis and contact allergy (de Groot 2013). Occupational exposure to propolis as well as local effects from these products have resulted in allergic stomatitis, labial and oral swelling, dyspnea, cheilitis, and perioral eczema, and skin eruptions have been described (Bellegrandi et al. 1996, de Groot 2013, Hay and Greig 1990). Mild, transient gastrointestinal adverse effects have been reported in children taking a combination botanical extract which included propolis (Cohen et al. 2004).

In vitro data has showed that caffeic acid phenethyl ester, a component of propolis, has a potent antiplatelet activity (Chen et al. 2007). It may theoretically increase the risk of bleeding in patients receiving antithrombotic agents. Caution should also be taken in patients with bleeding disorders or patients undergoing surgery. In addition, patients who have allergies to propolis and related compounds such as honey should avoid taking propolis.

12.6.2.5 Evidence

Few studies have evaluated the effectiveness of propolis in the treatment and prevention of upper respiratory tract infections.

Propolis has been shown to prevent respiratory tract infections in children. In a double-blind, placebo-controlled study, 430 children aged 1–5 years were randomly assigned to either 5 mL for children aged 1–3 years and 7.5 mL for children aged 4–5 years twice daily of preparation containing 50 mg/mL of echinacea, 50 mg/mL of propolis, and 10 mg/mL of vitamin C (n = 215) or placebo (n = 215) during the winter for 12 weeks. The objective was to evaluate the effectiveness of this product in the prevention of upper respiratory tract infections. The number of illness episodes was 138 in the treatment group compared to 308 in the control group representing a 55% reduction. The number of episodes per child was 0.9 ± 1.1 in the treatment group compared to 1.8 ± 1.3 in the placebo representing a 50% reduction ($p < 0.001$). The total number of illnesses, duration of the individual episode, and number of days with fever per child were also decreased (Cohen et al. 2004).

12.6.2.6 Clinical Application

Preliminary evidence supports the use of propolis for prevention and treatment of upper respiratory tract infections if patients do not have allergy to bee products.

12.6.3 Willow Bark

12.6.3.1 Background

Willow bark belongs to the family *Salicacea* and comes from the bark of several Salix species including *S. alba, S. nigra, S. fragilis,* and *S. purpurea.* It was first reported in the 18th century to have an antipyretic effect (Stone 1763). Salicin, the major active constituent of white willow bark has been used for pain and as an antipyretic since its discovery in 1831 (Nahrstedt et al. 2007; Uehleke et al. 2013). Salicin, one of two prominent salicylates in willow bark, is a prodrug that is metabolized in the gut and liver into salicylic acid which produces the analgesic, antipyretic, and anti-inflammatory activities (Shara and Stohs 2015, Uehleke et al. 2013). Acetylsalicylic acid is a chemical derivative of salicin and was first chemically synthesized in the late 1800s at Bayer in Germany by Felix Hoffman (Vane 2000).

12.6.3.2 Pharmacognosy

Like acetylsalicylic acid, salicin inhibits cyclooxygenases 1 and 2 (Uehleke et al. 2013). It has been proposed that salix extract, through compounds other than salicin or salicylate, inhibits cyclooxygenases-2-mediated prostaglandin E2 release (Fiebich and Chrubasik 2004). Other components of willow bark such as polyphenols, flavonoids, and proanthocyanidins may contribute significantly to the benefits from willow bark (Nahrstedt et al. 2007). Willow bark can also down-regulate the inflammatory mediators, tumor necrosis factor-α, and nuclear factor-kappa B (Shara and Stohs 2015).

12.6.3.3 Dosing and Preparations

Most trials of the treatment of pain or inflammatory conditions have used preparations that are standardized to salicin. These products provide salicin 240 mg as a daily dose, either willow bark extract two tablets twice daily for 6 weeks (Biegert et al. 2004) or four capsules per day of Assalix for 4 weeks (Chrubasik et al. 2001).

12.6.3.4 Safety

Similar to nonsteroidal anti-inflammatory drugs (NSAIDs), oral willow bark may cause gastrointestinal effects such as diarrhea, vomiting, dyspepsia, and heartburn but with a lower incidence (Biegert et al. 2004, Chrubasik et al. 2001, Schmid et al. 2001). Allergic reactions may occur in patients allergic to salicylates (Boullata et al. 2003).

Willow bark extract has antiplatelet effects but to a lesser extent than acetylsalicylic acid (Krivoy et al. 2001). Concomitant use of willow bark with antithrombotic agents may increase the risk of bleeding, especially in those with bleeding disorders or patients undergoing surgery. Due to its structural similarity with aspirin, caution should be taken in individuals with an aspirin allergy and its use avoided in children (Clauson et al. 2005).

12.6.3.5 Evidence

Studies for antipyretic effect of willow bark in humans are lacking. Most clinical data for willow bark in humans is for treatment of pain and inflammatory conditions such as arthritis. In rats with yeast-induced fever, after the oral administration of 5 mmol/kg of salicin delivered 6 hours following the yeast injection, the fever was significantly reduced. In addition, it prevented the development of fever when administered simultaneously with the yeast (Akao et al. 2002).

12.6.3.6 Clinical Application

Willow bark preparations can be used for treatment of chronic pain symptoms similarly to NSAIDs. In addition, it may play a role to reduce fever and myalgia in febrile conditions though human trials are lacking.

12.6.4 Meadowsweet

12.6.4.1 Background

Meadowsweet, or queen of the meadow, is also known as *Filipendula ulmaria* or *Spiraea ulmaria*, and belongs to the *Rosaceae* family (Katanic et al. 2016). Found in Europe, Asia, and the northeastern parts of the United States, it has been used since the 16th century as an anti-inflammatory, analgesic, antipyretic, and diuretic.

12.6.4.2 Pharmacognosy

Meadowsweet contains flavonoids, glycosylated flavonoids, hydrolysable tannins, and salicylates. Salicylic acid and its derivatives are responsible for its biologic activity (Bijttebier et al. 2016, Katanic et al. 2016). Flowers, leaves, and roots are all edible parts of the plant.

Excessive production of prostaglandins can sensitize pain receptors and induce fever and inflammation. Meadowsweet inhibits the synthesis of prostaglandins from arachidonic acid by inhibiting the cyclooxygenase enzymes 1 and 2. Salicylic acid and its derivatives are considered the major components responsible for these effects (Katanic et al. 2016). Meadowsweet has also shown to have bactericidal activity *in vitro* against *Staphylococcus aureus* and *Escherichia coli* (Rauha et al. 2000).

12.6.4.3 Dosing and Preparations

Clinical trials evaluating the safety and efficacy of a specific dosing regimen are not available. Recommendations are based on traditional use and expert opinion. A daily dose of 2.5–3.5 g meadowsweet flower or 4–5 g meadowsweet has been recommended (Blumenthal and Busse 2016).

12.6.4.4 Safety

Due to the salicylate content, oral meadowsweet may cause hypersensitivity and gastrointestinal effects such as diarrhea, vomiting, dyspepsia, and heartburn. Additive adverse effects may occur when taken with other salicylates such as aspirin. Caution should be taken in patients with aspirin allergy or asthma.

12.6.4.5 Evidence

Data is limited to assess the antipyretic effect of meadowsweet in humans.

12.6.4.6 Clinical Application

Based on *in vitro* and animal data and the fact that meadowsweet contains salicin, it will likely reduce fever. Due to limited data, other options for treating fever should be used.

12.6.5 Tea Tree Oil

12.6.5.1 Background

Tea tree oil, *Melaleuca alternifolia*, belongs to the *Myrtaceae* family and is native to Australia. It was first reported to have medicinal properties in 1920. The oil is extracted by steam distillation of the leaves and terminal branches with resultant separation of the oil from the aqueous layer (Carson et al. 2006). Historically, the Aborigines of northern New South Wales would crush tea tree leaves to inhale for coughs and colds, apply to wounds as a poultice, and make into an infusion for sore throats and skin conditions (Carson et al. 2006). *See Chapter 13 Dermatological Conditions for further discussion.*

12.6.5.2 Pharmacognosy

Tea tree oil contains terpene hydrocarbons which are volatile and aromatic. Over 100 components of tea tree oil have been described (Brophy et al. 1989). Terpinen-4-ol is the primary active antimicrobial constituent (Hammer et al. 1996). Tea tree oil has antibacterial, antifungal, antiviral, and antiprotozoal activities (Carson et al. 2006). Tea tree oil disrupts the structural integrity of the microbial cell membrane and consequently, microbial cells lose their chemiosmotic control (Cox et al. 2000). Tea tree is active *in vitro* against a wide range of bacteria and fungi including yeasts such as *Candida albicans,* dermatophytes, and other filamentous fungi (Carson et al. 2006, Catalan et al. 2008, Hammer et al. 1998). Alteration of the membrane permeability is the primary antifungal mechanism with *Candida albicans* being the most studied pathogen (Carson et al. 2006). Tea tree oil also exhibits antiviral activity against herpes simplex virus (Schnitzler et al. 2001).

12.6.5.3 Dosing and Preparation

For oropharyngeal candidiasis, 15 mL *Melaleuca alternifolia* oral solution (Breath-Away, Melaleuca, Inc., Idaho Falls, Idaho, USA) four times daily to swish in the mouth for 30–60 seconds before expelling and for a duration of 2–4 weeks has been studied (Jandourek et al. 1998). For onychomycosis, 100% tea tree oil applied to the affected nail twice daily for 6 months has been used (Buck et al. 1994). In addition, 10%, 25%, and 50% tea tree oil solution applied twice daily for 4 weeks has been used for tinea pedis (Satchell et al. 2002, Tong et al. 1992).

12.6.5.4 Safety

Tea tree oil is usually tolerated when used topically and appropriately. However, local adverse effects such as skin irritation, erythema, and allergic contact dermatitis have been reported (Bhushan and Beck

1997, Bruynzeel 1999, De Groot 1996, Khanna et al. 2000). Repeated topical exposure to lavender and tea tree oils has been reported to be a possible cause of prepubertal gynecomastia (Henley et al. 2007).

12.6.5.5 Evidence

Tea tree oil may be effective in the management of oropharyngeal candidiasis. A prospective, single center, open-labeled study enrolled 13 HIV patients with oropharyngeal candidiasis refractory or resistant to fluconazole. They received 15 mL *Melaleuca alternifolia* oral solution (Breath-Away®, Melaleuca, Inc., Idaho Falls, Idaho, USA) four times daily to swish in the mouth for 30–60 seconds for a duration of 2–4 weeks. The main outcome measure was the resolution of the oropharyngeal candidiasis lesions. After 2 weeks, seven patients had improved with no single case achieving cure and six cases had no changes. After 4 weeks, six participants had improved, two were cured, four did not respond, and one participant had deteriorated. These data suggest that tea tree oil might be effective to treat oropharyngeal candidiasis refractory or resistant to fluconazole (Jandourek et al. 1998).

In addition, a study enrolled 43 patients with terminal cancer where 22 received special mouth care with essential oil consisting of geranium, lavender, tea tree, and peppermint twice daily for one week and 21 received placebo. Subjective and objective measures were improved while numbers of colonizing *Candida albicans* decreased in the treatment group compared to placebo (Kang et al. 2010).

Positive results were also reported in an *in vitro* and *in vivo* study showing a total inhibition of the growth of *Candida albicans in vitro* when 1 mL of 20% *Melaleuca alternifolia* oil is mixed with tissue conditioners (Coe-Comfort, fitt, Lynal). A significant decrease in palatal inflammation and inhibition of *Candida albicans* growth were shown in patients with denture stomatitis treated with *Melaleuca alternifolia* mixed with Coe-Comfort compared to Coe-Comfort alone (Catalan et al. 2008).

Tea tree essential oil may be effective for treatment of onychomycosis. In a multicenter, double-blind, controlled trial, 117 patients with distal subungual onychomycosis were randomized to either 1% clotrimazole solution (n = 53) or 100% tea tree essential oil (n = 64) topical applications twice daily for 6 months. Microbiological cure and clinical improvement were achieved in 18% and 60%, respectively, in tea tree group compared to 11% and 61%, respectively, in clotrimazole group at 6 months, these changes were similar between the two groups. Three months after the end of therapy, 56% of patients in the tea tree group continued to improve or achieved resolution, similar to the clotrimazole group. (Buck et al. 1994).

The use of 5% *Melaleuca alternifolia* essential oil applied three times daily for 8 weeks did not show a favorable response, while 2% butenafine hydrochloride and 5% *Melaleuca alternifolia* cream three times daily for 8 weeks was effective in treating toenail onychomycosis (Syed et al. 1999).

Tea tree oil has demonstrated a beneficial effect in treating tinea pedis. In a double-blind, placebo-controlled study, 158 patients with tinea pedis were randomized to receive either placebo, 25%, or 50% tea tree oil solution applied twice daily for 4 weeks. Clinical response rates were 72%, 68%, and 39% in 25%, 50% tea tree oil solutions and placebo, respectively. Mycological cure rates were 55%, 64%, and 31% in 25% and 50% tea tree oil solutions and placebo, respectively, after 4 weeks of treatment (Satchell et al. 2002).

A 10% tea tree oil cream was comparable to 1% tolnaftate in clinical improvement of symptoms of tinea pedis, with both showing significant improvement compared to placebo. However, the 10% tea tree oil cream was no more effective than placebo in achieving mycological cure (Tong et al. 1992). *See Chapter 13 Dermatological Conditions for further discussion.*

12.6.5.6 Clinical Application

Minimal clinical data for topical tea tree oil exists in treating oropharyngeal candidiasis, onychomycosis or tinea pedis. Breath-Away® mouth rinse may be effective when swished in the mouth four times daily for 2–4 weeks in the treatment of oropharyngeal candidiasis. A trial of tea tree oil is reasonable for onychomycosis, although patients should be aware of the potential for dermatitis with its use.

12.7 Summary

Multiple botanicals have been used in the prevention, treatment, and symptomatic management of common infections. While some botanicals such as cranberry may offer an alternative to antimicrobials in low risk populations, additional research is needed to define their efficacy, optimal preparations, and drug interactions.

REFERENCES

Akao, T., T. Yoshino, K. Kobashi, and M. Hattori. 2002. "Evaluation of salicin as an antipyretic prodrug that does not cause gastric injury." *Planta Med* 68 (8):714–8. doi: 10.1055/s-2002-33792.

Allahverdiyev, A., N. Duran, M. Ozguven, and S. Koltas. 2004. "Antiviral activity of the volatile oils of Melissa officinalis L. against Herpes simplex virus type-2." *Phytomedicine* 11 (7–8):657–61. doi: 10.1016/j. phymed.2003.07.014.

Amoros, M., C. M. Simoes, L. Girre, F. Sauvager, and M. Cormier. 1992. "Synergistic effect of flavones and flavonols against herpes simplex virus type 1 in cell culture. Comparison with the antiviral activity of propolis." *Journal of Natural Products* 55 (12):1732–40.

Amroyan, E., E. Gabrielian, A. Panossian, G. Wikman, and H. Wagner. 1999. "Inhibitory effect of andrographolide from Andrographis paniculata on PAF-induced platelet aggregation." *Phytomedicine* 6 (1):27–31. doi: 10.1016/s0944-7113(99)80031-2.

Asher, G. N., A. H. Corbett, and R. L. Hawke. 2017. "Common herbal dietary supplement-drug interactions." *American Family Physician* 96 (2):101–107.

Astani, A., M. H. Navid, and P. Schnitzler. 2014. "Attachment and penetration of acyclovir-resistant herpes simplex virus are inhibited by Melissa officinalis extract." *Phytotherapy Res* 28 (10):1547–52. doi: 10.1002/ptr.5166.

Barak, V., T. Halperin, and I. Kalickman. 2001. "The effect of Sambucol, a black elderberry-based, natural product, on the production of human cytokines: I. Inflammatory cytokines." *European Cytokine Network* 12 (2):290–6.

Barbosa-Cesnik, C., M. B. Brown, M. Buxton, L. Zhang, J. DeBusscher, and B. Foxman. 2011. "Cranberry juice fails to prevent recurrent urinary tract infection: Results from a randomized placebo-controlled trial." *Clinical Infectious Disease* 52 (1):23–30. doi: 10.1093/cid/ciq073.

Barrett, B. 2003. "Medicinal properties of Echinacea: A critical review." *Phytomedicine* 10 (1):66–86. doi: 10.1078/094471103321648692.

Barrett, B., R. Brown, D. Rakel, D. Rabago, L. Marchand, J. Scheder, M. Mundt, G. Thomas, and S. Barlow. 2011. "Placebo effects and the common cold: A randomized controlled trial." *Annals of Family Medicine* 9 (4):312–22. doi: 10.1370/afm.1250.

Bauer, R., P. Remiger, K. Jurcic, and H. Wagner. 1989. "Effect of extracts of Echinacea on phagocytic activity." *Zeitschrift für Phytotherapie* 10:43–48.

Bellegrandi, S., G. D'Offizi, I. J. Ansotegui, R. Ferrara, E. Scala, and R. Paganelli. 1996. "Propolis allergy in an HIV-positive patient." *Journal of the American Academy of Dermatology* 35 (4):644.

Bhushan, M., and M. H. Beck. 1997. "Allergic contact dermatitis from tea tree oil in a wart paint." *Contact Dermatitis* 36 (2):117–8.

Biegert, C., I. Wagner, R. Ludtke, I. Kotter, C. Lohmuller, I. Gunaydin, K. Taxis, and L. Heide. 2004. "Efficacy and safety of willow bark extract in the treatment of osteoarthritis and rheumatoid arthritis: Results of 2 randomized double-blind controlled trials." *Journal Rheumatol* 31 (11):2121–30.

Bijttebier, S., A. Van der Auwera, S. Voorspoels, B. Noten, N. Hermans, L. Pieters, and S. Apers. 2016. "A first step in the quest for the active constituents in Filipendula ulmaria (Meadowsweet): Comprehensive phytochemical identification by liquid chromatography coupled to quadrupole-orbitrap mass spectrometry." *Planta Med* 82 (6):559–72. doi: 10.1055/s-0042-101943.

Blatherwick, N. R. 1914. "The specific role of foods in relation to the composition of the urine." *Archives of Internal Medicine* XIV (3):409–450. doi: 10.1001/archinte.1914.00070150122008.

Block, K. I., and M. N. Mead. 2003. "Immune system effects of echinacea, ginseng, and astragalus: A review." *Integrative Cancer Therapies* 2 (3):247–67. doi: 10.1177/1534735403256419.

Blumenthal, M., and W. R. Busse. 2016. The Complete German Commission E Monographs. *Austin, Texas: American Botanical Council.*

Bodinet, C., R. Mentel, U. Wegner, U. Lindequist, E. Teuscher, and J. Freudenstein. 2002. "Effect of oral application of an immunomodulating plant extract on Influenza virus type A infection in mice." *Planta Med* 68 (10):896–900. doi: 10.1055/s-2002-34919.

Boullata, J. I., P. J. McDonnell, and C. D. Oliva. 2003. "Anaphylactic reaction to a dietary supplement containing willow bark." *Annals of Pharmacotherapy* 37 (6):832–5. doi: 10.1345/aph.1D027.

Brahmi, Z., H. Niwa, M. Yamasato, S. Shigeto, Y. Kusakari, K. Sugaya, J. Onose, and N. Abe. 2011. "Effective cytochrome P450 (CYP) inhibitor isolated from thyme (Thymus saturoides) purchased from a Japanese market." *Bioscience Biotechnolology Biochemistry* 75 (11):2237–9. doi: 10.1271/bbb.110328.

Brophy, J., N. Davies, I. Southwell, I. A. Stiff, and L. R. Williams. 1989. Gas chromatographic quality control for oil of Melaleuca Terpinen-4-ol Type (Australian Tea Tree). *Journal f Agricultural Food Chemistry* 37 (5), 1330–35, doi: 10.1021/jf00089a027.

Bruynzeel, D. P. 1999. "Contact dermatitis due to tea tree oil." *Tropical Med Int Health* 4 (9):630.

Buck, D. S., D. M. Nidorf, and J. G. Addino. 1994. "Comparison of two topical preparations for the treatment of onychomycosis: Melaleuca alternifolia (tea tree) oil and clotrimazole." *Journal of Family Practice* 38 (6):601–5.

Burgos, R. A., J. L. Hancke, J. C. Bertoglio, V. Aguirre, S. Arriagada, M. Calvo, and D. D. Caceres. 2009. "Efficacy of an Andrographis paniculata composition for the relief of rheumatoid arthritis symptoms: A prospective randomized placebo-controlled trial." *Clinical Rheumatol* 28 (8):931–46. doi: 10.1007/s10067-009-1180-5.

Caceres, D. D., J. L. Hancke, R. A. Burgos, F. Sandberg, and G. K. Wikman. 1999. "Use of visual analogue scale measurements (VAS) to asses the effectiveness of standardized Andrographis paniculata extract SHA-10 in reducing the symptoms of common cold. A randomized double blind-placebo study." *Phytomedicine* 6 (4):217–23. doi: 10.1016/s0944-7113(99)80012-9.

Caceres, D. D., J. L. Hancke, R. A. Burgos, and G. K. Wikman. 1997. "Prevention of common colds with Andrographis paniculata dried extract. A Pilot double blind trial." *Phytomedicine* 4 (2):101–4. doi: 10.1016/s0944-7113(97)80051-7.

Carson, C. F., K. A. Hammer, and T. V. Riley. 2006. "Melaleuca alternifolia (Tea Tree) oil: A review of antimicrobial and other medicinal properties." *Clinical Microbiology Review* 19 (1):50–62. doi: 10.1128/cmr.19.1.50-62.2006.

Catalan, A., J. G. Pacheco, A. Martinez, and M. A. Mondaca. 2008. "In vitro and in vivo activity of Melaleuca alternifolia mixed with tissue conditioner on Candida albicans." *Oral Surgery Oral Medicine Oral Pathology Oral Radiolology Endod* 105 (3):327–32. doi: 10.1016/j.tripleo.2007.08.025.

CDC. 2013. "Antibiotic resistance threats in the United States, 2013." cdc.gov. http://www.cdc.gov/drugresistance/pdf/ar-threats-2013-508.pdf (accessed September 20, 2017).

CDC. 2015. "Nearly half a million Americans suffered from Clostridium difficile infections in a single year." cdc.gov. https://www.cdc.gov/media/releases/2015/p0225-clostridium-difficile.html (accessed September 20, 2017).

Chen, T. G., J. J. Lee, K. H. Lin, C. H. Shen, D. S. Chou, and J. R. Sheu. 2007. "Antiplatelet activity of caffeic acid phenethyl ester is mediated through a cyclic GMP-dependent pathway in human platelets." *Chin Journal of Physiology* 50 (3):121–6.

Choi, E. J., J. B. Park, K. D. Yoon, and S. K. Bae. 2014. "Evaluation of the in vitro/in vivo potential of five berries (bilberry, blueberry, cranberry, elderberry, and raspberry ketones) commonly used as herbal supplements to inhibit uridine diphospho-glucuronosyltransferase." *Food Chemistry Toxicology* 72:13–9. doi: 10.1016/j.fct.2014.06.020.

Chrubasik, S., O. Kunzel, A. Model, C. Conradt, and A. Black. 2001. "Treatment of low back pain with a herbal or synthetic anti-rheumatic: A randomized controlled study. Willow bark extract for low back pain." *Rheumatology (Oxford)* 40 (12):1388–93.

Clarke, T. C., L. I. Black, B. J. Stussman, P. M. Barnes, and R. L. Nahin. 2015. "Trends in the use of complementary health approaches among adults: United States, 2002-2012." *Nationall Health Statistics Report* (79):1–16.

Clauson, K. A., M. L. Santamarina, C. M. Buettner, and J. S. Cauffield. 2005. "Evaluation of presence of aspirin-related warnings with willow bark." *Annals of Pharmacotherapy* 39 (7–8):1234–7. doi: 10.1345/aph.1E650.

Cohen, H. A., I. Varsano, E. Kahan, E. M. Sarrell, and Y. Uziel. 2004. "Effectiveness of an herbal preparation containing echinacea, propolis, and vitamin C in preventing respiratory tract infections in children: A randomized, double-blind, placebo-controlled, multicenter study." *Arch Pediatrics Adolescent Medicine* 158 (3):217–21. doi: 10.1001/archpedi.158.3.217.

Coon, J. T., and E. Ernst. 2004. "Andrographis paniculata in the treatment of upper respiratory tract infections: A systematic review of safety and efficacy." *Planta Med* 70 (4):293–8. doi: 10.1055/s-2004-818938.

Cox, S. D., C. M. Mann, J. L. Markham, H. C. Bell, J. E. Gustafson, J. R. Warmington, and S. G. Wyllie. 2000. "The mode of antimicrobial action of the essential oil of Melaleuca alternifolia (tea tree oil)." *Journal of Applied Microbiology* 88 (1):170–5.

de Arriba, S. G., B. Naser, and K. U. Nolte. 2013. "Risk assessment of free hydroquinone derived from Arctostaphylos Uva-ursi folium herbal preparations." *International Journal of Toxicology* 32 (6):442–53. doi: 10.1177/1091581813507721.

De Groot, A. C. 1996. "Airborne allergic contact dermatitis from tea tree oil." *Contact Dermatitis* 35 (5):304–5.

de Groot, A. C. 2013. "Propolis: A review of properties, applications, chemical composition, contact allergy, and other adverse effects." *Dermatitis* 24 (6):263–82. doi: 10.1097/der.0000000000000011.

Dimitrova, Z., B. Dimov, N. Manolova, S. Pancheva, D. Ilieva, and S. Shishkov. 1993. "Antiherpes effect of Melissa officinalis L. extracts." *Acta Microbiology Bulg* 29:65–72.

EMA. 2012. "HMPC Community herbal monograph on Arctostaphylos uva-ursi (L.) Spreng, folium." ema. europa.eu. http://www.ema.europa.eu/docs/en_GB/document_ibrary/Herbal_-_HMPC_assessment_report/2011/07/WC500108750.pdf./ (accessed August 18, 2018).

Ernst, E. 2002. "The risk-benefit profile of commonly used herbal therapies: Ginkgo, St. John's Wort, Ginseng, Echinacea, Saw Palmetto, and Kava." *Annals of Internal Medicine* 136 (1):42–53.

Ernst, E., R. Marz, and C. Sieder. 1997. "A controlled multi-centre study of herbal versus synthetic secretolytic drugs for acute bronchitis." *Phytomedicine* 4 (4):287–93. doi: 10.1016/s0944-7113(97)80035-9.

ESCOP. 2012. "Arctostaphylos Uvae ursi folium, bearberry leaf." Exeter, United Kingdom. ISSN 2221-9021. 2012: 1–6./ www.escop.com (accessed August 18, 2018).

Fiebich, B. L., and S. Chrubasik. 2004. "Effects of an ethanolic salix extract on the release of selected inflammatory mediators in vitro." *Phytomedicine* 11 (2-3):135–8. doi: 10.1078/0944-7113-00338.

Foster, B. C., S. Vandenhoek, J. Hana, A. Krantis, M. H. Akhtar, M. Bryan, J. W. Budzinski, A. Ramputh, and J. T. Arnason. 2003. "In vitro inhibition of human cytochrome P450-mediated metabolism of marker substrates by natural products." *Phytomedicine* 10 (4):334–42. doi: 10.1078/094471103322004839.

Foxman, B., A. E. Cronenwett, C. Spino, M. B. Berger, and D. M. Morgan. 2015. "Cranberry juice capsules and urinary tract infection after surgery: Results of a randomized trial." *American Journal of Obstetrics and Gynecology* 213 (2):194.e1-8. doi: 10.1016/j.ajog.2015.04.003.

Fu, Z., D. Liska, D. Talan, and M. Chung. 2017. "Cranberry reduces the risk of urinary tract infection recurrence in otherwise healthy women: A systematic review and meta-analysis." *J Nutr* 147 (12):2282–2288. doi: 10.3945/jn.117.254961.

Gabrielian, E. S., A. K. Shukarian, G. I. Goukasova, G. L. Chandanian, A. G. Panossian, G. Wikman, and H. Wagner. 2002. "A double blind, placebo-controlled study of Andrographis paniculata fixed combination Kan Jang in the treatment of acute upper respiratory tract infections including sinusitis." *Phytomedicine* 9 (7):589–97. doi: 10.1078/094471102321616391.

Gertsch, J., R. Schoop, U. Kuenzle, and A. Suter. 2004. "Echinacea alkylamides modulate TNF-alpha gene expression via cannabinoid receptor CB2 and multiple signal transduction pathways." *FEBS Lett* 577 (3):563–9. doi: 10.1016/j.febslet.2004.10.064.

Gettman, M. T., K. Ogan, L. J. Brinkley, B. Adams-Huet, C. Y. Pak, and M. S. Pearle. 2005. "Effect of cranberry juice consumption on urinary stone risk factors." *Journal of Urology* 174 (2):590–4; quiz 801, doi: 10.1097/01.ju.0000165168.68054.f8.

Ghebrehewet, S., P. MacPherson, A. Ho. 2016. Influenza. *BMJ* 355:i6258. PMID: 27927672.

Goel, V., R. Lovlin, R. Barton, M. R. Lyon, R. Bauer, T. D. Lee, and T. K. Basu. 2004. "Efficacy of a standardized echinacea preparation (Echinilin) for the treatment of the common cold: A randomized, double-blind, placebo-controlled trial." *Journal of Clinical Pharmacology Therapy* 29 (1):75–83.

Goel, V., R. Lovlin, C. Chang, J. V. Slama, R. Barton, R. Gahler, R. Bauer, L. Goonewardene, and T. K. Basu. 2005. "A proprietary extract from the echinacea plant (Echinacea purpurea) enhances systemic immune response during a common cold." *Phytotherapy Res* 19 (8):689–94. doi: 10.1002/ptr.1733.

Gorski, J. C., S. M. Huang, A. Pinto, M. A. Hamman, J. K. Hilligoss, N. A. Zaheer, M. Desai, M. Miller, and S. D. Hall. 2004. "The effect of echinacea (Echinacea purpurea root) on cytochrome P450 activity in vivo." *Cliicaln Pharmacology Therapy* 75 (1):89–100. doi: 10.1016/j.clpt.2003.09.013.

Grange, J. M., and R. W. Davey. 1990. "Antibacterial properties of propolis (bee glue)." *J R Soc Med* 83 (3):159–60.

Grappe, F., G. Nance, L. Coward, and G. Gorman. 2014. "In vitro inhibitory effects of herbal supplements on tamoxifen and irinotecan metabolism." *Drug Metabol Drug Interact* 29 (4):269–79. doi: 10.1515/dmdi-2014-0017.

Grieve, M. and C. F. Leyel. 1980. *A modern herbal: The medicinal, culinary, cosmetic, and economic properties, cultivation and folklore of herbs, grasses, fungi, shrubs and trees with all their modern scientific uses.* Penguin, Harmondsworth, England.

Gruenwald, J., H. J. Graubaum, and R. Busch. 2005. "Efficacy and tolerability of a fixed combination of thyme and primrose root in patients with acute bronchitis. A double-blind, randomized, placebo-controlled clinical trial." *Arzneimittelforschung* 55 (11):669–76. doi: 10.1055/s-0031-1296916.

Gruenwald, J., H. J. Graubaum, and R. Busch. 2006. "Evaluation of the non-inferiority of a fixed combination of thyme fluid- and primrose root extract in comparison to a fixed combination of thyme fluid extract and primrose root tincture in patients with acute bronchitis. A single-blind, randomized, bi-centric clinical trial." *Arzneimittelforschung* 56 (8):574–81. doi: 10.1055/s-0031-1296754.

Guay, D. R. 2009. "Cranberry and urinary tract infections." *Drugs* 69 (7):775–807. doi: 10.2165/00003495-200969070-00002.

Gunning, K. 1999. "Echinacea in the treatment and prevention of upper respiratory tract infections." *West Journal of Medicine* 171 (3):198–200.

Gurley, B. J., S. F. Gardner, M. A. Hubbard, D. K. Williams, W. B. Gentry, J. Carrier, I. A. Khan, D. J. Edwards, and A. Shah. 2004. "In vivo assessment of botanical supplementation on human cytochrome P450 phenotypes: Citrus aurantium, Echinacea purpurea, milk thistle, and saw palmetto." *Clinical Pharmacology Therapy* 76 (5):428–40. doi: 10.1016/j.clpt.2004.07.007.

Gurley, B. J., A. Swain, M. A. Hubbard, D. K. Williams, G. Barone, F. Hartsfield, Y. Tong, D. J. Carrier, S. Cheboyina, and S. K. Battu. 2008a. "Clinical assessment of CYP2D6-mediated herb-drug interactions in humans: Effects of milk thistle, black cohosh, goldenseal, kava kava, St. John's wort, and Echinacea." *Mol Nutr Food Res* 52 (7):755–63. doi: 10.1002/mnfr.200600300.

Gurley, B. J., A. Swain, D. K. Williams, G. Barone, and S. K. Battu. 2008b. "Gauging the clinical significance of P-glycoprotein-mediated herb-drug interactions: Comparative effects of St. John's wort, Echinacea, clarithromycin, and rifampin on digoxin pharmacokinetics." *Mol Nutr Food Res* 52 (7):772–9. doi: 10.1002/mnfr.200700081.

Hammer, K. A., C. F. Carson, and T. V. Riley. 1996. "Susceptibility of transient and commensal skin flora to the essential oil of Melaleuca alternifolia (tea tree oil)." *American Journal of Infection Control* 24 (3):186–9.

Hammer, K. A., C. F. Carson, and T. V. Riley. 1998. "In-vitro activity of essential oils, in particular Melaleuca alternifolia (tea tree) oil and tea tree oil products, against Candida spp." *Journal of Antimicrobiology Chemotherapy* 42 (5):591–5.

Hay, K. D., and D. E. Greig. 1990. "Propolis allergy: A cause of oral mucositis with ulceration." *Oral Surgery Oral Medicine Oral Pathology* 70 (5):584–6.

Henley, D. V., N. Lipson, K. S. Korach, and C. A. Bloch. 2007. "Prepubertal gynecomastia linked to lavender and tea tree oils." *New England Journal of Medicine* 356 (5):479–85. doi: 10.1056/NEJMoa064725.

Hou, Y. D., G. L. Ma, S. H. Wu, Y. Y. Li, and H. T. Li. 1981. "Effect of Radix Astragali seu Hedysari on the interferon system." *Chinese Medical Journal (Engl)* 94 (1):35–40.

Howell, A. B. 2007. "Bioactive compounds in cranberries and their role in prevention of urinary tract infections." *Mol Nutr Food Res* 51 (6):732–7. doi: 10.1002/mnfr.200700038.

Hu, X. Y., R. H. Wu, M. Logue, C. Blondel, L. Y. W. Lai, B. Stuart, A. Flower, Y. T. Fei, M. Moore, J. Shepherd, J. P. Liu, and G. Lewith. 2017. "Andrographis paniculata (Chuan Xin Lian) for symptomatic relief of acute respiratory tract infections in adults and children: A systematic review and meta-analysis." *PLoS One* 12 (8):e0181780. doi: 10.1371/journal.pone.0181780.

Ibrahim, L. F., M. M. Marzouk, S. R. Hussein, S. A. Kawashty, K. Mahmoud, and N. A. Saleh. 2013. "Flavonoid constituents and biological screening of Astragalus bombycinus Boiss." *Nat Prod Res* 27 (4-5):386–93. doi: 10.1080/14786419.2012.701213.

Ikaheimo, R., A. Siitonen, T. Heiskanen, U. Karkkainen, P. Kuosmanen, P. Lipponen, and P. H. Makela. 1996. "Recurrence of urinary tract infection in a primary care setting: Analysis of a 1-year follow-up of 179 women." *Clinical Infectious Diseases* 22 (1):91–9.

Jandourek, A., J. K. Vaishampayan, and J. A. Vazquez. 1998. "Efficacy of melaleuca oral solution for the treatment of fluconazole refractory oral candidiasis in AIDS patients." *Aids* 12 (9):1033–7.

Jawad, M., R. Schoop, A. Suter, P. Klein, and R. Eccles. 2012. "Safety and efficacy profile of Echinacea purpurea to prevent common cold episodes: A randomized, double-blind, placebo-controlled trial." *Evidence-Based Complementary Alternative Medicine* 2012:841315. doi: 10.1155/2012/841315.

Jayakumar, T., C. Y. Hsieh, J. J. Lee, and J. R. Sheu. 2013. "Experimental and clinical pharmacology of andrographis paniculata and its major bioactive phytoconstituent andrographolide." *Evidence-Based Complementary Alternative Medicine* 2013:846740. doi: 10.1155/2013/846740.

Jefferson, T., M. Jones, P. Doshi, E. A. Spencer, I. Onakpoya, and C. J. Heneghan. 2014. "Oseltamivir for influenza in adults and children: Systematic review of clinical study reports and summary of regulatory comments." *BMJ: British Medical Journal* 348. doi: 10.1136/bmj.g2545.

Jellin, J. M. 2017. *Natural Medicines Comprehensive Database.* Stockton, CA: Therapeutic Research Faculty.

Jepson, R. G., and J. C. Craig. 2007. "A systematic review of the evidence for cranberries and blueberries in UTI prevention." *Mol Nutr Food Res* 51 (6):738–45. doi: 10.1002/mnfr.200600275.

Jepson, R. G., G. Williams, and J. C. Craig. 2012. "Cranberries for preventing urinary tract infections." *Cochrane Database System Review* 10:Cd001321. doi: 10.1002/14651858.CD001321.pub5.

Jukic, M., O. Politeo, M. Maksimovic, M. Milos, and M. Milos. 2007. "In vitro acetylcholinesterase inhibitory properties of thymol, carvacrol and their derivatives thymoquinone and thymohydroquinone." *Phytotherapy Res* 21 (3):259–61. doi: 10.1002/ptr.2063.

Kang, H. Y., S. S. Na, and Y. K. Kim. 2010. "[Effects of oral care with essential oil on improvement in oral health status of hospice patients]." *Journal of the Korean Academy of Nursing* 40 (4):473–81. doi: 10.4040/jkan.2010.40.4.473.

Karsch-Volk, M., B. Barrett, D. Kiefer, R. Bauer, K. Ardjomand-Woelkart, and K. Linde. 2014. "Echinacea for preventing and treating the common cold." *Cochrane Database System Review* (2):Cd000530. doi: 10.1002/14651858.CD000530.pub3.

Katanic, J., T. Boroja, V. Mihailovic, S. Nikles, S. P. Pan, G. Rosic, D. Selakovic, J. Joksimovic, S. Mitrovic, and R. Bauer. 2016. "In vitro and in vivo assessment of meadowsweet (Filipendula ulmaria) as anti-inflammatory agent." *Journal of Ethnopharmacology* 193:627–636. doi: 10.1016/j.jep.2016.10.015.

Kemmerich, B., R. Eberhardt, and H. Stammer. 2006. "Efficacy and tolerability of a fluid extract combination of thyme herb and ivy leaves and matched placebo in adults suffering from acute bronchitis with productive cough. A prospective, double-blind, placebo-controlled clinical trial." *Arzneimittelforschung* 56 (9):652–60. doi: 10.1055/s-0031-1296767.

Kennedy, D. O., A. B. Scholey, N. T. Tildesley, E. K. Perry, and K. A. Wesnes. 2002. "Modulation of mood and cognitive performance following acute administration of Melissa officinalis (lemon balm)." *Pharmacology Biochemical Behav* 72 (4):953–64.

Khanna, M., K. Qasem, and D. Sasseville. 2000. "Allergic contact dermatitis to tea tree oil with erythema multiforme-like id reaction." *American Journal of Contact Dermatitis* 11 (4):238–42.

Kong, F. 2009. "Pilot clinical study on a proprietary elderberry extract: Efficacy in addressing influenza symptoms." *Online Journal of Pharmacology and Pharmacokinetics* 5:32–43.

Koytchev, R., R. G. Alken, and S. Dundarov. 1999. "Balm mint extract (Lo-701) for topical treatment of recurring herpes labialis." *Phytomedicine* 6 (4):225–30. doi: 10.1016/s0944-7113(99)80013-0.

Krivoy, N., E. Pavlotzky, S. Chrubasik, E. Eisenberg, and G. Brook. 2001. "Effect of salicis cortex extract on human platelet aggregation." *Planta Med* 67 (3):209–12. doi: 10.1055/s-2001-12000.

Kucera, L. S., R. A. Cohen, and E. C. Herrmann, Jr. 1965. "Antiviral activities of extracts of the lemon balm plant." *Annals of the New York Academy of Sciences* 130 (1):474–82.

Langhammer, A. J., and O. G. Nilsen. 2014. "In vitro inhibition of human CYP1A2, CYP2D6, and CYP3A4 by six herbs commonly used in pregnancy." *Phytother Res* 28 (4):603–10. doi: 10.1002/ptr.5037.

Larsson, B., A. Jonasson, and S. Fianu. 1993. "Prophylactic effect of UVA-E in women with recurrent cystitis: A preliminary report." *Curr Ther Res* 53:441–443.

Li, X., L. Qu, Y. Dong, L. Han, E. Liu, S. Fang, Y. Zhang, and T. Wang. 2014. "A review of recent research progress on the astragalus genus." *Molecules* 19 (11):18850–80. doi: 10.3390/molecules191118850.

Lilja, J. J., J. T. Backman, and P. J. Neuvonen. 2007. "Effects of daily ingestion of cranberry juice on the pharmacokinetics of warfarin, tizanidine, and midazolam–probes of CYP2C9, CYP1A2, and CYP3A4." *Clinical Pharmacology Ther* 81 (6):833–9. doi: 10.1038/sj.clpt.6100149.

Linde, K., B. Barrett, K. Wolkart, R. Bauer, and D. Melchart. 2006. "Echinacea for preventing and treating the common cold." *Cochrane Database System Review* (1):Cd000530,10.1002/14651858.CD000530.pub2.

Lindenmuth, G. F., and E. B. Lindenmuth. 2000. "The efficacy of echinacea compound herbal tea preparation on the severity and duration of upper respiratory and flu symptoms: A randomized, double-blind placebo-controlled study." *Journal of Alternative Complementary Medicine* 6 (4):327–34. doi: 10.1089/10755530050120691.

Ma, J., A. Peng, and S. Lin. 1998. "Mechanisms of the therapeutic effect of astragalus membranaceus on sodium and water retention in experimental heart failure." *Chinese MedicalJournal (Engl)* 111 (1):17–23.

Mahmood, N., C. Pizza, R. Aquino, N. De Tommasi, S. Piacente, S. Colman, A. Burke, and A. J. Hay. 1993. "Inhibition of HIV infection by flavanoids." *Antiviral Res* 22 (2-3):189–99.

Malik, T. A., A. N. Kamili, M. Z. Chishti, S. Ahad, M. A. Tantry, P. R. Hussain, and R. K. Johri. 2017. "Breaking the resistance of Escherichia coli: Antimicrobial activity of Berberis lycium Royle." *Microb Pathog* 102:12–20. doi: 10.1016/j.micpath.2016.11.011.

Marchese, A., I. E. Orhan, M. Daglia, R. Barbieri, A. Di Lorenzo, S. F. Nabavi, O. Gortzi, M. Izadi, and S. M. Nabavi. 2016. "Antibacterial and antifungal activities of thymol: A brief review of the literature." *Food Chemistry* 210:402–14. doi: 10.1016/j.foodchem.2016.04.111.

Marzian, O. 2007. "[Treatment of acute bronchitis in children and adolescents. Non-interventional postmarketing surveillance study confirms the benefit and safety of a syrup made of extracts from thyme and ivy leaves]." *MMW Fortschr Med* 149 (27–28 Suppl):69–74.

Matkovic, Z., V. Zivkovic, M. Korica, D. Plavec, S. Pecanic, and N. Tudoric. 2010. "Efficacy and safety of Astragalus membranaceus in the treatment of patients with seasonal allergic rhinitis." *Phytother Res* 24 (2):175–81. doi: 10.1002/ptr.2877.

Mellen, C. K., M. Ford, and J. P. Rindone. 2010. "Effect of high-dose cranberry juice on the pharmacodynamics of warfarin in patients." *British Journal of Clinical Pharmacology* 70 (1):139–42. doi: 10.1111/j.1365-2125.2010.03674.x.

Nagai, T., Y. Miyaichi, T. Tomimori, Y. Suzuki, and H. Yamada. 1990. "Inhibition of influenza virus sialidase and anti-influenza virus activity by plant flavonoids." *Chem Pharm Bull (Tokyo)* 38 (5):1329–32.

Nagoor Meeran, M. F., H. Javed, H. Al Taee, S. Azimullah, and S. K. Ojha. 2017. "Pharmacological properties and molecular mechanisms of thymol: Prospects for its therapeutic potential and pharmaceutical development." *Front Pharmacol* 8:380. doi: 10.3389/fphar.2017.00380.

Nahrstedt, A., M. Schmidt, R. Jaggi, J. Metz, and M. T. Khayyal. 2007. "Willow bark extract: The contribution of polyphenols to the overall effect." *Wien Med Wochenschr* 157 (13-14):348–51. doi: 10.1007/s10354-007-0437-3.

Panossian, A., T. Davtyan, N. Gukassyan, G. Gukasova, G. Mamikonyan, E. Gabrielian, and G. Wikman. 2002. "Effect of andrographolide and Kan Jang–fixed combination of extract SHA-10 and extract SHE-3–on proliferation of human lymphocytes, production of cytokines and immune activation markers in the whole blood cells culture." *Phytomedicine* 9 (7):598–605. doi: 10.1078/094471102321616409.

Pao, L. H., O. Y. Hu, H. Y. Fan, C. C. Lin, L. C. Liu, and P. W. Huang. 2012. "Herb-drug interaction of 50 Chinese herbal medicines on CYP3A4 activity in vitro and in vivo." *American Journal of Chinese Medicine* 40 (1):57–73. doi: 10.1142/s0192415x1250005x.

Parnham, M. J. 1996. "Benefit-risk assessment of the squeezed sap of the purple coneflower (Echinacea purpurea) for long-term oral immunostimulation." *Phytomedicine* 3 (1):95–102. doi: 10.1016/s0944-7113(96)80020-1.

Poolsup, N., C. Suthisisang, S. Prathanturarug, A. Asawamekin, and U. Chancharoen. 2004. "Andrographis paniculata in the symptomatic treatment of uncomplicated upper respiratory tract infection: Systematic review of randomized controlled trials." *Journal of Clinical Pharmacology Ther* 29 (1):37–45.

Puri, A., R. Saxena, R. P. Saxena, K. C. Saxena, V. Srivastava, and J. S. Tandon. 1993. "Immunostimulant agents from Andrographis paniculata." *Journal of Natural Products* 56 (7):995–9.

Rauha, J. P., S. Remes, M. Heinonen, A. Hopia, M. Kahkonen, T. Kujala, K. Pihlaja, H. Vuorela, and P. Vuorela. 2000. "Antimicrobial effects of Finnish plant extracts containing flavonoids and other phenolic compounds." *International Journal of Food Microbiology* 56 (1):3–12.

Reiter, M., and W. Brandt. 1985. "Relaxant effects on tracheal and ileal smooth muscles of the guinea pig." *Arzneimittelforschung* 35 (1a):408–14.

Sambucus nigra. 2014. http://www.cbif.gc.ca/eng/species-bank/canadian-poisonous-plants-information-system/all-plants-scientific-name/sambucus-nigra/?id=1370403266999 (accessed December 05, 2018).

Satchell, A. C., A. Saurajen, C. Bell, and R. S. Barnetson. 2002. "Treatment of interdigital tinea pedis with 25% and 50% tea tree oil solution: A randomized, placebo-controlled, blinded study." *Australas J Dermatol* 43 (3):175–8.

Saxena, R. C., R. Singh, P. Kumar, S. C. Yadav, M. P. Negi, V. S. Saxena, A. J. Joshua, V. Vijayabalaji, K. S. Goudar, K. Venkateshwarlu, and A. Amit. 2010. "A randomized double blind placebo controlled clinical evaluation of extract of Andrographis paniculata (KalmCold) in patients with uncomplicated upper respiratory tract infection." *Phytomedicine* 17 (3–4):178–85. doi: 10.1016/j.phymed.2009.12.001.

Schapowal, A., D. Berger, P. Klein, and A. Suter. 2009. "Echinacea/sage or chlorhexidine/lidocaine for treating acute sore throats: A randomized double-blind trial." *European Journal of Med Res* 14 (9):406–12.

Schappert, S. M. 1999. "Ambulatory care visits to physician offices, hospital outpatient departments, and emergency departments: United States, 1997." *Vital Health Stat*istics 13 (143)i–iv: 1–39.

Schindler, G., U. Patzak, B. Brinkhaus, A. von Niecieck, J. Wittig, N. Krahmer, I. Glockl, and M. Veit. 2002. "Urinary excretion and metabolism of arbutin after oral administration of Arctostaphylos uvae ursi extract as film-coated tablets and aqueous solution in healthy humans." *Journal of Clinical Pharmacology* 42 (8):920–7.

Schmid, B., R. Ludtke, H. K. Selbmann, I. Kotter, B. Tschirdewahn, W. Schaffner, and L. Heide. 2001. "Efficacy and tolerability of a standardized willow bark extract in patients with osteoarthritis: Randomized placebo-controlled, double blind clinical trial." *Phytother Res* 15 (4):344–50.

Schnitzler, P., K. Schon, and J. Reichling. 2001. "Antiviral activity of Australian tea tree oil and eucalyptus oil against herpes simplex virus in cell culture." *Pharmazie* 56 (4):343–7.

Schnitzler, P., A. Schuhmacher, A. Astani, and J. Reichling. 2008. "Melissa officinalis oil affects infectivity of enveloped herpesviruses." *Phytomedicine* 15 (9):734–40. doi: 10.1016/j.phymed.2008.04.018.

Sengupta, K., K. V. Alluri, T. Golakoti, G. V. Gottumukkala, J. Raavi, L. Kotchrlakota, S. C. Sigalan, D. Dey, S. Ghosh, and A. Chatterjee. 2011. "A randomized, double blind, controlled, dose dependent clinical trial to evaluate the efficacy of a proanthocyanidin standardized whole cranberry (Vaccinium macrocarpon) powder on infections of the urinary tract." *Current Bioactive Compounds* 7 (1):39–46. doi: 10.2174/157340711795163820.

Shah, S. A., S. Sander, C. M. White, M. Rinaldi, and C. I. Coleman. 2007. "Evaluation of echinacea for the prevention and treatment of the common cold: A meta-analysis." *Lancet Infect Dis* 7 (7):473–80. doi: 10.1016/s1473-3099(07)70160-3.

Shao, B. M., W. Xu, H. Dai, P. Tu, Z. Li, and X. M. Gao. 2004. "A study on the immune receptors for polysaccharides from the roots of Astragalus membranaceus, a Chinese medicinal herb." *Biochem Biophys Res Commun* 320 (4):1103–11. doi: 10.1016/j.bbrc.2004.06.065.

Shara, M., and S. J. Stohs. 2015. "Efficacy and safety of white Willow bark (Salix alba) extracts." *Phytother Res* 29 (8):1112–6. doi: 10.1002/ptr.5377.

Siegers, C., C. Bodinet, S. S. Ali, and C. P. Siegers. 2003. "Bacterial deconjugation of arbutin by Escherichia coli." *Phytomedicine* 10 (Suppl 4):58–60.

Speciale, A., R. Costanzo, S. Puglisi, R. Musumeci, M. R. Catania, F. Caccamo, and L. Iauk. 2006. "Antibacterial activity of propolis and its active principles alone and in combination with macrolides, beta-lactams and fluoroquinolones against microorganisms responsible for respiratory infections." *Journal of Chemotherapy* 18 (2):164–71. doi: 10.1179/joc.2006.18.2.164.

Stone, E. 1763. "XXXII. An account of the success of the bark of the willow in the cure of agues. In a letter to the Right Honourable George Earl of Macclesfield, President of R. S. from the Rev. Mr. Edward Stone, of Chipping-Norton in Oxfordshire." *Philosophical Transactions* 53:195–200. doi: 10.1098/rstl.1763.0033.

Sun, Y., E. M. Hersh, S. L. Lee, M. McLaughlin, T. L. Loo, and G. M. Mavligit. 1983. "Preliminary observations on the effects of the Chinese medicinal herbs Astragalus membranaceus and Ligustrum lucidum on lymphocyte blastogenic responses." *J Biol Response Mod* 2 (3):227–37.

Syed, T. A., Z. A. Qureshi, S. M. Ali, S. Ahmad, and S. A. Ahmad. 1999. "Treatment of toenail onychomycosis with 2% butenafine and 5% Melaleuca alternifolia (tea tree) oil in cream." *Trop Med Int Health* 4 (4):284–7.

Tan, M. L., and L. E. Lim. 2015. "The effects of Andrographis paniculata (Burm.f.) Nees extract and diterpenoids on the CYP450 isoforms' activities, a review of possible herb-drug interaction risks." *Drug Chemistry Toxicolog* 38 (3):241–53. doi: 10.3109/01480545.2014.947504.

Taylor, J. A., W. Weber, L. Standish, H. Quinn, J. Goesling, M. McGann, and C. Calabrese. 2003. "Efficacy and safety of echinacea in treating upper respiratory tract infections in children: A randomized controlled trial." *Jama* 290 (21):2824–30. doi: 10.1001/jama.290.21.2824.

Thamlikitkul, V., T. Dechatiwongse, S. Theerapong et al. 1991. "Efficacy of Andrographis paniculata, Nees for pharyngotonsillitis in adults." *Journal of the Medical Association of Thailand* 74 (10):437–42.

Tognolini, M., E. Barocelli, V. Ballabeni, R. Bruni, A. Bianchi, M. Chiavarini, and M. Impicciatore. 2006. "Comparative screening of plant essential oils: Phenylpropanoid moiety as basic core for antiplatelet activity." *Life Sciences* 78 (13):1419–32. doi: 10.1016/j.lfs.2005.07.020.

Tong, M. M., P. M. Altman, and R. S. Barnetson. 1992. "Tea tree oil in the treatment of tinea pedis." *Australas J Dermatol* 33 (3):145–9.

Tong, X., D. Xiao, F. Yao, and T. Huang. 2014. "Astragalus membranaceus as a cause of increased CA19-9 and liver and kidney cysts: A case report." *Journal of Clinical Pharmacology Ther* 39 (5):561–3. doi: 10.1111/jcpt.12173.

Trill, J., C. Simpson, F. Webley et al. 2017. "Uva-ursi extract and ibuprofen as alternative treatments of adult female urinary tract infection (ATAFUTI): Study protocol for a randomised controlled trial." *Trials* 18 (1):421. doi: 10.1186/s13063-017-2145-7.

Turi, M., E. Turi, S. Koljalg, and M. Mikelsaar. 1997. "Influence of aqueous extracts of medicinal plants on surface hydrophobicity of Escherichia coli strains of different origin." *Apmis* 105 (12):956–62.

Turner, R. B., R. Bauer, K. Woelkart, T. C. Hulsey, and J. D. Gangemi. 2005. "An evaluation of Echinacea angustifolia in experimental rhinovirus infections." *New England Journal of Medicine* 353 (4):341–8. doi: 10.1056/NEJMoa044441.

Uehleke, B., J. Muller, R. Stange, O. Kelber, and J. Melzer. 2013. "Willow bark extract STW 33-I in the long-term treatment of outpatients with rheumatic pain mainly osteoarthritis or back pain." *Phytomedicine* 20 (11):980–4. doi: 10.1016/j.phymed.2013.03.023.

Van Den Broucke, C. O., and J. A. Lemli. 1983. "Spasmolytic activity of the flavonoids from Thymus vulgaris." *Pharm Weekbl Sci* 5 (1):9–14.

Vane, J. R. 2000. "The fight against rheumatism: From willow bark to COX-1 sparing drugs." *Journal of Physiology Pharmacology* 51 (4 Pt 1):573–86.

Vlachojannis, J. E., M. Cameron, and S. Chrubasik. 2010. "A systematic review on the sambuci fructus effect and efficacy profiles." *Phytother Res* 24 (1):1–8. doi: 10.1002/ptr.2729.

Wang, L., and L. V. Del Priore. 2004. "Bull's-eye maculopathy secondary to herbal toxicity from uva ursi." *American Journal of Ophthalmology* 137 (6):1135–7. doi: 10.1016/j.ajo.2004.01.004.

Wang, R. T., B. E. Shan, and Q. X. Li. 2002. "[Extracorporeal experimental study on immuno-modulatory activity of Astragalus memhranaceus extract]." *Zhongguo Zhong Xi Yi Jie He Za Zhi* 22 (6):453–6.

WHO. 2004. "Folium Uvae Ursi." WHO.int. http://apps.who.int/medicinedocs/en/d/Js4927e/32. html#Js4927e.32/ (accessed August 18, 2018).

WHO. 2016. "Influenza (seasonal)-fact sheets." WHO.int. www.who.int/mediacentre/factsheets/fs211/en/ (accessed May 24, 2017).

WHO. 2017a. "Herpes simplex virus." WHO.int. http://www.who.int/mediacentre/factsheets/fs400/en/#hsv1 (accessed May 24, 2017).

WHO. 2017b. "WHO publishes list of bacteria for which new antibiotics are urgently needed." WHO.int. http://www.who.int/mediacentre/news/releases/2017/bacteria-antibiotics-needed/en/ (accessed September 20, 2017).

Wing, D. A., P. J. Rumney, C. W. Preslicka, and J. H. Chung. 2008. "Daily cranberry juice for the prevention of asymptomatic bacteriuria in pregnancy: A randomized, controlled pilot study." *J Urol* 180 (4):1367–72. doi: 10.1016/j.juro.2008.06.016.

Woelkart, K., W. Xu, Y. Pei, A. Makriyannis, R. P. Picone, and R. Bauer. 2005. "The endocannabinoid system as a target for alkamides from Echinacea angustifolia roots." *Planta Med* 71 (8):701–5. doi: 10.1055/s-2005-871290.

Wolbling, R. H., and K. Leonhardt. 1994. "Local therapy of herpes simplex with dried extract from Melissa officinalis." *Phytomedicine* 1 (1):25–31. doi: 10.1016/s0944-7113(11)80019-x.

Wu, X., G. Cao, and R. L. Prior. 2002. "Absorption and metabolism of anthocyanins in elderly women after consumption of elderberry or blueberry." *J Nutr* 132 (7):1865–71.

Yale, S. H., and K. Liu. 2004. "Echinacea purpurea therapy for the treatment of the common cold: A randomized, double-blind, placebo-controlled clinical trial." *Arch Intern Med* 164 (11):1237–41. doi: 10.1001/archinte.164.11.1237.

Yamamoto, J., K. Yamada, A. Naemura, T. Yamashita, and R. Arai. 2005. "Testing various herbs for antithrombotic effect." *Nutrition* 21 (5):580–7. doi: 10.1016/j.nut.2004.09.016.

Zakay-Rones, Z., E. Thom, T. Wollan, and J. Wadstein. 2004. "Randomized study of the efficacy and safety of oral elderberry extract in the treatment of influenza A and B virus infections." *J Int Med Res* 32 (2):132–40. doi: 10.1177/147323000403200205.

Zakay-Rones, Z., N. Varsano, M. Zlotnik, O. Manor, L. Regev, M. Schlesinger, and M. Mumcuoglu. 1995. "Inhibition of several strains of influenza virus in vitro and reduction of symptoms by an elderberry extract (Sambucus nigra L.) during an outbreak of influenza B Panama." *J Altern Complement Med* 1 (4):361–9. doi: 10.1089/acm.1995.1.361.

Zava, D. T., C. M. Dollbaum, and M. Blen. 1998. "Estrogen and progestin bioactivity of foods, herbs, and spices." *Proc Soc Exp Biol Med* 217 (3):369–78.

Zhang, C., M. Kuroyangi, and B. K. Tan. 1998. "Cardiovascular activity of 14-deoxy-11,12-didehydroandrographolide in the anaesthetised rat and isolated right atria." *Pharmacol Res* 38 (6):413–7. doi: 10.1006/phrs.1998.0373.

Zhang, L. F., W. D. Cheng, M. M. Gui, X. Y. Li, and D. F. Wei. 2012. "[Comparative study of Radix Hedyseri as sulstitute for Radix Astragali of yupingfeng oral liquid on cellular immunity in immunosuppressed mice]." *Zhong Yao Cai* 35 (2):269–73.

Zhao, H. Y., and W. Y. Fang. 1991. "Antithrombotic effects of Andrographis paniculata nees in preventing myocardial infarction." *Chin Med J (Engl)* 104 (9):770–5.

13

Dermatologic Conditions

Emily M. Ambizas and Celia P. MacDonnell

CONTENTS

13.1 Introduction

The skin is the body's largest organ accounting for almost 15% of total body weight. Consisting of the epidermis, dermis, and the subcutaneous fat layer, the skin serves as the body's first line of defense and acts as a two-way barrier. The skin works to block toxic chemicals and microbes from entering the circulation as well as shielding internal organs from mechanical damage. It also serves to maintain body fluids, prevent dehydration, and helps with thermal regulation. The integumentary system is significantly involved in the body's immune and sensory systems as well. Over the past 10 years, interest in the use of botanicals in the cosmetic industry has increased (Stallings and Lupo 2009). During this time, public attention has also been increasingly focused on options for dermatologic preparations that are "naturally occurring."

13.2 Aloe Vera

13.2.1 Background

Aloe vera, also known as *Aloe barbadensis Miller*, is a cactus-like succulent plant belonging to the Liliaceae family. Aloe vera likely originated in the upper Nile area, but it has become indigenous to dry subtropical and tropical climates, including dry regions of Asia, Europe, and the southern United States (Grindlay and Reynolds 1986). It is characterized by large, thick, stemless leaves that are lacerated and have a sharp apex and a spiny margin (Dat et al. 2012).

Aloe vera has been used for centuries for its medicinal and beauty benefits. It has been used for healing of wounds, stomach ailments, alopecia, skin irritations, and oral manifestations. The ancient Egyptians referred to aloe as "the plant of immortality." The Greeks referred to it as a universal panacea. The first authentic recording of aloe's healing properties was found on Mesopotamian clay tablets dated 2100 BCE; the first detailed descriptions of aloe's use was discovered in the Papyrus Ebers, identifying aloe as an ingredient in preparations for both internal and external ailments (Foster et al. 2011). More recently, topical aloe gel has been used for dermatological conditions including skin and wound healing. *See Chapter 7 Gastrointestinal Diseases for further discussion.*

13.2.2 Pharmacognosy

The aloe vera plant has two medicinal components including aloe vera latex or aloe juice and aloe vera gel. The yellow latex is found just beneath the outer green rind and contains anthraquinones, which contributes to aloe's laxative effect (Foster et al. 2011; Hamman 2008). Aloe vera gel, located in the parenchyma, has a water content ranging between 99% and 99.5% (Hamman 2008). The remaining 1% consists of over 75 ingredients including water-soluble and fat-soluble vitamins, minerals, enzymes, polysaccharides, and low-molecular weight substances (Hamman 2008; Atherton 1998; Choi and Chung 2003).

13.2.3 Dosing and Preparation

Aloe is available in many products in varying compositions and potencies. These products include various gels, creams, and hair products; aloe can also been found in tissues and paper products. It is also commonly used as an inactive ingredient in many nonprescription topical medications. Most preparations are derived from the internal gel of the aloe leaf and not the sap (Davis and Perez 2009).

13.2.4 Safety

The topical application of aloe vera is considered generally safe and well tolerated when used appropriately. Aloe has been associated with rash and mild skin irritations, including burning, itching, and erythema. (Cosmetic Ingredient Review Expert Panel 2007) Although rare, there have been several case reports describing hypersensitivity reactions and contact dermatitis which are most likely attributable to anthraquinone contamination of the topical preparation. (Morrow et al. 1980; Shoji 1982; Nakamura and Kotajima 1984; Hunter and Frumkin 1991; Ferreira et al. 2007; Short et al. 2014) This may be more common in individuals who have a known hypersensitivity to members of the Liliaceae family such as lilies, garlic, or onions.

13.2.5 Evidence

Aloe's potential immunomodulatory and anti-inflammatory effects suggest that it may be beneficial in wound healing (Gallagher and Gray 2003). A 2012 Cochrane review evaluated seven randomized controlled trials that included 347 subjects using aloe or aloe-derived products to determine the effectiveness of aloe in acute and chronic wound healing (Dat et al. 2012). Aloe treatments included topical creams, mucilage, gel dressings, and gels. They were applied from three times a day to every 3 days for 2–19 weeks or until wound healing occurred. The primary outcome measures included time to complete wound healing and the percentage of patients with complete wound healing. Three trials evaluated the efficacy of aloe in patients with burns. One trial compared aloe vera mucilage to silver sulfadiazine; no difference in burn healing duration was demonstrated. Another trial evaluated aloe vera cream to framycetin cream. Although not statistically significant, wound healing occurred faster, with a 12.9-day difference in favor of the aloe vera group. When used after a hemorrhoidectomy, aloe vera significantly reduced healing time when compared to placebo (RR 16.33 days, 95% CI 3.46 to 77.15).

Another systematic review evaluated four trials with a total of 371 patients (Maenthaisong et al. 2007). Treatment products included aloe vera mucilage, gauze saturated with 85% aloe vera gel, aloe vera cream and 1% aloe vera powder wrapped with Vaseline gauze with application of treatment ranging from twice daily to every 3 days. The primary outcome measure was duration of burn wound healing. The studies were combined and analyzed using weight mean differences (WMD) and confidence intervals on healing time. The summary WMD in healing time was reduced in the aloe vera group by 8.79 days when compared to the control group (p = 0.0006; 95% CI: 2.51, 15.07). *See Chapter 7 Gastrointestinal Diseases for further discussion.*

13.2.6 Clinical Application

Aloe vera is safe and generally well tolerated when used topically. There is some evidence that it may be beneficial to burn and wound healing but data is conflicting. Most published trials are not of high quality, having methodological flaws. Standardization of aloe products is lacking in studies. Until further well-designed trials with standardized products are conducted, aloe may be considered as adjunctive therapy in burn and wound healing.

13.3 Alpha-Hydroxy Acids

13.3.1 Background

Alpha hydroxy acids (AHAs) are organic carboxylic acids with one hydroxyl group attached to the α-position of the carboxyl group (Green et al. 2009; Kornhauser et al. 2010). They can be found naturally in many foods and fruits; glycolic acid occurs in sugar cane, lactic acid is found in fermented milk products and tomato juice, fermented grapes are a source of tartaric acid, apples are a source of malic acid, citric acid can be found in citrus fruits, mandelic acid occurs in bitter almonds, and ascorbic acid is widely distributed in fruits, vegetables, and other plants (Babilas et al. 2012; Van Scott et al. 1996). Although AHAs are present naturally, they are also synthetically produced.

The effects of AHAs on the skin have been known for centuries. It was said that the ancient Egyptians, and in particular Queen Cleopatra, bathed in spoiled donkey milk, which contains lactic acid, to help improve the appearance and texture of their skin (Clark 1996; Rajanala and Vashi 2017). The ladies of the French court also benefitted from washing their faces in spoiled wine which contains tartaric acid (Clark 1996). It wasn't until 1974 when AHAs were recognized to have significant effects on hyperkeratinization due to ichthyosis when applied topically (Van Scott and Yu 1974). Since then, AHAs, commonly lactic acid and glycolic acid, have been used to treat skin disorders such as dry skin, acne, and photoaging. In 2014, the FDA reported that glycolic acid was used in 339 formulations and lactic acid was used in 1,092 cosmetic formulations (Fiume 2017).

13.3.2 Pharmacognosy

AHAs have effects on the epidermal and dermal levels of the skin (Van Scott et al. 1996). When used topically, AHAs stimulate exfoliation of the stratum corneum by interfering with intercellular ionic bonding; calcium ion concentration in the epidermis is reduced which disrupts cellular adhesions, allowing for exfoliation to occur (Van Scott and Yu 1984; Wang 1999). The degree of exfoliation is dependent on the concentration and pH of the AHA; epidermolysis may occur at higher concentrations and low pH (Van Scott and Yu 1989). These agents also increase cutaneous hyaluronic acid affecting skin appearance, texture and function by improving the stratum corneum barrier function, increasing epidermal proliferation and thickness, and restoring hydration (Bernstein et al. 2001).

13.3.3 Dosing and Preparation

Lactic acid and glycolic acid are found in many skincare products including creams, lotions, gels, and facial peels. Typically, the AHA concentrations range from 2% to 70%. AHAs are classified as cosmetics with the exception of a 12% ammonium lactate cream/lotion, which is FDA approved for the treatment of dry, scaly skin and ichthyosis vulgaris. These products can be applied two to three times a day for management of dry skin disorders. Chemical peels are typically conducted under the supervision of a trained professional and are performed in intervals of generally 2–4 weeks (Tung et al. 2000; Sharad 2013).

13.3.4 Safety

The safety of AHAs is dependent on the concentration and pH of the preparations (Babilas et al. 2012). These agents are associated mild skin irritation, pain and erythema. At lower concentrations and higher pHs, the risk of experiencing these effects is decreased. The optimal pH for AHA-based products is between 4 and 5.5; erythema is reduced to its minimum in this range (Morganti 1996). Topical application of AHAs has been associated with increased risk of photosensitivity for the duration of use and up to one week after discontinuation (Kaidbey et al. 2003). In 2005, the FDA recommended labeling of all topical cosmetic products containing AHAs bear a statement conveying the risk of increased sun sensitivity and the importance of using sunscreen and protective clothing. The Cosmetic Ingredient Review Expert Panel concluded that products containing an AHA concentration of 10% or less, a pH of 3.5 or greater, and formulated to avoid photosensitivity were safe for use (Nutrition n.d.).

13.3.5 Evidence

13.3.5.1 Dry Skin

Lactic acid is effective in relieving dry skin (Kempers et al. 1998; Wehr et al. 1986). One study evaluated 20 patients with a range of dry skin conditions, including xerosis, epidermolytic hyperkeratosis, and ichthyosis (Kempers et al. 1998). Subjects applied either regular strength or extra strength AHA cream for 4 weeks to a test site. This was compared to a non-AHA moisturizer lotion applied on a control site. After 2 weeks of treatment, symptoms were reduced, and cosmetic appearance improved. These changes were significant when compared to baseline and sites treated with a non-AHA moisturizer.

13.3.5.2 Acne and Acne Scars

The efficacy of AHAs in the management of acne has been demonstrated in a few studies (Baldo et al. 2010; Abels et al. 2011). A multicenter, open-label study evaluating 248 patients with mild to moderate acne showed that an AHA-based cream applied twice daily, alone or in combination with other drug therapy for 60 days improved acne severity in 64% of patients (Baldo et al. 2010). Another study investigated the effect of an oil-in-water emulsion containing 10% glycolic acid compared to placebo (Abels et al. 2011). This double-blind, randomized trial demonstrated the clinical efficacy of this mixture. Altogether, 120 patients suffering from mild acne applied either the preparation or placebo to their facial skin once daily before bedtime for 90 days. At day 45, there was a significant improvement in the treatment group and this effect was seen throughout the 90-day study period.

Glycolic peels, also known as fruit peels, are also used in the management of acne. They are often applied in dermatologic offices. In a randomized, double-blind, placebo-controlled study, 26 patients with moderate acne were treated with 40% glycolic acid on half the face and placebo on the other half (Kaminaka et al. 2014). Patients were treated for five times at 2-week intervals. The side of the face treated with glycolic acid demonstrated a significant reduction in acne lesions, at least by 50%, compared to placebo.

In another study, 40 Asian patients with moderate to moderately severe acne were divided into two groups, Group A and Group B, and were treated with four series of a 35% and 50% glycolic peel respectively in conjunction with a 15% glycolic acid home care product (C. M. Wang et al. 1997). Significant reductions were seen in the appearance of comedones, papules, and pustules with improved skin texture and reduction in follicular pore size in all patients. Overall, patients had brighter and lighter looking skin. Consistent and repetitive use of 15% glycolic acid was needed for the improvement of acne scars and lesions. However, a single blind, placebo controlled, randomized study determined that a 70% glycolic acid peel performed every 2 weeks improved atrophic scarring as compared to a 15% glycolic acid cream used daily (Erbağci and Akçali 2000). The authors concluded that glycolic peels were effective for the management of atrophic scars, but repetitive peels were necessary to see improvements. Consistent use with a low concentration product may also have some useful effects and should be recommended to those who cannot tolerate the peeling procedure.

13.3.5.3 Photoaging

Studies have shown the positive effect AHAs have on photoaged skin (Stiller et al. 1996; Piacquadio et al. 1996; Ditre et al. 1996; Thibault et al. 1998; Newman et al. 1996). The use of glycolic acid 5%–8% cream or lactic acid 8% cream for up to 5 months showed improvements in roughness and mottled pigmentation when compared to placebo and vehicle creams (Stiller et al. 1996; Thibault et al. 1998). In a pilot study of 17 patients with severe photoaged skin, AHAs applied twice daily demonstrated a statistically significant increase in skin thickness, along with a reversal of epidermal and dermal markers of photoaging (Ditre et al. 1996). Another study compared a 50% glycolic acid peel to a vehicle gel. The application of the 50% glycolic acid once weekly for 4 weeks improved mild photoaging of the skin, including decreases in rough texture, fine wrinkling, fewer solar keratoses, and slight lightening of solar lentigines (Newman et al. 1996).

13.3.6 Clinical Application

Alpha hydroxy acids are incorporated into skincare products due to their many benefits. Studies have shown their effectiveness in reversing the signs of photoaging and dry skin. These compounds have possible effects in the management of acne. They are generally safe although risk of photosensitivity may be increased.

13.4 Arnica

13.4.1 Background

Arnica is a perennial herb belonging to the Asteraceae/Compositae family. Arnica is a native plant to the meadows and mountainous regions of Europe and western North America. It is characterized by orange-yellow daisy-like flower heads (Kouzi and Nuzum 2007).

Arnica montana, also known as mountain daisy, mountain tobacco, wolf's bane, and leopard's bane has been used as a healing agent since the Middle Ages ("Traditional and Historic Uses of Arnica" 2015). Europeans and Native Americans have used this plant to reduce the inflammation and pain associated with sprains, bruises, and wounds. It is commonly used as a homeopathic remedy for acne, bruises, sprains, muscle aches, and as a general counterirritant (Kouzi and Nuzum 2007). Topical arnica is approved by the German Commission E for the treatment of injuries, conditions as a consequence of accidents (hematomas, contusions, dislocations, edema due to fracture) and for rheumatic muscle and joint problems. The FDA has classified pure arnica as an unsafe botanical ("Final Report on the Safety Assessment of Arnica Montana Extract and Arnica Montana" 2001).

13.4.2 Pharmacognosy

The dried flower head is the most widely used portion of the plant, but the roots and rhizomes may be used as well. Sesquiterpene lactones are the active constituents with the highest levels found in the flowers and the lowest in the stem (Douglas et al. 2004). They possess anti-inflammatory, antimicrobial, analgesic, antirheumatic, and uterus-stimulating properties (Adkison et al. 2010).

13.4.3 Dosage and Preparation

The most common arnica formulation is a 1:10 hydroalcoholic extract of the flower heads, containing 92% of the active sesquiterpene lactones (Kouzi and Nuzum 2007). This tincture is diluted three to 10 times with water and applied externally. Other dosage forms include cream, ointment and gel; they contain 20%–25% arnica tincture or 15% arnica oil which is usually prepared as a 1:5 extract of the botanical in vegetable oil (Kouzi and Nuzum 2007). There is no consensus as to the topical dosing (Dinman 2007). Oral dosage forms are also available, including capsules, tablets, and pellets.

13.4.4 Safety

When used topically or in homeopathic medicine, arnica is considered generally safe due to the low concentrations present. Topical use has been associated with itching, rash, petechiae, and dry skin (Kouzi and Nuzum 2007). Many cases of contact dermatitis have also been reported (Paulsen 2002). The sesquiterpene lactones, specifically helenalin and its derivatives, are strong sensitizers and irritants (Paulsen 2002; Hausen 1978). Patients who are allergic to other members of the Asteraceae/Compositae family, including ragweed, chrysanthemums, daisies, and marigolds, should avoid arnica.

Orally, arnica can result in serious adverse effects. One case report describes toxic optic neuropathy, causing acute, bilateral and severe vision loss after the consumption of a large quantity of homeopathic Arnica-30 (Venkatramani et al. 2013). Taken internally, arnica has been known to cause cardiotoxicity, arrhythmia, tachycardia, shortness of breath, severe gastroenteritis, hepatic failure, intense muscular weakness, and death ("Final Report on the Safety Assessment of Arnica Montana Extract and Arnica Montana" 2001; Dinman 2007).

13.4.5 Evidence

13.4.5.1 Bruising

Arnica is a classic remedy for bruising and related soft tissue damage, but clinical trials have not supported its efficacy. Systematic reviews of homeopathic arnica demonstrated no benefit of arnica in preventing or treating ecchymosis when compared to placebo (Ernst and Pittler 1998; Ho et al. 2016). Other studies have indicated a potential benefit from arnica. Topical application of a 20% arnica ointment to laser-induced bruising may be more effective than placebo (Leu et al. 2010). Arnica may also be beneficial in reducing bruising associated with rhinoplasty (Simsek et al. 2016; Chaiet and Marcus 2016).

13.4.5.2 Osteoarthritis

The efficacy of topical arnica in the management of osteoarthritis (OA) was evaluated in two clinical trials. In a 6-week open multicenter trial *Arnica montana* was evaluated in 79 patients with OA of the knee (Knuesel et al. 2002). Participants applied a thin layer of *Arnica montana* gel containing 50 g of an arnica fresh plant tincture to the affected knee(s) every morning and evening for 3 weeks. Efficacy was evaluated using the Western Ontario and McMaster Universities Osteoarthritis Index (WOMAC), a validated instrument for OA. Total scores decreased at 21 days and 42 days (p < 0.0001). A statistically significant decrease in pain, stiffness, and restriction of function was also reported. Three-quarters of patients stated that they would use the *Arnica montana* gel again.

A randomized, double-blind, equivalence trial evaluated the efficacy of arnica gel compared to ibuprofen gel 5% in the treatment of OA in the fingers of 204 patients (Widrig et al. 2007). A 4 cm strip of either 5% ibuprofen gel or a 50 g/100 g (1:20 drug-to-extract ratio) arnica gel was rubbed onto the affected joints three times daily for 3 weeks. Participants were also given a preset number of acetaminophen tablets for breakthrough use. At the end of the 21 days, the two groups were similar in terms of pain and hand function improvement, demonstrating that arnica was similar to ibuprofen in the treatment of OA of the hands.

13.4.6 Clinical Application

Although arnica has been used for centuries, data supporting its use has been limited with studies having small patient populations and short durations. Topical use studies of osteoarthritis and bruising provide some support with one showing similar benefits to topical ibuprofen. With its known toxicities when orally ingested, arnica can be potentially fatal.

13.5 Calendula

13.5.1 Background

Calendula officinalis or pot marigold is a common plant belonging to the Asteraceae/Compositae family. It is an annual flower native to Asia and southern Europe. It produces large yellow or orange flowers and grows up to 60 cm in height. The name calendula is derived from the Latin word "calends," which means the first day of each month; this was when the flowers bloom. It has also been referred to as the "herb of the sun," blooming in the morning and closing in the evening (Basch et al. 2006).

The flower petals of calendula have been used medicinally since the 12th century. Its medicinal properties have been mentioned in Ayurvedic and Unani system of medicine, indicating that the leaves and flowers of the plant contain antipyretic, anti-inflammatory, antiepileptic, and antimicrobial properties (Arora et al. 2013). Traditionally it has been used to treat stomach upset, peptic ulcers, menstrual cramps, and dermatologic disorders although data is insufficient for most of these conditions. Calendula is approved by the German Commission E as a wound healing agent (Blumenthal and Busse 1998).

13.5.2 Pharmacognosy

The therapeutic activities of calendula include anti-inflammatory, antibacterial, antifungal, antioxidant, and the ability to stimulate angiogenesis (Basch et al. 2006; Pereira and Bártolo 2016). The anti-inflammatory and diuretic effects can be mostly attributed to the triterpenoids and flavonoids found in the petals of the plant (Basch et al. 2006). Other substances include steroids, carbohydrates, lipids, quinones, carotenes, essential oils, fatty acids, and minerals (Pereira and Bártolo 2016).

13.5.3 Dosing and Preparation

According to German Commission E and the European Scientific Cooperative on Phytotherapy (ESCOP), a 2%–5% ointment is commonly used (Blumenthal and Busse 1998; ESCOP 2009). Topical preparations may be applied three to four times a day as needed. A 1:1 tincture in 40% alcohol or 1:5 in 90% alcohol may be diluted to at least 1:3 with freshly boiled water for compresses (Blumenthal and Busse 1998).

13.5.4 Safety

When used topically, calendula is generally safe and well tolerated. Patients who have a known allergy or hypersensitivity to other species in the Asteraceae/Compositae family, such as ragweed, chrysanthemum, and daisy, should avoid the use of calendula (Paulsen 2002).

13.5.5 Evidence

One trial compared the effectiveness of twice daily applications of 7.5% Calendula ointment to daily applications of saline dressings in 34 patients with venous leg ulcers (Duran et al. 2005). After 3 weeks, the total surface area of the ulcer decreased by 41.7%, with seven patients achieving complete epithelization in the treatment group and by 14.5% with four patients achieving complete epithelization in the control group ($p < 0.05$).

A more recent study evaluated the therapeutic benefits of Plenusdermax® *Calendula officinalis* spray on pressure ulcer healing (Buzzi et al. 2016). This was a prospective, observational study of 41 patients with a diagnosis of pressure ulcers that have been stable in size for over 3 months. The spray was applied twice daily after cleaning the wound with sterile saline. The patients were observed every 2 weeks over a 30-week period for reduction of the wound area, infection control, types of tissue and exudate, and ulcer microbiology. Eighty-eight percent of patients achieved complete response with a mean healing time of 12 weeks with a significant reduction in odor, edema, erythema, and bacterial count observed.

13.5.6 Clinical Application

Data on the use of calendula as a wound healing agent is of lower quality. While calendula may be beneficial, evidence from well conducted human trials are needed to support its use as an effective wound healing agent.

13.6 Chamomile

13.6.1 Background

Chamomile is an annual herbaceous flowering plant belonging to the Asteraceae/Compositae family. The ancient Egyptians believed the plant to be sacred and considered it a gift from the sun god (Salamon 2004). The chamomile species originated in southern Europe, North Africa, and West Asia, where it is still grown today. It is also cultivated in many other parts of the world, including North and South America (Salamon 2004; Singh et al. 2011).

The two most common types of chamomile are German chamomile (*Matricaria chamomilla)* and Roman chamomile (*Chamaemelum nobile)*. They have similar physical appearances, chemical properties, and uses. They both have a yellow center and white petals, giving an appearance similar to daisies (Sharafzadeh and Alizadeh 2011). Traditionally, chamomile has been used for its sedative, antispasmodic, anti-inflammatory, and wound healing properties (O'Hara et al. 1998). The German Commission E has acknowledged German chamomile's benefits when used externally for inflammatory skin and mucous membrane conditions as well as bacterial skin diseases (Blumenthal and Busse 1998).

13.6.2 Pharmacognosy

Most of chamomile's medicinal effect is determined by the essential oil content (Salamon et al. 2010). Over 120 active constituents have been identified (Mann and Staba 1986). These compounds include terpenes, phenols, flavonoids, flavones, coumarins, and polysaccharides. One of the primary active ingredients is the terpenoid α-bisabolol, an antispasmodic for intestinal smooth muscles and azulenes, including chamazulene which gives the oil its light blue color (McKay and Blumberg 2006; Sharafzadeh and Alizadeh 2011). Other components include apigenin and luteolin which possess anti-inflammatory and antispasmodic properties, the spiroethers with antifungal, antispasmodic and anti-inflammatory properties, and the coumarins herniarin and umbelliferone which possess antispasmodic, antibacterial and antifungal properties (McKay and Blumberg 2006; Sharafzadeh and Alizadeh 2011). Apigenin may also produce a mild sedative effect.

13.6.3 Dosing and Preparation

Chamomile is used in a variety of preparations. In the United States, it is commonly used as a tea or compress (O'Hara et al. 1998). Externally it can be used as a bath additive, as an inhalant, a poultice, and rinse. As a bath additive it may provide relief from anogenital inflammation at a dose of 50 g per liter of hot water (WHO Monographs on Selected Medicinal Plants; Blumenthal and Busse 1998). As an inhalant, 6 grams of chamomile or 0.8 g of alcoholic extract per liter of hot water is mixed and inhaled to relieve anxiety and general depression (WHO Monographs on Selected Medicinal Plants; Blumenthal and Busse 1998). Research also suggests dissolving 13–39 mL of a German chamomile product (Kneipp Kamillen-Konzentrat) in one liter of hot water and inhale the steam for 10 minutes (Saller et al. 1990).

For compresses, rinses and gargles, 3%–10% w/v infusion or 1% fluid extract or 5% tinctures are used (WHO Monographs on Selected Medicinal Plants; Blumenthal and Busse 1998). A commercially available cream, Kamillosan®, containing 2% ethanolic extract of German chamomile flowers is available, applied up to three times a day for 4 weeks for eczema (Patzelt-Wenczler and Ponce-Pöschl 2000; Aertgeerts et al. 1985). In addition, a topical German chamomile product (Kamille Spitzner) applied three times daily for up to 14 days has been used for wound healing (Glowania et al. 1987).

13.6.4 Safety

Contact dermatitis or irritation has been reported with the use of chamomile (Denizli et al., n.d.; Pereira et al. 1997). The content of sensitizing sesquiterpene lactones such as anthecotulide is important. (Paulsen 2002) Other possible allergens include the coumarins and bisabolol (Paulsen et al. 2010; Wilkinson et al. 1995). Only a low percentage of patients who are Asteraceae/Compositae-sensitive will develop dermatitis from chamomile (Paulsen 2002). Chamomile is on the generally recognized as safe (GRAS) list (FDA n.d.). Some allergic reactions may be due to contamination by "dog chamomile" (*Anthemis cotula*), a highly allergenic plant that is similar in appearance to chamomile (Paulsen 2002).

13.6.5 Evidence

13.6.5.1 Eczema

A cream containing chamomile extract (Kamillosan®) from German chamomile of the Manzana type improved pruritus, erythema, and desquamation in a partially double-blind, randomized trial carried out as a half-size comparison (Patzelt-Wenczler and Ponce-Pöschl 2000). Kamillosan® cream was compared to 0.5% hydrocortisone cream and placebo in patients with medium-degree atopic eczema. After a two-week treatment period, this cream demonstrated a modest superiority over hydrocortisone and a marginal difference compared to placebo.

13.6.5.2 Wound Healing

Chamomile's effect on wound healing was evaluated in a double-blind trial evaluating 14 patients who underwent dermabrasion of tattoos (Glowania et al. 1987). Chamomile produced wound drying and speeding epithelialization. Wound size was reduced by day 4 of treatment compared to placebo although healing was similar after 18 days. *See Chapter 12 Psychiatric Conditions for further discussion.*

13.6.6 Clinical Application

Limited data is available to support chamomile's use in the management of eczema and wound healing. Although generally safe, the potential for allergic reactions exists.

13.7 Echinacea

13.7.1 Background

See Chapter 12 Botanicals for Common Infections.

13.7.2 Pharmacognosy

See Chapter 12 Botanicals for Common Infections.

13.7.3 Dosing and Preparation

See Chapter 12 Botanicals for Common Infections.

13.7.4 Safety

See Chapter 12 Botanicals for Common Infections.

13.7.5 Evidence

Echinacea's effectiveness in the treatment of warts is due to its immunomodulating effects. One study compared conventional standard therapy consisting of salicylic acid and lactic acid or liquid nitrogen cryotherapy to the combination of standard therapy with an oral supplement containing echinacea, methionine, zinc, probiotics, antioxidants, and immunostimulants (Cassano et al. 2011). After 6 months of therapy, the combination group had a lower number of warts compared to standard therapy alone. Remission was achieved in 86% of patients in the combination group compared to 54% in the control group (p < 0.001). Another study suggested taking 600 mg of echinacea for 3 months provided no advantage over placebo in treating common and plane warts (Zedan et al. 2009).

13.7.6 Clinical Application

Echinacea should not be routinely recommended for the treatment of warts as data on its efficacy is insufficient at this time.

13.8 Lemon Balm

See Chapters 6 Endocrine Disorders, 11 Pyschiatric Conditions, and 12 Botanicals for Common Infections.

13.9 Licorice Root

13.9.1 Background

Licorice root (*Glycyrrhiza glabra*.) is indigenous to southeast Europe, Turkey, and Asia. The main root, or taproot, can descend over 3 feet into the ground, sending out spiny brown and yellow rhizomes. Both roots and rhizomes, harvested ever 3–5 years, are used medicinally (Skidmore-Roth 2010). *See Chapter 7 Gastrointestinal Disease for further discussion.*

13.9.2 Pharmacognosy

The dermatologic actions of licorice are related to glycyrrhizin, isoflavonoids hispaglabridin A and B, and glabridin. The viral inhibitory action is attributed to glycyrrhizin, which increases interferon formation. The antimicrobial activity is conferred by the plant's isoflavonoids hispaglabridin A and B and glabridin (Saeedi et al. 2003).

13.9.3 Dosage Form and Preparation

The 1% and 2% gel should be applied to the affected area three times daily for 2 weeks.

13.9.4 Safety

See Chapter 7 *Gastrointestinal Disease.*

13.9.5 Evidence

Gel preparations containing both 1% and 2% glycyrrhizinic acid were used in a double-blind clinical trial. Sixty patients (30 in each group) treated fortwo weeks, after which they were evaluated for erythema, edema, and itching. Both preparations reduced the markers, however the 2% preparation showed a greater reduction in scores (Saeedi et al. 2003).

Glycyrrhiza glabra, along with its anti-inflammatory properties, has also demonstrated its effectiveness in the treatment of acne. Studies report a similar antibacterial effect against *P. acnes* as erythromycin, although bacterial resistance to the botanical formulation does not occur (Nam et al. 2003, Nasri et al. 2015).

Licorice root has been studied to treat melasma. When used topically, licorice extract inhibits the production of melanocytes. In a comparative trial with hydroquinone, a significant improvement occurred in patients treated with a combination of licorice, emblica, and belides extracts (Costa et al. 2010, Fisk et al. 2014). *See Chapters 7 Gastrointestinal Disease and 11 Psychiatric Conditions for further discussion.*

13.9.6 Clinical Application

Data is generally limited for dermatologic conditions. Topical licorice extract may have efficacy in treating acne, though has not been compared to other treatments.

13.10 Marshmallow

13.10.1 Background

Marshmallow (*Althaea officinalis*) native to Europe is now cultivated in Poland. The large leaves of the plant have a similarity to Maple leaves and the roots are yellow, thick and elongated (Skidmore-Roth 2010). Topically, marshmallow has some value when used to treat minor skin conditions (Skidmore-Roth 2010).

13.10.2 Pharmacognosy

The extract of the root of marshmallow stimulates phagocytosis and the release of leukotrienes and cytokines resulting in potential anti-inflammatory activity (Dawid-Pać 2013).

13.10.3 Dosage and Preparation

The root is dried, pulverized, and generally compounded with other botanical extracts for the treatment of abscesses, atopic dermatitis, and inflammation (Zerehsaz et al. 1999, Cravotto et al. 2010).

13.10.4 Safety

Safety data on the topical use of marshmallow is not available.

13.10.5 Evidence

Limited evidence on the efficacy of marshmallow for minor irritations has been published. An ointment formulation containing a 20% extract of marshmallow root demonstrated a moderate reduction in irritation caused by ultraviolet radiation (Dawid-Pać 2013). When combined in an ointment also containing 0.05% dexamethasone, the anti-inflammatory activity increases. It can also be used locally, applied as a warm poultice for furunculosis. (ESCOP 2009)

13.10.6 Clinical Application

Topical marshmallow root has demonstrated anti-inflammatory effects though clinical data on use is limited. Safety of topical marshamallow root is unknown.

13.11 Papain

13.11.1 Background

Papain is an enzyme that is found in the fluid from papaya pulp. The proteolytic enzyme is released when the papaya plant is damaged. It grows naturally in Mexico, Central America, and other tropical regions (Skidmore-Roth 2010). Papain is commonly identified as a medicinal fruit. It contains a mixture of enzymes known as "vegetable pepsin" due to the similarity of the proteolytic enzymes it contains with pepsin. Orally it has been used to treat intestinal parasites (Alum et al. 2010).

13.11.2 Pharmacognosy

Papain is developed as a dried, purified latex that is obtained from the unripe fruit of *Carica papaya*. It is used topically to treat wounds as the enzyme released contains cysteine proteinases, which degrades proteins, and when combined with other agents is reported to have positive effects on wound healing. It can also be combined with bromelain, a plant enzyme extracted from the juice of macerated pineapple.

13.11.3 Dosage and Preparation

Papain is combined with urea commercially, in a 10% hydrophilic ointment base for topical use. When this combination is used for wound debridement, it is applied directly to the damaged area of the skin and covered, one or two times daily (Alvarez et al. 2002).

13.11.4 Safety

Papain is generally well tolerated. A transient stinging sensation has been reported upon application.

13.11.5 Evidence

Papain has been studied in children for burn treatment, in which the pulp was mashed and applied directly to full thickness (formerly known as third-degree) burns. The overall effect was debridement of the wound, and increased granulation of the wound site allowing for skin grafting (Starley et al. 1999). Papain has also been used for debridement of pressure ulcers. A 4-week study compared the use of collagenase with a combination papain-urea product in patients with pressure ulcers. The papain- urea group had a clinically significant greater degree of granulation of the wound (Alvarez et al. 2002). It should be noted that papain is often combined with other proteolytic enzymes. In this case it was combined with urea which is also a keratolytic.

13.11.6 Clinical Application

Topical application of papain is well tolerated. A combination of papain and urea has been effectively used for the debridement of wounds. Data comparing to current treatment protocols is lacking.

13.12 Rhubarb

13.12.1 Background

While used for centuries in China for centuries, the rhubarb plant (*Rheum officinale, Rheum Emodi*) was reportedly brought to Europe by Marco Polo, via the "Silk Road" (DerMarderosian 2014). The plant gained acceptance as a medicinal throughout Europe in the 1700s, prompting the British East India Company to set up the *Rhubarb Commission*, allowing them to import the best root at a fixed price (Malik et al. 2016).

13.12.2 Pharmacognosy

The roots contain anthraquinone derivatives, flavonoids, oxalic acid and sennosides, which are responsible for its effect on gastrointestinal motility (Malik et al. 2016). Rhubarb also contains tannins which have been shown to be useful in treating dermatitis caused by leaking and coagulation of surface proteins on inflamed skin. Tannins in Chinese rhubarb reportedly decrease cell permeability and secretions (Bedi and Shenefelt 2002).

13.12.3 Dosage and Preparation

The prepared cream containing 23 mg/gram each of rhubarb extract and sage extract is applied every 2–4 hours while awake. The treatment should start within one day of the appearance of symptoms and continue for 10–14 days for cold sores (Saller et al. 2004).

13.12.4 Safety

The leaves of the rhubarb plant contain oxalic acid and irritant contact dermatitis has been reported (Malik et al. 2016).

13.12.5 Evidence

A double blind, randomized trial of 145 patients compared the efficacy of a compound containing rhubarb and sage extracts with acyclovir cream (50 mg/gm) as the control for treatment of herpes simplex virus 1 (HSV1) infection. The mean time to healing with the acyclovir group was 6.7 days and 7.6 days with rhubarb/sage treatment (Saller et al. 2004).

13.12.6 Clinical Application

The use of rhubarb as a topical agent has not extensively been studied. Rhubarb's tannins have astringent properties, and because of reported antimicrobial and antiviral activity, it may have a role in treatment of acne and HSV1.

13.13 St. John's Wort

13.13.1 Background

St. John's wort (*Hypericum perforatum*) is found in both sunny and partially shaded areas around the world. The distinctive flowers whose petals are yellow with black rims are dried along with their leaves and used for medicinal purposes. Its active constituents include volatile oils and flavonoids, as well as anthraquinones (Bongiorno and Murray 2013). Topical St. John's wort has been used in Europe for the treatment of minor wounds, ulcers, abrasions, sunburns, and contusions (Wölfle et al. 2014).

13.13.2 Pharmacognosy

Hypericum perforatum extracts possess antibacterial activity against both gram positive and gram negative bacteria including *Staphylococcus aureus* and *Escherichia coli* (Schempp et al. 1999). Tannins from the plant also have astringent activity, which may be responsible for wound healing.

13.13.3 Dosage and Preparation

Formulations for external application come as a cream, oil and tincture, although no standard dosage form is recommended. Both 5% cream and oil extracts have been used two to three times daily for up to 4 weeks. Longer treatment increases the risk of adverse effects and drug interactions (Wölfle et al. 2014).

13.13.4 Safety

St. John's wort is well recognized to cause multiple serious drug interactions, although it is likely to be rare with topical use. Topical application can cause photosensitivity and excessive sun exposure should be avoided. *See Chapters 2 Pharmacokinetic and Pharmacogenomic Considerations and 11 Psychiatric Disorders for further discussion.*

13.13.5 Evidence

St. John's wort has been studied in a double-blind, placebo-controlled trial of atopic dermatitis of 21 patients with mild to moderate disease. The patients served as their own control. They were randomized to application of the placebo treatment to lesions affecting one side of the body, and the hyperforin cream to lesions on the opposite side. The patients" disease severity was evaluated by means of a clinical Severity of Atopic Dermatitis (SCORAD) assessment tool which allowed for an objective measurement of disease (Schäfer et al. 1997). The indices, or measurement of the severity of the lesions, were reported on days 7, 14, and 28. Significant improvement was observed in the treated areas. The hyperforin extract showed excellent skin tolerability, increased hydration to the area, and decreased scaliness (Schempp et al. 2003).

Another study compared a topical formulation containing copper sulfate and St. John's wort, to topical acyclovir for the treatment of HSV1 and HSV2. The study was designed to assess efficacy and tolerability. The product containing the St. John's wort showed no adverse effects and was beneficial in treating the symptoms such as pain and erythema, related to HSV 1 and 2 (Clewell et al. 2012). *See Chapters 11 Psychiatric Disorders and 15 Obesity and Weight Loss for further discussion.*

13.13.6 Clinical Application

Evidence suggests some benefits from topical St. John's wort in atopic dermatitis and HSV1 and 2. Unlike oral St. John's wort, drug interactions and safety would be expected to be less likely with the topical formulation.

13.14 Tea Tree Oil

13.14.1 Background

See Chapter 12 Botanicals for Common Infections.

13.14.2 Pharmacognosy

See Chapter 12 Botanicals for Common Infections.

13.14.3 Dosage and Preparation

As a nasal cream, 4%–10% can be applied three times daily for 5 days. For use as a body wash, use 5% use daily for 5 days. A 5% gel applied for 20 minutes then wash off, twice daily for the treatment of acne vulgaris. For the treatment of onychomycosis, 100% tea tree oil should be applied to the nail daily for 6 months. Tinea pedis treatment 25%–50% tea tree oil applied daily for 4 weeks. (Carson et al. 2006)

13.14.4 Safety

Tea tree oil should only be used topically. Contact dermatitis have been reported with tea tree oil, with one study indicating that almost 100 allergic patients have been described in the literature (deGroot and Schmidt 2016). Ascaridole, terpinolene, and alpha-terpinene among others are major sensitizers in tea tree oil (deGroot and Schmidt 2016).

13.14.5 Evidence

The use of tea tree oil as an antibacterial agent, in particular against *P acnes,* has long been established. A comparison trial evaluated 5% tea tree oil gel to 5% benzoyl peroxide lotion, which was the preferred treatment at the time. They compared efficacy and tolerance of each treatment in 124 patients with mild to moderate acne. While both agents were equally effective in improving lesions, the tea tree oil had a slower onset of action (Bassett et al. 1990). Other studies supporting the use of tea tree oil for mild to moderate acne have been published (Walton et al. 2004; Malhi et al. 2016).

More recently a worldwide epidemic of skin diseases caused by ectoparasites such as *Scaroptes scabiei (scabies)* has prompted researchers to evaluate tea tree oil for this purpose. The studies have demonstrated a reduction in mite survival time with tea tree oil (Walton et al. 2004; Thomas et al. 2016).

Tea tree oil has also been studied for use against HSV 2. Participants with recurrent herpes labialis applied 6% tea tree oil gel to the affected areas. The tea tree oil appeared not only to penetrate the skin but the epithelial cells as well, blocking viral replication. The tea tree oil group reported similar reductions in lesions as those produced by other topical therapies (Koch et al. 2008). *See Chapter 12 Botanicals for Common Infections for further discussion.*

13.14.6 Clinical Application

Tea tree oil has demonstrated efficacy in treating various skin diseases and may be less expensive and more readily available to the public. It is commonly found in many topical preparations for acne and has potential use in the treatment of mild to moderate acne. Dermatitis may occur with higher concentrations.

13.15 Witch Hazel

13.15.1 Background

Witch hazel (*Hamamelis virginiana*) comes from a deciduous shrub. The plant originated in Japan and China, but now grows throughout the continental United States and Canada, as well as central and southern Europe. The seedpods, when ripe, do not drop but explode, scattering them a greater distance. The bark of the shrub and seedpods can be made into a decoction from 5–10 g of the botanical in a cup of warm water and then strained (Bedi and Shenefelt 2002).

Witch hazel is used traditionally for the topical treatment for skin disorders including hemorrhoids, burns, diaper rash and symptomatic relief of itching and minor irritations. (Brown and Dattner 1998).

13.15.2 Pharmacognosy

The therapeutic properties of topical witch hazel are due to a shared effect with other tannins. Tannins are effective in the treatment of dermatitis by fusing cell surface proteins, which results in a reduction of secretions and cell permeability. The coagulated proteins form a protective layer on the skin (Brown and Dattner 1998).

13.15.3 Dosage and Preparations

Topical witch hazel is used as an astringent, wet dressing, ointment, suppository and gel. Over-the-counter distilled witch hazel extract is available in the United States and contains virtually no tannins. As such, it does not act as an astringent (Awang 2009). It is available as a solution and wipes, as well as an ingredient in hemorrhoidal creams and suppositories. Witch hazel bark can be prepared as a decoction from 5–10 g of bark in 1 cup of water.

13.15.4 Safety

Witch hazel is considered safe to use topically.

13.15.5 Evidence

The role of witch hazel in the treatment of atopic dermatitis had been limited to its use as an astringent. Due to the disease related suppression of the immune system of patients with atopic dermatitis, more than 90% demonstrate bacterial colonization of the skin with *S. aureus* (Bieber 2008). In one small study, the antimicrobial effect of a topical formulation containing distillate of witch hazel combined with urea for patients with atopic dermatitis. The formulation demonstrated significant antimicrobial activity when applied to 15 healthy volunteers (Gloor et al. 2002). This formulation was not effective for moderately severe disease and should therefore be recommended only for mild forms of the disease.

13.15.6 Clinical Application

Witch hazel is an effective topical anti-inflammatory agent. It also has established hydrating properties and works as a barrier-stabilizing agent, thus making it a possible alternative for maintenance therapy of atopic dermatitis.

13.16 Summary

Multiple botanicals have been used topically for dermatologic conditions ranging from atopic dermatitis to skin infections. The clinical evidence supporting their use is variable and much of the use is based on traditional medicine. Although generally very safe, contact dermatitis is a potential adverse effect in susceptible individuals.

REFERENCES

Abels, C., A. Kaszuba, I. Michalak, D. Werdier, U. Knie, and A. Kaszuba. 2011. "A 10% glycolic acid containing oil-in-water emulsion improves mild acne: A randomized Double-Blind Placebo-Controlled Trial." *Journal of Cosmetic Dermatology* 10(3): 202–209.

Adkison, J. D., D. W. Bauer, and T. Chang. 2010. "The effect of topical arnica on muscle pain." *The Annals of Pharmacotherapy* 44(10): 1579–1584.

Aertgeerts, P., M. Albring, F. Klaschka, T. Nasemann, R. Patzelt-Wenczler, K. Rauhut, and B. Weigl. 1985. "Comparative testing of Kamillosan cream and steroidal (0.25% hydrocortisone, 0.75% fluocortin butyl ester) and non-steroidal (5% bufexamac) dermatologic agents in maintenance therapy of eczematous diseases." *Zeitschrift Fur Hautkrankheiten* 60 (3): 270–277.

Alvarez, O. M., A. Fernandez-Obregon, R. S. Rogers, L. Bergamo, J. Masso, and M. Black. 2002. "A prospective, randomized, comparative study of collagenase and papain-urea for pressure ulcer debridement." *Wounds* 14(8): 293–301.

Alum, A., J. R. Rubino, and M. K. Ijaz. 2010. "The global war against intestinal parasites—Should we use a holistic approach?" *International Journal of Infectious Diseases* 14(9): e732–e738.

Arora, D., A. Rani, and A. Sharma. 2013. "A review on phytochemistry and ethnopharmacological aspects of genus calendula." *Pharmacognosy Reviews* 7(14): 179–187.

Atherton, P. 1998. "Aloe vera: Magic or medicine?" *Nursing Standard (Royal College of Nursing (Great Britain): 1987)* 12(41): 49–52, 54.

Awang, D. V. C. "Chapter 8." In *Tyler's Herbs if Choice The Therapeutic Use of Phytomedicinals*, 151–152. 3rd ed. Boca Raton, FL: CRC Press, 2009.

Babilas, P., U. Knie, and C. Abels. 2012. "Cosmetic and dermatologic use of alpha hydroxy acids." *Journal Der Deutschen Dermatologischen Gesellschaft = Journal of the German Society of Dermatology: JDDG* 10(7): 488–491.

Baldo, A., P. Bezzola, S. Curatolo et al. 2010. "Efficacy of an alpha-hydroxy acid (AHA)-based cream, even in monotherapy, in patients with mild-moderate acne." *Giornale Italiano Di Dermatologia E Venereologia: Organo Ufficiale, Societa Italiana Di Dermatologia E Sifilografia* 145(3): 319–322.

Basch, E., S. Bent, I. Foppa et al. 2006. "Marigold (calendula officinalis L.): An evidence-based systematic review by the natural standard research collaboration." *Journal of Herbal Pharmacotherapy* 6(3–4): 135–159.

Bassett, I. B., D. L. Pannowitz, and R. S. Barnetson. 1990. "A comparative study of tea-tree oil versus benzoylperoxide in the treatment of acne." *Medical Journal of Australia* 153(8): 455–458.

Bedi, M. K. and P. D. Shenefelt. 2002. "Herbal therapy in dermatology." *Archives of Dermatology* 138: 232–242.

Bernstein, E. F., J. Lee, D. B. Brown, R. Yu, and E. Van Scott. 2001. "Glycolic acid treatment increases type I collagen MRNA and hyaluronic acid content of human Sskin." *Dermatologic Surgery: Official Publication for American Society for Dermatologic Surgery* 27(5): 429–433.

Bieber, T. 2008. "Mechanisms of disease: Atopic dermatitis." *New England Journal of Medicine* 358: 1483–1494.

Blumenthal, M. and W. R. Busse. *The Complete German Commission E Monographs*. Austin (Texas): American Botanical Council, 1998.

Bongiorno, P. B. and M. T. Murray. 2013. "Hypericum perforatum (St. John's Wort)." in *Textbook of Natural Medicine*, 833–841. St. Louis, MO: Elsevier/Saunders.

Brown, D. J. and A. M. Dattner. 1998. "Phytotherapeutic approaches to common dermatologic conditions." *Archives of Dermatology* 134(11): 1401–1404.

Buzzi, M., F. de Freitas, and M. de Barros Winter. 2016. "Pressure ulcer healing with plenusdermax® calendula officinalis L. extract." *Revista Brasileira De Enfermagem* 69(2): 250–257.

Carson, C. F., K. A. Hammer, and T. V. Riley. 2006. "Melaleuca alternifolia (tea tree) oil: A review of antimicrobial and other medicinal properties." *Clinical Microbiology Reviews* 19(1): 50–62.

Cassano, N., A. Ferrari, D. Fai et al. 2011. "Oral supplementation with a nutraceutical containing echinacea, methionine and antioxidant/immunostimulating compounds in patients with cutaneous viral warts." *Giornale Italiano Di Dermatologia E Venereologia: Organo Ufficiale, Societa Italiana Di Dermatologia E Sifilografia* 146(3): 191–195.

Chaiet, S. R. and B. C. Marcus. 2016. "Perioperative arnica montana for reduction of ecchymosis in rhinoplasty surgery." *Annals of Plastic Surgery* 76(5): 477–482.

Choi, S. and M.-H. Chung. 2003. "A review on the relationship between aloe vera components and their biologic effects." *Seminars in Integrative Medicine* 1(1): 53–62.

Clark, C. P. 1996. "Alpha hydroxy acids in skin care." *Clinics in Plastic Surgery* 23(1): 49–56.

Clewell, A. M. Barnes, J. R. Endres, M. Ahmed, and D. K. Ghambeer. 2012. "Efficacy and tolerability assessment of a topical formulation containing copper sulfate and hypericum perforatum on patients with herpes skin lesions." *Journal of Drugs and Dermatology* 11(2): 209–215.

Cosmetic Ingredient Review Expert Panel. 2007. "Final report on the safety assessment of aloeandongensis extract, aloe andongensis leaf juice, aloe arborescens leaf extract, aloe arborescens leaf juice, aloe arborescens leaf protoplasts, aloe barbadensis flower extract, aloe barbadensis leaf, aloe barbadensis leaf extract, aloe barbadensis leaf juice, aloe barbadensis leaf polysaccharides, aloe barbadensis leaf water, aloe ferox leaf extract, aloe ferox leaf juice, and aloe ferox leaf juice extract." *International Journal of Toxicology* 26(Suppl 2): 1–50.

Costa A., T. A. Moises, T. Cordero, C. R. Alves, and J. Marmirori. 2010. "The association of emblica, licorice, and belides is an effective alternative to hydroquinone for the clinical treatment of melasma." *An Bras of Dermatology* 85(5):613–620.

Cravotto, G., L. Boffa, L. Genzini, and D. Garella. 2010. "Phytotherapeutics: An evaluation of the potential of 1,000 plants." *Journal of Clinical Pharmacy and Therapeutics* 35(1): 11–48.

Dat, A. D., F. Poon, K. B. T. Pham, and J. Doust. 2012. "Aloe vera for treating acute and chronic wounds." *The Cochrane Database of Systematic Reviews* February 15(2): CD008762.

Dawid-Pać, R. 2013. "Medicinal plants used in treatment of inflammatory skin diseases." *Advances in Dermatology and Allergology* 3: 170–177.

Davis, S. C. and R. Perez. 2009. "Cosmeceuticals and natural products: Wound healing." *Clinics in Dermatology* 27(5): 502–506.

deGroot, A. C. and E. Schmidt. 2016. "Tea tree oil: Contact allergy and chemical composition." *Contact Dermatitis* 75(3): 129–143.

Denizli, H., M. G. Özden, F. Aydın, N. Şentürk, T. Cantürk, and A. Y. Turanlı. n.d. "Allergic contact dermatitis from chamomile plant." *Journal of Experimental and Clinical Medicine*, 26.

DerMarderosian, A. *The Review of Natural Products*. Saint Louis, MO: Clinical Drug Information, LLC, 2014.

Dinman, S. 2007. "Arnica." *Plastic Surgical Nursing: Official Journal of the American Society of Plastic and Reconstructive Surgical Nurses* 27(1): 52–53.

Ditre, C. M., T. D. Griffin, G. F. Murphy, H. Sueki, B. Telegan, W. C. Johnson, R. J. Yu, and E. J. Van Scott. 1996. "Effects of alpha-hydroxy acids on photoaged skin: A pilot clinical, histologic, and ultrastructural study." *Journal of the American Academy of Dermatology* 34(2 Pt 1): 187–195.

Douglas, J. A., B. M. Smallfield, E. J. Burgess, N. B. Perry, R. E. Anderson, M. H. Douglas, and V. LeAnne Glennie. 2004. "Sesquiterpene lactones in arnica montana: A rapid analytical method and the effects of flower maturity and simulated mechanical harvesting on quality and yield." *Planta Medica* 70(2): 166–170.

Duran, V., M. Matic, M. Jovanović, N. Mimica, Z. Gajinov, M. Poljacki, and P. Boza. 2005. "Results of the clinical examination of an ointment with marigold (calendula officinalis) extract in the treatment of venous leg ulcers." *International Journal of Tissue Reactions* 27(3): 101–106.

Erbağci, Z. and C. Akçali. 2000. "Biweekly serial glycolic acid peels vs. long-term daily use of topical low-strength glycolic acid in the treatment of atrophic acne scars." *International Journal of Dermatology* 39(10): 789–794.

Ernst, E. and M. H. Pittler. 1998. "Efficacy of homeopathic arnica: A systematic review of placebo-controlled clinical trials." *Archives of Surgery (Chicago, Ill.: 1960)* 133(11): 1187–1190.

ESCOP Monographs. *The scientific foundation for herbal medicinal products.* 2nd ed. New York: ESCOP, 2009.

Ferreira, M., M. Teixeira, E. Silva, and M. Selores. 2007. "Allergic contact dermatitis to aloe vera." *Contact Dermatitis* 57(4): 278–279.

"Final report on the safety assessment of arnica montana extract and arnica montana." 2001. *International Journal of Toxicology* 20(Suppl 2): 1–11.

Fisk, W. A., O. Agbai, H. A. Lev-Tov, and R. K. Sivamani. 2014. "The use of botanically derived agents for hyperpigmentation: A systematic review." *Journal of the American Academy of Dermatology* 70(2): 352–365.

Fiume, M. M. 2017. "Alpha hydroxy acids." *International Journal of Toxicology* 36(5_suppl2): 15S–21S.

Foster, M., D. Hunter, and S. Samman. 2011. "Evaluation of the Nutritional and Metabolic Effects of Aloe Vera." In *Herbal Medicine: Biomolecular and Clinical Aspects*, Iris F. F. (ed). Benzie and Sissi Wachtel-Galor, 2nd ed. Boca Raton (FL): CRC Press/Taylor & Francis.

Gallagher, J. and M. Gray. 2003. "Is aloe vera effective for healing chronic wounds?" *Journal of Wound, Ostomy, and Continence Nursing* 30(2): 68–71.

Gloor, M., J. Reichling, B. Wasik, and H.E. Holzgang. 2002. "Antiseptic effect of a topical dermatological formulation that contains hamamelis distillate and urea." *Complementary Medicine Research* 9(3): 153–159.

Glowania, H. J., C. Raulin, and M. Swoboda. 1987. "Effect of chamomile on wound healing--A clinical double-blind study." *Zeitschrift Fur Hautkrankheiten* 62(17): 1262, 1267–1271.

Green, B. A., R. J. Yu, and E. J. Van Scott. 2009. "Clinical and cosmeceutical uses of hydroxyacids." *Clinics in Dermatology* 27(5): 495–501.

Grindlay, D. and T. Reynolds. 1986. "The aloe vera phenomenon: A review of the properties and modern uses of the leaf parenchyma gel." *Journal of Ethnopharmacology* 16(2–3): 117–151.

Hamman, J. H. 2008. "Composition and applications of aloe vera leaf gel." *Molecules (Basel, Switzerland)* 13(8): 1599–1616.

Hausen, B. M. 1978. "Identification of the allergens of arnica montana L." *Contact Dermatitis* 4(5): 308.

Ho, D., J. Jagdeo, and H. A. Waldorf. 2016. "Is there a role for arnica and bromelain in prevention of post-procedure ecchymosis or edema? A systematic review of the literature." *Dermatologic Surgery: Official Publication for American Society for Dermatologic Surgery* 42(4): 445–463.

Hunter, D. and A. Frumkin. 1991. "Adverse reactions to vitamin E and aloe vera preparations after dermabrasion and chemical peel." *Cutis; Cutaneous Medicine for the Practitioner* 47(3): 193–196.

Kaidbey, K., B. Sutherland, P. Bennett, W. G. Wamer, C. Barton, D. Dennis, and A. Kornhauser. 2003. "Topical glycolic acid enhances photodamage by ultraviolet light." *Photodermatology, Photoimmunology and Photomedicine* 19(1): 21–27.

Kaminaka, C., M. Uede, H. Matsunaka, F. Furukawa, and Y. Yamomoto. 2014. "Clinical evaluation of glycolic acid chemical peeling in patients with acne vulgaris: A randomized, double-blind, placebo-controlled, split-face comparative study." *Dermatologic Surgery: Official Publication for American Society for Dermatologic Surgery* 40(3): 314–322.

Kempers, S., H. I. Katz, R. Wildnauer, and B. Green. 1998. "An evaluation of the effect of an alpha hydroxy acid-blend skin cream in the cosmetic improvement of symptoms of moderate to severe xerosis, epidermolytic hyperkeratosis, and ichthyosis." *Cutis; Cutaneous Medicine for the Practitioner* 61(6): 347–350.

Knuesel, O., M. Weber, and A. Suter. 2002. "Arnica montana gel in osteoarthritis of the knee: An open, multicenter clinical trial." *Advances in Therapy* 19(5): 209–218.

Koch, C., J. Reichling, J. Schneele, and P. Schnitzler. 2008. "Inhibitory effect of essential oils against herpes simplex virus type 2." *Phytomedicine* 15(1–2): 71–78.

Kornhauser, A., S. G. Coelho, and V. J. Hearing. 2010. "Applications of hydroxy acids: Classification, mechanisms, and photoactivity." *Clinical, Cosmetic and Investigational Dermatology* 3: 135–142.

Kouzi, S. A. and D. S. Nuzum. 2007. "Arnica for bruising and swelling." *American Journal of Health-System Pharmacy* 64(23): 2434–2443.

Leu, S., J. Havey, L. E. White, N. Martin, S. S. Yoo, A. W. Rademaker, and M. Alam. 2010. "Accelerated resolution of laser-induced bruising with topical 20% arnica: A rater-blinded randomized controlled trial." *The British Journal of Dermatology* 163(3): 557–563.

Maenthaisong, R., N. Chaiyakunapruk, S. Niruntraporn, and C. Kongkaew. 2007. "The efficacy of aloe vera used for burn wound healing: A systematic review." *Burns: Journal of the International Society for Burn Injuries* 33(6): 713–718.

Malhi, H. K., J. Tu, T. V. Riley, S. P. Kumarasinghe, and K. A. Hammer. 2016. "Tea tree oil gel for mild to moderate acne: A 12-week uncontrolled, open-label phase II pilot study." *Australasian Journal of Dermatology* 58(3): 205–210.

Malik, M. A., S. A. Bhat, B. Fatima, S. B. Ahmad, S. Sidiqui, and P. Shrivastava. 2016. "Rheum emodi as a valuable medicinal plant." *International Journal of General Medicine and Pharmacy* 5(4): 35–44.

Mann, C., and E. J. Staba. 1986. "The Chemistry, Pharmacology, and Commercial Formulation in Chamomile." In *Herbs, Spices, and Medicinal Plants: Recent Advances in Botany, Horticulture, and Pharmacology*, 1:235–280. Phoenix: Oryx Press.

McKay, D. L. and J. B. Blumberg. 2006. "A review of the bioactivity and potential health benefits of chamomile tea (matricaria recutita L.)." *Phytotherapy Research: PTR* 20(7): 519–530.

Morganti, P. 1996. "Alpha hydroxy acids in cosmetic dermatology." *Journal of Applied Cosmetology* 14(2): 35–41.

Morrow, D. M., M. J. Rapaport, and R. A. Strick. 1980. "Hypersensitivity to aloe." *Archives of Dermatology* 116(9): 1064–1065.

Nakamura, T. and S. Kotajima. 1984. "Contact dermatitis from aloe arborescens." *Contact Dermatitis* 11(1): 51.

Nam, C., S. Kim, Y. Sim, and I. Chang. 2003. "Anti-acne effects of oriental herb extracts: A novel screening method to select anti-acne agents." *Skin Pharmacology and Physiology* 16(2): 84–90.

Nasri, H., M. Bahmani, N. Shahinfard, A. M. Nafchi, S. Saberianpour, and M. R. Kopaei. 2015. "Medicinal plants for the treatment of acne vulgaris: A review of recent evidences." *Jundishapur Journal of Microbiology* 8(11): e25580.

Newman, N., A. Newman, L. S. Moy, R. Babapour, A. G. Harris, and R. L. Moy. 1996. "Clinical improvement of photoaged skin with 50% glycolic acid. A double-blind vehicle-controlled study." *Dermatologic Surgery: Official Publication for American Society for Dermatologic Surgery* 22(5): 455–e25460.

Nutrition, Center for Food Safety and Applied. n.d. "Ingredients—Alpha Hydroxy Acids." WebContent. Accessed April 25, 2018. https://www.fda.gov/Cosmetics/ProductsIngredients/Ingredients/ucm107940.htm.

O'Hara, M., D. Kiefer, K. Farrell, and K. Kemper. 1998. "A review of 12 commonly used medicinal herbs." *Archives of Family Medicine* 7(6): 523–536.

Patzelt-Wenczler, R. and E. Ponce-Pöschl. 2000. "Proof of efficacy of kamillosan cream in atopic eczema." *European Journal of Medical Research* 5(4): 171–175.

Paulsen, E. 2002. "Contact sensitization from compositae-containing herbal remedies and cosmetics." *Contact Dermatitis* 47(4): 189–198.

Paulsen, E., A. Otkjaer, and K. E. Andersen. 2010. "The coumarin herniarin as a sensitizer in german chamomile [chamomilla recutita (L.) rauschert, compositae]." *Contact Dermatitis* 62(6): 338–342.

Pereira, F., R. Santos, and A. Pereira. 1997. "Contact dermatitis from chamomile tea." *Contact Dermatitis* 36(6): 307.

Pereira, R. F. and P. J. Bártolo. 2016. "Traditional therapies for skin wound healing." *Advances in Wound Care* 5(5): 208–229.

Piacquadio, D., M. Dobry, S. Hunt, C. Andree, G. Grove, and K. A. Hollenbach. 1996. "Short contact 70% glycolic acid peels as a treatment for photodamaged skin. A pilot study." *Dermatologic Surgery: Official Publication for American Society for Dermatologic Surgery* 22(5): 449–452.

Rajanala, S. and N. A. Vashi. 2017. "Cleopatra and sour milk—The ancient practice of chemical peeling." *JAMA Dermatology* 153(10): 1006.

Saeedi, M., K. Morteza-Semnani, and M.-R. Ghoreishi. 2003. "The treatment of atopic dermatitis with licorice gel." *Journal of Dermatological Treatment* 14(3): 153–157.

Salamon, I. 2004. "The slovak gene pool of german chamomile (matricaria recutita L.) and comparison in its parameters." *Horticultural Science* 31(2): 70–75.

Salamon, I., M. Ghanavati and H. Khazaei. 2010. "Chamomile biodiversity and essential oil qualitative-quantitativecharacteristics in egyptian production and iranian landraces." *Emirates Journal of Food and Agriculture* 22(1): 59–64.

Saller, R., M. Beschorner, D. Hellenbrecht, and M. Bühring. 1990. "Dose-dependancy of symptomatic relief of complaints by chamomile steam inhalation in patients with common cold." *European Journal of Pharmacology* 183(3): 728–729.

Saller, R., S. Büechi, R. Meyrat, and C. Schmidhauser. 2004. "Combined herbal preparation for ttopical treatment of herpes labialis." *Forschende Komplementärmedizin / Research in Complementary Medicine* 8(6): 373–382.

Schäfer, T., D. Dockery, U. Krämer, H. Behrendt, and J. Ring. 1997. "Severity scoring of atopic dermatitis (SCORAD)." *Allergo Journal* 6(8): 410.

Schempp, C., K. Pelz, A. Wittmer, E. Schöpf, and J. C. Simon. 1999. "Antibacterial activity of hyperforin from St. John's wort, against multiresistant staphylococcus aureus and gram-positive bacteria." *The Lancet* 353(9170): 2129.

Schempp, C. M., T. Windeck, S. Hezel, and J. C. Simon. 2003. "Topical treatment of atopic dermatitis with St. John's wort cream – a randomized, placebo controlled, double blind half-side comparison." *Phytomedicine* 10: 31–437.

Sharad, J. 2013. "Glycolic acid peel therapy – A current review." *Clinical, Cosmetic and Investigational Dermatology* 6(November): 281–288.

Sharafzadeh, S. and O. Alizadeh. 2011. "German and roman chamomile." *Journal of Applied Pharmaceutical Science* 1(10): 1–5.

Shoji, A. 1982. "Contact dermatitis to aloe arborescens." *Contact Dermatitis* 8(3): 164–167.

Short, J., A. Ehrlich, and K. Dodds. 2014. "Aloe vera gel as a culprit of allergic contact dermatitis: A case report." *Journal of the American Academy of Dermatology* 70(5): AB67.

Simsek, G., E. Sari, R. Kilic, and N. B. Muluk. 2016. "Topical application of arnica and mucopolysaccharide polysulfate attenuates periorbital edema and ecchymosis in open rhinoplasty: A randomized controlled clinical study." *Plastic and Reconstructive Surgery* 137(3): 530e–535e.

Singh, O., Z. Khanam, N. Misra, and M. K. Srivastava. 2011. "Chamomile (matricaria chamomilla L.): An overview." *Pharmacognosy Reviews* 5(9): 82–95.

Skidmore-Roth, L. *Mosby Elsevier.* 4th ed. St. Louis, MO: Mosby Elsevier, 2010.

Stallings, A. F. and M. P. Lupo. 2009. "Practical uses of botanicals in skin care." *J Clin Aesthet Dermatol* 2(1): 36–40.

Starley, I. F., P. Mohammed, G. Schneider, and S. W. Bickler. 1999. "The treatment of paediatric burns using topical papaya." *Burns* 25(7): 636–639.

Stiller, M. J., J. Bartolone, R. Stern, S. Smith, N. Kollias, R. Gillies, and L. A. Drake. 1996. "Topical 8% glycolic acid and 8% L-lactic acid creams for the treatment of photodamaged skin. A double-blind vehicle-controlled clinical trial." *Archives of Dermatology* 132(6): 631–636.

Thibault, P. K., J. Wlodarczyk, and A. Wenck. 1998. "A Double-blind randomized clinical trial on the effectiveness of a daily glycolic acid 5% formulation in the treatment of photoaging." *Dermatologic Surgery: Official Publication for American Society for Dermatologic Surgery* 24(5): 573–577; discussion 577–578.

Thomas, J., C. F. Carson, G. M. Peterson et al. 2016. "Therapeutic potential of tea tree oil for scabies." *American Journal of Tropical Medicine and Hygiene* 94(2): 258–266.

"Traditional and Historic Uses of Arnica." 2015. *Arnica.Com* (blog). July 18, 2015. http://www.arnica.com/about-arnica/arnicas-humble-beginnings/.

Tung, R. C., W. F. Bergfeld, A. T. Vidimos, and B. K. Remzi. 2000. "Alpha-hydroxy acid-based cosmetic procedures. Guidelines for patient management." *American Journal of Clinical Dermatology* 1(2): 81–88.

Van Scott, E. J., C. M. Ditre, and R. J. Yu. 1996. "Alpha-hydroxyacids in the treatment of signs of photoaging." *Clinics in Dermatology* 14(2): 217–226.

Van Scott, E. J. and R. J. Yu. 1974. "Control of keratinization with alpha-hydroxy acids and related compounds. I. topical treatment of ichthyotic disorders." *Archives of Dermatology* 110(4): 586–590.

Van Scott, E. J. and R. J. Yu. 1984. "Hyperkeratinization, corneocyte cohesion, and alpha hydroxy acids." *Journal of the American Academy of Dermatology* 11(5 Pt 1): 867–879.

Van Scott, E. J. and R. J. Yu. 1989. "Alpha hydroxy acids: Procedures for use in clinical practice." *Cutis; Cutaneous Medicine for the Practitioner* 43(3): 222–228.

Venkatramani, D. V., S. Goel, V. Ratra, and R. A. Gandhi. 2013. "Toxic optic neuropathy following ingestion of homeopathic medication arnica-30." *Cutaneous and Ocular Toxicology* 32(1): 95–97.

Walton, S. F., M. Mckinnon, S. Pizzutto, A. Dougall, E. Williams, and B. J. Currie. 2004. "Acaricidal activity of melaleuca alternifolia (tea tree) oil." *Archives of Dermatology* 140(5): 563–566.

Wang, C. M., C. L. Huang, C. T. Hu, and H. L. Chan. 1997. "The effect of glycolic acid on the treatment of acne in asian skin." *Dermatologic Surgery: Official Publication for American Society for Dermatologic Surgery* 23(1): 23–29.

Wang, X. 1999. "A theory for the mechanism of action of the alpha-hydroxy acids applied to the skin." *Medical Hypotheses* 53(5): 380–382.

Wehr, R., L. Krochmal, F. Bagatell, and W. Ragsdale. 1986. "A controlled two-center study of lactate 12 percent lotion and a petrolatum-based creme in patients with xerosis." *Cutis; Cutaneous Medicine for the Practitioner* 37(3): 205–207, 209.

"WHO Monographs on Selected Medicinal Plants—Volume 1: Flos Chamomillae." n.d. Accessed August 19, 2018. http://apps.who.int/medicinedocs/en/d/Js2200e/11.html#Js2200e.11.

Widrig, R., A. Suter, R. Saller, and J. Melzer. 2007. "Choosing between NSAID and arnica for topical treatment of hand osteoarthritis in a randomised,double-blind study." *Rheumatology International* 27(6): 585–591.

Wilkinson, S. M., B. M. Hausen, and M. H. Beck. 1995. "Allergic contact dermatitis from plant extracts in a cosmetic." *Contact Dermatitis* 33(1): 58–59.

Wölfle, U., G. Seelinger, and C. Schempp. 2014. "Topical application of St. John's wort (hypericum perforatum)." *Planta Medica* 80(02/03): 109–120.

Zedan, H., E. R. M. Hofny, and S. A. Ismail. 2009. "Propolis as an alternative treatment for cutaneous warts." *International Journal of Dermatology* 48(11): 1246–1249.

Zerehsaz F., R. Salmanpour, F. Handjani, S. Ardehali, M. R. Panjehshahin, Z. S. Tabei, H. R. Tabatabaee. 1999. "A double-blind randomized clinical trial of a topical herbal extract (Z-HE) vs. systemic meglumine antimoniate for the treatment of cutaneous leishmaniasis in iran." *International Journal of Dermatology* 38(8): 610–612.

14

Musculoskeletal Conditions

Lana Gettman, Melissa Max, Christine Eisenhower, and Robin Lane Cooke

CONTENTS

14.1 Introduction

According to the World Health Organization, musculoskeletal disorders are the second leading cause of disability globally (WHO 2018). In the United States, as many people have these disorders as do individuals with cardiovascular or respiratory diseases (WHO 2018). Botanical products have been used to relieve pain, joint stiffness/immobility, and functional discomfort associated with multiple musculoskeletal conditions. This chapter will focus on the available evidence for botanicals for osteoarthritis, osteopenia, gout, and fibromyalgia.

14.2 Osteoarthritis

Osteoarthritis is a common disease associated with aging that involves the degeneration and breakdown of joint cartilage and underlying bone. The primary pathological feature of the condition is progressive loss of articular cartilage that results in remodeling of subchondral bone. This leads to whole joint failure with deterioration in joint structures that can include cartilage, bone, muscle, synovial, and the joint capsule. Risk factors for osteoarthritis include age, sex, and genetic factors. Assessments of the potential efficacy of both drugs and botanicals should ideally be made using standard instruments such as the Western Ontario and McMaster Universities Osteoarthritis Index (WOMAC). The WOMAC tool includes 24 items that assess pain, joint stiffness, and physical function. A visual analogue (WOMAC-VAS) version also exists, with a larger range of points.

14.2.1 Avocado-Soybean Unsaponifiables (ASU)

14.2.1.1 Background

Avocado-soybean unsaponifiables (ASU) have been used in patients with knee and/or hip osteoarthritis to reduce pain and joint stiffness, and as a means of reducing the need for analgesics. ASU exhibits its major biological activity through its sterol components and is believed to have chondroprotective effects (Christiansen et al. 2015).

14.2.1.2 Pharmacognosy

In vitro studies of ASU have demonstrated stimulatory effects on collagen synthesis, collagen II mRNA, aggrecan proteoglycan, transforming growth factor-beta 3, and osteocalcin. Radiographic evaluation has suggested delayed destruction of joints. In vitro studies have shown inhibitory effects of ASU on inflammatory and catabolic mediators of osteoarthritis including interleukin, macrophage inhibitory proteins, matrix metalloproteinases, cyclooxygenase-2 (COX-2), alkaline phosphatase, and prostaglandin E-2 (Christiansen et al. 2015).

14.2.1.3 Preparation and Dosing

ASU is prepared from unsaponifiable natural extracts in a proportion of 1/3 avocado oil to 2/3 soybean oil. Commercially available ASU products contain phytosterols and possibly fat-soluble vitamins, green tea extract, manganese, iron, chondroitin sulfate, and/or glucosamine sulfate. Most studies evaluate the Piascledine® preparation, which is supplied internationally as 300 mg capsules. Maximize Avocado® 300 SU with SierraSil® is available from a U.S. manufacturer and contains calcium carbonate and dicalcium phosphate 168 mg/ASU 300 mg/SierraSil 600 mg per two tablets. SierraSil may contain about 1.1 mg of iron. Piascledine dosing is one 300 mg capsule by mouth daily, whereas labelling for Maximize Avocado 300 SU suggests two tablets (300 mg) by mouth three times daily (Christiansen et al. 2015).

14.2.1.4 Safety

Variability in the major sterol components of commercially available ASU products has been demonstrated (Christiansen et al. 2015). Due to patents, ASU manufacturers did not provide information regarding exact ingredients and preparation to the authors (Christiansen et al. 2015). Lack of standardization may contribute to dermatologic, hepatic, gastrointestinal, and hematologic adverse effects (Christiansen et al. 2015). However, when compared to placebo, results from four studies ranging from 3–12 months have shown no difference in adverse events, withdrawals due to adverse events, and/or serious adverse events (Cameron and Chrubasik 2014). In addition, a 6-month trial did not show a difference in adverse events with ASU versus chondroitin sulfate (Pavelka et al. 2010).

14.2.1.5 Evidence

In a 2014 Cochrane systematic review, four studies evaluating piascledine versus placebo over 3–12 months (Cameron and Chrubasik 2014). The results indicated that use of ASU 300 mg daily resulted in small improvements in pain and physical function without a significant difference in adverse events. Two studies lasting 24 and 36 months in duration evaluated change in overall joint width space from baseline with ASU versus placebo, but significant differences were not observed (Cameron and Chrubasik 2014).

Piascledine has also been compared to chondroitin sulfate in a prospective, controlled, double-blind, multinational study. Patients with knee osteoarthritis were randomized to receive piascledine 300 mg daily (n = 183) or chondroitin sulfate 400 mg three times daily (n = 178) for six months, with a two-month follow-up period. The primary outcome was change in baseline WOMAC score at 6 months. The average patient was 62 years old with a body mass index (BMI) of 28–29 kg/m² and a baseline total WOMAC-VAS score of 1,174–1,176, and had had knee osteoarthritis for more than 6 months, with pain and functional discomfort. Results were similar in both groups; WOMAC scores decreased in about 50% of patients and the daily intake of rescue analgesics decreased, with more than 80% of patients rating efficacy as excellent or good (Pavelka et al. 2010).

14.2.1.6 Clinical Application

ASU 300 mg by mouth daily may provide small improvements in pain and physical function in patients with hip or knee osteoarthritis. Adverse events are similar to placebo or chondroitin sulfate. ASU has shown efficacy similar to chondroitin sulfate with a more convenient dosing schedule.

14.2.2 Boswellia Serrata

14.2.2.1 Background

The gum resin of *Boswellia serrata* has long been used in Ayurvedic medicine for the treatment of inflammatory disorders such as arthritis (Dragos et al. 2017). It contains boswellic acids, which undergo an enrichment process and are present in varying amounts in commercially available *Boswellia serrata* products.

14.2.2.2 Pharmacognosy

The bioactivity of *Boswellia serrata* is exerted by boswellic acids, particularly acetyl-11-keto-beta boswellic acid (AKBA). In vitro studies have demonstrated inhibitory effects of *Boswellia serrata* on matrix metalloproteinases, COX-2, nitric oxide, prostaglandin E-2, and intercellular adhesion molecule 1. As a result, the inflammatory process and degradation of cartilage and collagen is reduced. A combination of *Boswellia serrata*, *Uncaria tomentosa* (cat's claw), *Lepidium meyenii* (maca), and L-leucine was shown to reduce interleukin-mediated nitric oxide production and cartilage deterioration in chondrocytes while promoting aggrecan and collagen (Dragos et al. 2017).

14.2.2.3 Preparation and Dosing

Boswellia serrata is the main active ingredient in WokVel® 333 mg capsules (40% AKBA), 5-Loxin® 125 mg capsules (30% AKBA), and Aflapin® 50 mg capsules (20% AKBA). Aflapin contains a non-volatile oil that is prepared by selective removal of boswellic acids and removal of volatiles under a high vacuum (Sengupta et al. 2010). Movardol® combination tablets contain *Boswellia serrata* (180 mg; 65% AKBA), N-acetyl-D-glucosamine (500 mg), and *Zingiber officianle* (250 mg; 8% gingerols) (Bolognesi et al. 2016).

14.2.2.4 Safety

The use of 5-Loxin 100 mg/day or 250 mg/day did not result in a significant difference in adverse events compared to placebo over 12 weeks (Cameron and Chrubasik 2014). Adverse events were not associated with Movardol in a 6-month trial, and general gastrointestinal complications were lower for patients receiving the botanical versus those who did not (−78% versus −23% at 6 months). The authors concluded that this was likely due to a significant reduction in the use of nonsteroidal anti-inflammatory drugs (NSAIDS) (Bolognesi et al. 2016).

14.2.2.5 Evidence

The 2014 Cochrane systematic review also analyzed the efficacy of *Boswellia serrata* extract products using five randomized controlled trials (Cameron and Chrubasik 2014). The WokVel product was compared to placebo in a crossover trial of 30 patients with two 8-week intervention periods. Statistically significant improvements in pain and function were demonstrated, as measured by the VAS and WOMAC. The 5-Loxin product has been compared to placebo, as well as an alternative Boswellia product, Aflapin. Pain and function were improved versus placebo with both high-dose (250 mg/day) and low-dose (100 mg/day) 5-Loxin over 12 weeks. More study participants reported improvements with the high dose, but a difference in clinical outcomes was not detected (Cameron and Chrubasik 2014).

A double-blind trial of 60 patients with symptomatic mild to moderate knee osteoarthritis compared the safety and efficacy of two *Boswellia serrata* products to placebo (Sengupta et al. 2010). Patients who were already taking a prescription dose of NSAID for at least 30 days or acetaminophen 1,200–4,000 mg/day regularly were randomized to receive 5-Loxin 50 mg twice daily (n = 20), Aflapin 50 mg twice daily (n = 20) or placebo (n = 20) for 90 days. All patients were prescribed ibuprofen 400 mg three times daily as needed for pain. Fifty-seven patients completed the trial and dropouts were only due to poor follow-up availability. Most patients were women with an average age of 51–53 years, BMI of 25 kg/m², and total baseline WOMAC score of 126.2–128.7. The results demonstrated statistically significant improvements in pain, joint stiffness, and function using the VAS and WOMAC at 90 days in all groups, but greater reductions were observed with the use of 5-Loxin and Aflapin (Sengupta et al. 2010).

The efficacy of the combination product, Movardol, plus standard osteoarthritis management versus standard management alone was evaluated in a 6-month registry study (Bolognesi et al. 2016). Details regarding standard management were not provided by the authors. Fifty-four patients with symptomatic, moderate knee osteoarthritis on x-ray were included and allowed to choose their study group. Twenty-six received Movardol in a dosage of 3 tablets daily for 1 week, then 2 tablets daily, plus standard management and 28 received standard management alone. Outcomes included changes in functional impairment as measured using the Karnofsky Performance Scale Index, pain, stiffness, and physical, social, and emotional functioning using the WOMAC score, total and pain-free walking distance, and inflammatory and oxidative stress biomarkers. Most patients were men and the average age was 52–53 years. Results showed statistically significant improvements in pain, stiffness, and physical, social, and emotional function at 1 month for patients receiving Movardol plus standard management; this was sustained at 6 months. In terms of total and pain-free walking distance, statistically significant improvements with use of the product were observed at 6 months. In addition, use of NSAIDS or other analgesics was reduced for the Movardol plus standard management group at the end of the study (−68% versus −12%, p < 0.05) (Bolognesi et al. 2016). *See Chapter 10 Neurologic Conditions for further discussion.*

14.2.2.6 Clinical Application

Despite differences in AKBA, both 5-Loxin and Aflapin formulations improve pain, joint stiffness, and physical function from knee osteoarthritis over three months without adverse events. Current evidence does not support a need for high-dose (250 mg/day) 5-Loxin over low-dose (100 mg/day). Use of the combination product Movardol may improve symptoms as early as 1 month.

14.2.3 Cat's Claw

14.2.3.1 Background

Cat's claw is a medicinal plant that refers to the Uncaria species *U. guianensis* and *U. tomentosa*. It has been widely used for centuries in South America to treat chronic inflammatory disorders including arthritis (Piscoya et al. 2001).

14.2.3.2 Pharmacognosy

U. tomentosa has been shown to inhibit peroxynitrite, UV radiation, and cytotoxicity induced by free radicals, specifically, 1,1-diphenyl-2-picrylhydrazyl (DPPH). It also inhibits nuclear factor-kappa beta and tumor necrosis factor-alpha gene expression. Free radical scavenging assay and enzyme-linked immunosorbent assay demonstrated *in vitro* equivalence between *U. tomentosa and U. guianensis* for reducing DPPH radicals and inhibiting TNF-alpha production (Piscoya et al. 2001).

14.2.3.3 Preparation and Dosing

A preparation of *U. guianensis* was produced using an aqueous extraction of cat's claw bark that was boiled for 30 minutes and decanted (Piscoya et al. 2001). The solids formed were separated by filtration and then freeze-dried. Tablets were prepared using 100 mg of freeze-dried cat's claw with excipients (Piscoya et al. 2001). The *U. guianensis* extract is also manufactured in the U.S. as Vincaria® and available in combination Reparagen® products with *Lepidium meyenii* (maca), glucosamine, and/or *Croton palanostigma*. Reparagen capsules contain Vincaria 300 mg and RNI 249 (*L. meyenii*) 1500 mg (Mehta et al. 2007).

14.2.3.4 Safety

A 4-week study of *U. guianensis* 100 mg daily versus placebo had similar adverse events. A few patients in each group reported dizziness or headache (Piscoya et al. 2001). An 8-week study comparing glucosamine to Reparagen did not report any serious adverse events, including on vital signs and/or complete blood count (Mehta et al. 2007).

14.2.3.5 Evidence

U. guianensis has been evaluated as a single agent and in combination with other anti-inflammatory botanicals. Forty-five men with symptomatic knee osteoarthritis requiring NSAIDS for at least three months prior to enrollment were randomized to receive placebo (n = 15) or one capsule daily of 100 mg freeze-dried cat's claw (*U. guianensis*) for four weeks. Patients were allowed to use acetaminophen as needed and asked to record its dosage and duration. The results demonstrated a statistically significant difference in reduction of pain between cat's claw and placebo beginning at week 1 and continuing at week 4. Small but nonsignificant reductions in pain at rest and at night were observed (Piscoya et al. 2001).

An 8-week, double-blind, multicenter study randomized patients with mild to moderate osteoarthritis to receive glucosamine sulfate 1,500 mg/day (n = 47) or Reparagen 1,800 mg/day (n = 48) (Mehta et al. 2007). The treatments were administered as two capsules by mouth twice daily before meals. Patients were allowed to take acetaminophen 1,500 mg/day for the first 4 weeks and 1,000 mg/day for the last 4 weeks as a rescue analgesic. The average patient was female and 52–55 years of age, with a total baseline WOMAC score of 47.1–50.1. Average baseline WOMAC pain scores were 8.1–8.9. The primary outcome measure was a 20% reduction in WOMAC pain and was observed in 89% of patients receiving glucosamine and 94% receiving Reparagen. Patients receiving Reparagen used less of the rescue analgesic throughout the study compared to those receiving glucosamine (Mehta et al. 2007).

Vincaria was also studied in combination with SierraSil in an 8-week, double-blind, multicenter trial in patients with mild to moderate osteoarthritis (Miller et al. 2005).

Patients were randomized to SierraSil 3 g/day (high dose), SierraSil 2 g/day (low dose), SierraSil 2 g/day plus Vincaria 100 mg/day, or placebo. Each treatment was administered as two capsules by mouth twice daily with meals. Acetaminophen 2000 mg/day was allowed as the rescue medication. Most patients were female, 50–52 years of age, and had a baseline total WOMAC score of 46.4–51.1. Starting at week 2, statistically significant improvements in pain, physical function, and total WOMAC scores were observed for the three active treatment groups. At week 4, joint stiffness was also improved in those groups. These results were sustained at week 8; however, at that time, statistically significant improvements were also observed in the placebo group (Miller et al. 2005). *See Chapter 17 Supportive and Palliative Care for Cancer for further discussion.*

14.2.3.6 Clinical Application

Cat's claw extract may provide improvements in pain, joint stiffness, and physical function for a short period of time, and could be considered an alternative to glucosamine sulfate. Studies are needed to confirm long-term efficacy and to also compare 100 mg/day of *U. guianensis* to larger doses from the Reparagen products.

14.2.4 Devil's Claw

14.2.4.1 Background

Devil's claw (*Harpagophytum procumbens*) belongs to Pedaliaceae family and is native to the Kalahari region of southern Africa. Dried and powdered tubers (root) of this plant have been used for centuries for alleviation of pain and complications during pregnancy, and also to heal sores and other skin problems. Data also exists on the clinical efficacy of its extract and crude powder to treat the inflammation and pain in rheumatoid arthritis and osteoarthritis. Laboratory studies of this plant as early as in 1950s were mainly done in Germany where *H. procumbens* is a licensed medicine (Abdelouahab and Heard 2008).

14.2.4.2 Pharmacognosy

Studies indicate that *H. procumbens* has analgesic, antioxidant, antidiabetic, anti-epileptic, antimicrobial and antimalarial activities (Mncwangi et al. 2012). Phytochemical analysis of *H. procumbens* indicates that it contains iridoid glycosides, acetylated phenolic glycosides, and terpenoids. The effects of *H. procumbens* are attributed to iridoid and phenylethanoid glycosides (harpagoside, harpagide, 8-coumaroylharpagide, verbascoside) present in the tubers of the plant. Although anti-inflammatory activity of *H. procumbens* is not clearly understood, it is proposed to inhibit arachidonic, cyclooxygenase-2, lipo-oxygenase, and thromboxane pathways (Abdelouahab and Heard 2008).

14.2.4.3 Preparation and Dosing

H. procumbens is used in the forms of infusions, decoctions, tinctures, powders, and extracts (Mncwangi et al. 2012). Current European Pharmacopeia monograph for *H. procumbens* tuber extracts requires at least 1.2% of the iridoid glycoside harpagoside, which is calculated with reference to the dried drug (Abdelouahab and Heard 2008). Extracts containing more than 50 mg/day of the active constituent, harpagoside, have shown efficacy for knee and hip osteoarthritis (Vitetta et al. 2008).

14.2.4.4 Safety

A systematic review of trials using botanicals including *Harpagophytum* preparations in osteoarthritis have reported that serious adverse events have not occurred with botanical preparation (Chrubasik et al. 2007b). However, in a study evaluating efficacy and tolerance of *Harpagophytum procumbens* in patients with osteoarthritis, diarrhea occurred in 8.1% of patients taking the botanical (Chantre et al. 2000). Harpagophytum procumbens contains bitter ingredients which stimulate secretion of gastrointestinal juices. As a result, patients may have discomfort when consuming a *Harpagophytum procumbens* product. Therefore, patients with stomach or duodenal ulcers should not use *H. procumbens* (Chantre et al. 2000, Vlachojannis et al. 2008). Due to *Harpagophytum procumbens'* ability to reduce cyclooxygenase-2 and thromboxane pathways activity, reduction in platelet activation and aggregation and thus a bleeding risk might be of concern. In addition, allergic skin reactions, dysmenorrhea, and hemodynamic instability have been observed (Chrubasik et al. 2002).

14.2.4.5 Evidence

A French double-blind, randomized controlled trial in which 50 patients with osteoarthritis were randomized to 400 mg *Harpagophytum* extract (1.5% iridoid content) or placebo at a dose of two capsules three times daily for 3 weeks demonstrated significant reduction in pain severity at 4 weeks

(Long et al. 2001). In a similar study, patients were given capsules containing 335 mg of powdered *Harpagophytum* (3% iridoid content) at a dose of two capsules three times daily for 2 months. Pain intensity was significantly decreased and spinal and coxofemoral mobility was improved in the treated group (Long et al. 2001).

A systematic review identified trials which assessed the effectiveness of *H. procumbens* for the treatment of musculoskeletal pain of diverse origin (Gagnier et al. 2004). Data on effectiveness was limited at dosages less than 30 mg harpagoside daily. Moderate evidence supported the use of *Harpagophytum* powder at 60 mg harpagoside for osteoarthritis (Gagnier et al. 2004).

14.2.4.6 Clinical Application

Evidence from several controlled trials has shown that *H. procumbens* in doses greater than 60 mg per day may be beneficial for the management of osteoarthritis and pain.

14.2.5 Ginger

14.2.5.1 Background

See Chapter 7 Gastrointestinal Disease for discussion.

14.2.5.2 Pharmacognosy

More than 400 compounds have been isolated in extracts of ginger rhizomes, with gingerols, shogaols, and paradols accounting for its anti-inflammatory properties (Grzanna et al. 2005). In vitro studies have shown that ginger extracts inhibit the activation of cyclooxygenase-2 and tumor necrosis factor alpha (White 2007). *See Chapter 7 Gastrointestinal Disease for further discussion.*

14.2.5.3 Preparation and Dosing

Most studies have used from 250 mg to 1 gram of the powdered root in a capsule form, taken 1 to 4 times per day. Rubbing ginger oil into painful joints and inhaling the fumes in steamed water have been suggested, however these techniques have not been studied (White 2007). *See Chapter 7 Gastrointestinal Disease for further discussion.*

14.2.5.4 Safety

See Chapter 7 Gastrointestinal Disease for discussion.

14.2.5.5 Evidence

Some studies have shown that ginger may be safe and effective for osteoarthritis. A randomized, double-blind, double-dummy, cross-over study of ginger extract and ibuprofen was conducted in 67 patients with knee or hip osteoarthritis (Bliddal et al. 2000). The mean age of patients was 66 years and the mean duration of the disease was 7.7 years. Prior to the start of the study, all patients had a 1-week washout period which required discontinuation of analgesics and NSAIDs. Patients were randomized to 170 mg ginger extract, 400 mg ibuprofen, or placebo administered three times a day for 3 weeks and were crossover to the other treatments. Acetaminophen up to 3 g daily was given to patients as a rescue drug for pain during washout period and for duration of the study. A visual analogue scale (VAS) was used for pain assessment, while the disease severity was evaluated using the Lequesne index (LI). In terms of efficacy, ibuprofen had greater effects than the ginger extract and placebo. A similar trend was documented for acetaminophen consumption and the LI. No significant adverse reactions were recorded (Bliddal et al. 2000).

A meta-analysis of randomized placebo-controlled trials has also evaluated the safety and efficacy of ginger (Bartels et al. 2015). Five trials including 593 patients were included and the average age of patients was between 47 and 66 years. The daily dose of ginger ranged from 500 to 1,000 mg/day. Trial durations ranged from 3–12 weeks. Most trials had adequate randomization and blinding, but their analyses were inadequate. Pain and disability were reduced with ginger, demonstrating modest efficacy (Bartels et al. 2015).

See Chapters 7 Gastrointestinal Disease and 17 Supportive and Palliative Care for Cancer for further discussion.

14.2.5.6 Clinical Application

Ginger appears to be effective in reducing osteoarthritis symptoms and potentially joint swelling (Grzanna et al. 2005). Adverse effects primarily include heartburn, diarrhea, and mouth irritation (White 2007).

14.2.6 Turmeric

14.2.6.1 Background

Turmeric, *curcumin longa* L., is a member of the Zingiberacea family like ginger. In modern time, it is a popular botanical medicine and spice for cooking with distinctive yellow coloring; however, it's culinary and religious use dates back approximately 4,000 years. Over 130 species of this perennial plant have been identified. Native to Southeast Asia, several tropical countries grow turmeric with India supplying the majority of product. Turmeric has been used to treat various health conditions, including respiratory, gastrointestinal, cardiovascular, and inflammatory diseases, cancer, and topically as an antibacterial or anti-inflammatory agent, or even sunscreen (Prasad and Aggarwal 2011).

14.2.6.2 Pharmacognosy

Curcuminoids are present in turmeric which include curcumin, demethoxycurcumin, and bidemothoxycurcumin. Curcumin, a lipophilic polyphenol, is the most prevalent (77%) and biologically active component of the curcuminoids. Curcurmin has demonstrated potential anticancer, antioxidant, and anti-inflammatory activities (Kocaadam and Şanlier 2017).

Anti-inflammatory properties contribute to curcumin's potential use in musculoskeletal conditions. It impacts activity of pro-inflammatory interleukins such as IL-1, IL-2, IL-6, IL-8, and IL-12, along with cytokines tumor necrosis factor-alpha and monocyte chemoattractant protein-1. This results in a downregulation of the signaling pathway janus kinase and signal transducer and activator of transcription (JAK/STAT). Curcurmin also may suppress NF-KB by down-regulation of other inflammatory mediators by downregulation of cyclooxygenase-2 (COX-2), inducible nitric oxide (iNOS), lipoxygenase, and xanthine oxidase (Kocaadam and Şanlier 2017).

14.2.6.3 Preparation and Dosing

To produce the final powder product, plant rhizomes are boiled and steamed, then dried and ground (Prasad and Aggarwal 2011). Bioavailability of curcurmin is low due to poor absorption, rapid metabolism, and rapid clearance from the body. Advancements in nanoformulations, such as liposomes, phospholipid complexes, microemulsions, nanoparticles, or polymer micelles, may enhance bioavailability (Liu et al. 2016) Piperine, from black pepper, paired with curcumin has demonstrated an increase in bioavailability by up to 20 times (Patil et al. 2016). Commercially available products are labeled as turmeric or curcumin, and some combine with piperine.

Fresh turmeric root dosed at 8–60 g three times a day has been recommended for treatment of arthritis (Prasad and Aggarwal 2011). Randomized clinical trials have administered approximately 1 g per day of curcumin.

14.2.6.4 Safety

Turmeric is generally recognized as safe (GRAS) and has been consumed at high doses of 12 gram per day without safety concern (Kocaadam and Şanlier 2017). Most common adverse effects association with use are GI related, including heartburn, nausea, and diarrhea. Patients taking antiplatelet or antithrombotic medications should be cautioned about an increased risk of bleeding, especially with high doses of turmeric (Ulbricht et al. 2008).

14.2.6.5 Evidence

A systematic review and meta-analysis evaluated clinical trials using turmeric/curcumin for arthritis. Included in the analysis were eight randomized controlled trials (1 rheumatoid arthritis, 7 osteoarthritis) which met criteria using assessment measures of pain visual analogue score (PVAS) or WOMAC (Daily et al. 2016). Compared to placebo, turmeric/curcumin demonstrated significant difference in PVAS ($p < 0.00001$) in three studies and no significant difference compared to NSAIDs in five studies. An overall decrease in WOMAC ($p < 0.009$) was also noted in four studies. Authors concluded approximately 1 g of curcumin per day appears to be efficacious in the treatment of arthritis symptoms, though results are limited by the number of studies and participants, as well as overall quality (Daily et al. 2016).

Combined with boswella, curcumin been studied for osteoarthritis symptoms compared to curcumin alone and placebo in a parallel group, double-blind, randomized trial with 201 subjects. Curamin® 500 mg capsules, a combination of 350 mg curcuminoids and 150 mg boswellic acid, or Curamed® 500 mg capsules, consisting of 333 mg curcuminoids, were administered over 12 weeks, along with a placebo group. Subjects were assessed using WOMAC scores, physical function performance-based tests, limits of physical function, morning stiffness, and patients' global assessment of disease severity. Both curcumin groups demonstrated significant efficacy in WOMAC scores compared to placebo, only Curamin showed significant results in physical performance tests. Boswella and curcumin may act synergistically to improve osteoarthritis symptoms (Haroyan et al. 2018).

14.2.6.6 Clinical Application

Popularity for turmeric has been growing as a dietary supplement. Turmeric is well tolerated and generally safe, adverse effects are GI-related with the possibility of increased risk of bleeding at high doses. Curcurmin (approximately 1 g per day) has demonstrated potential benefit in the treatment of osteoarthritis symptoms, however, studies have been limited.

14.3 Osteopenia

The development of osteopenia or osteoporosis occurs commonly in women after the menopausal transition. Vertebral and hip fractures from falls in people with osteoporosis result in multiple hospitalizations, impaired mobility and potentially a significant decline in their quality of life.

14.3.1 Soy Isoflavones

14.3.1.1 Background

Soy isoflavones are biologically active phytoestrogens found in leguminous plants such as soybeans, seeds, and grains. Soy isoflavones have been used with black cohosh and other botanicals for vasomotor and other postmenopausal symptoms. Additionally, they have been studied for the prevention of bone resorption. *See Chapter 8 Women's Health for more discussion.*

14.3.1.2 Pharmacognosy

Soy isoflavones exhibit weak estrogen agonist/antagonist effects and may also produce antioxidant effects, induction of cell differentiation and apoptosis, and inhibition of tyrosine kinase and topoisomerases (Zheng et al. 2016). Genistein and daidzein are the major isoflavones. Genistein has been shown to reduce viability of osteoclasts, upregulate insulin-like growth factor (IGF)-1 and estrogen receptor-1, and downregulate interleukin and matrix metalloproteinases (Zheng et al. 2016). Daidzein is converted to equol, which is more potent and is selective for bone estrogen receptor (ER)-beta. An estimated 30%–60% of people are equol-producers, and prevalence is higher in those who are Asian and/or vegetarian (Zheng et al. 2016). Individual gut microflora may play a role in the ability of patients to convert daidzein to equol, as isoflavones are activated after removal of glucose residue by gastrointestinal bacterial enzymes (Pawlowski et al. 2015, Lagari and Levis 2013). *See Chapter 8 Women's Health for more discussion.*

14.3.1.3 Preparation and Dosing

The ratio and content of soy isoflavones may vary significantly between products (Pawlowski et al. 2015). Novasoy® may be found in several over-the-counter products that generally contain 60 mg of 40% soy isoflavone extract per tablet. Genistein-enriched products may contain 250 mg of 80% soy isoflavone extract per serving size of two vegetarian capsules.

See Chapter 8 Women's Health for more discussion.

14.3.1.4 Safety

Patients with a soy allergy should not use these products. Most long-term studies have not demonstrated adverse effects of soy isoflavones on endometrial thickness. One 3-year, double-blind study evaluated the safety of two dosages, 80 and 120 mg daily, of soy isoflavones in 224 postmenopausal women. Patients had a median age of 54.3 years and had been postmenopausal for 2.8 years. Serious adverse events during the study were not attributed to soy isoflavone use. A higher number of genitourinary adverse effects occurred with the 80 mg dose versus 120 mg. Endometrial thickness or circulating hormones were similar (Alekel et al. 2015). *See Chapter 8 Women's Health for more discussion.*

14.3.1.5 Evidence

A randomized, blinded, crossover study of 24 women who had been postmenopausal for more than four years evaluated the efficacy of five soy isoflavone supplements. These included mixed isoflavones with low-dose soy (Novasoy), mixed isoflavones with high-dose soy, mixed isoflavones enriched with genistein, low-dose genistein, and high-dose genistein. At the start of the trial, bone was labeled with the rare isotope tracer ^{41}Ca to determine the effects of patient ability to convert daidzein to equol, which was hypothesized to enhance prevention of bone resorption by soy isoflavones. It was found that eight patients were equol-producers. All patients received Novosoy, and then could choose to receive one of the other four supplements followed by risedronate 5 mg by mouth daily (n = 14), or just risedronate 5 mg by mouth daily alone (n = 19). Each treatment period was 50 days followed by a 50-day washout. The average patient was 59 years old with a BMI of 27.4 kg/m^2, and a dietary calcium intake of 961 mg/day. The prevention of bone resorption did not differ between patients who were equol-producers and those who were not. Novasoy produced the greatest increase in bone calcium retention among the supplements (7.6%; p < 0.0001). The other supplements also showed statistically significant increases, with the exception of high-dose genistein (Pawlowski et al. 2015).

A review of two large prospective studies of Chinese patients examined the relationship between dietary intake of soy and fracture. The first study included more than 63,000 men and women who provided information about soy food intake for about 7 years. Hospital discharge databases were used to collect information about hip fractures. A statistically significant fracture risk reduction (21%–36%) was shown in the women who consumed soy. A second study of more than 24,000 women also provided information about soy intake for 4 years. Fractures at all skeletal sites were reported by patients. The results also showed a statistically significant reduction in fracture with soy (Lagari and Levis 2013).

14.3.1.6 Clinical Application

Supplemental intake of soy isoflavones can be beneficial for increasing bone calcium retention, particularly with products that contain Novasoy containing mixed isoflavones with low-dose soy. Additional information about the amount of dietary and/or supplemental soy isoflavones to reduce fracture risk in postmenopausal women is needed. Long-term studies have not shown adverse effects on endometrial thickness and/or circulating hormones.

14.4 Gout

Gout is common disorder is middle-aged and older adults. The typical attack of gouty arthritis is characterized by onset of pain, swelling, and inflammation of the first metatarsophalangeal joint. Botanical medicines may offer an effective alternative for management of patients with acute and chronic gout.

14.4.1 *Apium Graveolens*

14.4.1.1 *Background*

Apium graveolens (celery plant) belongs to the family Apiaceae and is found in Europe, the Mediterranean, and parts of Asia. The plant was first cultivated as a food in France in 1623 (Fazal and Singla 2012). It is annual or biennial botanical that is in flower from January to August, and the seed ripens between August to September (Tyagi et al. 2013). The leaves, stalks, and seeds can be ingested and it has been used medicinally since the Middle Ages. The plant has a broad spectrum of uses including as a urinary antiseptic, antifungal, antihypertensive, hypolipidemic, and anticancer among others (Fazal and Singla 2012).

14.4.1.2 *Pharmacognosy*

Celery is rich in vitamins A, B1, B2, B6, C, E, and K, as well as flavonoids and minerals such as iron, calcium, phosphorus, magnesium, and zinc (Tyagi et al. 2013). Its diuretic effect promotes excretion of uric acid and other unwanted waste products (Asif et al. 2011). It also consists of an essential oil that contains limonene and various sesquiterpenes.

14.4.1.3 *Preparation and Dosing*

Celery oil/oil extract, ground seed, or root tinctures are dietary supplements which are advertised to promoted healthy blood pressure, joint health, and uric acid levels. A suggested dose for celery seed extract is 20 mg (Fazal and Singla 2012).

14.4.1.4 *Safety*

If the plant is infected with the fungus *Sclerotinia sclerotiorum*, in sensitive people who are more likely Caucasians, skin contact can cause dermatitis. Allergic responses can include anaphylaxis in some individuals. Possible cross allergenicity between celery, cucumber, carrot, and watermelon.

14.4.1.5 *Evidence*

Human studies are lacking. *See Table 14.1 Multi-Ingredient Botanical Products for Gout for discussion involving celery.*

14.4.1.6 *Clinical Application*

Although well-designed human studies are lacking, celery has been shown to have anti-inflammatory properties that decrease swelling and pain around joints, and therefore, it has been used as a therapy for arthritis, rheumatism, and gout.

TABLE 14.1

Multi-Ingredient Botanical Products for Gout

Practitioners have reported that certain botanicals used in clinical practice help eliminate uric acid (*Apium graveolens*, *Urtica* spp., *Taraxacum officinale*) or have an anti-inflammatory effect (*Harpagophytum procumbens*, *Filipendula ulmaria*, *Salix* spp., *Betula* spp., *Curcuma longa* and *Guaiacum* spp.). Among the botanicals most frequently mentioned for the treatment of gout are *Apium graveolens* and *Urtica* spp. *In vitro* studies with these botanicals have been shown to inhibit xanthine oxidase and *in vivo* animal studies support their analgesic and anti-inflammatory activities (Chrubasik et al. 2007a, Marrassini et al. 2010, Bonaterra et al. 2010, Dyah Iswantini et al. 2012). Clinical trials with *Curcuma longa* and *Harpagophytum procumbens* support their benefit in inflammatory and painful musculoskeletal conditions (Chrubasik et al. 2007b, Denner 2007, Mobasheri et al. 2012, Ramadan et al. 2011).

A clinical study conducted at Shifa ul Mulk Memorial Hospital in Pakistan between 2007 and 2009 compared serum uric acid levels in patients taking a botanical medicine Gouticin which contained different medicinal botanicals including *A. graveolens* 100 mg and allopurinol 300 mg once daily. The trial included 100 patients with hyperuricemia (serum uric acid level >8 mg/dL), 50 patients in Gouticin group and 50 patients in allopurinol group. The study was conducted according to the principles of good clinical practice. Gouticin 500 mg was administered orally three times per day for 18 weeks to 50 patients between ages of 35–75 years with gouty arthritis. At the end of therapy, patients on Gouticin had statistically significant reduction in mean serum uric acid level from 10.03 to 4.74 mg/dL. In allopurinol group, mean serum uric acid level at baseline was 10.18 mg/dL and decreased to 5.27 mg/dL at the end of therapy. It was concluded that Gouticin was effective for the treatment of acute gout (Akram et al. 2010).

14.4.2 Cherry

14.4.2.1 Background

Cherries have been used for cancer, cardiovascular diseases, and osteoarthritis. In the past decade, cherries gained public attention as a potential option in preventing and managing gout. Small human and animal studies have demonstrated that consumption of cherries lowers serum uric acid levels and possess anti-inflammatory and antioxidant properties (Zhang et al. 2012). Herbalists recommend eating cherries or drinking cherry juice as their consumption has been shown to relieve arthritic pain and gout (Kelley et al. 2018).

14.4.2.2 Pharmacognosy

Sweet and tart cherries are rich in antioxidants, anthocyanins, catechins, chlorogenic acid, flavonal glycosides, fiber, and melatonin. Anthocyanins have shown to have anti-inflammatory properties by inhibiting cyclooxygenase activity, scavenging reactive nitric oxide radicals, inhibiting nitric oxide production, and modulating secretion of tumor necrosis factor alpha (Jacob et al. 2003).

14.4.2.3 Preparation and Dosing

Studies have used 10–60 pitted cherries or one tablespoon twice a day of cherry juice concentrate.

14.4.2.4 Safety

The fruit is safe when it is consumed in the amounts commonly found in foods (Serrano et al. 2005). No drug interactions have been reported.

14.4.2.5 Evidence

Human studies involving cherries have assessed changes in plasma urate concentrations and other markers, as well as the number of gouty attacks (Kelley et al. 2018). In one small study, plasma and urinary urate levels were measured in 10 healthy women between the ages of 22–40 years who consumed within 10 minutes two servings (280 g; about 45 cherries) of Bing sweet cherries after an overnight fast. Inflammatory markers such as plasma C-reactive protein, tumor necrosis factor-α, and nitric oxide were also measured. Blood and urine samples were collected before the dose, and at 1.5, 3, and 5 hours after the dose. Subjects were required to empty their bladder for the predose urine collection and were instructed to avoid any food or drink except a 237 mL bottle of water given after a 1.5 hour draw. Results showed a statistically significant reduction in plasma urate and increased urinary urate excretion compared to the baseline. Five hours after the dose, mean plasma urate decreased to 183 μmol/L compared to baseline of 214 μmol/L. Three hours after the dose, urinary urate excretion increased to 350 μmol/mmol compared to 202 μmol/mmol at baseline. Plasma C-reactive protein and nitric oxide concentrations decreased 3 hours after dose although this did not achieve statistical significance (Jacob et al. 2003).

Another case-crossover study consisted of 633 individuals with gout who were followed for 1 year (Zhang et al. 2012). The results suggested that intake of one (10–12 cherries) or more servings of cherries or cherry extract was associated with lower risk of gout attacks. Individuals who consumed cherries over a 2-day period had 35% lower risk of gout attacks compared to individuals who did not consume cherries. Similar results were observed in individuals who consumed cherry extract with a 45% lower risk of gout attacks. Risk of gout attacks was 75% lower in patients who consumed cherries and were taking concurrent allopurinol (Zhang et al. 2012). An additional study revealed that the consumption of one tablespoon cherry juice concentrate (equivalent to 45–60 cherries) twice a day for 4 or more months had an anti-inflammatory effect and reduced frequency of acute gout flare-ups (Schlesinger et al. 2012).

14.4.2.6 Clinical Application

Small clinical trials show that cherry consumption may be beneficial for management of gout since it increases urinary urate excretion and reduces plasma inflammatory markers.

14.5 Fibromyalgia

Fibromyalgia is a syndrome characterized by chronic widespread pain, proposed to be of neurogenic origin. Fatigue and sleep disturbances are common symptoms, as well as tenderness, mood disturbances, and cognitive difficulties. Fibromyalgia may result in a significant reduction in quality of life for patients.

14.5.1 Cannabis Sativa or Cannabis Indica

14.5.1.1 Background

Cannabinoid use in patients with chronic pain and fibromyalgia remains controversial. Phytocannabinoid-dense botanicals include the schedule I medicinal plants *Cannabis sativa* or *Cannabis indica*. As discussed in this book, the use of cannabis may have value in managing seizures, muscle spasms, and for supportive care in cancer as well as other conditions.

14.5.1.2 Pharmacognosy

See Chapter 18 Therapeutic Potential of Cannabis chapter for discussion.

14.5.1.3 Preparation and Dosing

See Chapter 18 Therapeutic Potential of Cannabis chapter for discussion.

14.5.1.4 Safety

Dizziness is the most commonly reported adverse effect. Concomitant use of cannabinoids and opioids requires careful evaluation as both agents have effects on mood and cognition (Ste-Marie et al. 2012). Symptoms of fatigue, mood disorder, and cognitive function in patients with fibromyalgia raises potential concerns about its use (Ste-Marie et al. 2012). *See Chapter 18 Therapeutic Potential of Cannabis chapter for more discussion.*

14.5.1.5 Evidence

In an observational study of 56 patients with fibromyalgia, the 28 cannabis users reported significant relief of pain, stiffness, relaxation, somnolence, and perception of well-being. This assessment was based on using a VAS before and two hours after self-administration of cannabis (Fiz et al. 2011). The Fibromyalgia Impact Questionnaire, the Pittsburgh Sleep Quality Index and the SF-36 were also used in the study, but only the mental health component of the latter instrument was improved with cannabis use.

In a study of nine patients with fibromyalgia, orally administered delta-9-tetrahydrocannabinol reduced electrically-induced pain and daily reports of pain, but not axon-induced flare. Five of the nine patients withdrew because of adverse effects (Schley et al. 2006).

14.5.1.6 Clinical Application

The formal evaluation of cannabinoids for fibromyalgia has been limited to date. Based on available evidence, their roles in fibromyalgia are unclear.

14.6 Conclusion

Musculoskeletal conditions are common worldwide. Although prescription drugs are widely available, significant adverse effects have been associated with their use. Many botanicals including *Boswellia serrata*, cat's claw extract, devil's claw, ginger, turmeric, and cherry products may reduce pain and inflammation and improve functional status.

REFERENCES

Abdelouahab, N. and C. Heard. 2008. Effect of the major glycosides of *Harpagophytum procumbens* (devil's claw) on epidermal cyclooxygenase-2 (COX-2) *in vitro*. *Journal of Natural Products* 71, no. 5:746–49. doi: 10.1021/np070204u.

Akram M., E. Mohiuddin, A. Hannan, and K. Usmanghani. 2010. Comparative study of herbal medicine with allopathic medicine for the treatment of hyperuricemia. *Journal of Pharmacognosy and Phytotherapy* 2, no. 6:86–90.

Alekel, D.L., U. Genschel et al. 2015. Soy isoflavones for reducing bone loss study. "*Menopause (New York, N. Y.)*" 22, no. 2: 185–97. doi: 10.1097/gme.0000000000000280.

Asif, H.M., M. Akram et al. 2011. Monograph of *Apium graveolens* Linn. *Journal of Medicinal Plants Research* 5, no. 8 (Apr):1494–6.

Bartels, E.M., V.N. Folmer et al. 2015. Efficacy and safety of ginger in osteoarthritis: a meta-analysis of randomized placebo-controlled trials. *Osteoarthritis and Cartilage* 23, no. 1 (Jan):13–21. doi: 10.1016/j.joca.2014.09.024.

Bliddal, H., A. Rosetzsky et al. 2000. A randomized, placebo-controlled, cross-over study of ginger extracts and ibuprofen in osteoarthritis. *Osteoarthritis and Cartilage* 8, no. 1 (Jan):9–12.

Bonaterra, G.A., E.U. Heinrich, O. Kelber, D. Weiser, J. Metz, and R. Kinscherf. 2010 Anti-inflammatory effects of the willow bark extract STW 33-I (Proaktiv®) in LPS-activated human monocytes and differentiated macrophages. *Phytomedicine* 17, no. 14 (Jan):1106–13.

Bolognesi, G., G. Belcaro, B. Feragalli, U. Cornelli, R. Cotellese, S. Hu, and M. Dugall. 2016. Movardol® (N-acetylglucosamine, *Boswellia serrata*, Ginger) supplementation in the management of knee osteoarthritis: Preliminary results from a 6-month registry study. *European Review for Medical and Pharmacological Sciences* 20, no. 24 (Dec):5198–204.

Cameron, M. and S. Chrubasik. 2014. Oral herbal therapies for treating osteoarthritis. *Cochrane Database of Systematic Reviews* 5 (May): CD002947. doi: 10.1002/14651858.cd002947.pub2.

Chantre, P., A. Cappelaere, D. Lebian, D. Guedon, J. Vandermander, and B. Fournie. 2000. Efficacy and tolerance of Harpagophytum procumbens versus diacerhein in treatment of osteoarthritis. *Phytomedicine* 7, no. 3 (June):177–83.

Christiansen, B.A., B. Simrit, R. Goudarzi, and S. Emami. 2015. Management of Osteoarthritis with Avocado/Soybean Unsaponifiables. *Cartilage* 6, no. 1 (Jan):30–44. doi: 10.1177/194760351455992.

Chrubasik, J.E., B.D. Roufogalis, H. Wagner, and S.A. Chrubasik. 2007a. A comprehensive review on nettle effect and efficacy profiles, part I: Herba urticae. *Phytomedicine* 14, no. 6 (Jun):423–35.

Chrubasik, J.E., B.D. Roufogalis, and S. Chrubasik. 2007b. Evidence of effectiveness of herbal anti-inflammatory drugs in the treatment of painful osteoarthritis and chronic low back pain. *Phytotherapy Research* 21, no. 7 (Jul):675–83.

Chrubasik, S., J. Thanner et al. 2002. Comparison of outcome measures during treatment with the proprietary Harpagophytum extract doloteffin in patients with pain in the lower back, knee or hip. *Phytomedicine* 9, no. 3 (Apr):181–94.

Daily, J.W., M. Yang, and S. Park. 2016. Efficacy of turmeric extracts and curcumin for alleviating the symptoms of joint arthritis: A systematic review and meta-analysis of randomized clinical trials. *Journal of Medicinal Food* 19, no. 8 (Aug):717–29. doi: 10.1089/jmf.2016.3705.

Denner, S.S. 2007. A review of the efficacy and safety of devil's claw for pain associated with degenerative musculoskeletal diseases, rheumatoid, and osteoarthritis. *Holistic Nursing Practice* 21, no. 4 (Jul):203–7.

Dragos, D., M. Gilca, L. Gaman, A. Vlad, L. Iosif, I. Stoian, and O. Lupescu. 2017. Phytomedicine in Joint Disorders. *Nutrients* 9, no. 1 (Jan):70. doi: 10.3390/nu9010070.

Dyah Iswantini, N., L.K. Darusman, and Trivadila. 2012. Inhibition kinetic of *Apium graveolens* L. ethanol extract and its fraction on the activity of xanthine oxidase and its active compound. *Journal of Biological Sciences* 12:51–6. doi: 10.3923/jbs.2012.51.56.

Fazal, S.S. and R.K. Singla. 2012. Review on the Pharmacolognostical & Pharmacological Characterization of *Apium Graveolens* Linn. *Indo Global Journal of Pharmaceutical Sciences* 2, no. 1:36–42.

Fiz, J., M. Durán, D. Capellà, J. Carbonell, and M. Farré. 2011. Cannabis use in patients with Fibromyalgia: Effect on symptoms relief and health-related quality of life. *PLoS ONE* 6, no. 4:e18440. doi: 10.1371/journal.pone.0018440.

Gagnier, J.J., S. Chrubasik, and E. Manheimer. 2004. *Harpgophytum procumbens* for osteoarthritis and low back pain: A systematic review. *BMC Complementary and Alternative Medicine* 4 no. 13 (Sep):1–10.

Grzanna, R., L. Lindmark, and C.G. Frondoza. 2005. Ginger – an herbal medicinal product with broad anti-inflammatory actions. *Journal of Medicinal Food* 8, no. 2:125–32.

Haroyan, A., V. Mukuchyan et al. 2018. Efficacy and safety of curcumin and its combination with boswellic acid in osteoarthritis: a comparative, randomized, double-blind, placebo-controlled study. *BMC Complementary and Alternative Medicine* 18, no. 7 (Jan): doi: 10.1186/s12906–017-2062-z.

Jacob, R.A., G.M. Spinozzi et al. 2003. Consumption of cherries lowers plasma urate in healthy women. *The Journal of Nutrition* 133, no. 6 (Jun):1826–9.

Kelley, D.S., Y. Adkins, and K.D. Laugero. 2018. A review of the health benefits of cherries. *Nutrients* 10, no. (3). pii: E368. doi: 10.3390/nu10030368.

Kocaadam, B. and N. Şanlier. 2017. Curcumin, an active component of turmeric (*Curcuma longa*), and its effects on health. *Critical Reviews in Food Science and Nutrition* 57, no. 13 (Sept):2889–95. doi: 10.1080/10408398.2015.1077195.

Lagari, V.S. and S. Levis. 2013. Phytoestrogens in the prevention of postmenopausal bone loss. *Journal of Clinical Densitometry* 16, no. 4 (Oct):445–49. doi: 10.1016/j.jocd.2013.08.011.

Long L., K. Soeken, and E. Ernst. 2001. Herbal medicines for the treatment of osteoarthritis: A systematic review. *Rheumatology* 40, no. 7 (Jul):779–93.

Liu, W., Y. Zhai et al. 2016. Oral bioavailability of curcumin: Problems and advancements. *Journal of Drug Targeting* 24, no. 8 (Feb):694–702. doi: 10.3109/1061186X.2016.1157883.

Marrassini, C., C. Acevedo, J. Mino, G. Ferraro, and S. Gorzalczany. 2010. Evaluation of antinociceptive, antinflammatory activities and phytochemical analysis of aerial parts of *Urtica urens* L. *Phytotherapy Research* 24, no. 12 (Dec):1807–12.

Mehta, K., J. Gala, S. Bhasale, S. Naik, M. Modak, H. Thakur, N. Deo, and M.J.S. Miller. 2007. Comparison of glucosamine sulfate and a polyherbal supplement for the relief of osteoarthritis of the knee: A randomized controlled trial [ISRCTN25438351]. *BMC Complementary and Altnerative Medicine* 7, no. 34. doi: 10.1186/1472-6882-7-34.

Miller, M.J.S., K. Mehta et al. 2005. Early relief of osteoarthritis symptoms with a natural mineral supplement and a herbomineral combination: A randomized controlled trial [ISRCTN38432711]. *Journal of Inflammation* 2, no. 11 (Oct). doi: 10.1186/1476-9255-2-11.

Mncwangi, N., W. Chen, I. Vermaal, A.M. Viljoen, and N. Gericke. 2012. Devil's claw: A review of the ethnobotany, phytochemistry and biological activity of *Harpagophytum procumbens*. *Journal of Ethnopharmacology* 143, no. 3 (Oct):755–71.

Mobasheri, A., Y. Henrotin, H.K. Biesalski, and M. Shakibaei. 2012. Scientific evidence and rationale for the development of curcumin and resveratrol as nutraceutricals for joint health. *International Journal of Molecular Sciences* 13, no. 4 (Mar):4202–32.

Patil, V.M., S. Das, and K. Balasubramanian. 2016. Quantum chemical and docking insights into bioavailability enhancement of curcumin by piperine in pepper. *The Journal of Physical Chemistry A* 120, no. 20 (May):3643–53. doi: 10.1021/acs.jpca.6b01434.

Pavelka, K., P. Coste, P. Géher, and G. Kreici. 2010. Efficacy and safety of piascledine 300 versus chondroitin sulfate in a 6 months treatment plus 2 months observation in patients with osteoarthritis of the knee. *Clinical Rheumatology* 29, no. 6 (Jun):659–70. doi: 10.1007/s10067-010-1384-8.

Pawlowski, J.W., R. Berdine et al. 2015. Impact of equol-producing capacity and soy-isoflavone profiles of supplements on bone calcium retention in postmenopausal women: A randomized crossover trial. *American Journal of Clinical Nutrition* 102, no. 3 (Sep):695–703. doi: 10.3945/ajcn.114.093906.

Piscoya, J., Z. Rodriguez, S.A. Bustamante, N.N. Okuhama, M.J.S. Miller, and M. Sandoval. 2001. Efficacy and safety of freeze-dried cat's claw in osteoarthritis of the knee: Mechanisms of action of the species Uncaria guianensis. *Inflammation Research* 50, no. 9:442–48. doi: 10.1007/pl00000268.

Prasad, S. and B.B. Aggarwal. 2011. Turmeric, the Golden Spice: From Traditional Medicine to Modern Medicine. In: Benzie, I.F.F., Wachtel-Galor, S., editors. *Herbal Medicine: Biomolecular and Clinical Aspects*. 2nd edition. Boca Raton (FL): CRC Press/Taylor & Francis. Chapter 13. Available from: https://www.ncbi.nlm.nih.gov/books/NBK92752/

Ramadan, G., M.A. Al-Kahtani, and W.M. El-Sayed. 2011. Anti-inflammatory and anti-oxidant properties of Curcuma longa (turmeric) versus *Zingiber officinale* (ginger) rhizomes in rat adjuvant-induced arthritis. *Inflammation* 34, no. 4 (Aug):291–301. doi: 10.1007/s10753-010-9278-0.

Serrano, M., F. Guillen et al. 2005. Chemical constiuents and antioxidant activity of sweet cherry at different ripening stages. *Journal of Agriculture and Food Chemistry* 53, no. 7 (Apr):2741–5.

Schlesinger, N., R. Rabinowitz, and M. Schlesinger. 2012. Pilot studies of cherry juice concentrate for gout flare prophylaxis. *Journal of Arthritis* 1:101. doi: 10.4172/2167-7921.1000101.

Schley, M., A. Legler, G. Skopp, M. Schmelz, C. Konrad, and R. Rukwied. 2006. Delta-9-THC based monotherapy in fibromyalgia patients on experimentally induced pain, axon reflex flare, and pain relief. *Current Medical Research and Opinion* 22, no. 7 (May):1269–76. doi: 10.1185/030079906x112651.

Sengupta, K., A.V. Krishnaraju, A.A. Vishal et al. 2010. Comparative efficacy and tolerability of 5-Loxin® and Aflapin® against osteoarthritis of the knee: A double blind, randomized, placebo controlled clinical study. *International Journal of Medical Sciences* 7, no. 6:366–77. doi: 10.7150/ijms.7.366.

Ste-Marie, P.A., M. Fitzcharles, A. Gamsa, M.A. Ware, and Y. Shir. 2012. Association of herbal cannabis use with negative psychosocial parameters in patients with fibromyalgia. *Arthritis Care & Research*, 64, no. 8 (July):1202–8. doi: 10.1002/acr.21732.

Tyagi, S., P. Chirag, M. Dhruv et al. 2013. Medical benefits of *Apium graveolens* (celery herb). *Journal of Drug Discovery and Therapeutics* 1, no. 5:36–8.

Ulbricht, C., W. Chao, D. Costa, E. Rusie-Seamon, W. Weissner, and J. Woods. 2008. Clinical evidence of herb-drug interactions: A systematic review by the natural standard research collaboration. *Current Drug Metabolism* 9, no. 10 (Dec):1063–120.

Vitetta, L., F. Cicuttini, and A. Sali. 2008. Alternative therapies for musculoskeletal conditions. *Best Practice and Research Clinical Rheumatology* 22, no. 3(Jun):499–522. doi: 10.1016/j.berth2007.12.007

Vlachojannis, J., B.D. Roufogalis, and S. Chrubasik. 2008. Systematic review on the safety of Harpagophytum preparations for osteoarthritic and low back pain. *Phytotherapy Research* 22, no. 2 (Feb):149–52. doi: 10.1002/ptr.2314.

White, B. 2007. Ginger: An overview. *American Academy of Family Physicians* 75, no. 11 (Jun):1689–91.

World Health Organization. Musculoskeletal conditions. Fact sheet. February 2018, http://www.who.int/mediacentre/factsheets/musculoskeletal/en/ (Accessed June 14, 2018).

Zhang, Y., T. Neogi et al. 2012. Cherry consumption and decreased risk of recurrent gout attacks. *Arthritis and Rheumatism* 64, no. 12 (Dec):4004–11. doi: 10.1002/art.34677.

Zheng, X., L. Sun-Kyeong, and O.K. Chun. 2016. Soy isoflavones and osteoporotic bone loss: A review with an emphasis on modulation of bone remodeling. *Journal of Medicinal Food* 19, no. 1 (Jan):1–14. doi: 10.1089/jmf.2015.0045.

15

Obesity and Weight Loss

Monika Nuffer and Wesley Nuffer

CONTENTS

15.1 Background

Obesity continues to pose a major health problem to the United States (U.S.) and across the world. Over 65% of the U.S. adult population is overweight or obese. With the prevalence of obesity defined by a body mass index ≥ 30 kg/m^2 approximately 36.5%, or more than 1/3 of the adult population (Centers of Disease Control 2015). The incidence of childhood obesity has tripled in the U.S. since the 1970s (Hill 2006). The rates of obesity in the U.S. are higher among women than in men (38.3% compared to 34.3%), and more common in minority populations, with African Americans demonstrating the highest rates (48.1%), followed by the Hispanic white population (42.5%) (Centers of Disease Control 2015).

The cost of medical care for obesity in the U.S. was estimated at $147 billion for 2008, or approximately 10% of all medical spending for that year (Hammond and Levine 2010). An economic analysis from 2006 demonstrated that compared with expenditures on healthy-weight individuals, medical spending was 41.5% higher due to obesity (Hammond and Levine 2010). Obesity has been shown to contribute to heart disease, type 2 diabetes, and cancer, all of which are among the top leading causes of death in the U.S (Jensen et al. 2014).

As a result, the development of agents to help facilitate weight loss or prevent further weight gain is essential. The 2013 Consensus Obesity Guidelines developed by the American Heart Association (AHA), American College of Cardiology (ACC), and the Obesity Society (TOS) indicated that patients with a body mass index (BMI) greater than 35 kg/m^2, or those with a BMI of >27 kg/m^2 with comorbid conditions could benefit from the addition of drug therapy to help manage their weight (Jensen et al. 2014).

Research has shown that many American consumers are seeking nonprescription weight loss products, and that the market for weight loss supplements is a multi-billion dollar industry. As of 2004, more than 50 individual dietary supplements and more than 125 commercial combination products were marketed for weight loss. Estimates from 2010 showed a total weight loss industry of over $60 billion, with over-the-counter/herbal product sales estimated at $3.04 billion (Marketdata Enterprises, 2011).

TABLE 15.1

Weight Loss Botanical Products by Category

Class	Botanical Products							
Appetite Suppressants	Hoodia *(Hoodia gordonii)*	Caralluma *(Caralluma fibriata)*		St. John's Wort *(Hypericum perforatum)*				
Digestion Inhibitors	Fiber • Barley *(Hordeum vulgare)* • Bean Pod *(Phaseolus vulgaris)* • Blonde Psyllium *(Plantago ovata)* • Fenugreek *(Trigonella foenum-graecum)* • Glucomannan *(Amorphophallus konjac)* Guggul *(Commiphora mukul)*							
Thermogenic Agents	Ephedra *(Ephedra sinica)*	Bitter Orange *(Citrus aurantium)*		Capsaicin *(Capsicum genus)*				
Miscellaneous Agents	Aristolochia *(Aristolochia auricularia)*	Cha de Bugra *(Cordia ecalycuata)*	Forskolin *(Coleus forskohlii)*	Gracinia *(Garcinia cambogia)*	Usnea *(Usnea barbata)*	Irvingia *(Irvingia gabonensis)*	Green Tea *(Camellia sinensis)*	Green Coffee *(Coffea arabica)*

15.2 Botanical Products Used in the Treatment of Obesity

Many botanical products have been explored for weight management and the treatment of obesity. Natural Medicines, a reputable tertiary literature source for integrative health, has developed a categorization system for the botanical products used for these purposes (Natural Medicines 2016). For consistency, that categorization has been maintained for presenting these agents in this chapter. Botanical products, by category, are presented in Table 15.1.

15.3 Appetite Suppressants

The appetite suppressant class are associated with central activity in the brain, where they affect appetite signaling to either inhibit hunger or promote fullness. These substances have also been called *anorectics* or *anorexients*, and can affect various neurotransmitters in the central nervous system or disrupt brain signaling regarding eating and hunger. Some of these substances are also known as *stimulants* due to the increased activity they may have on epinephrine and norepinephrine neurotransmitters involved in the fight-or-flight response.

15.3.1 Hoodia Extract (*Hoodia gordonii*)

15.3.1.1 Background

Hoodia refers to a genus of over 20 related species of plants. *Hoodia gordonii* is a leafless, spiny succulent cactus plant indigenous of the Kalahari Desert region of Africa. This plant was often chewed by natives in the area and was reported to stave off hunger for long periods of time, such as during tribal animal hunts (Whelan et al. 2010).

15.3.1.2 Pharmacognosy

The medicinal parts of the plant are the stems, root, and latex. The active ingredient, coined "P57," was identified and isolated by the Council of Scientific and Industrial Research (CSIR) in South Africa, and was patented in 1996 (Van Heerden 2008). P57 is theorized to increase adenosine triphosphate in the hypothalamus to regulate food intake (Whelan et al. 2010). Hoodia species in South Africa are currently protected and permits are required for collection and cultivation of this desert plant (Van Heerden 2008). Due to the limited number of these plants and the slow-growing nature of the species, adulteration of hoodia products has been a major concern (Van Heerden 2008).

15.3.1.3 Dosing and Preparation

As mentioned, adulteration of commercial Hoodia products is a concern. Early studies which randomly tested preparations of Hoodia demonstrated as little as 30% of commercial products contained sufficient amounts of the active ingredient (Lee and Balick 2007). Similar testing performed in 2006 brought this number up to 60%, but still demonstrated the presence of mislabeled and/or adulterated products (Lee and Balick 2007).

15.3.1.4 Safety

Safety is an important consideration with *Hoodia gordonii,* due to P57's low overall bioavailability, leading to relatively high doses being administered to produce any effects. A developmental toxicity study performed in pregnant rabbits showed no effects in embryonic or fetal development with doses up to 12 mg/kg/day (Dent et al. 2012a). The same researchers performed a similar study, using higher concentrations of the active botanical and found similar results, with only the highest dose of 50 mg/kg/day demonstrating low fetal weight mass (Dent et al. 2012b). A toxicity study with *Hoodia gordonii* showed no genotoxicity in doses up to 400 mg/kg/day in mice (Scott et al. 2012). This study reported that doses greater than 350 mg/kg/day demonstrated signs of toxicity, including swelling in the abdomen, weight loss, and death within 48 hours (Scott et al. 2012). The human trial utilizing *Hoodia gordonii* performed extensive monitoring, and noted that no severe adverse events were reported by either group across the 15-day treatment period. The most common adverse events in the active treatment group were disturbances in skin sensation, headache, dizziness, giddiness, and nausea (Blom et al. 2011).

15.3.1.5 Evidence

Animal data, primarily with rats, have shown positive effects on decreased food intake and body mass with the use of Hoodia. In regards to human trials, data are more limited. A small double-blind, placebo, randomized control trial (RCT) of 49 healthy, overweight women demonstrated no difference in body weight changes or energy intake between the active group using *Hoodia gordonii* extract at 1110 mg/dose (n = 25) and the placebo (n = 24) (Blom et al. 2011). Women in the active treatment group, however, reported higher rates of nausea and vomiting, as well as statistically significant increases in blood pressure, pulse, and heart rate ($p < 0.05$) (Blom et al. 2011).

Another RCT with 103 participants evaluated a different Hoodia species, *Hoodia parviflora,* compared with placebo across 40 days. The study showed a statistically significant change in body weight (-0.58 kg for Hoodia vs $+0.2$ kg for placebo, $p = 0.04587$) (Landor et al. 2015). Of the participants, 55% within the study group lost weight at the end of the study. Two other unpublished trials with small numbers of participants and short durations are mentioned in a review of *Hoodia gordonii,* one conducted by a British pharmaceutical company, Phytopharm, that owned rights to the P57 compound, and another utilizing a formulation of 500 mg capsules, which reported results on the internet (Whelan et al. 2010). While both of these reported successful decreased body mass and lowered energy intake with Hoodia use, it is difficult to draw conclusions regarding validity without access to these trials' designs and methods.

15.3.1.6 Clinical Application

At this time, whether *Hoodia gordonii* has a role in the area of obesity and weight loss is uncertain, due to limited human data. Of interest, Pfizer entered into a partnership to further evaluate P57, but ended up releasing the rights in 2003, due to toxicity concerns and difficulty in synthesizing the compound (Lee et al. 2007). The available human evidence suggest that any effects are modest in obesity and that the compound may be hard to tolerate.

15.3.2 Caralluma (*Caralluma fimbriata*)

15.3.2.1 Background

Caralluma fimbriata is an edible succulent cactus used by tribes in India to suppress appetite and increase endurance. The plant grows wild in India, Africa, and parts of Europe (Kuriyan et al. 2007).

15.3.2.2 Pharmacognosy

The medicinal value comes from the aerial parts of the plant. Potential active ingredients include flavone glycosides, pregnane glycosides, and saponins. These glycosides are thought to inhibit citrate lyase, and enzyme involved in formulating fat from fatty acids through the Kreb cycle. Caralluma may also work centrally, suppressing appetite in the central nervous system (Astell et al. 2013).

15.3.2.3 Dosing and Preparation

The plant can be consumed raw or cooked in boiling water. It is often dried into a powder or formulated into an extract. Extract doses up to 500 mg twice daily have been studied, but there is currently not a consensus on an effective dose (Astell et al. 2013).

15.3.2.4 Safety

Caralluma is generally well tolerated, with gastrointestinal symptoms being the most common, including moderate acidity, constipation, and flatulence.

15.3.2.5 Evidence

Several studies have evaluated caralluma in humans. A randomized, placebo-controlled trial with 50 subjects evaluated caralluma's effects on weight and appetite, where subjects were given 1 gram of extract or placebo daily over 60 days (Kuriyan et al. 2007). The study showed decrease in waist circumference (-3.0 inches vs -0.8 inches, $p < 0.001$) and hunger levels (visual analog scale, decrease in hunger by 19.7% compared to 1.2% in placebo, $p < 0.001$). Changes in total weight, BMI, energy intake, and body fat did not achieve statistical significance. An Australian study evaluated 43 adults with metabolic syndrome, giving 1 g of extract or placebo over 12 weeks (Astell et al. 2013). The active group showed greater waist circumference reductions that did not achieve statistical significance, but did demonstrate significant changes in waist to hip ratio, total body weight, and BMI reductions ($p < 0.05$).

15.3.2.6 Clinical Application

Based on these data, caralluma may have some weight loss effects, but more data are needed to confirm efficacy and determine a therapeutic dose.

15.3.3 St. John's Wort (*Hypericum perforatum*)

15.3.3.1 Background

St. John's Wort (SJW), or *Hypericum perforatum*, is a yellow flower-producing plant that has a long history of use for medicinal purposes. The name of the plant may refer to John the Baptist, as the plant's flowers bloom around the time of John the Baptist's feast in late June (National Center for Complementary and

Integrative Health 2016). Many medicinal claims have been made for the use of SJW, including the treatment of depression and mood, menopause symptoms, smoking cessation, fibromyalgia, pain, and weight loss.

15.3.3.2 Pharmacognosy

The medicinal parts of SJW are thought to be the flowers and leaves. Both hypericin and hyperforin are considered to be active compounds found from the plant (Apaydin et al. 2016). Other ingredients, such as flavonoids and naphthodianthrones, have also been studied (Apaydin et al. 2016).

15.3.3.3 Dosing and Preparation

See Chapter 11 Psychiatric Disorders for discussion on SJW.

15.3.3.4 Safety

Sufficient evidence exists from its use in humans, mostly evaluating its effects on psychiatric disorders. A review article pooled 35 SJW studies enrolling almost 7,000 patients (Apaydin et al. 2016). Across the studies, patients using SJW were no more likely to experience adverse effects than those on placebo (OR 0.83; CI 0.62, 1.13) (Apaydin et al. 2016). Patients using SJW were more likely to experience adverse events related to the nervous system or to eye, ear, liver, renal, and reproductive organ systems. The authors did note, however, that there was high variability across trials on adverse event reporting, which was inadequate for detecting rare adverse events and lowered the quality of evidence (Apaydin et al. 2016). Concerns exist about the effects of SJW on the cytochrome P450 system of metabolism, leading to drug interactions with drugs, such as warfarin, phenytoin, and oral contraceptives. *See Chapter 2 Pharmacokinetic and Pharmacogenomic Considerations for further discussion.*

15.3.3.5 Evidence

Little evidence exists regarding SJW and its role in the treatment of obesity, as most of the data are on depression. No human trials focused on obesity and weight loss were identified, although some animal studies were found. One 2-week rodent study demonstrated that SJW may improve insulin sensitivity and increase adiponectin levels, while having no net effect on overall body weight or food intake (Fuller et al. 2014). A study performed on Wistar rats in Mexico examined oral administration of two ingredients, *Hypericum silenoides* and *Hypericum philonotis*, working with various extracts of these ingredients, specifically evaluating their effects on lipids and weight reduction (Garcia-de la Cruz et al. 2013). After 35 days, the researchers demonstrated a 24.6% higher body weight in the control rats compared to the treatment group ($p < 0.05$). The aqueous extract showed the greatest reduction in weight gain, whereas the methanol extract demonstrated no weight effects. Of note, two of the extracts (hexane, dichloromethane) were toxic to the rats, causing diarrhea and premature deaths. Both active ingredients demonstrated a dose-dependent reduction in glucose, ranging from 48%–75% ($p < 0.05$). The preparations had variable effects on the lipid panel components (Garcia-de la Cruz et al. 2013).

15.3.3.6 Clinical Application

Evidence is insufficient to recommend SJW for the treatment of obesity.

15.4 Digestion Inhibitors

Digestion inhibitors have been investigated to evaluate their impact on weight loss, modeled after the lipase inhibitor orlistat, which blocks the breakdown and absorption of dietary fat. The mechanism of this drug led to the evaluation of other digestion inhibitors as potential weight loss products.

15.4.1 Fiber Products

15.4.1.1 Background

Fiber products including barley, bean pod, blonde psyllium, fenugreek, and glucomannan have shown efficacy in their ability to bind fat and reduce the severity of some of the adverse effects from orlistat. This prompted researchers to investigate whether the fat-binding properties of these fibers may actually produce weight loss or help to treat obesity. While many nonabsorbable fiber products available, products highlighted here are most commonly used for this purpose.

15.4.1.2 Safety

Adverse effects from the use of fiber supplements are similar and primarily are gastrointestinal in nature. Patients experience abdominal discomfort, diarrhea, fecal urgency, and cramping. Fat-soluble vitamins such as A, D, E, and K have decreased absorption when taken at the same time as fiber supplements.

15.4.1.3 Evidence

A review article sponsored by Proctor and Gamble categorized dietary fiber as soluble and insoluble fibers, as well as viscous (gel-forming) and non-viscous types (Chutkan et al. 2012). This article listed wheat bran and β-glucan (oatmeal) as having probable positive effects on weight, listing psyllium as having a modest effect and guar gum as having no effects on weight. Several large epidemiologic studies have evaluated dietary fiber's effects on weight as well. A prospective cohort study of over 74,000 women age 12 and older showed that subjects with the highest quintile of dietary fiber consumption had a 49% lower risk of major weight gain compared to subjects in the lowest quintile (Liu et al. 2003). Another prospective cohort study in Europe with almost 900,000 participants followed for more than 6 years associated dietary fiber consumption with reduced waist circumference and lower weight (Du et al. 2010).

Multiple RCTs have evaluated fibers' effects on fat. A meta-analysis evaluating 16 RCTs, which examined various fiber products' effects on weight, demonstrated significant reductions of weight at 4 and 8 weeks, with a 4.9% reduction in body weight from baseline at 8 weeks, compared to a 2.9% reduction in the placebo group (Anderson et al. 2009).

Whole-grain barley *(Hordeum vulgare)* has been studied for its effects on fat and obesity both in animal models and in humans. Barley is qualified by the Food and Drug Administration (FDA) as having beneficial health claims to reduce the risk of heart disease (United States Food and Drug Administration 2006). Animal studies with barley have shown decreased food intake but not weight loss with the supplement. In humans, a randomized crossover study was performed in 46 overweight women, using whole-grain barley and legumes to evaluate their impact on cardiometabolic risk (Tovar et al. 2014). Both diets had a favorable impact on total cholesterol, low-density lipoprotein (LDL) cholesterol, and high-density lipoprotein (HDL) cholesterol, but the barley group also showed positive reductions in apolipoprotein B (apoB) ($p < 0.001$), γ-glutamyl transferase ($p < 0.05$), diastolic blood pressure ($p < 0.05$), and Framingham heart risk estimates ($p < 0.05$) (Tovar et al. 2014). The BMI increased slightly with both diets, and there were no significant differences in BMI or waist circumference. Another randomized crossover trial, conducted in Japan, studied the effects of high β-glycan barley on appetite and energy intake in 21 healthy women on two separate days, separated by a 7-day washout period (Aoe et al. 2014). The barley and control meals were given at breakfast, with similar meal composition in both diets for lunch and dinner. The barley diet significantly reduced scores of hunger ($p = 0.032$), prospective food consumption ($p = 0.019$), and increased fullness ($p = 0.038$) Energy intake for subsequent lunch and dinner were significantly lower with the barley diet ($p = 0.035$) (Aoe et al. 2014). *See Chapter 7 Gastrointestinal Disease for more discussion on barley.*

Bean pod, or *Phaseolus vulgaris,* refers to the common bean, and includes many bean varieties such as pinto beans, kidney beans, green beans, and refried beans. The bean pod is used without the seeds, and has a high fiber content. Most of the research for medicinal uses of bean pod are specific to a white kidney bean extract. A RCT performed with 101 people in China demonstrated weight reduction after 60 days of supplementation (−1.9 kg compared to −0.4 kg in placebo, p < 0.001) (Wu et al. 2010). Another study with 39 subjects evaluated the same white bean extract over 8 weeks, and while the active group lost more weight than placebo, it did not reach clinical significance (Udani et al. 2004).

The seed and seed husk of blonde psyllium (*Plantago ovat*) has modest beneficial effects on weight. Adding psyllium fiber to the diet may promote satiety and decrease food intake. A 2003 review article evaluated the evidence of psyllium's use in improving metabolic control in obese children and adolescents (Moreno et al. 2003). In regards to weight, the authors noted a ∼2 kg reduction in weight with increased dietary fiber across the RCTs performed in children. An Australian study assessed the acute effects of psyllium on lipids and thermogenesis in ten overweight and obese men, providing either a low amount of fiber or high amount on two distinct days, separated by a one week washout period (Khossousi et al. 2008). The researchers reported significantly lower triglycerides and apoB levels after consumption of the high-fiber meal, but no difference in resting energy expenditure or diet-induced thermogenesis between the groups.

Another Australian study evaluated the effects of psyllium on weight and metabolic risk factors with four groups. Two groups were given a healthy diet, one of which received psyllium, and two groups who had no dietary intervention, one of which received psyllium (Pal et al. 2011). Both psyllium groups demonstrated significant reductions in weight, BMI, and total body fat percentage compared to the control group with no dietary intervention. *See Chapter 7 Gastrointestinal Disease for more discussion on psyllium.*

Fenugreek (*Trigonella foenum-graecum*) has shown good results on its effects on weight gain and obesity in animal studies. Little human evidence exists for the use of this fiber for weight loss. One study with 18 subjects used either 4 grams or 8 grams of fenugreek and recorded ratings of hunger and fullness every 30 minutes for 3.5 hours (Mathern et al. 2009). Energy intake was measured for the remainder of the day. The eightgram dose demonstrated increased satiety and fullness and reduced hunger and food consumption (p < 0.05). A review article evaluating 4-hydroxyisoleucine, thought to be the active ingredient in fenugreek, cited hypoglycemic and antihyperlipidemic effects when given orally, based on both animal and human data (Avalos-Soriano et al. 2016). They concluded a potential exists for fenugreek's use for both diabetes and obesity. *See Chapter 6 Endocrine Disorders and Chapter 8 Women's Health for more discussion on fenugreek.*

Glucomannan *(Amorphophallus konjac)* is a soluble fiber obtained from the roots of the konjac plant. It is used as a food additive to enrich noodles in traditional Japanese food. A 2015 review article evaluated glucomannan's effects on body weight in overweight or obese children and adults (Zalewski et al. 2015). Six RCTs were selected for inclusion, three of which demonstrated a significant reduction in body weight at some point in the trial (between 2 and 5 weeks), but none of which showed a significant impact on BMI. This suggests that glucomannan may have favorable impact on weight in the short-term. A 2014 meta-analysis of RCTs involving glucomannan identified 18 trials, of which nine were included for analysis. The result was a non-significant impact on weight of −0.22 kg (95% CI −0.62, 0.19), suggesting that any effects are modest at best (Onakpoya et al. 2013). *See Chapter 6 Endocrine Disorders for more discussion on glucomannan.*

15.4.1.4 Clinical Application

The collective evidence with fiber products suggest a modest positive impact on weight. It should be noted that positive effects have also been documented with dietary fibers on diabetes glucose control and on cholesterol and lipids, two comorbid conditions that often accompany obesity. With that consideration, increasing dietary fiber could represent an easy clinical intervention for an overweight or obese patient.

15.4.2 Guggul (*Commiphora mukul*)

15.4.2.1 Background

Guggul, also known as guggulsterone or guggulipid, is the gum resin of the *Commiphora mukul* tree, which is native to India (Mithila and Khanum 2014). Guggul is of the same genus as *Commiphora myrrha*, which is the source of myrrh, referenced in the Holy Bible. This resin extract is common within Ayurvedic medicine practices, used to treat ailments such as obesity and dyslipidemia (Mithila and Khanum 2014).

15.4.2.2 Pharmacognosy

The yellow resin produced from the stem is commonly used as the extract formulation. The extract contains guggulsterones, which are steroid compounds that function as antioxidants. These compounds are also thought to increase the degradation and excretion of cholesterol, while inhibiting cholesterol formation, leading to a net weight loss effect. They also increase the formation of thyroid hormones, which can increase metabolism.

15.4.2.3 Dosing and Preparation

Most guggul preparations utilize the extract from the resin. Dosing for obesity has ranged between 1,500 and 4,000 mg per day (Yamada and Sugimoto 2016).

15.4.2.4 Safety

Guggul is safe and well tolerated. Adverse effects in human trials have included headache, nausea, vomiting, diarrhea and hiccups (Sidhu et al. 1976, Bhatt et al. 1995, Szapary et al. 2003). A few patients had hypersensitivity to the resin. Due to guggul's ability to bind to estrogen receptors, this supplement should not be combined with estrogen therapy, as it may worsen estrogenic adverse effects.

15.4.2.5 Evidence

A double-blind, placebo-controlled pilot study performed on 20 patients with a BMI ≥ 25 kg/m^2 over 6 weeks demonstrated a significant decrease in body weight (-3.2%) and fat mass 20.6% compared to 8.6% in placebo (Antonio et al. 1999). Of note, the supplement evaluated in the active group also included phosphate, L-tyrosine, and *Garcinia cambogia*. Another RCT, however, evaluating the effects of 3,000 mg or 6,000 mg/day of guggul on hyperlipidemia across 8 weeks with a secondary outcome of effects on weight, failed to demonstrate any beneficial weight loss effects (Szapary et al. 2003). Two older trials specifically examining guggul's effects on weight also did not demonstrate significant changes to weight with treatment, although one did show a nonsignificant weight loss of 3.2% in patients weighing over 90 kg (Sidhu et al. 1976, Bhatt et al. 1995). Of note, the authors concluded that larger, carefully designed trials would be needed to clarify any weight loss effects of guggul.

The effects that guggul may have on lipids are interesting, but evidence is lacking to make a recommendation for supplementation.

15.4.2.6 Clinical Application

Evidence evaluating guggul for weight loss and the treatment of obesity is limited. Most of the available research centers around its effects on lipids and possible protection from cardiovascular disease.

15.5 Thermogenic Agents

Thermogenic agents increase metabolism or increase energy output, thereby consuming calories and burning fat. These agents often affect neurotransmitters that are "excitable," such as epinephrine and norepinephrine. Of note, no prescription medications are considered thermogenic. The over-the-counter diet aid, phenylpropanolamine, also known as "*PPA*," was removed from the market in 2005 due to safety concerns, most notably due to an increased risk of stroke in young women (United States Food and Drug Administration 2005).

15.5.1 Ephedrine (*Ephedra sinica*)

15.5.1.1 Background

The most well-known thermogenic supplement previously available on the U.S. market is ephedra, also known as ephedrine or *ma huang* in Chinese medicine. The dietary aid *Metabolife 356®* contained ephedra, along with caffeine and several other botanicals, and gained popularity in the late 1990s (United States Food and Drug Administration 2003).

15.5.1.2 Pharmacognosy

Ephedra comes from the plant *Ephedra sinica*, with the stem and leaf containing ephedra alkaloids. The plant is dried and undergoes an extraction process to produce the alkaloids.

15.5.1.3 Dosing and Preparation

Ephedrine has been evaluated by itself and combined with various formulations of caffeine. Studied doses range from 5–50 mg daily.

15.5.1.4 Safety

Safety is a major concern with the use of ephedra. A meta-analysis evaluated the safety of ephedra across 22 trials. (Shekelle et al. 2003a) The authors estimated a 2.2–3.6 fold increased risk of adverse events that included psychiatric symptoms, gastrointestinal distress, autonomic dysfunction, and heart palpitations. Odds ratios (OR) for cardiac adverse effects included 2.29 for heart palpitations (95% CI 1.27–4.32) and 2.19 for hypertension (95% CI 0.49–13.34). The authors also cited a case-control study that associated ephedra use with an increased risk of hemorrhagic stroke with doses over 32 mg/day (OR 3.59, 95% CI 0.70–18.35).

A review evaluated 140 reports of adverse events associated with ephedra use between 1997 and 1999, applying a standardized rating system to evaluate causality (Haller and Benowitz 2000). The authors found that 31% of the reports were classified as either definitely or probably related to ephedra treatment, with another 31% being ranked as possibly related. Across these reports linked to ephedra, a total of 47% were associated with cardiovascular events, with another 18% related to the central nervous system. In addition, multiple case reports of psychosis and mania associated with ephedra use have been published, correlating with the psychiatric symptoms seen from the meta-analysis (Doyle and Kargin 1996, Whitehouse and Duncan 1987).

Not all evidence suggests that ephedrine shows serious cardiovascular risks. A Danish registry-based case-control study evaluated the risk of serious cardiovascular events associated with ephedrine/caffeine combination products (Hallas et al. 2008). The authors analyzed data on over 250,000 people using prescribed ephedrine/caffeine between 1995 and 2002, with a composite endpoint of death outside a hospital, myocardial infarction, and stroke. The analysis showed an odds ratio for this endpoint of 0.84 (95% CI 0.71, 1.00), and after adjusting for length of use of the product showed a slightly higher OR of 0.95 (95% CI 0.79, 1.16). The authors concluded that no substantial increased risks of cardiovascular events were associated with prescribed use of ephedrine and caffeine.

Safety concerns regarding ephedrine use prompted the FDA to examine the supplement as early as 1993. In 2002, the United States Department of Health and Human Services commissioned the RAND Corporation to evaluate the safety and efficacy of ephedrine specifically for weight loss and athletic performance. Their findings stated that ephedrine and ephedrine with caffeine, promoted modest short-term weight loss, but lacked any long-term weight loss data (Shekelle et al. 2003b). The report further stated that ephedrine was associated with an increased risk of gastrointestinal, psychiatric, and autonomic adverse events, and identified enough case reports for adverse cardiovascular and psychiatric adverse events, some of which included death, that the report recommended further studies be done to establish potential causality. This report prompted the FDA to publish a final rule, stating that ephedrine alkaloids present an unreasonable risk in February 2004, effectively withdrawing all products containing ephedrine from the U.S. market (United States Food and Drug Administration 2004).

15.5.1.5 Evidence

Some studies have suggested that ephedra can effectively produce weight loss in humans. One RCT involving 90 patients over 24 weeks examined the use of ephedra plus caffeine, ephedra/caffeine and leptin, or leptin alone (Liu et al. 2013). Both the ephedra/caffeine and the ephedra/caffeine/leptin groups demonstrated weight reductions compared to the leptin-alone group ($-5.9 \pm 1.2\%$ and $-6.5 \pm 1.1\%$ respectively, $p < 0.05$). Whole body fat mass was also reduced ($-9.6 \pm 2.4\%$ and $-12.4 \pm 2.3\%$ respectively, $p < 0.05$) (Liu et al. 2013). Another RCT evaluated a product containing ephedrine, caffeine, salicin, and other botanical ingredients, given to 102 patients over 12 weeks (Coffey et al. 2004). Subjects receiving the active treatment lost an average of 1.5 kg compared to control, reductions in BMI (-0.82 kg/m^2 compared to -0.18 kg/m^2, $p = 0.001$) and waist circumference (-2.57 cm versus -0.91 cm, $p = 0.006$) (Coffey et al. 2004).

A meta-analysis published evaluated the safety and efficacy of ephedrine and ephedra, including 22 trials in the analysis (Shekelle et al. 2003a,b). The trials were all of short duration, generally 6 months or less, and many combined ephedra or ephedrine with other supplements, such as caffeine. The pooled results demonstrated weight loss of between 0.6–1 kg per month of treatment, when compared to placebo (Shekelle et al. 2003a,b). The authors concluded that ephedra has modest short-term weight loss effects, which appear to be greater when combined with sources of caffeine.

15.5.1.6 Clinical Application

While ephedrine has been established as efficacious in producing modest weight loss, the cardiovascular safety concerns outweigh any potential benefits from the supplement.

15.5.2 Bitter Orange (*Citrus aurantium*)

15.5.2.1 Background

Bitter orange is the fruit from a citrus tree endogenous to Southeast Asia, now found in locations across the world (Stohs et al. 2012).

15.5.2.2 Pharmacognosy

The active ingredients of bitter orange are the synephrine alkaloids, of which the p-synephrine has shown to be the safest. These alkaloids are thought to have effects on metabolic processes, increasing basal metabolism and lipolysis, as well as suppressing the appetite (Stohs et al. 2012).

15.5.2.3 Dosing and Preparation

The evidence on bitter orange suggests that isolating the p-synephrine alkaloid is important to limit the activity the supplement has on adrenergic receptors and the central nervous system. Other alkaloid isomers are present in the natural fruit form. Usual dosing is around 50–100 mg, although studies have evaluated doses up to almost 1,000 mg.

15.5.2.4 Safety

The safety of bitter orange appears to be specific to the source of the synephrine. Two reviews evaluated p-synephrine's effects on cardiovascular function and on stimulatory neurotransmitters, and found no significant adverse cardiovascular effects (Stohs et al. 2011, 2012). These reviews note that p-synephrine has significantly lower lipid solubility when compared to ephedrine, restricting its passage through the blood-brain barrier and limiting its activity on central nervous system. Another study conducted in 75 people evaluated p-synephrine's safety across 60 days, giving either bitter orange extract alone, in combination with naringin and hesperidin, or placebo (Kaats et al. 2013). The authors found no changes in blood pressure or blood cell counts with active treatments, and only a small increase in heart rate with the active groups, concluding that dosages up to 98 mg daily were without serious adverse effects when used for 2 months. A 2012 study conducted due to the close similarity in structure of synephrine to ephedrine, specifically evaluated the safety of two different extracts (6% and 95%) of synephrine in rats over 28 days (Hansen et al. 2012). Of note, this study used an extract of *C. aurantium*, but did not isolate the p-synephrine enantiomer. In this trial, the rats did not demonstrate any appreciable weight loss, but the synephrine did increase both heart rate and blood pressure, effects that were more pronounced with the addition of caffeine. This supports earlier findings in rats where synephrine 4% and 6% extracts did decrease food consumption and body weight, but increased mortality, blood pressure and produced ECG abnormalities after 15 days (Calapai et al. 1999). The authors also cited a number of human case reports which associated synephrine with cardiovascular adverse events, including myocardial infarction, stroke, Q-T prolongation, angina, and ventricular fibrillation. The authors called for longer-term studies to better evaluate the safety of synephrine use.

15.5.2.5 Evidence

A review article evaluating human clinical studies using bitter orange associated the supplement with modest short-term weight loss and increased metabolic rate and energy expenditure. The article considered both published and unpublished data, and included studies that used p-synephrine alone, along with combinations of caffeine and other botanical products for durations up through 12 weeks. Due to the fact that many studies include bitter orange in combination with multiple botanicals, it is difficult to determine what effects the supplement has on weight when used alone.

15.5.2.6 Clinical Application

Currently the use of p-synephrine may result in modest weight loss over a short period of time. To better determine its role in weight loss, larger studies evaluating p-synephrine alone and over a longer interval of time are needed. Formulations that are not specific to the p-synephrine alkaloid may carry cardiovascular risks similar to ephedrine.

15.5.3 Capsaicin (*Capsicum genus*)

15.5.3.1 Background

Capsaicin comes from the Cayenne pepper, a spice that has been used for cooking throughout the world.

15.5.3.2 Pharmacognosy

Capsaicin has demonstrated medicinal value in several areas, and has been studied for its effects on weight, with theorized activation of brown fat thermogenesis, increasing energy expenditure. Animal models have demonstrated activity in activating the transient receptor potential cation channel, or TRPV1 receptors, leading to increased energy expenditure (Snitker et al. 2009).

15.5.3.3 Dosing and Preparation

Capsaicin has been used in both topical and oral formulations for various medicinal properties. Weight loss effects have been studied using oral formulations, with doses around 1,000 mg/day.

15.5.3.4 Safety

Capsaicin holds Generally Recognized as Safe (GRAS) status with the FDA. It has been shown to be safe both as a food additive and when used as an oral supplement. The product does produce local irritation, and can burn if used topically or intranasally.

15.5.3.5 Evidence

A 13-week study examined 80 subjects randomized to receive either *Capsicum annum* extract delivered in capsules or placebo before the morning and evening meals. Both groups lost similar amounts of weight, but capsaicin demonstrated a greater reduction in abdominal adiposity ($-1.11 \pm .83\%$ versus $-0.18 \pm 1.94\%$) (Snitker et al. 2009). Two other studies showed that people who regularly consume chili peppers showed decreased weight compared to controls (Henry and Emery 1986, Yoshioka et al. 1998).

15.5.3.6 Clinical Application

There is limited evidence in humans evaluating capsaicin's effects on weight. More data are needed to clarify capsaicin's modest effects on obesity.

15.6 Miscellaneous Agents

15.6.1 Aristolochic Acid (*Aristolochia auricularia*)

15.6.1.1 Background

Aristolochia, or aristolochic acid, is a traditional medicinal botanical popular in many Chinese formulations. It has been used as an analgesic, anti-inflammatory, antitussive, and for the treatment of obesity (Yang et al. 2007). The *Aristolochia* genus comprises over 800 plant species, which grow in both temperate and tropical regions.

15.6.1.2 Pharmacognosy

Aristolochia contains many alkaloids and flavonoids that are likely the active components of the supplement. With over 800 different species in the genus, there is a high degree of variability in which alkaloids/plant steroids are the most active.

15.6.1.3 Dosing and Preparation

There is no known standardization of aristolochia, nor is there an accepted dose for the supplement, due to safety concerns occurring across a spectrum of doses.

15.6.1.4 Safety

Safety concerns have limited research to explore aristolochia as a weight loss agent. Since the 1990s, warnings from international regulatory agencies have been issued identifying risks for cancer and end-stage renal disease (Gold and Slone 2003). A review of Chinese botanical slimming regimens in 2002 identified aristolochia contributing to case report toxicities, with renal failure as the primary outcome (Ioset et al. 2003). Reports from the United Kingdom and the United States prompted the FDA to issue a consumer warning in April of 2001 to avoid all botanical products that contain aristolochia (United States Food and Drug Administration 2001). These severe adverse reactions limit any therapeutic use.

15.6.1.5 Evidence

Efficacy data is limited on the *Aristolochia* species, as the botanical has nephrotoxicity and carcinogenic properties. Laboratory evidence in mice has suggested that Aristolochia affects adipocyte differentiation by down-regulating key transcription factors in the adipogenesis pathway, resulting in lower serum triglyceride and cholesterol concentrations (Kwak et al. 2012).

15.6.1.6 Clinical Application

The nephrotoxicity of aristolochia restricts its clinical usefulness at this time and this supplement should be avoided.

15.6.2 Cha de Bugre (*Cordia ecalycuata*)

15.6.2.1 Background

Cha de Bugre is a Brazilian plant that is known to produce energy, appetite suppression, and weight loss. The tree produces red fruits similar to a coffee bean, which has been roasted and brewed as a tea or coffee preparation. In Brazil, it is also called café do mato, or "coffee of the woods." Many products, marketed as "Brazilian diet pills" contain Cha de Bugre along with other ingredients. Some of these products may be adulterated with amphetamine-like compounds.

15.6.2.2 Pharmacognosy

The fruit of the plant appears to have the medicinal properties, but it is not known what the actual active components may be at this time, or what medicinal value they may hold.

15.6.2.3 Dosing and Preparation

There is currently no established dose of Cha de Bugre. Preparations are often drinks, such as teas.

15.6.2.4 Safety

Due to a lack of evidence, the safety profile of Cha de Bugre is difficult to ascertain. More research is needed to evaluate the safety of this product.

15.6.2.5 Evidence

Little evidence exists regarding Cha de Bugre either in animal models or in humans. One Japanese study suggested that the plant had antiviral activities against the herpes simplex virus (Hayashi et al. 1990).

15.6.2.6 Clinical Application

Many testimonials regarding the product's stimulant properties exist on the internet, but until studies are conducted, little can be concluded regarding this product.

15.6.3 Forskolin (*Coleus forskohlii*)

15.6.3.1 Background

Coleus forskohlii is a plant native to India, belonging to the *Labiatae* family, better known as mint.

15.6.3.2 Pharmacognosy

Forskolin is isolated from the roots of *Coleus forskohlii*, and has been shown to have activity on adeylate cyclase. Forskolin increases the levels of cyclic AMP (cAMP), leading to increased lipolysis and potential weight loss (Godard et al. 2005).

15.6.3.3 Dosing and Preparation

Forskolin extract is most commonly used in research, with doses between 250 and 700 mg daily.

15.6.3.4 Safety

Coleus forkohlii has been evaluated in doses up to 1.5 g daily, with no serious adverse events associated with its use. Evidence exists for the use of forskolin topically, orally, and intravenously, all of which have been well tolerated (Henderson et al. 2005).

15.6.3.5 Evidence

A study evaluating 23 women across 12 weeks randomized to receive 500 mg of forskolin extract or placebo showed no differences in caloric intake, changes in fat mass, or body fat (Henderson et al. 2005). Subjects in the active group reported less fatigue ($p = 0.07$), hunger ($p = 0.02$), and more fullness ($p = 0.04$). Another study followed 30 obese men for 12 weeks, receiving either 500 mg of 10% forskolin extract or placebo daily (Godard et al. 2005). The active treatment group showed a significant decrease in body fat percentage ($-4.14 \pm 4.47\%$ compared with $-0.96 \pm 1.66\%$) at 12 weeks.

15.6.3.6 Clinical Application

Both of these studies were small and of short in duration, so further data are needed to clarify the effects forskolin has on weight.

15.6.4 Garcinia (*Garcinia cambogia*)

15.6.4.1 Background

Garcinia, also called *Malabar tamarind,* is a plant native to Southeast Asia whose dried rind has been used as a food preservative or flavoring agent. Many dietary supplement blends for weight loss contain this botanical. Garcinia has been studied for weight loss, exercise performance, joint pain, and as an antiparasitic agent.

15.6.4.2 Pharmacognosy

The primary acid in the fruit rinds, hydroxycitric acid (HCA), has been demonstrated to reduce body fat accumulation and suppress appetite in animal models (Greenwood et al. 1981, Ishihara et al. 2000). HCA may decrease fatty acid synthesis by inhibiting ATP-citrate lyase in a variety of tissues.

15.6.4.3 Dosing and Preparation

Daily doses of 2,000–5,000 mg of garcinia have been evaluated for its effects on weight loss. Standardization of garcinia products focuses on the HCA content of the supplement.

15.6.4.4 Safety

Garcinia has been well tolerated, with rates of adverse effects similar to placebo. Headache and upper respiratory tract symptoms have been most commonly reported. A review article summarized garcinia's safety from both animal and human trials (Soni et al. 2004). Evaluating 15 clinical studies with over 900 subjects, garcinia was well tolerated and did not produce severe adverse effects. The authors concluded that taking garcinia or the active ingredient HCA, at levels up to 2,800 mg/day, was safe for human consumption.

15.6.4.5 Evidence

Evidence examining garcinia use in humans is available. A randomized placebo-controlled study in Thailand assessed garcinia's effects on adipose tissue and body weight in 50 obese women over two months (Roongpisuthipong et al. 2007). The researchers demonstrated significant weight loss in the garcinia group over the placebo group (2.8 kg versus 1.4 kg, $p < 0.05$), as well as a decrease in fat storage, as evidenced by decreased tricep skinfold thickness. Another randomized placebo-controlled trial evaluated garcinia's effects on body weight and fat mass loss in 135 subjects across 12 weeks (Heymsfield et al. 1998). Patients in both study arms demonstrated significant weight loss from baseline, however the difference was similar between the treatment and placebo group for weight loss or fat mass reduction. This trial cited four other randomized controlled trials published only in abstract form, with three of the four demonstrating significant weight loss with garcinia compared to placebo, including one with 200 subjects where the active group demonstrated a significant weight loss using 1,500 mg of garcinia compared to placebo (2.8 kg versus 1.4 kg, $p < 0.01$) (Heymsfield et al. 1998). Finally, a randomized, placebo-controlled crossover trial examined garcinia's effects on metabolic parameters in sedentary men over 3 days and showed no changes in energy expenditure or fat oxidation, as proposed by animal models (Kriketos et al. 1999).

15.6.4.6 Clinical Application

Based upon this established safety, with some efficacy data in humans, garcinia is an option that can be considered for mild to moderate weight loss benefits.

15.6.5 Irvingia (*Irvingia gabonensis*)

15.6.5.1 Background

Irvingia gabonensis, or the African bush mango, is a forest tree indigenous to West Africa. Medicinal properties are attributed to the fruit and seeds. *Irvingia gabonensis* has been used for weight loss, diabetes, dyslipidemia, and pain management.

15.6.5.2 Pharmacognosy

Irvingia gabonensis is believed to inhibit adipogenesis and may also affect the secretion of gut hormones, increasing levels of adiponectin, and reducing levels of leptin by adipocytes.

15.6.5.3 Dosing and Preparation

Usual dosing for *Irvingia* that has been studied in weight loss and in diabetes is 3–4 g of crude seed extract per day, given in divided doses.

15.6.5.4 Safety

Irvingia gabonensis has been generally well tolerated. Of note, the studies in one review used widely varying dosing, with one trial using almost 10-fold greater amounts of *Irvingia gabonensis* compared to the other two trials. This suggests a relatively wide therapeutic window for the botanical. Adverse effects included headache, sleep disturbances, and flatulence, and occurred at similar rates as placebo (Onakpoya et al. 2013).

15.6.5.5 Evidence

A review article evaluating the effects of *Irvingia gabonensis* on weight loss in obese and overweight individuals had difficulties in its assessment due to poor study design and reporting across trials, starting with 431 initially screened studies and after applying criteria including only three trials (Onakpoya et al. 2013). Based on these studies, the authors concluded that *Irvingia gabonensis* supplementation had significant effects on reductions in body weight and waist circumference, but noted that poor study design and reporting of methodology limited the ability to definitively recommend the product for weight management. These studies, which were all of short duration, showed weight reduction in the active group, compared with placebo (12.8 kg versus 0.7 kg, p < 0.01 for the Ngondi 2009 trial, 4.1 kg versus 0.1 kg, p < 0.01 for the Ngondi 2005 trial, and 11.9 kg versus 2.1 kg, p < 0.001 for the Oben 2008 trial) (Onakpoya et al. 2013). The authors used a 10-week time point across these trials to yield weight loss percentages of over 5% across all three trials, suggesting clinically relevant weight loss. Waist circumference was also reduced in the active groups compared to placebo, at −16.2 cm versus −5.3 cm (p < 0.05), −6.2 cm versus +5.5 cm (p < 0.01), and −21.9 cm versus 1.0 cm, (p < 0.0001) respectively.

15.6.5.6 Clinical Application

While more evidence over longer time periods are needed to determine the role of *Irvingia gabonensis* in weight loss, the safety data suggest it is a potential option for the treatment of obesity.

15.6.6 Green Coffee (*Coffea arabica*)

15.6.6.1 Background

Green coffee refers to the green, unroasted coffee beans originating from the coffea fruits. These fruits are processed in different ways to yield the green coffee beans.

15.6.6.2 Pharmacognosy

The active ingredients from the green coffee bean are caffeine and chlorogenic acid, a potent antioxidant (Marcason 2013).

15.6.6.3 Dosing and Preparation

Green coffee extracts are standardized based upon the chlorogenic acids, usually containing between 30% and 60%.

15.6.6.4 Safety

See Chapter 5 Cardiovascular Disease for more discussion on green coffee.

15.6.6.5 Evidence

Green coffee extract was associated with significant weight loss in a crossover study presented at the American Chemical Society in 2012, where a cohort of 16 patients without notable diet and exercise demonstrated a 7.7 kg reduction in body weight from baseline, or 10.5% reduction in weight over 22 weeks (Vinson et al. 2012). These results were highlighted on a popular talk host show, and popularity for the product surged. Unfortunately, the authors later retracted the publication, stating that the sponsors of the study were unable to assure the validity of the data, and the Federal Trade Commission settled with the company, fining them $3.5 million dollars and requiring substantial evidence in human subjects prior to the company marketing any further products (Federal Trade Commission 2014).

15.6.6.6 Clinical Application

No trials are currently available examining green coffee extract for the treatment of obesity or weight loss. Since the earlier data are unsubstantiated, this product should not be recommended.

15.6.7 Green Tea (*Camellia sinensis*)

15.6.7.1 Background

Green tea originates from the *Camellia sinensis* plant, where the dried leaves are made into various teas, including green tea. It has been associated with multiple health benefits, and has been studied for its effects on obesity and weight loss in both human and animal trials.

15.6.7.2 Pharmacognosy

The active ingredient in green tea is thought to be epigallocatechin-3-gallate (EGCG). For obesity, doses between 500 and 1,000 mg are most commonly used, although there are data for other indications where over 2 g of EGCG have been studied.

15.6.7.3 Dosing and Preparation

See Chapter 5 Cardiovascular Disease for more discussion on green tea.

15.6.7.4 Safety

Green tea is well tolerated in both extract pill form and consumed as tea. The major adverse effects reported include stimulant effects, likely due to caffeine, including tachycardia, restlessness, and insomnia, as well as allergic reactions.

15.6.7.5 Evidence

Overall, the data regarding green tea's effects on obesity and weight are mixed. Some studies suggest that the weight loss effects are linked to the catechins and caffeine content in the tea or supplement. Some specific extract formulations have shown positive results, whereas others have not shown effects on weight. Multiple animal trials including mice, rats, and chickens have evaluated green tea's effects on metabolism and weight. Studies have demonstrated weight loss benefits, with proposed mechanisms including effects on the peroxisome proliferator-activated receptors, and regulation of metabolism-related genes and transcription factor expression (Huang et al. 2013, Yan et al. 2013, Xu et al. 2015).

In humans, results have been mixed regarding green tea's efficacy in weight loss. A study evaluating the supplement's effects on body composition and energy in 83 obese women over 12 weeks demonstrated no significant changes in body weight, fat mass, or energy (Mielgo-Ayuso et al. 2014). A randomized, controlled trial evaluated the effects of both green tea extract capsules as well as drinking green tea in 35 subjects across 8 weeks, standardizing both groups based on EGCG content (Basu et al. 2010). This study showed a decrease in BMI with the extract of -1.9 kg $\pm$ 0.6, $p < 0.05$, and with the tea itself a decrease of -2.5 kg $\pm$ 0.7, $p < 0.01$.

A Cochrane review evaluated weight loss effects of green tea, identifying 72 articles and, after exclusions, evaluated 14 RCTs, eight of which were conducted in Japan (Jurgens et al. 2012). The meta-analysis of these 14 trials showed an average weight loss of -0.95 kg (95% CI -1.75 to -0.15, $p = 0.02$), but also showed a high degree of heterogeneity across the trials. This was most prominent in the trials conducted in Japan, where there were fewer details regarding how the outcome measures were performed, such as how/when weight was measured. Performing a meta-analysis on the studies outside of Japan showed better heterogeneity, but still did not demonstrate significant weight loss effects. The authors concluded that green tea preparations produced small, nonsignificant weight loss in overweight or obese adults.

15.6.7.6 Clinical Application

Additional data are needed to further clarify green tea's role for the management of obesity.

15.6.8 Usnea (*Usnea barbata*)

15.6.8.1 Background/Pharmacognosy

Usnea, or usnic acid, is a metabolite from lichen that grow on a variety of tree species. It has been used for weight loss, pain relief, wound healing, and as an expectorant. Usnea was included in nonprescription diet aids, with proposed mechanisms to increase metabolism and raise basal metabolic rates.

15.6.8.2 Safety

A review article referred to 21 reports of hepatotoxicity with usnea received by the FDA, prompting the agency to issue a warning on one commercial product line (Guo et al. 2008). The review cited *in vitro* studies conducted on usnea, which demonstrated clear effects increasing liver enzymes (ALT and AST), reducing glutathione content, and causing a loss of cell membrane integrity. One study compared usnea to a known hepatotoxin, carbon tetrachloride, and demonstrated similar detrimental cellular responses to both substances (Pramyothin et al. 2004). *In vivo* evidence involving guinea pigs, rats, and mice also demonstrated hepatotoxicity with usnea use (Guo et al. 2008). Based upon this established toxicity, usnea should not be recommended.

15.6.8.3 Evidence/Clinical Application

There is no scientific data evaluating usnea's use as a weight loss agent, likely due to its toxicity.

15.7 Conclusions

With the continued problem of obesity in the United States, and the large number of consumers trying to lose weight, numerous botanical products have been explored for their weight loss properties. Many of these have shown some efficacy in helping facilitate weight loss, or reduction in adipose tissue, but definitive data are lacking. Weight loss trials are challenging even with prescription drugs, which include well-designed studies and excellent follow-up. Dietary changes and exercise regimens have dramatic effects on both reducing weight and on the maintenance of that weight loss, so these changes should be considered when evaluating weight loss data. Nevertheless, some potential products could be recommended as an adjunct to diet and exercise modifications, as well as highlighting products with little to no evidence and those that have known toxicities and should be avoided. Health care professionals should remember that the best evidence for sustained weight loss include multifactorial approach that emphasizes diet and exercise in an overall weight reduction plan.

REFERENCES

Anderson J, Baird P, Davis H et al. 2009. Health benefits of dietary fiber. *Nutrition Review* 67 (4):188–205.
Antonio J, Colker C, Torina G et al. 1999. Effects of a standardized guggulsterone phosphate supplement on body composition in overweight adults: A pilot study. *Current Therapeutic Research- Clinical and Experimental* 60 (4):220–7.
Aoe S, Ikenaga T, Noguchi H et al. 2014. Effect of cooked white rice with high beta-glucan barley on appetite and energy intake in healthy Japanese subjects: A randomized controlled trial. *Plant Foods and Human Nutrition* 69 (4):325–30.
Apaydin E, Maher A, Shanman R et al. 2016. A systematic review of St. John's wort for major depressive disorder. *System Review* 5 (1):148.
Astell K, Mathai M, McAinch A, Stathis C et al. 2013. A pilot study investigating the effect of Caralluma fimbriata extract on the risk factors of metabolic syndrome in overweight and obese subjects: A randomised controlled clinical trial. *Complementary Therapeutic Medicine* 21 (3):180–9.
Avalos-Soriano A, De la Cruz-Cordero R, Rosado J, Garcia-Gasca T. 2016. 4-Hydroxyisoleucine from fenugreek (Trigonella foenum-graecum): Effects on insulin resistance associated with obesity. *Molecules* 21 (11).

Basu A, Sanchez K, Leyva MJ et al. 2010. Green tea supplementation affects body weight, lipids, and lipid peroxidation in obese subjects with metabolic syndrome. *Journal of American Collective Nutrition* 29(1):31–40.

Bhatt A, Dalal G, Shah S et al. 1995. Conceptual and methodologic challenges of assessing the short-term efficacy of Guggulu in obesity: Data emergent from a naturalistic clinical trial. *Journal of Postgraduate Medicine* 41 (1):5–7.

Blom W, Abrahamse L, Bradford R et al. 2011. Effects of 15-d repeated consumption of Hoodia gordonii purified extract on safety, ad libitum energy intake, and body weight in healthy, overweight women: A randomized controlled trial. *American Journal of Clinical Nutrition* 94 (5):1171–81.

Calapai G, Firenzuoli F, Saitta A et al. 1999. Antiobesity and cardiovascular toxic effects of Citrus aurantium extracts in the rat: A preliminary report. *Fitoterapia* 70 (6):586–92.

Centers of Disease Control and Prevention. 2015. Prevalence of Obesity Among Adults and Youth: United States, 2011–2014. https://www.cdc.gov/nchs/data/databriefs/db219.pdf (accessed April 18, 2017).

Chutkan R, Fahey G, Wright W, McRorie J. 2012. Viscous versus nonviscous soluble fiber supplements: Mechanisms and evidence for fiber-specific health benefits. *Journal of American Academy of Nurse Practitioners* 24 (8):476–87.

Coffey C, Steiner B, Baker A, Allison D. 2004. A randomized double-blind placebo-controlled clinical trial of a product containing ephedrine, caffeine, and other ingredients from herbal sources for treatment of overweight and obesity in the absence of lifestyle treatment. *International Journal of Obesity Related Metabolic Disorders* 28 (11):1411–9.

Dent M, Wolterbeek A, Russell P, Bradford R. 2012a. Safety profile of Hoodia gordonii extract: Mouse prenatal developmental toxicity study. *Food Chemical Toxicology* 50 Suppl 1:S20–5.

Dent M, Wolterbeek A, Russel P, Bradford R. 2012b. Safety profile of Hoodia gordonii extract: Rabbit prenatal developmental toxicity study. *Food Chemical Toxicology* 50 Suppl 1:S26–33.

Doyle H, Kargin, M. 1996. Herbal stimulant containing ephedrine has also caused psychosis. *British Medical Journal* 313 (7059):756.

Du H, Van der D, Boshuizen H et al. 2010. Dietary fiber and subsequent changes in body weight and waist circumference in European men and women. *American Journal of Clinical Nutrition* 91 (2):329–36.

Federal Trade Commission. 2014. Federal Trade Commission vs Applied Food Sciences Incorporated. https://www.ftc.gov/system/files/documents/cases/140908afscmpt.pdf (accessed April 18th, 2017).

Fuller S, Richard A, Ribnicky DM, Mynatt RL, Beyl R, Stephens JM. 2014. St. John's Wort has metabolically favorable effects on adipocytes in vivo. *Evidence Based Complementary Alternative Medicine*, Article ID 862575. PMCID: PMC4054923.

Garcia-de la Cruz L, Galvan-Goiz Y, Caballero-Caballero S et al. 2013. Hypericum silenoides Juss. and Hypericum philonotis Cham. & Schlecht. extracts: In-vivo hypolipidaemic and weight-reducing effects in obese rats. *Journal of Pharmacy Pharmacology* 65 (4):591–603.

Godard M, Johnson B, Richmond S. 2005. Body composition and hormonal adaptations associated with forskolin consumption in overweight and obese men. *Obesity Res* 13(8):1335–43.

Gold LS, Slone, TH. 2003. Aristolochic acid, an herbal carcinogen, sold on the Web after FDA alert. *New England Journal of Medicine* 349 (16):1576–7.

Greenwood M, Cleary M, Gruen R et al. 1981. Effect of (-)-hydroxycitrate on development of obesity in the Zucker obese rat. *American Journal of Physiology* 240 (1):E72–78.

Guo L, Shi Q, Fang J et al. 2008. Review of usnic acid and Usnea barbata toxicity. *Journal of Environmental Science and Health Care Environmental Carcinogenic Ecotoxicology Review* 26 (4):317–38.

Hallas J, Bjerrum L, Stovring H, Andersen M. 2008. Use of a prescribed ephedrine/caffeine combination and the risk of serious cardiovascular events: A registry-based case-crossover study. *American Journal of Epidemiology* 168(8):966–73.

Haller C, Benowitz N. 2000. Adverse cardiovascular and central nervous system events associated with dietary supplements containing ephedra alkaloids. *New England Journal of Medicine* 343 (25):1833–8.

Hammond R, Levine R. 2010. The economic impact of obesity in the United States. *Diabetes, Metabolic Syndromes and Obesity* 3:285–95.

Hansen D, George N, White G et al. 2012. Physiological effects following administration of Citrus aurantium for 28 days in rats. *Toxicology Appl Pharmacology* 261 (3):236–47.

Hayashi K, Hayashi T, Morita N, Niwayama S. 1990. Antiviral activity of an extract of Cordia salicifolia on herpes simplex virus type 1. *Planta Med* 56 (5):439–43.

Henderson S, Magu B, Rasmussen C et al. 2005. Effects of coleus forskohlii supplementation on body composition and hematological profiles in mildly overweight women. *Journal of International Society of Sports Nutrition* 2:54–62.

Henry C, Emery B. 1986. Effect of spiced food on metabolic rate. *Human Nutrition and Clinical Nutrition* 40 (2):165–8.

Heymsfield S, Allison B, Vasselli J, Pietrobelli A et al. 1998. Garcinia cambogia (hydroxycitric acid) as a potential antiobesity agent: A randomized controlled trial. *JAMA* 280 (18):1596–600.

Hill J. 2006. Understanding and addressing the epidemic of obesity: An energy balance perspective. *Endocrinology Review* 27 (7):750–61.

Huang J, Zhang Y, Zhou Y et al. 2013. Green tea polyphenols alleviate obesity in broiler chickens through the regulation of lipid-metabolism-related genes and transcription factor expression. *Journal of Agricultural Food Chemistry* 61 (36):8565–72.

Ioset J, Raoelison G, Hostettmann K. 2003. Detection of aristolochic acid in Chinese phytomedicines and dietary supplements used as slimming regimens. *Food Chem Toxicology* 41 (1):29–36.

Ishihara K, Oyaizu S, Onuki K, Lim K, Fushiki T. 2000. Chronic (-)-hydroxycitrate administration spares carbohydrate utilization and promotes lipid oxidation during exercise in mice. *Journal of Nutrition* 130 (12):2990–5.

Jensen M, Ryan D, Apovian M et al. 2014. Guidelines American College of Cardiology/American Heart Association Task Force on Practice, and Society Obesity. 2013 AHA/ACC/TOS guideline for the management of overweight and obesity in adults: A report of the American College of Cardiology/American Heart Association Task Force on Practice Guidelines and The Obesity Society. *Circulation* 129 (25 Suppl 2):S102–38.

Jurgens T, Whelan A, Killian L, Doucette S, Kirk S, Foy E. 2012. Green tea for weight loss and weight maintenance in overweight or obese adults. *Cochrane Database System Review* 12.

Kaats G, Miller H, Preuss H, Stohs S. 2013. A 60day double-blind, placebo-controlled safety study involving Citrus aurantium (bitter orange) extract. *Food Chem Toxicology* 55:358–62.

Khossousi A, Binns C, Dhaliwal S, Pal S. 2008. The acute effects of psyllium on postprandial lipaemia and thermogenesis in overweight and obese men. *British Journal of Nutrition* 99 (5):1068–75.

Kriketos A, Thompson H, Greene H, Hill, J. 1999. (-)-Hydroxycitric acid does not affect energy expenditure and substrate oxidation in adult males in a post-absorptive state. *International Journal of Obesity Related Metabolic Disorders* 23 (8):867–73.

Kuriyan R, Raj T, Srinivas S, Vaz M et al. 2007. Effect of Caralluma fimbriata extract on appetite, food intake and anthropometry in adult Indian men and women. *Appetite* 48 (3):338–44.

Kwak D, Lee J, Kim T et al. 2012. Aristolochia manshuriensis Kom inhibits adipocyte differentiation by regulation of ERK1/2 and Akt pathway. *PLoS One* 7 (11):e49530.

Landor M, Benami A, Segev N, Loberant B. 2015. Efficacy and acceptance of a commercial Hoodia parviflora product for support of appetite and weight control in a consumer trial. *Journal of Medical Food* 18 (2):250–8.

Lee R, Balick M. 2007. Indigenous use of Hoodia gordonii and appetite suppression. *Explore (NY)* 3 (4):404–6.

Liu A, Smith S, Fujioka K, Greenway F. 2013. The effect of leptin, caffeine/ephedrine, and their combination upon visceral fat mass and weight loss. *Obesity (Silver Spring)* 21 (10):1991–6.

Liu S, Willett W, Manson J et al. 2003. Relation between changes in intakes of dietary fiber and grain products and changes in weight and development of obesity among middle-aged women. *American Journal of Clinical Nutrition* 78 (5):920–7.

Marcason W. 2013. What is green coffee extract? *Journal of Acad Nutritional Diet* 113 (2):364.

Marketdata Enterprises. 2011. U.S. weight-loss market tops $60 billion. http://www.dietscam.org/reports/market.shtml (accessed May 31st, 2017).

Mathern J, Raatz S, Thomas W, Slavin J. 2009. Effect of fenugreek fiber on satiety, blood glucose and insulin response and energy intake in obese subjects. *Phytotherapy Resserves* 23 (11):1543–8.

Mielgo-Ayuso J, Barrenechea L, Alcorta P et al. 2014. Effects of dietary supplementation with epigallocatechin-3-gallate on weight loss, energy homeostasis, cardiometabolic risk factors and liver function in obese women: Randomised, double-blind, placebo-controlled clinical trial. *British Journal of Nutrition* 111 (7):1263–71.

Mithila M, Khanum F. 2014. The appetite regulatory effect of guggulsterones in rats: A repertoire of plasma hormones and neurotransmitters. *Journal of Dietary Supplements* 11 (3):262–71.

Moreno L, Tresaco B, Bueno G et al. 2003. Psyllium fibre and the metabolic control of obese children and adolescents. *Journal of Physiology Biochemistry* 59 (3):235–42.

National Center for Complementary and Integrative Health. 2016. St John's Wort. https://nccih.nih.gov/health/stjohnswort/ataglance.htm. (accessed April 18th, 2017).

Natural Medicines. 2016. https://naturalmedicines.therapeuticresearch.com/ (accessed April 18th, 2017).

Onakpoya I, Davies L, Posadzki P, Ernst E. 2013. The efficacy of Irvingia gabonensis supplementation in the management of overweight and obesity: A systematic review of randomized controlled trials. *Journal of Dietary Supplements* 10 (1):29–38.

Pal S, Khossousi A, Binns C, Dhaliwal S, Ellis V. 2011. The effect of a fibre supplement compared to a healthy diet on body composition, lipids, glucose, insulin and other metabolic syndrome risk factors in overweight and obese individuals. *British Journal of Nutrition* 105 (1):90–100.

Pramyothin P, Janthasoot W, Pongnimitprasert N, Phrukudom S, Ruangrungsi N. 2004. Hepatotoxic effect of (+)usnic acid from Usnea siamensis Wainio in rats, isolated rat hepatocytes and isolated rat liver mitochondria. *Journal of Ethnopharmacology* 90 (2–3):381–7.

Roongpisuthipong C, Kantawan R, Roongpisuthipong W. 2007. Reduction of adipose tissue and body weight: Effect of water soluble calcium hydroxycitrate in Garcinia atroviridis on the short term treatment of obese women in Thailand. *Asia Pacific Journal of Clinical Nutrition* 16 (1):25–9.

Scott A, Orsi A, Ward C, Bradford R. 2012. Genotoxicity testing of a Hoodia gordonii extract. *Food Chem Toxicology* 50 Suppl 1:S34–40.

Shekelle P, Hardy M, Morton S et al. 2003a. Efficacy and safety of ephedra and ephedrine for weight loss and athletic performance: A meta-analysis. *JAMA* 289 (12):1537–45.

Shekelle P, Hardy M, Morton S et al. 2003b. Ephedra and ephedrine for weight loss and athletic performance enhancement: Clinical efficacy and side effects. *Evid Rep Technol Assess (Summ)* (76):1–4.

Sidhu L, Sharma K, Puri A et al. 1976. Effect of gum guggul on body weight and subcutaneous tissue folds. *J Res Indian Med Yoga Hom* 2 (11):16–22.

Snitker S, Fujishima Y, Shen H et al. 2009. Effects of novel capsinoid treatment on fatness and energy metabolism in humans: Possible pharmacogenetic implications. *American Journal of Clinical Nutrition* 89 (1):45–50.

Soni M, Burdock G, Preuss H, Stohs S, Ohia S, Bagchi D. 2004. Safety assessment of (-)-hydroxycitric acid and Super CitriMax, a novel calcium/potassium salt. *Food Chem Toxicology* 42(9):1513–29.

Stohs S, Preuss H, Shara M. 2011. A review of the receptor-binding properties of p-synephrine as related to its pharmacological effects. *Oxid Med Cell Longevity* 2011:1–9.

Stohs S, Preuss H, Shara M. 2012. A review of the human clinical studies involving Citrus aurantium (bitter orange) extract and its primary protoalkaloid p-synephrine. *International Journal of Medical Science* 9 (7):527–38.

Szapary P, Wolfe M, Bloedon L, Cucchiara A et al. 2003. Guggulipid for the treatment of hypercholesterolemia—A randomized controlled trial. *JAMA* 290 (6):765–72.

Tovar J, Nilsson A, Johansson M, Bjorck I. 2014. Combining functional features of whole-grain barley and legumes for dietary reduction of cardiometabolic risk: A randomised cross-over intervention in mature women. *British Journal of Nutrition* 111 (4):706–14.

Udani J, Hardy M, Madsen D. 2004. Blocking carbohydrate absorption and weight loss: A clinical trial using Phase 2 brand proprietary fractionated white bean extract. *Alternative Medicine Review* 9 (1):63–9.

United States Food and Drug Administration. 2001. Aristolochic Acid: FDA Warns Consumers to Discontinue Use of Botanical Products that Contain Aristolochic Acid. https://www.fda.gov/Food/RecallsOutbreaksEmergencies/SafetyAlertsAdvisories/ucm096388.htm (accessed April 18th, 2017).

United States Food and Drug Administration. 2003. Ephedrine Alkaloid-Containing Dietary Supplements. http://www.fda.gov/NewsEvents/Testimony/ucm115044.htm (accessed April 18th, 2017).

United States Food and Drug Administration. 2004. Final Rule Declaring Dietary Supplements Containing Ephedrine Alkaloids Adulterated Because They Present an Unreasonable Risk. https://www.fda.gov/ohrms/dockets/98fr/04-2912.htm (accessed April 18th, 2017).

United States Food and Drug Administration. 2005. Phenylpropanolamine (PPA) Information Page. https://www.fda.gov/Drugs/DrugSafety/InformationbyDrugClass/ucm150738.htm (accessed May 31st, 2017).

United States Food and Drug Administration. 2006. Barley Betafiber and Coronary Heart Disease. https://www.fda.gov/ohrms/dockets/dockets/06p0393/06p-0393-cp00001-002-vol1.pdf (accessed April 18th, 2017).

Van Heerden F. 2008. Hoodia gordonii: A natural appetite suppressant. *Journal of Ethnopharmacology* 119 (3):434–7.

Vinson J, Burnham R, Nagendran M. 2012. Randomized, double-blind, placebo-controlled, linear dose, crossover study to evaluate the efficacy and safety of a green coffee bean extract in overweight subjects. *Diabetes, Metabolic Syndromes, and Obesity* 5:21–7.

Whelan A, Jurgens M, Szeto V. 2010. Case report. Efficacy of Hoodia for weight loss: Is there evidence to support the efficacy claims? *J Clin Pharm Ther* 35 (5):609–12.

Whitehouse A, Duncan J. 1987. Ephedrine psychosis rediscovered. *British Journal of Psychiatry* 150:258–61.

Wu X, Xu X, Shen J, Perricone N, Preuss H. 2010. Enhanced Weight Loss From a Dietary Supplement Containing Standardized Phaseolus vulgaris Extract in Overweight Men and Women. *Journal of Applied Research* 10 (2):73–9.

Xu Y, Zhang M, Wu T, Dai S, Xu J, Zhou Z. 2015. The anti-obesity effect of green tea polysaccharides, polyphenols and caffeine in rats fed with a high-fat diet. *Food Functions* 6 (1):297–304.

Yamada T, Sugimoto K. 2016. Guggulsterone and its role in chronic diseases. *Drug Dis Mother Nat* 929:329–61.

Yan J, Zhao Y, Zhao B. 2013. Green tea catechins prevent obesity through modulation of peroxisome proliferator-activated receptors. *Sci China Life Sci* 56 (9):804–10.

Yang L, Li X, Wang H. 2007. Possible mechanisms explaining the tendency towards interstitial fibrosis in aristolochic acid-induced acute tubular necrosis. *Nephrology Dial Transplant* 22 (2):445–56.

Yoshioka M, St-Pierre S, Suzuki M, Tremblay A. 1998. Effects of red pepper added to high-fat and high-carbohydrate meals on energy metabolism and substrate utilization in Japanese women. *British Journal of Nutrition* 80 (6):503–10.

Zalewski B, Chmielewska A, Szajewska H. 2015. The effect of glucomannan on body weight in overweight or obese children and adults: A systematic review of randomized controlled trials. *Nutrition* 31 (3):437–42.

16

Cancer Prevention and Treatment

Margaret M. Charpentier, Britny Rogala, Rachel Ryu, and Jordan O'Leary

CONTENTS

16.1 Introduction

Oncology is the primary area of medicine which has benefited from the development of drugs derived from a range of plants. Common plant-based therapies include the taxanes, podophyllotoxins, camptothecans, and the vinca alkyloids which remain core treatments in diverse malignancies. The National Cancer Institute supports CAM research, with an annual budget of 120 million dollars available for research proposals (Jia 2012). Evidence for the use of botanicals using well-designed studies is needed. The botanicals with the best evidence for the treatment and/or prevention of cancer are discussed in this chapter.

16.2 Turmeric

16.2.1 Background

See Chapter 14 Musculoskeletal Conditions for discussion.

16.2.2 Pharmacognosy

See Chapter 14 Musculoskeletal Conditions for discussion.

16.2.3 Dosing and Preparation

Curcumin is typically given in large doses to achieve adequate serum concentrations. Dosages of 4–8 g daily in three divided doses have been administered (Kanai et al. 2011; Golombick et al. 2012; Ryan et al. 2013). A proprietary pharmacokinetically-boosted formulation of curcumin (Meriva®) is available (Belcaro et al. 2014; Panahi et al. 2014) and is dosed 300–1,000 mg of curcumin three times daily after meals.

16.2.4 Safety

Several trials have indicated that doses ranging between 2–8 g per day were not feasible given the large number of patients who discontinued treatment due to gastrointestinal (GI) toxicity (Epelbaum et al. 2010; Carroll et al. 2011). However, other trials with doses up to 8 g per day have concluded that GI adverse effects are manageable, given their low grade and that patients were able to continue therapy (Kanai et al. 2011; Panahi et al. 2014).

Due to concerns for the bleeding risk with curcumin, some trials have excluded patients who have recently undergone surgery (Belcaro et al. 2014). In addition, similar concerns exist if patients that are receiving concomitant antithrombotic therapy (Ryan et al. 2013).

In terms of drug interactions, curcumin has been shown to reduce the efficacy of doxorubicin and cyclophosphamide in human breast cancer cell lines (Somasundaram et al. 2002). It also has been shown *in vitro* to inhibit CYP3A4 (Zhang and Lim 2008) and CYP1A2 (Chen et al. 2010) and induce CYP2D6 (Chen et al. 2010); thus, caution is advised when coadministering with agents that are metabolized via these enzymes.

16.2.5 Evidence

16.2.5.1 Chemoprevention

In a phase IIa trial, 41 patients at risk for colon cancer underwent screening endoscopy and thereafter received either 2 or 4 grams daily of curcumin for 30 days. The number of aberrant crypt foci (ACF), which are thought to be the precursor to an adenomatous polyp, were counted at baseline and after treatment. Four grams per day of curcumin (n = 19) significantly reduced the number of ACF (p < 0.005). The same result was not found in 21 patients taking 2 g daily (Carroll et al. 2011).

In patients with myeloma precursor disease (monoclonal gammopathy of undetermined significance [MGUS] or smoldering multiple myeloma [SMM]), an abnormal free light chain ratio (rFLC) is an independent predictor of the risk of progression to symptomatic multiple myeloma (Golombick et al. 2012). In a randomized, double-blind, placebo-controlled cross-over study in patients with MGUS or SMM, curcumin 4 g daily decreased the rFLC. Likely due to a small sample size (n = 25), this result was not statistically significant. In the open-label extension study that followed, patients received curcumin 4 g twice daily (n = 18), and a significant decrease in the rFLC was noted after 3 months of therapy. There was a trend towards significance in patients receiving 4 g daily. Further study is warranted in a larger population of patients to validate these findings prior to implementation of its use to prevent the progression to symptomatic multiple myeloma in the MGUS/SMM population.

16.2.5.2 Chemotherapy Treatment

16.2.5.2.1 Pancreatic Cancer

A nonrandomized, open-label, phase II trial assigned 25 patients with metastatic pancreatic cancer to receive single-agent curcumin 8 g per day (Dhillon et al. 2008). Of the 21 evaluable patients, one continued to have stable disease over 18 months, along with a decreased CA125 level. Another patient had a radiographically-proven marked response (73% reduction in tumor size) that lasted one month and correlated with increases in serum cytokine levels (IL-6, IL-8, IL-10, and IL-1 receptor antagonists). A third patient remained in the study for about 8 months with progression in nontarget lesions. The response to curcumin may have been limited by a lack of adequate exposure, given that the range of curcumin levels at steady state was 22–41 ng/mL. Antiproliferative effects *in vitro* require blood concentrations in microgram amounts have been shown *in vitro* to be the most efficacious in terms of antiproliferative effects.

In a phase I trial, 19 patients with pancreatic cancer receiving gemcitabine 1,000 mg/m^2 took 8 g per day of curcumin at dosing intervals of their own discretion and two patients received single-agent gemcitabine (Kanai et al. 2011). Among the patients taking curcumin, no complete or partial responses were noted and 28% (n = 5) had stable disease. Given the small enrollment in this trial, the authors concluded that curcumin supplementation was safe and feasible, but could not comment on efficacy.

16.2.5.2.2 Prostate Cancer

Curcumin has been studied as an adjunct to radiation therapy in patients with prostate cancer (Hejazi et al. 2016). One trial of 40 patients was single-center, randomized, and double-blinded. Patients received either 3 g of curcumin (Biocurcumin) as two 500 mg capsules with each meal daily or placebo. No significant differences in prostate specific antigen (PSA) or imaging were noted between the two groups.

A study of 203 patients with prostate cancer on active surveillance or watchful waiting were randomized to a whole food formulation containing 100 mg broccoli powder, 100 mg turmeric powder, 100 mg pomegranate whole food powder, and 20 mg green tea extract or placebo three times daily in a double-blinded trial (Thomas et al. 2014). Over a period of six months, the PSA level increased significantly less in the intervention group versus placebo (14.7% versus 78.5%, respectively, P = 0.0008).

A phase II, nonrandomized, single-arm study treated 26 patients with castration-resistant prostate cancer with docetaxel, the standard of care, and curcumin 6,000 mg per day (Mahammedi et al. 2016). The objective response rate was 40%, with a PSA response of 59%. These preliminary results warrant further investigation with a randomized, controlled trial in which comparison to patients without the intervention can be made.

See Chapter 17 Supportive and Palliative Care for Cancer for further discussion.

16.2.6 Clinical Application

Given the lack of statistically significant survival data, as well as the risk of rendering anticancer therapy ineffective, turmeric should not be used as a substitution or adjunct to standard of care chemotherapy or radiation. Similarly, it should not be used for adverse effect management after chemotherapy or radiation. In the absence of risk factors for bleeding, turmeric can be considered for chemoprevention, with the most evidence for the prevention of colorectal cancer.

16.3 Glycine Max L Soy Isoflavones

16.3.1 Background

Soybeans (Glycine Max L) are legumes which were first cultivated as a domesticated crop in Asia more than 5,000 years ago (He and Chen 2013). Soybeans were not grown in the Americas until the 1940s. Soybeans are processed for use as soy milk, soy fiber, soy protein and soybean oil, and used in many foodstuffs (Graham and Vance 2003). Soy is a major source for isoflavones (He and Chen 2013), however the isoflavone content varies by region in which it is grown, with U.S. soy having significantly lower isoflavone content per gram of soy than Asian soybeans. Although soy is a major component of the Asian diet, only recently has soy been incorporated into U.S. diets, and is typically in much lower quantities (He and Chen 2013; Mahmoud et al. 2014).

16.3.2 Pharmacognosy

Glycine max L is used as both foods and as a supplement. The main isoflavones consist of genistein, daidzein, and glycitien. Isoflavones exhibit estrogenic-like effects, through weak binding to estrogenic receptors. In addition, geistein and daidzein may provide additional anticancer activity such as decreased cell proliferation, cell cycle regulation, cell death, anti-angiogenesis, inhibition of tumor cell invasion, and metastasis (Zand et al. 2000; Mahmoud et al. 2014).

The isoflavone content in various soy products is available; however, consideration of the phytoestrogen content must also be determined since this varies greatly among soy foods based on environmental factors such as harvest time, growing environment and processing (Harnly et al. 2006; Kuhnle et al. 2009). Another important consideration is equol which is a metabolite of daidzein, produced by intestinal microflora. Equol may have higher estrogenic activity than daidzein, although only about a third of people are believed to be able to produce equol. The ability to produce equol varies in individuals, and by region of the world: Japanese, Chinese and Korean populations are more likely to be equol producers (50%–60%) than Americans (25%–30%) (Lampe et al. 1998; Setchell et al. 2002; Sonoda et al. 2004; Setchell and Clerici 2010).

16.3.3 Dosing and Preparation

As noted, soy is processed into many different products. Soy consumption in cancer is most often based on the isoflavone component, where typical doses range from 10 to 120 mg daily (Dong and Qin 2011). Studies evaluating the dietary consumption of soy used different dosages and formulations of soy, although one meta-analysis used 10 mg as a cut off between high (10 mg or more), and less than 10 mg for a low consumption of isoflavones (Nechuta et al. 2012). One recently published trial evaluating dietary isoflavone intake in North American populations for breast cancer survival defined a high intake of isoflavone, based on food frequency questionnaires, as >1.5 mg/day (Zhang et al. 2017). There was no consistency across trials for these definitions (Chi et al. 2013). Of note, typically in Asian populations, 1 g of soy is equivalent to 3.5 mg of isoflavones (Messina et al. 2006).

16.3.4 Safety

In general, soy is well tolerated and has received "generally recognized as safe" (GRAS) status from the FDA (Archer Daniels Midland Company 1998). Soy has been a major component on the Asian diet for generations. The most common adverse effect is constipation, in one trial up to 50% of patients reported this (Albertazzi et al. 1998); however, most trials do not report this nearly as commonly, if at all. The other adverse effect in that same trial, bloating, was reported in about 11% of patients. Allergies have been reported rarely to soy. Concern regarding cross allergy with peanuts has been investigated, since soybeans and peanuts are phylogenetically and antigenically similar. Fortunately, cross reactivity is rare, and the evidence is insufficient to warrant avoiding soy in patients with a peanut allergy (Sicherer et al. 2000).

16.3.5 Evidence

16.3.5.1 Breast Cancer Prevention

Soy has been studied for breast cancer prevention based on epidemiologic data comparing high soy diets versus low soy diets. A meta-analysis of trials has shown that diets high in soy appear to lower breast cancer risk in Asian countries (RR 0.76; 95% CI 0.65, 0.86), yet not in Western countries (RR 0.97, 95% CI 0.87, 1.06) (Dong and Qin 2011). These differences may be due to the type of soy consumed such as glycosides versus aglycons, equol producer status, differences in breast cancer risk based on ethnicity, and dietary survey accuracy (Setchell and Clerici 2010). Of note, this meta-analysis of trials included studies using a variety of soy dosages with inconsistent definitions for low dose and high dose of soy, and a dose response effect with soy was not demonstrated. Based on current evidence, it is premature to conclude that diets high in soy lower breast cancer risk in Non Asian populations.

16.3.5.2 Breast Cancer Recurrences

A study evaluated 9,514 patients diagnosed with breast cancer using combined dietary survey information from two trials conducted in US and one trial in a Chinese population. High soy diets, defined as at least

10 mg soy isoflavones daily, were compared with low soy diets for their effects on recurrence and survival in breast cancer (Nechuta et al. 2012). The US populations who consumed a high soy diet had a lower body mass index (BMI), were more likely to exercise, were more highly educated, ate more cruciferous vegetables, and were less likely to smoke. In China, those who consumed a high soy diet were more likely to eat cruciferous vegetables and to exercise, however these patients had a higher BMI. A reduction in recurrence in breast cancer (HR 0.75, 95% CI 0.65–0.92) without a statistically significant benefit in survival was observed in patients consuming a high soy diet. The reduction in recurrence was similar in both populations. This trial followed patients for 7.4 years which may not be long enough nor powered adequately to evaluate actual survival.

A more recent study evaluating dietary isoflavone intake in 6,235 female breast cancer survivors in North America did identify a 22% reduction in all-cause mortality with higher intake of isoflavone (defined as >1.5 mg/day) compared to lower intakes (Zhang et al. 2017). This study was of a long duration, about 9.4 years; however confounders in the ethnically diverse population were many. Women who consumed higher levels of isoflavones in this study were more likely to be Asian Americans, younger, pre-menopausal, physically active, less likely to smoke, not overweight or obese, and drank less alcohol than the low soy intake. Additionally the women in the high isoflavone intake also had a higher diet quality index compared to other quartiles. None of these potential confounders were adjusted for in the findings.

A meta-analysis of trials evaluating soy consumption after the diagnosis of breast cancer, and the risk of breast cancer recurrence identified a reduction in mortality with soy intake (HR 0.7, 95% CI 0.58–0.85), as well as a reduction in recurrence (HR 0.77, 95% CI 0.63–0.95). The effects of soy did not vary based on menopausal status, estrogen receptor (ER) status or tamoxifen use (Chi et al. 2013).

16.3.5.3 Gynecologic Cancer Prevention

A meta-analysis of the effects of soy on the prevention of gynecologic cancer included both case-control and cohort studies (Myung et al. 2009). Randomized controlled trials were not available to include. A total of seven trials were identified, including five case-controlled trials. The odds ratio (OR) for the highest soy intake was 0.61 (95% CI 0.53–0.71). The analysis reported an OR for endometrial cancer of 0.70 (95% CI 0.57–0.86) and an OR of 0.52 for ovarian cancer (95% CI 0.36–0.90). Although these results are significant, they warrant should be verified by prospective controlled trials. Potential biases from these results include a lack of definitions across trials of what constituted high dose of soy compared to lower doses, recall bias from the case-control trials. Of note, populations included in the trial were U.S. published trials (3), China (2), Italy (1) and Japan (1). The results from the U.S. trials were similar to those the Asian countries. The authors did not report on publication bias or heterogeneity.

16.3.5.4 Prostate Cancer

The available data on soy supplementation or diets high in soy in prostate cancer is inconclusive. The evidence is primarily from small trials of short duration. The assessed outcomes have included effects on sex hormonal levels, indicating no change with short term use. An effect on PSA levels has not been identified (van Die MD et al. 2014). Soy supplementation may be beneficial in prevention of prostate cancer in patients with high risk based on the limited data from two small studies enrolling a total of 116 patients (Hamilton-Reeves et al. 2008; Miyanaga et al. 2012), with follow up for 6–12 months. Caution should be used when extrapolating from the studies, as one showed no significant benefit, while the second trial of 58 patients, reported a RR of 0.16, based on 6 months of follow up (Hamilton-Reeves et al. 2008; Miyanaga et al. 2012; van Die et al. 2014).

See Chapters 6 Endocrine Disorders, 8 Women's Health, 14 Musculoskeletal Diseases, and 17 Supportive and Palliative Care for Cancer for further discussion in other conditions.

16.3.6 Clinical Application

A diet rich in soy may protect Asian women from developing breast cancer, and also protect against recurrence in Asian women diagnosed with breast cancer. Data is inconclusive if this benefit exists in Western women. Factors such as the type of soy consumed (grown in Asia vs grown in the West), harvesting and processing of soy, a patient's equol production, and ethnicity may be important in determining the effects of soy on breast cancer. Published evidence thus far indicates that a diet rich in isoflavones does not increase mortality in breast cancer in U.S. populations. It is premature to state that soy can decrease mortality or recurrence of breast cancer in U.S. populations.

Similarly, data is lacking on the use of soy supplementation or increased soy consumption for prevention or treatment of prostate cancer. No recommendations can be made based on the published data, although consumption of higher soy diets appears safe and well tolerated.

16.4 Green Tea

16.4.1 Background

See Chapter 5 Cardiovascular Disease for discussion.

16.4.2 Pharmacognosy

See Chapter 5 Cardiovascular Disease for discussion.

16.4.3 Dosing and Preparation

See Chapter 5 Cardiovascular Disease for discussion.

16.4.4 Safety

Due to its antioxidant properties, green tea can counteract the therapeutic effect of bortezomib and other anticancer proteasome inhibitors (Golden et al. 2009). It also affects the metabolism and transport of tamoxifen, irinotecan, UGT substrates, and CYP 3A4 substrates and thus concomitant use should be avoided (Lin et al. 2008; Shin and Choi 2009; Wanwimolruk et al. 2009; Mohamed et al. 2011). *See Chapter 5 Cardiovascular Disease for further safety discussion.*

16.4.5 Evidence

16.4.5.1 Prevention

16.4.5.1.1 Colorectal Cancer

In a Japanese multicenter trial, 133 patients with a previous endoscopic resection of at least one colorectal adenoma were randomized to receive 1.5 grams of green tea extract (GTE) daily or placebo (Shimizu et al. 2008). Each 500 mg tablet is equal to two Japanese-size cups of green tea, meaning patients were taking the equivalent of six cups daily as a supplement. This dose was selected based on epidemiologic studies that suggested at least 10 cups of green tea daily may delay onset of cancer and that the average daily green tea consumption in Japan is six cups. Patients requiring aspirin or nonsteroidal anti-inflammatory drugs were excluded from the trial. Enrollment began one year after resection, after confirmation of absence of polyps. The primary endpoint was a reduction in recurrent adenomas. At one year following enrollment, GTE supplementation resulted in a decreased risk of metachronous adenomas (15 versus 31%, $p < 0.05$). No serious adverse effects were noted in the intervention arm.

16.4.5.1.2 Oral Premalignant Lesions

A phase II, randomized, placebo-controlled trial examined the effect of GTE in patients with high-risk oral premalignant lesions (OPL) (Tsao et al. 2009). Patients were randomized in a double-blinded manner to one of four treatment arms including placebo (n = 11), GTE 500 mg/m^2 (n = 11), 750 mg/m^2 (n = 9), or 1,000 mg/m^2 (n = 10) given three times daily. Patients had follow-up biopsies 12 weeks after enrollment. A pooled analysis of response to GTE revealed a response rate, defined as at least a 50% reduction in

OPL, of 50% versus 18.2% in patients receiving placebo (P = 0.09). The response was dose-dependent, with the highest doses (750–1,000 mg/m²) resulting in greatest response (58%) as compared with a 36% response rate in the 500 mg/m² group and 18% in the placebo arm (P = 0.03). However, after over 2 years of follow up, the GTE and placebo groups were similar in terms of oral cancer-free survival.

16.4.5.1.3 Prostate Cancer

Sixty white men with high-grade prostate intraepithelial neoplasia at high risk for prostate cancer were randomly assigned in a double-blinded fashion to green tea catechins (GTCs) or placebo at a single institution in Italy (Bettuzzi et al. 2006). Patients received three 200 mg GTC capsules daily. After one year, the incidence of prostate cancer was significantly reduced (30% versus 3%, control versus experimental, respectively). This correlated with a 90% reduction in risk (p < 0.01). A reduction in International Prostate Symptom Score was also noted (11.12–9.12, p < 0.05), indicating a potential link between GTCs and reduction in symptoms of benign prostate hyperplasia.

16.4.5.1.4 Endometrial Carcinoma

A meta-analysis comprised of two cohort and five case-control studies evaluated the effect of tea consumption on the risk of primary endometrial cancer (Tang et al. 2009). Both green and black tea studies were included with a total of 3,487 cases and 104,643 controls of endometrial carcinoma. Definitions for non/low consumption varied, but generally fell within a range of 0–2 cups of tea per day. A subgroup analysis was conducted and found a benefit with green tea consumption, but not black tea. The relative risk (RR) of endometrial cancer was 0.79 (95% CI, 0.69–0.90), showing a 21% reduction in risk of endometrial carcinoma for patients consuming green tea versus those who were not or had minimal consumption. Both heterogeneity and sensitivity analyses were conducted and neither was found to be significant. The authors concluded that green tea may be associated with a decreased risk of endometrial carcinoma but acknowledged that findings should be validated with a large, prospective, well-controlled study.

16.4.5.1.5 Ovarian Cancer

A case-control study was conducted in China to examine the effect of tea consumption on the incidence of ovarian cancer (Zhang et al. 2002). Two hundred fifty-four cases with confirmed epithelial ovarian cancer and 652 controls were enrolled into the study and evaluated for green tea consumption. Patients who had confirmed ovarian cancer were interviewed about tea consumption 5 years prior to their diagnosis. Controls were asked similarly to report tea consumption 5 years prior to the interview. The risk of ovarian cancer decreased with increasing amounts and duration of consumption. In patients who drink tea daily, the odds ratio was 0.39 (95% CI, 0.27–0.57) and for those who drank for over 30 years, the odds ratio was 0.23 (p < 0.001; 95% CI, 0.13–0.41).

A meta-analysis of 11 case-control and seven cohort studies was recently conducted to evaluate the effect of tea consumption on the risk of ovarian cancer (Zhan et al. 2017). Trials were evaluated for methodological quality using the Jadad score, with trials scoring less than 3 being excluded from the analysis. Patients were reported to have consumed various teas, including green, black, and red tea. The relative risks adjusted for confounders were used for final analysis. A total of 8,683 cases and 693,174 controls were included. Tea consumption was found to have a protective effect against ovarian cancer, with a relative risk of 0.86 (95% CI, 0.76–0.96). The effect was sustained when adjusted for risk factors including family history of cancer, menopausal status, education, BMI, smoking, and Jadad score of 3 or 5. Unfortunately, the authors did not separately analyze the effect of different types of teas, nor did they report on relative dosages.

16.4.5.2 Treatment

16.4.5.2.1 Chronic Lymphocytic Leukemia

A phase II, single-arm trial was conducted in 42 patients with previously untreated, asymptomatic, Rai stage 0-II chronic lymphocytic leukemia (CLL) who did not meet criteria to initiate chemotherapy (Shanafelt et al. 2013). All patients received Polyphenon E 2,000 mg capsules, each containing approximately 200 mg of epigallocatechin gallate (EGCG). Patients received one capsule (2,000 mg) twice daily for up to 6 months. Thirteen patients (31%) had a sustained reduction in absolute lymphocyte count (ALC) and 20 patients (69%) with palpable adenopathy had at least a 50% reduction in the sum of the products of all nodal areas. No statistical analysis was conducted. Adverse effects were rare, with one report each of hepatic transaminitis, abdominal pain, and fatigue. The authors concluded that a randomized trial would be required to confirm these promising results.

16.4.5.2.2 Ovarian Cancer

Patients with stage III to IV ovarian cancer who had a complete response to debulking surgery and platinum and taxane-based chemotherapy were enrolled in a single-arm trial to drink 500 mL of double brewed green tea daily and to assess the risk for recurrent disease (Trudel et al. 2013). After 18 months, only 5 of the 16 women remained disease-free. The study was then terminated due to a lack of response to treatment. Based on this evidence, green tea likely does not have a protective effect against ovarian cancer recurrence.

See Chapters 5 Cardiovascular Disease, 6 Endocrine Disorders, and 15 Obesity and Weight Loss for further discussion of other conditions.

16.4.6 Clinical Application

Some evidence suggests that green tea may have a role in the prevention and treatment of malignancies, most notably ovarian and endometrial cancers. Given its safety and tolerability, the use of green tea for the prevention of cancer is reasonable. Larger, prospective, randomized, placebo-controlled trials with standardized dosing schemes are needed to validate these preliminary results before implementing into cancer treatment.

16.5 Guarana (*Paullinia cupana*)

16.5.1 Background

Guarana is a monoecious fruit native to Brazil, Venezuela, and Costa Rica (Schimpl et al. 2013). The fruit of guarana can range in color from yellow to bright red when ripe. Each fruit contains one to four seeds that contain high quantities of caffeine. Guarana, varana, or uarana translates to "vine," which describes its tendrils that can be up to 10 meters in length. Historically, guarana was used as a tonic, stimulant, and aphrodisiac since pre-Columbian times. Medicinal uses included treatment of fever, headache, and cramps. Recently, guarana is most commonly used as a soft and energy drink. The fruit is also used for metabolic and mood disorders, along with cancer-related fatigue (Smith and Atroch 2007; Schimpl et al. 2013).

16.5.2 Pharmacognosy

Guarana seeds contain caffeine that ranges from 2.5% to 6%, which is higher than that of coffee, tea, and yerba mate (Schimpl et al. 2013). The caffeine content is dependent on the type of plant tissue and organ, genetic variability, climate, and soil conditions. Other xanthine alkaloids may be present including theophylline and theobromine; these compounds are primarily responsible for the psychostimulant properties of guarana. Other constituents in guarana include terpenes, flavonoids such as epicatechin and catechin, starch, saponins, tannins like proanthocyanidins, and resinous substances (Schimpl et al. 2013; Hertz et al. 2015).

16.5.3 Dosing and Preparation

Guarana can be prepared as a suspension, powder, extract, syrup, and capsules (de Oliveira Campos et al. 2011a). Doses of 75 mg were well tolerated when used for the improvement of cognition and memory. In studies of cancer patients, dosages between 75 and 100 mg daily are safe in the treatment of cancer-related fatigue.

16.5.4 Safety

Guarana is considered GRAS by the FDA when used as a food additive in minimal amounts necessary to produce the desired effect (CFR - Code of Federal Regulations Title 21 2016). Reported adverse effects include those attributed to caffeine, such as palpitation, insomnia, nausea, and anxiety (de Oliveira Campos et al. 2011b; del Giglio et al. 2013). Pregnant women should be cautioned, since increasing doses of caffeine have been associated with a higher risk of miscarriage and spontaneous abortion (Klebanoff et al. 1999; Weng et al. 2008).

16.5.5 Evidence

In a Portuguese double-blind, placebo-controlled crossover trial, patients with any stage breast cancer with no history of anticancer therapy were initially screened for fatigue. Those with severe baseline fatigue rated as over seven on the Brief Fatigue Inventory were excluded (de Oliveira Campos et al. 2011b). Fatigue was again assessed after the first cycle of chemotherapy and patients were excluded if their fatigue severity failed to increase. Only patients who had a new or worsening fatigue after chemotherapy were enrolled and received guarana. Women were randomized to dry crude guarana extract (n = 32) or placebo (n = 43). Capsules of 50 mg guarana or placebo were administered twice daily for 21 days. The two groups had similar baseline characteristics. Portuguese language questionnaires that had been previously validated were used. Fatigue was measured by the Functional Assessment of Chronic Illness Therapy – Fatigue (FACIT-F) and Chalder Fatigue Scale. Other questionnaires included the Functional Assessment of Chronic Illness Therapy – Endocrine Symptoms for menopausal symptoms, the Hospital Anxiety and Depression Scale (HADS), and the Pittsburgh Sleep Quality Index (PSQI). Evaluation was conducted on the first day and after the second and third cycles of chemotherapy on days 21 and 49, respectively. After day 21, patients had a 7-day washout period before crossing over to the other experimental arm. Dropouts included eight patients who received placebo in the first phase and seven who received guarana in the first phase. Adverse effects that led to discontinuation included tachycardia and rash. All results on the fatigue scales showed significance on days 21 and 49 ($p < 0.01$), except for the Chalder Fatigue Score on day 49 ($p = 0.27$). Adverse effects included insomnia, palpitation, nausea, anxiety, and dermatologic reaction. Anxiety, depression, and sleep quality were similar between the two arms. The same investigators conducted a phase II, double-blind, placebo-controlled study in which patients with any stage head and neck tumors receiving chemoradiation were randomized to the treatment (n = 31) or control (n = 29) group (dos Santos Martins et al. 2017). Patients in the treatment group received a dry extract of guarana at a dose of 50 mg twice daily during 6 weeks of chemoradiation, in which three cycles of chemotherapy were administered on days 1, 21, and 42. The two arms did not cross over during the study. Data on general demographics and initial fatigue using the FACT-F tool were collected at baseline. Additional questionnaires were used, the Functional Assessment of Cancer Therapy: Head and Neck (FACT-HN), European Organization for Research and Treatment of Cancer Core Quality of Life Questionnaire C30 (EORTC QLQ-C30), and the Quality of Life Head and Neck module on days 1, 21, 42, and 63, along with toxicity assessments on days 21 and 43. After two cycles of chemotherapy, changes in quality of life were significantly worsened for women in the treatment group on the FACT-F questionnaire in the overall ($p = 0.0054$), functional ($p = 0.018$), and symptom ($p = 0.0042$) domains. However, differences were not significant at baseline and at the end of treatment. On the FACT-HN questionnaire, the treatment group showed significant improvement after one cycle of chemotherapy in pain ($p = 0.0133$), weight loss ($p = 0.012$), social eating ($p = 0.0227$), swallowing ($p = 0.0254$), and coughing ($p = 0.0107$). After the third cycle, there was a significant worsening of weight loss and a greater need for nasogastric tubing and analgesics for the guarana group. On the EORTC QLQ-C30, improvement in all three domains of quality of life were seen. The two groups were similar in reported toxicity. The authors concluded that guarana did not provide benefit in this patient group.

A lower dose of guarana has also been used in patients with breast cancer who were receiving adjuvant radiation in a double-blind pilot study (da Costa Miranda et al. 2009). Women were randomized to receive either guarana 75 mg (n = 17) or placebo (n = 19). Guarana or placebo was taken once daily until the end of radiation therapy, which was approximately 35 days. Halfway through the course of radiation treatment, women were crossed over to the other arm. The groups were similar at baseline for age, race, stage, and initial fatigue intensity. Fatigue was assessed before radiation, during the crossover phase, and after radiation with validated questionnaires using the Chalder Fatigue Scale, the MD Anderson Brief Fatigue Inventory (BFI), and the Beck Inventory Depression Scale II. Dropouts did not occur. No differences were reported in fatigue, depression, or toxicity between the groups. The lower guarana dose could be associated with the lack of significant improvement in the treatment group. In addition, the study may have been underpowered to detect any significant differences due to its small sample size.

Another study initially administered a standardized purified dry extract of guarana in an open study to 40 patients with various tumors in the induction phase (del Giglio et al. 2013). Guarana was dosed at 37.5 mg twice daily for 21 days. Only patients who showed improvement in fatigue afterward were randomized to either guarana (n = 17) or placebo (n = 16). The same guarana dose and regimen were used for 3 weeks in the maintenance phase. The BFI was used before and after induction. The FACIT-F, Chalder Fatigue Scale, HADS, and PSQI were used at the beginning and end of the maintenance phase. All the validated questionnaires were in Portuguese. Dropouts included two patients in the treatment group and one in the placebo group. No improvements in fatigue, anxiety, depression, and sleep were observed. Two grade 3 toxicities that were unique to the treatment group were dizziness and depression. Insomnia and dry skin were observed in both groups.

A meta-analysis of three double-blind trials by the same authors included 137 cancer patients receiving either chemotherapy (74%) or radiation (26%) (Giglio et al. 2011). Of the total, 85% were patients with breast cancer. In the trials, patients were randomized to either guarana or placebo, and subsequently crossed over to the other treatment. Two studies did not require fatigue to be present at baseline, whereas the third did after one cycle of chemotherapy. The dose of guarana ranged from 75 to 100 mg daily. Women who received guarana had significant improvement in fatigue on the global (p = 0.0007), physical (p = 0.05), and mental (p = 0.006) Chalder Fatigue Scale. When examined individually, the two studies that did not require the presence of fatigue at baseline showed no significant improvement in fatigue, whereas the third that required fatigue presence after one cycle of chemotherapy showed benefit. No grade 3 or 4 adverse events occurred. Quality of sleep, anxiety, and depression were not worsened in one of the studies that addressed adverse events. Larger studies are needed to confirm the efficacy of guarana in this patient population.

16.5.6 Clinical Application

Available studies show conflicting results regarding the use of guarana to treat fatigue in cancer patients. Pregnant women should be cautioned of guarana's caffeine content and all patients should avoid the concomitant use of guarana with other stimulant-like drugs. Patients with uncontrolled hypertension, cardiovascular disease, angina, insomnia, and other neurologic disorders should avoid its use (del Giglio et al. 2013).

16.6 Maitake (*Grifola frondosa*)

16.6.1 Background

Native to northern Japan, maitake has long been treasured as a rare and valuable mushroom with potent health benefits (Nanba 1996). Maitake means "dancing mushroom," for one would "start dancing with joy" upon discovering it. In feudal times, people traded maitake for its weight in silver (Mayell 2001). Its weight can sometimes exceed 50 pounds. The mushroom is found on deciduous oak trees and has a large fruiting body made of overlapping caps. Historically, it has been used in Asia for human immunodeficiency virus (HIV), hepatitis, and arthritis. The Japan National Institute of Health and the U.S. National Cancer Institute in 1992 confirmed maitake's anti-HIV activity (Preuss and Konno 2002). As such, practitioners began administering maitake in HIV/ AIDS patients. In addition, the maitake D-fraction extract is used topically for the treatment of lesions from Kaposi's sarcoma, a common cancer in patients with AIDS. Maitake is also used in hypertension, hyperlipidemia, obesity, diabetes, cancer, and immune deficiency (Nanba 1996; Preuss and Konno 2002; Ulbricht et al. 2009).

16.6.2 Pharmacognosy

D-fraction is derived from the polysaccharides of maitake's fruiting body and the MD-fraction is obtained from further purification, which was patented in the United States (Mayell 2001). Other constituents of maitake include polysaccharide-peptides, triterpenoids, nucleosides, and complex starches (Preuss and Konno 2002; Ulbricht et al. 2009). Various mechanisms have been proposed for maitake's anticancer activity, with polysaccharide-induced immunomodulation being the most studied. In cancer patients, D-fraction increased concentrations of IL-12, enhancing NK cell activity and cytotoxicity in tumor cells, subsequently increasing TNF-α and IFN-γ concentrations as well as suppressing tumor growth (Kodama et al. 2002b). Another reported property of D-fraction was the *in vivo* induction of angiogenesis and *in vitro* proliferation of human vascular endothelial cells and growth factor (Matsui et al. 2001). Based on *in vitro* data, maitake polysaccharides induced apoptosis of various cancer cells by causing oxidative stress and mitochondrial dysfunction (Fullerton et al. 2000; Shomori et al. 2009; Soares et al. 2011).

16.6.3 Dosing and Preparation

Doses vary depending on fraction and type of formulation, which includes liquid extracts, tablets, capsules, and dried powder (Ulbricht et al. 2009). In breast cancer, 0.1–5 mg/kg of maitake liquid extract was given twice daily (Deng et al. 2009). In studies with cancer patients, doses ranged from 35 to 150 mg of MD-fraction per day as caplets or liquid extracts, and 4–6 g of whole maitake powder per day in the form of capsules and tablets (Nanba 1996; Kodama et al. 2002a; Preuss and Konno 2002; Ulbricht et al. 2009). For immune support, 1–3 g maitake tablets are recommended and up to 7 g is recommended for therapeutic purposes (Preuss and Konno 2002).

16.6.4 Safety

Maitake in low doses is presumed to be safe based on hundreds of years of experience as a food (Ulbricht et al. 2009). In addition, because of its safety, a phase I test for toxicology was exempt by the FDA for maitake D-fraction (Preuss and Konno 2002). However, hypoglycemic properties of maitake has been suggested although data is limited (Konno et al. 2001). As a result, patients with diabetes should use caution. Patients allergic to maitake mushroom should avoid use since there have been reports of hypersensitivity (Deng et al. 2009; Wesa et al. 2015). Safety has not yet been determined in pregnant or lactating women (Ulbricht et al. 2009).

16.6.5 Evidence

In a Japanese case series, 36 patients with stage II-IV cancers were given a mixture of isolated beta-glucan polysaccharides (MD-fraction) and whole maitake powder after discontinuing chemotherapy (Kodama et al. 2002a). The dosages of MD-fraction ranged from 40 to 150 mg daily, and whole Maitake powder ranged from 4–6 g daily. A positive response was considered to be one of the following: tumor reduction on a CT or MRI scan by 50%–75%, decrease in tumor markers by 33%–50%, reduction or maintenance of TNM staging, increase to normal levels of immune parameters (T lymphocytes, macrophages, NK cells, etc.), or increase in cytokine (IL-1 and IL-2) production. The baseline characteristics were not clearly stated. After treatment, cancer regression was significant, especially among cancers of the liver (7/12), breast (11/16), and lung (5/8), but not for leukemia and cancers of the brain and stomach. Significant symptom improvement occurred, although specific symptoms were not identified. Unclear definitions of symptom improvement and tumor regression were used and therefore, data must be interpreted with caution. Clinical outcomes such as duration of response, time to progression, or overall survival could not be evaluated.

In a nonrandomized, single-arm, multicenter study, maitake D-fraction was administered to 165 patients with various types of stage III-IV tumors in western Japan (Nanba 1996). The dose of the tablets containing crude maitake powder was unclear with the exception of six patients in whom the daily doses of D-fraction and maitake caplet ranged from 35 to 100 mg, and 4 to 6 g, respectively. It is uncertain which patients took maitake alone or in combination with chemotherapy. The duration of treatment was not defined and baseline characteristics were only provided for six patients. A positive response was defined one of the following: reduction or maintenance of tumor on a CT or MRI scan, decrease in tumor markers, reduction or maintenance of TNM staging, or extension of prognosis by a minimum of 4-fold. Tumor regression or significant improvement occurred in breast cancer patients (11/15), lung cancer patients (12/18), and liver cancer patients (7/15). Symptoms such as anorexia, leukopenia, alopecia, nausea, and vomiting were improved in 90% of patients and pain reduction in 83% of patients. The authors noted that compared to maitake alone, maitake with chemotherapy had a synergistic effect in breast, lung, and liver cancer, but not in bone cancer, stomach cancer, and leukemia. Limitations of the study included inadequate descriptions of patient characteristics and treatment received, along with ambiguous definitions of symptom improvement and tumor regression.

A single-arm, nonrandomized, phase II trial administered maitake extract to patients (n = 21) with low to intermediate-1 risk myelodysplastic syndromes based on the International Prognostic Scoring System (Wesa et al. 2015). A dose of 3 mg/kg was given twice a day for 12 weeks. Three dropouts occurred, one of which was caused by grade one diarrhea and the others were due to disease progression. Neutrophil count and function were compared with those of healthy controls that were matched for age. Results were significant for increase in neutrophil count (p = 0.005), increase in monocyte function (p = 0.021), production of reactive oxygen species (p = 0.03), decrease in monocyte response pre-treatment compared to healthy controls (p = 0.002), and increase in monocyte response post-treatment compared to healthy controls (p = 0.03). Adverse effects included four cases of grade one eosinophilia (p = 0.014), three cases of diarrhea, and one case of nausea. Limitations include lack of a control group and unknown clinical significance.

16.6.6 Clinical Application

Limited evidence exists regarding the role of maitake in tumor regression, symptom improvement, and immune enhancement in cancer patients. In addition, the dosages, preparation, and administration schedules for maitake are not standardized. Studies have not examined clinical endpoints such as response rate, duration of response, or survival. Some studies permitted the use of chemotherapy, with no standardization of background therapy. The trials did not evaluate specific cancer types or stages, making its application in patients difficult. Because of the immunomodulating properties of maitake, patients taking immunosuppressive medications should avoid its use. Any use of maitake in cancer patients should be limited to clinical trials.

16.7 Pomegranate (*Punica granatum L*)

16.7.1 Background

Pomegranate, from the family Lythraceae, originated in Persia and has been cultivated through the Mediterranean region and Northern India since ancient times (Langley 2000). Pomegranate has been used as a symbol for royalty and for fertility (Langley et al. 2000). The fruit has been used to treat hypertension, myocardial infarction, congestive heart failure, atherosclerosis; all believed to benefit from the antioxidant polyphenols. Pomegranate may have chemopreventive, and anticancer effects from the punicalagin component. Pomegranate can interfere with cell proliferation, cell cycle, angiogenesis and invasion in skin, prostate, and other cancer cells lines (Seidi et al. 2016). The antioxidant capacity of pomegranate is three times greater than those of red wine and green tea (Turrini et al. 2015).

16.7.2 Pharmacognosy

The seed, juice, peel, leaf, flower, bark and roots contain phenolics, flavonoids, ellagitannins, gallic acid, ellagic acid, gallocatechin, delphinidin, cyanidin, pelargonidin, sitosterol, proanthocyanidin compounds, hydrolysable tannins, and anthocyanins (Seidi et al. 2016; Sharma et al. 2017). Punicalagin is a large polyphenol that includes the minor tannins punicalagin and ellagic acid. Punicalagin represents the bioactive constituent responsible for more than 50% of antioxidant activity (Turrini et al. 2015). Pomegranate affects multiple pathways involved in inflammation, cellular transformation, hyperproliferation, angiogenesis, initiation of tumorigenesis, and suppressing the final steps of tumorigenesis and metastasis (Sharma et al. 2017). Some studies have shown that pomegranate use can prolong PSA doubling time (PSADT), thereby possibly blocking prostate cancer growth (Malik et al. 2005).

16.7.3 Dosing and Preparation

The formulation with the highest antioxidant activity is the juice, followed by the total pomegranate tannin, punicalagin, and lastly ellagic acid (Seeram et al. 2005). There is no general consensus on dosage for pomegranate. In some studies pomegranate ellagitannin-enriched polyphenol providing 710–1,420 mg of extract has been used for up to 4 weeks (Pantuck et al. 2006). In another trial a dose of 8 ounces of pomegranate juice has been administered daily for more than 13 years (Paller et al. 2017).

16.7.4 Safety

Pomegranate is generally well tolerated. Rarely, pomegranate can cause hypersensitivity reactions, especially in people with other plant allergies. Other rare reactions include pruritus, angioedema, bronchospasm, cardiac-related adverse effects, and gastrointestinal issues including diarrhea, reflux disease, nausea, abdominal pain, constipation, frequent bowel movements, stomach discomfort, and vomiting (Paller et al. 2013). In one case report, pomegranate reportedly caused rhabdomyolysis in a patient receiving rosuvastatin (Sorokin et al. 2006). Patients with diabetes should use caution when using this product because of sugar content (Adams et al. 2006).

Drug interactions include medications metabolized through 3A4, 2D6, and 2C9, such as warfarin, carbamazepine, and oncology agents metabolized through these pathways. (Srinivas 2013). Clinically, these findings appear to be weak (Abdlekawy et al. 2017). Pomegranate may low blood pressure, and therefore use with caution in patients on antihypertensive medication (Adams et al. 2006). Another potential concern is that pomegranate has a mild angiotensin converting enzyme (ACE) inhibitor effect; therefore, in patients who cannot tolerate ACE inhibitors, or are already receiving ACE inhibitors, these patients should be aware of this (Aviram and Dornfeld 2001).

Since pomegranate is a strong antioxidant, supplements of pomegranate should not be used in patients receiving radiation therapy and chemotherapy such as anthracyclines, bleomycin, and alkylating agents that relies on free radical formation for its cell killing.

16.7.5 Evidence

In a trial of 48 men with biochemically recurrent prostate cancer, all participants received 8 ounces of pomegranate juice daily (Pantuck et al. 2006). Patients were enrolled after initial surgery or radiation treatment and had a PSA less than 5 ng/mL and a Gleason score of 7 or less at baseline. At 33 months, in 46 evaluable patients, PSADT rose from a mean of 15 months at baseline to a mean of 54 months ($p < 0.001$). Thirteen years later, 10% of the patients have still not met the PSADT criteria and continue receiving pomegranate juice (Paller et al. 2017). No serious adverse events were reported. While these results appear promising, this study has few participants and requires additional details on enrollees, such as age at enrollment and responses based on Gleason score. Without a placebo-control and risk stratification, it is difficult to determine if these results are due to pomegranate intake or if participants were simply at low risk of prostate cancer progression.

A trial using pomegranate phenols extract powder randomized 104 patients to 1–3 g of the extract daily (Paller et al. 2013). Of note, the study authors indicated that 1 g of extract is equivalent to antioxidant effect of 8 ounces of pomegranate juice. Men could be enrolled with any PSA or Gleason score at baseline. The patients' PSA baseline score was not reported. A total of 92 evaluable patients were presented. Baseline characteristics reveal that 76% had a Gleason score of 6 or less. While no dose effect relationship was identified, the median PSADT increased from the patient baseline of 11.9 months to 18.5 months (p < 0.001). Serious adverse events were not reported. This trial lacked information on patients with higher Gleason score and their risk for a PSADT versus patients with lower Gleason scores, information regarding other treatments and its effect on PSADT.

Both trials were sponsored by POM Wonderful. Neither study included a control arm, and both lacked information regarding effects of other treatments received for prostate cancer on the effects of PSADT. Using PSADT is not the most reliable or relevant marker for prostate cancer since there can be variations in PSA over time. Without a control group, no conclusions regarding pomegranate can be made.

A phase III randomized, placebo-controlled, multicenter trial was conducted to answer these questions (Pantuck et al. 2015). This trial evaluated 8 ounces liquid pomegranate extract to placebo. A total of 183 men were enrolled with 64 treated with placebo. The primary endpoint was PSADT which was similar between the treatment arm and the placebo arm. A planned subset analysis in men with manganese superoxide dismutase (MnSOD) AA genotype demonstrated a significantly improved PSADT from 13.6 months at baseline to 25.6 months with pomegranate extract (p = 0.03) compared to no improvements observed in the placebo arm (10.9 months to 12.7 months, p = 0.22). The AA genotype of MnSOD codes for a more aggressive prostate cancer than the VA or VV genotype of MnSOD. While this finding is interesting, it requires validation in future clinical trials. In this trial, pomegranate extract was safe over at least 2 years.

16.7.6 Clinical Application

Pomegranate may be used for lengthening PSADT in men who underwent radical prostatectomy, brachytherapy, or cryotherapy. Whether pomegranate offers any benefit in prostate cancer is unclear, although it does appear safe. Patients with diabetes should use pomegranate juice with caution.

16.8 European Mistletoe (*Viscum album L*)

16.8.1 Background

Mistletoe is a semiparasitic shrub that grows on other trees including elm, pine, apple, oak, poplar, and spruce. Its leaves are small, yellowish green, the flowers are a yellowish color, while the berries are white and waxy. Mistletoe has been used for its healing powers for millennia, first described by Pliny during the first century BC, where he noted its use for inflammation, scrofulous sores, wounds, and for "dispersing tumors." Mistletoe is also included in Nordic mythology for its magical qualities, and is believed to be an antidote to poisons (Kandela 2001). During the 1920s mistletoe began to be more widely used as a subcutaneous injection to treat tumors, particularly in Europe (Ostermann et al. 2009).

16.8.2 Pharmacognosy

The parts of the plant used for extraction include the berry, and fresh leafy shoots. The plant is harvested in summer and winter, and the extract is prepared using a combination of these juices prepared as aqueous solution of water and alcohol and are non-fermented or a fermented extract. The extract is typically identified by the source of the host tree: M = apple, P = pine, U = elm, Qu = oak, and A = spruce. The quantities of the active moiety will vary by season extracted, host tree, and preparation methods. Active components of mistletoe include lectins (MLI, II and III), which are the most investigated; viscotoxins, low molecular weight proteins, oligosaccharides and polysaccharides, flavonoids, and others. The lectins are biologic response modifiers that stimulate the immune system resulting in leukocytosis; increasing neutrophils and natural killer cells. An increase in release of cytokines, such as interleukin (IL) 1, IL2, IL 6, and tumor necrosis factor alpha has been observed. Tachyphylaxis to immune stimulation results from repeated administration, requiring a dose escalation to maintain response (Huber et al. 2000; Heinzerling et al. 2006). A DNA stabilizing effect on mononuclear cells in the periphery is described (Büssing et al. 1995). Some data suggest that mistletoe induces apoptosis related to the effects of lectins and viscotoxins (Ostermann et al. 2009).

16.8.3 Dosing and Preparation

The dose and the formulations used in cancer vary, based on host plant, harvest time, and extraction methods used. Some formulations are manufactured to provide a consistent quantity of mistletoe lectin. Other formulations are manufactured are using standardized pharmaceutical processes (Horneber et al. 2008). The most widely used formulation, and best studied in cancer patients, is the IscatorÒ extract, made from fermentation, using the summer and winter harvest of the leafy shoots and berry (Ostermann et al. 2009). Dosing involves subcutaneous injections of the extract two to three times per week. The doses and the formulations used varied in studies; mistletoe dosing is based on patient tolerance and response. Therefore, the dose is continually increased over time. Mistletoe has also been injected directly into tumors and administered intrapleurally and intravesically.

16.8.4 Safety

Mistletoe extract appears to be well tolerated. In a Cochrane review, 12 studies reported on safety and was evaluated as moderate evidence to suggest it is well tolerated. Most commonly reported reactions were local injection site reactions, dose-related, which occurred in up to a third of patients. These were described as rubor, prurigo, and induration. Systemic reactions are dose dependent. In one retrospective analysis of adverse events with mistletoe, lower doses, ≤ 0.02 mg, the rate of adverse reactions was 0.8%, while with higher initial doses, 20.7% of patients experienced a reaction (Schad et al. 2017). Pyrexia was reported most commonly, up 62% of the reported adverse effects. Local reactions were about 30%. Most reactions were mild to moderate; however 1.2% of the reactions were deemed severe; consisting of severe pyrexia, one report of syncope, and one of a hypersensitivity reaction. Another study on adverse events related to mistletoe injection in over 1,300 patients reported similar findings, with about 8% of patients reporting any reaction. The reactions were mild to moderate in severity, and were largely redness, irritation, itching, and induration, and were dose related (Steele et al. 2014).

16.8.5 Evidence

Studies of mistletoe in cancer are generally smaller, of poor methodological design, with inconsistent dosing, formulation, and often used unclear enrollment criteria. Many of the trials used matched pair designs, but the criteria for matching was not well defined. In a Cochrane database review, 21 studies were identified, of which 13 reported on survival. A survival benefit was not identified in any population including breast cancer, colorectal, renal cell, head and neck, non-small cell lung cancer, malignant melanoma, malignant glioma, gastric cancer, and urinary bladder. Of the trials identified, six reported a survival benefit, while seven did not. Of these 13 trials, four were deemed to be of high quality methodology, all of these reported no survival benefit (Horneber et al. 2008). A total of 16 studies were identified that evaluated quality of life, performance status, psychological measures, and 11 of these evaluated the effects of mistletoe extract in reducing adverse events from chemotherapy. Fourteen of these studies found a benefit in improving QOL with significant heterogeneity in study design and results. Two studies, in breast cancer patients, had a high quality of methodology. Overall, the studies lacked consistent methods to evaluate quality of life, baseline assessments, and were unclear as to the evaluator. In addition, when evaluating if mistletoe reduced adverse effects of chemotherapy, the assessment was conducted weeks following the administration of the regimen (Horneber et al. 2008).

A meta-analysis of four studies in patients with various cancers evaluated the survival benefit of mistletoe extract (Ostermann and Bussing 2012). The studies used a retrolective method in which treatment had already begun before the start of the study. An overall positive survival benefit was noted with mistletoe, although major methodological issues were present. The limitations included a lack of randomization, no blinding in patient selection, problems with endpoint criteria, diversity in extracts, and different treatment regimens. These major issues made the systematic analysis difficult and the results suspect. *See Chapter 17 Supportive and Palliative Care for Cancer for further discussion.*

16.8.6 Clinical Application

The use of mistletoe extract in cancer patients is likely well tolerated, however evidence on its usefulness is lacking. A survival benefit has not been identified, and the effects of mistletoe extract to improve quality of life are unclear. With many different formulations and a lack of specific dosing, further research into mistletoe extract's role in cancer treatment is warranted.

16.9 Reishi (*Ganoderma lucidum*)

16.9.1 Background

Reishi is a mushroom found on deciduous trees in temperate regions throughout Asia, North and South America, and Europe (Wasser 2010). *Lucidus* means "shiny" in Latin, which is characteristic of its fruiting body. The mushroom has been used for thousands of years and is mentioned as early as 221 B.C. Historic uses include treatment of neurasthenia, coronary heart disease, hypertension, hypercholesterolemia, chronic hepatitis, insomnia, and cancer.

16.9.2 Pharmacognosy

Active components of *G. lucidum* are found in its spores, mycelia, and fruiting body (Wasser 2010). These include polysaccharides, triterpenoids, sterols, steroids, fatty acids, nucleotides, proteins and peptides, and trace elements. A proposed mechanism of action for antitumor activity is through immune system potentiation by polysaccharides, particularly active β-D-glucans. This polysaccharide may bind to the surfaces of leukocytes and proteins, activating T-helper cells, natural killer (NK) cells, macrophages, and other effector cells. The subsequent result would be an increase in the production of cytokines including interleukins (IL) and interferons, tumor necrosis factor (TNF-α), nitric oxide, and antibodies. Ultimately, vascular damage to the tumor would occur, causing necrosis and tumor regression.

16.9.3 Dosing and Preparation

G. lucidum is available as tablets, capsules, tinctures, syrups, teas, foods, and boluses (Wasser 2010). Doses include 10 mL tinctures (20%) three times a day and 1 g tablets three times a day. For advanced cancer, Ganopoly® 600 mg was given as three capsules three times daily before meals (Gao et al. 2003; Gao et al. 2005; Chen et al. 2006). Published cancer studies have used varied preparations, dosing, and administration (Wasser 2010; Jin et al. 2016).

16.9.4 Safety

β-glucans derivatives of *G. lucidum* are not GRAS by the FDA. Overall, adverse effects are temporary and mild, such as bloating, rashes, thirst, polyuria, and loose stools (Wasser 2010). Because *G. lucidum* has potentiating effects on the immune system, patients receiving immunosuppressive therapy should be cautioned. In addition, bleeding is a potential risk with the concomitant use of antithrombotic drugs (Wasser 2010; Jin et al. 2016).

16.9.5 Evidence

16.9.5.1 Lung Cancer

In a Chinese double-blind, multicenter, placebo-controlled study, standardized Ganopoly® capsules containing 600 mg extract of *G. lucidum* (equal to 30 g fruiting body) was administered as three capsules three times daily before meals for 12 weeks to patients with advanced lung cancer (Gao et al. 2003). Patients received only Ganopoly® or placebo. Baseline characteristics were similar between the treatment (n = 37) and placebo groups (n = 31) for chemotherapy history, tumor histology, smoking status, gender, and age. The extent of disease (WHO criteria, 1979) and Karnofsky performance status (KPS), along with biochemical, hematologic, and immunological studies were evaluated at baseline and after 12 weeks of treatment. There were five dropouts in the treatment group and three in the placebo group. The number of patients with stable disease was significantly higher in the Ganopoly® group compared to the placebo group (35.1% vs 22.6%). Statistical analysis was not conducted for the clinical response.

In addition, 50% of patients who received Ganopoly® had significant increases in KPS score (over 10) compared to 14% of those that received placebo ($p < 0.05$). Increases in immune parameters such as lymphocyte transformation, CD3 percentage, and NK cell activity ($p < 0.05$) were found in the intervention group. Patients in the Ganopoly® group had improvement of cancer-related symptoms such as fever, sweating, weakness, anorexia, weight loss, and insomnia ($p < 0.05$). Mild adverse effects included two episodes of insomnia and one episode of nausea in the treatment group. The authors concluded that adjunct Ganopoly® may be beneficial in the treatment of advanced lung cancer (Gao et al. 2003). The study limitations included a lack of information on survival benefits, duration of effect, or other outcomes. This trial was of a short duration and in a small population of lung cancer patients with a mixed pathology, limiting its applicability.

A Chinese trial with a less rigorous design reported conflicting results on the effects of *G. lucidum* on immune response in 36 patients with advanced lung cancer (Gao et al. 2005) In a noncontrolled, single-arm, open-label study, Ganopoly® 1,800 mg, equal to 27 g fruiting body of *G. lucidum*, was administered three times daily prior to meals for 12 weeks. *G. lucidum* was the only intervention that was administered during the study period. Immune parameters including phytohemagglutinin-induced mitogenic reactivity; lymphocyte counts of CD3, CD4, CD8, and CD56; and plasma concentrations of IL-1, IL-2, IL-6, IFN-γ, TNF-α, and NK activity were measured at baseline and after 12 weeks in 30 assessable patients. Six patients dropped out due to nonadherence, loss to follow-up, and death from disease complications. The mean immune variables were not significantly different before and after treatment with Ganopoly®. However, in a subsequent correlation analysis, significant relationships were identified between the changes of immune variables after treatment with *G. lucidum*. Changes in IL-1 correlated with those for IL-6, IFN-γ, CD3, CD4, CD8, and NK activity ($p < 0.05$). Other correlations were also seen with changes for IL-2, TNF-α, IFN-γ, CD3, and CD4.

16.9.5.2 Breast Cancer

In a Chinese randomized, placebo-controlled pilot trial, breast cancer patients who completed or were receiving endocrine therapy with cancer-related fatigue were enrolled (Zhao et al. 2012). Patients were excluded if they had other diseases that could contribute to fatigue such as chronic fatigue syndrome and fibromyalgia. *G. lucidum* spore powder 1,000 mg (n = 25) or placebo (n = 23) was administered three times daily for 4 weeks. The FACT-F, HADS, and European Organization for Research and Treatment of Cancer Core Quality of Life Questionnaire C30 (EORTC QLQ-C30) were used at baseline and after 4 weeks. Immune markers including TNF-α and IL-6, along with hepatic and renal function, were assessed before and after the study. Baseline characteristics were similar between the groups, including fatigue. On the fatigue subscale, patients in the treatment group scored 39.76 ± 5.10 on the FACT-F and 43.7 ± 17.9 on the EORTC QLQ-C30. All women were post-surgical patients with stage I-IIIA breast cancer. The average age in the treatment group and control group was 51 and 53 years, respectively. Results for women receiving *G. lucidum* improved on the FACT-F scale for physical well-being ($p < 0.01$), emotional well-being ($p < 0.05$), functional well-being ($p < 0.05$), fatigue ($p < 0.01$), and total score ($p < 0.01$). The difference in scores for social/family well-being between the two groups was similar. On the HADS scale, women in the treatment group had less depression ($p < 0.01$), anxiety ($p < 0.05$), and total score ($p < 0.01$). Compared to women in the control group, those in the treatment group had higher scores for fatigue ($p < 0.01$), physical functioning ($p < 0.01$), emotional functioning ($p < 0.01$), cognitive functioning ($p < 0.05$), global quality of life ($p < 0.01$), as well as lower scores for appetite loss ($p < 0.05$) and sleep disturbance ($p < 0.01$) on the EORTC QLQ-C30. The two groups were similar for role functioning, social functioning, pain, constipation, and diarrhea. At the end of the study, women in the treatment group also showed significantly lower TNF-α ($p < 0.01$) and IL-6 ($p < 0.05$) concentrations than at baseline. Hepatic and renal function was similar during the study Mild adverse effects including dry mouth and dizziness occurred in 12% and 16% of participants, respectively.

16.9.5.3 Colorectal Cancer

16.9.5.3.1 Prevention

In a Japanese study, 1.5 g of *G. lucidum* was administered daily for 12 months to 123 patients with colorectal adenomas (Oka et al. 2010). The authors selected 102 patients from the same institution to serve as controls: the selection criteria was not defined. Baseline characteristics were comparable between the two groups; however, the number of adenomas was higher in the treatment group ($p = 0.05$). Colonoscopy was performed at baseline in all patients and after 12 months in 96 and 102 accessible patients in the treatment group and control group, respectively, to measure the site, size, and macroscopic classification of adenomas. Of the 27 dropouts in the treatment group, six were due to adverse events related to diarrhea, stomach discomfort, and poor health. After 12 months, patients in the control group had an increased number of adenomas (0.66 ± 0.10), whereas this number decreased for those in the treatment group (-0.42 ± 0.10) ($p < 0.01$). The difference in number of polypoid-type adenomas was significant ($p < 0.01$) but not for superficial-type adenomas. Also, the size of adenomas increased in the control group (1.73 ± 0.28 mm) while it decreased in the treatment group (-1.40 ± 0.64 mm) ($p < 0.01$). Changes were significant for adenomas on the left and right side between the two groups ($p < 0.01$) but not for changes in the rectum. The authors suggested that *G. lucidum* prevents the development of colorectal adenomas. The study was limited by lack of placebo-control, randomization, blinding, and duration of follow up to determine if these findings ultimately result in the prevention of cancer.

16.9.5.3.2 Treatment

In a nonrandomized, open-label study, Ganopoly® was administered orally to 47 patients with advanced colorectal cancer to monitor immune response (Chen et al. 2006). A dose of 1,800 mg, equal to 27 g fruiting body of *G. lucidum*, was taken three times daily for 12 weeks and no other intervention was administered. The same immune parameters as a previous study (Gao et al. 2005) were measured at baseline and after 12 weeks in 41 assessable patients. Six patients dropped out due to cancer-related death, nonadherence, and loss to follow-up. Treatment with Ganopoly® resulted in small increases in counts of CD3, CD4, CD8, and CD56, concentrations of IL-2, IL-6, and IFN-γ, and NK activity; and a small decrease in concentrations of IL-1 and TNF-α. None of these changes between baseline and after treatment reached statistical significance. The authors found correlations between IL-1 changes and those for IL-6, IFN-γ, CD3, CD4, CD8, and NK activity ($p < 0.05$). IL-2 changes also correlated with those for IL-6, CD8, and NK activity. While these findings are interesting, there is no information on clinical data such as response, survival, or adverse effects.

16.9.5.4 Hepatocellular Carcinoma

A case series of three patients with advanced hepatocellular carcinoma (HCC) reported on the use of *G. lucidum* (Gordan et al. 2011). Patient 1 initiated *G. lucidum* shortly after beginning chemotherapy. After 8 months of taking *G. lucidum*, decreases in α-fetoprotein (AFP) level (from 13,074 to 15.2 μg/L) and retroperitoneal lymphadenopathy were observed. Disease progression was not evident for 2 years, until the development of peritoneal carcinomatosis and death soon after. Patient 2 took *G. lucidum* and Gan Fu Le, another traditional Chinese medicine (TCM), shortly after diagnosis. His liver mass, which was initially 8.9×4 cm, progressively decreased in size for 10 years until remaining stable at 4.2×1.8 cm. He received no other anticancer treatment and still took TCM as of the authors' publication. Patient 3 took *G. lucidum* and Pian Zhi Huang, another TCM which also includes *G. lucidum*. After taking these products, the AFP level decreased from 1,899 to 7.2 μg/L and the major hepatic lesion reduced in size from $11.8 \times 9.3 \times 12.7$ cm to a diameter of 5.4 cm on the longest side 10 months later. She continued to remain asymptomatic and took TCM for an additional 9 months, at time of publication. These cases show promise in the treatment of the highly aggressive HCC and warrant a clinical trial to explore the effect of *G. lucidum* in this population.

TABLE 16.1

PC-SPES

PC-SPES was a commonly used combination botanical for the treatment of prostate cancer marketed from 1996 to 2002 (DiPaola et al. 1998). The name represents prostate cancer (PC), and *spes* is Latin for hope. PC-SPES consists of eight compounds: *Ganoderma lucidum, Sutellaria baicalensis, Rabdosia rubescens, Isatis indigotica, Dendranthema morifolium, Seronoa repens* (saw palmetto) *Panax pseudoginseng* and *Glycyrrhiza uralensis* (licorice root).

PC-SPES has been evaluated for the treatment of androgen–insensitive prostate cancer (AIPC) in small phase II trials (de la Taille et al. 2000; Small et al. 2000; Kosty 2004; Oh et al. 2004). Response rate, defined as a 50% or greater reduction in the PSA level was high in these trials, 50%–80%. These results are similar to those reported in trials evaluating estrogen and chemotherapy. Adverse effects were similar to the use of estrogen, including gynecomastia (over 90% of patients), leg cramps (69%), nausea and vomiting (14%), and thromboembolism (5%). Observations and reports of estrogenic therapeutic activity and adverse effects, in addition to its widespread use in patients with prostate cancer, prompted an exploration of the estrogenic activity of PC-SPES (Kosty 2004).

Adulteration of PC-SPES with multiple ingredients has been identified. Analysis of four lots of PC-SPES used in one phase II trial identified both diethylstilbesterol and ethinyl estradiol, which was confirmed by two additional independent laboratories (Oh et al 2004); (Guns et al. 2002; Sovak et al 2002). Warfarin has also been detected, prompting a public health alert from the State of California in 2002, along with a product recall by the manufacturer, Botanic Labs. Botanic labs moved the production of PC-SPES to China, announcing that this move was to be closer to the raw ingredients used and to improve quality control. An analysis of the first batch revealed poor quality. Ultimately, Botanic labs ceased production in June 2002.

16.9.5.5 Cancers Combined

A Cochrane review of five randomized controlled trials examined *G. lucidum* as the intervention in 373 cancer patients (Jin et al. 2016). Although the evidence was insufficient to show improvements in tumor shrinkage and increases in NK cell activity, increases in T-cell subsets, attenuation of leukocyte depletion, and improvement in quality of life were significant. The trials used different designs, preparations, dosages, or administration schedules. Adverse events were limited to one study that described three cases of adverse events which included insomnia and nausea (Gao et al. 2003). The authors concluded that while evidence does not support *G. lucidum* as first-line therapy or monotherapy in cancer, there may be an adjuvant role in some patients. Doses used in the studies are considered safe in cancer patients.

16.9.6 Clinical Application

Reishi has been used in cancer patients for improving immune parameters, although the clinical relevance is not clear. Limited evidence exists for the effects of reishi on tumor response, and safety; however, no published evidence supports reishi for clinical outcomes such as recurrence rate, overall response rate, time to progression, and survival. The FDA does not consider β-glucans derivatives of *G. lucidum* as GRAS (Center for Food Safety and Applied Nutrition 2014). Caution should be taken for patients receiving immunosuppressive therapy and antithrombotic agents, along with for patients with severe thrombocytopenia (Wasser 2010). Reishi should not be used outside of a clinical trial in the treatment of cancer (Table 16.1).

16.10 Summary

Botanicals are widely used to treat cancers. Many patients are interested in using natural products to treat their cancer. Caution must be exercised however, since most of the trials of any botanical do not use comparisons with current standards of care. Additionally, since data must be of a long duration to determine the effects on survival, very few botanicals provide this level of evidence. Of concern, a recent case-control trial of alternative therapy in treatment of early stages of cancer patients reported a worse survival than standard treatment (Johnson et al. 2018). Whether complementary therapy is beneficial in cancer is yet to be proven for most marketed agents. Caution should be used when considering botanicals in cancer patients. A careful review of the evidence, with close scrutiny of the formulations, the sources of botanicals, as well as the methods to evaluate efficacy, is of vital importance prior to recommending use.

REFERENCES

Abdlekawy, K. S., A. M. Donia, and F. Elbarbry. "Effects of grapefruit and pomegranate juices on the pharmacokinetic properties of dapoxetine and midazolam in healthy subjects." *European Journal of Drug Metabolism and Pharmacokinetics* 42, no. 3 Jun, 2017: 397–405. doi:10.1007/s13318-016-0352-3.

Adams, L. S., N. P. Seeram, B. B. Aggarwal, Y. Takada, D. Sand, and D. Heber. "Pomegranate juice, total pomegranate ellagitannins, and punicalagin suppress inflammatory cell signaling in colon cancer cells." *Journal of Agricultural and Food Chemistry* 54, no. 3 Feb 08, 2006: 980–985. doi:10.1021/jf052005r.

Albertazzi, P., F. Pansini, G. Bonaccorsi, L. Zanotti, E. Forini, and D. De Aloysio. "The effect of dietary soy supplementation on hot flushes." *Obstetrics and Gynecology* 91, no. 1 Jan, 1998: 6–11.

Archer Daniels Midland Company (4 February 1998). "GRAS Notification for Isoflavones Derived from Soybeans" (PDF). *US Food and Drug Administration*. Retrieved September 3, 2017.

Aviram, M. and L. Dornfeld. "Pomegranate juice consumption inhibits serum angiotensin converting enzyme activity and reduces systolic blood pressure." *Atherosclerosis* 158, no. 1 Sep, 2001: 195–198.

Belcaro, G., M. Hosoi, L. Pellegrini, G. Addendino, E. Ippolito, and A. Ricci. "A controlled study of a lecithinized delivery system of curcumin (Meriva®) to alleviate the adverse effects of cancer treatment." *Phytother Res* Mar; 28(3); 2014: 440–450. doi.10.1002/ptr.5014

Bettuzzi, S., M. Brausi, F. Rizzi, G. Castagnetti, G. Peracchia, and A. Corti. "Chemoprevention of human prostate cancer by oral administration of green tea catechins in volunteers with high-grade prostate intraepithelial neoplasia: A preliminary report from a one-year proof-of-principle study." *Cancer Research* 66, no. 2 (Jan 15, 2006): 1234–1240. doi:10.1158/0008-5472.CAN-05-1145.

Büssing, A., A. Regnery, and K. Schweizer. "Effects of viscum album L. on cyclophosphamide-treated peripheral blood mononuclear cells in vitro: Sister chromatid exchanges and activation/proliferation marker expression." *Cancer Letters* 94, no. 2 Aug 01, 1995: 199–205.

Carroll, R. E., R. V. Benya, D. K. Turgeon et al. "Phase IIa clinical trial of curcumin for the prevention of colorectal neoplasia." *Cancer Prevention Research (Philadelphia, Pa.)* 4, no. 3 (Mar, 2011): 354–364. doi:10.1158/1940-6207.CAPR-10-0098.

Center for Food Safety and Applied Nutrition, Food and Drug Administration. "GRAS Notice Inventory— Agency Response Letter GRAS Notice no. GRN 000413." *Center for Food Safety and Applied Nutrition*, August 10, 2012 last modified Dec 23, 2014. Accessed July 17, 2017, https://www.fda.gov/Food/IngredientsPackagingLabeling/GRAS/NoticeInventory/ucm319626.htm

Chen, X., Z. P. Hu, X. X. Yang et al. "Monitoring of immune responses to a herbal immuno-modulator in patients with advanced colorectal cancer." *International Immunopharmacology* 6, no. 3 2006: 499–508.

Chen, Y., W-H. Liu, B-L. Chen et al. "Plant polyphenol curcumin significantly affects CYP1A2 and CYP2A6 activity in healthy, male chinese volunteers." *The Annals of Pharmacotherapy* 44, no. 6 Jun, 2010: 1038–1045. doi:10.1345/aph.1M533.

Chi, F., R. Wu, Y-C. Zeng, R. Xing, Y. Liu, and Z-G. Xu. "Post-diagnosis soy food intake and breast cancer survival: A meta-analysis of cohort studies." *Asian Pacific Journal of Cancer Prevention: APJCP* 14, no. 4 2013: 2407–2412.

"CFR - Code of Federal Regulations Title 21." *U.S. Food and Drug Administration*. September 21, 2016. Accessed July 14, 2017. https://www.accessdata.fda.gov/scripts/cdrh/cfdocs/cfcfr/CFRSearch.cfm?fr=172.510.

da Costa Miranda, V., D. C. Trufelli, J. Santos et al. "Effectiveness of Guaraná (Paullinia Cupana) for Postradiation Fatigue and Depression: Results of a Pilot Double-Blind Randomized Study." *Journal of Alternative and Complementary Medicine* 15, no. 4 2009: 431–433.

de la Taille, A., R. Buttyan, O. Hayek, E. Bagiella, A. Shabsigh, M. Burchardt, T. Burchardt, D. K. Chopin, and A. E. Katz. "Herbal therapy PC-SPES: In vitro effects and evaluation of its efficacy in 69 patients with prostate cancer." *The Journal of Urology* 164, no. 4 (Oct, 2000): 1229–1234.

de Oliveira Campos, M. P., B. J. Hassan, R. Riechelmann, and A. Del Giglio. "Cancer-Related Fatigue: A Review." *Revista da Associação Médica Brasileira* 57, no. 2 2011a: 211–219.

de Oliveira Campos, M. P., R. Riechelmann, L. C. Martins, B. J. Hassan, F. B. Casa, A. Del Giglio. "Guarana (paullinia cupana) improves fatigue in breast cancer patients undergoing systemic chemotherapy." *Journal of Alternative and Complementary Medicine* 17, no. 6 2011b: 505–512.

del Giglio, A. B., I. Cubero Dde, T. G. Lerner et al. "Purified dry extract of paullinia cupana (guarana) (PC-18) for chemotherapy-related fatigue in patients with solid tumors: An early discontinuation study." *Journal of Dietary Supplements* 10, no. 4 2013: 325–334.

Deng, G., H. Lin, A. Seidman et al. "A phase I/II trial of a polysaccharide extract from grifola frondosa (maitake mushroom) in breast cancer patients: Immunological effects." *Journal of Cancer Research and Clinical Oncology* 135, no. 9 2009: 1215–1221.

Dhillon, N., B. Aggarwal, R. Newman et al. "Phase II trail of curcumin in patients with advanced pancreatic cancer." *Clinical Cancer Research* 14 no. 14 Jul 15 2008: 4491–4499. doi:10.1158/1078-0432CCR-08-0024.

DiPaola, R. S., H. Zhang, G. H. Lambert et al. "Clinical and biologic activity of an estrogenic herbal combination (PC-SPES) in prostate cancer." *The New England Journal of Medicine* 339, no. 12 Sep 17, 1998: 785–791. doi:10.1056/NEJM199809173391201

Dong, J-Y. and L-Q. Qin. "Soy isoflavones consumption and risk of breast cancer incidence or recurrence: A meta-analysis of prospective studies." *Breast Cancer Research and Treatment* 125, no. 2 Jan, 2011: 315–323. doi:10.1007/s10549-010-1270-8.

dos Santos Martins, S. P., C. L. Ferreira, and A. del Giglio. "Placebo-controlled, double-blind, randomized study of a dry guarana extract in patients with head and neck tumors undergoing chemoradiotherapy: Effects on fatigue and quality of life." *Journal of Dietary Supplements* 14, no. 1 2017: 32–41.

Epelbaum, R., M. Schaffer, B. Vizel, V. Badmaev, and G. Bar-Sela. "Curcumin and gemcitabine in patients with advanced pancreatic cancer." *Nutrition and Cancer* 62, no. 8 Nov 5, 2010: 1137–1141. doi:10.1080/01635581.2010.513802. http://www.tandfonline.com/doi/abs/10.1080/01635581.2010.513802.

Fullerton, S. A., A. A. Samadi, D. G. Tortorelis, M. S. Choudhury, C. Mallouh, H. Tazaki, and S. Konno. "Induction of apoptosis in human prostatic cancer cells with beta-glucan (maitake mushroom polysaccharide)." *Molecular Urology* 4, no. 1 2000: 7–13.

Gao, Y. H., W. B. Tang, X. H. Dai et al. "Effects of water-soluble ganoderma lucidum polysaccharides on the immune functions of patients with advanced lung cancer." *Journal of Medicinal Food* 8, no. 2 2005: 159–168.

Gao, Y., X. Dai, G. Chen, J. Ye, and S. Zhou. "A randomized, placebo-controlled, multicenter study of ganoderma lucidum (W.Curt.:Fr.) loyd (Aphyllophoromycetideae) polysaccharides (ganopoly(R)) in patients with advanced lung cancer." *International Journal of Medicinal Mushrooms* 5, no. 4 2003: 369–381.

Giglio, A. del., A. Serpa, D. Cubero, R. Riechelmann, and M. Paschoin. "Paulinia cupana (guarana) For the treatment of cancer-related fatigue in patients undergoing radiation therapy or chemotherapy: A meta-analysis of three clinical Ttrials." *Journal of Clinical Oncology: Official Journal of the American Society of Clinical Oncology* 29, (15_suppl) 2011: e19706.

Golden, E. B., P. Y. Lam, A. Kardosh, K. J. Gaffney, E. Cadenas, S. G. Louie, N. A. Petasis, T. C. Chen, and A. H. Schönthal. "Green tea polyphenols block the anticancer effects of bortezomib and other boronic acid-based proteasome inhibitors." *Blood* 113, no. 23 (Jun 04, 2009): 5927–5937. doi:10.1182/blood-2008-07-171389.

Golombick, T., T. H. Diamond, A. Manoharan, and R. Ramakrishna. "Monoclonal gammopathy of undetermined significance, smoldering multiple myeloma, and curcumin: A randomized, double-blind placebo-controlled cross-over 4 g study and an open-label 8 g Extension Study." *American Journal of Hematology* 87, no. 5 (May, 2012): 455–460. doi:10.1002/ajh.23159.

Gordan J. D., W. Y. Chay, R. K. Kelley, A. H. Ko, and S. P. Choo, A. P. Venook. "And whatother medications are you taking?" *Journal of Clinical Oncology* 29, no. 11 2011: e288–291.

Graham, P. H. and C. P. Vance. "Legumes: Importance and constraints to greater use." *Plant Physiology* 131, no. 3 Mar, 2003: 872–877. doi:10.1104/pp.017004.

Guns, E. S., S. L. Goldenberg, and P. N. Brown. "Mass spectral analysis of PC-SPES confirms the presence of diethylstilbestrol." *The Canadian Journal of Urology* 9, no. 6 Dec, 2002: 1688; discussion 1689.

Hamilton-Reeves, J. M., S. A. Rebello, W. Thomas, M. S. Kurzer, and J. W. Slaton. "Effects of soy protein isolate consumption on prostate cancer biomarkers in men with HGPIN, ASAP, and low-grade prostate cancer." *Nutrition and Cancer* 60, no. 1 2008: 7–13. doi:10.1080/01635580701586770.

Harnly, J. M., R. F. Doherty, G. R. Beecher, J. M. Holden, D. B. Haytowitz, S. Bhagwat, and S. Gebhardt. "Flavonoid content of U.S. fruits, vegetables, and nuts." *Journal of Agricultural and Food Chemistry* 54, no. 26 Dec 27, 2006: 9966–9977. doi:10.1021/jf061478a.

He, F-J. and J-Q. Chen. Consumption of soybean, soy foods, soy isoflavones and breast cancer incidence: Differences between chinese women and women in western countries and possible. *Mechanisms* 2, 2013: 146–161. doi://dx.doi.org/10.1016/j.fshw.2013.08.002.

Heinzerling, L., V. von Baehr, C. Liebenthal, R. von Baehr, and H-D. Volk. "Immunologic effector mechanisms of a standardized mistletoe extract on the function of human monocytes and lymphocytes in vitro, ex vivo, and in vivo." *Journal of Clinical Immunology* 26, no. 4 Jul, 2006: 347–359. doi:10.1007/s10875-006-9023-5.

Hejazi, J., R. Rastmanesh, F. Taleban et al. "Effect of curcumin supplementation during radiotherapy on oxidative status of patients with prostate cancer: a double blinded, randomized, placebo-controlled study." *Nutrition and Cancer* 68 no. 1 2016: 77–85. doi:10.1080/01635581.2016.1115527.

Hertz, E., F. C. Cadona, A. K. Machado et al. "Effect of paullinia cupana on MCF-7 breast cancer cell response to chemotherapeutic drugs." *Molecular and Clinical Oncology* 3, no. 1 2015: 37–43.

Horneber, M. A., G. Bueschel, R. Huber, K. Linde, and M. Rostock. "Mistletoe therapy in oncology." *The Cochrane Database of Systematic Reviews* no. 2 (Apr 16, 2008): CD003297. doi:10.1002/14651858.CD003297.pub2.

Huber, R., H. Barth, A. Schmitt-Gräff, and R. Klein. "Hypereosinophilia induced by high-dose intratumoral and peritumoral mistletoe application to a patient with pancreatic carcinoma." *Journal of Alternative and Complementary Medicine (New York, N.Y.)* 6, no. 4 (Aug, 2000): 305–310. doi:10.1089/act.2000.6.305.

Jia, L. "Cancer complementary and alternative medicine research at the U.S. national cancer institute." *Chinese Journal of Integrative Medicine* 18, no. 5 (May, 2012): 325–332. doi:10.1007/s11655-011-0950-5.

Jin, X., B. J. Ruiz, D. M. Sze, and G. C. Chan. 2016. "Ganoderma lucidum reishi mushroom) for cancer treatment." *The Cochrane Database of Systematic Reviews* (4):CD007731. doi (4):CD007731.

Johnson, S. B., H. S. Park, C. P. Gross, and J. B. Yu. "Use of alternative medicine for cancer and its impact on survival. *Journal of the National Cancer Institute* 1, no. 110 Jan 1 2018: 1–4.

Kandela, P. "Mistletoe." *The Lancet* 358 (Dec 22/29) 2001.

Kanai, M., K. Yoshimura, M. Asada et al. "A phase I/II study of gemcitabine-based chemotherapy plus curcumin for patients with gemcitabine-resistant pancreatic cancer." *Cancer Chemotherapy and Pharmacology* 68, no. 1 (Jul, 2011): 157–164. doi:10.1007/s00280-010-1470-2. http://www.ncbi.nlm.nih.gov/pubmed/20859741.

Klebanoff, M. A., R. J. Levine, R. DerSimonian et al. "Maternal serum paraxanthine, a caffeine metabolite, and the risk of spontaneous abortion." *New England Journal of Medicine* 341, no. (22) 1999: 1639–1644.

Kodama, N., K. Komuta, and H. Nanba. "Can maitake MD-fraction aid cancer patients?" *Alternative Medicine Review* 7, no. 3 2002a: 236–239.

Kodama, N., K. Komuta, N. Sakai, and H. Nanba. "Effects of D-fraction, a polysaccharide from grifola frondosa on tumor growth involve activation of NK cells." *Biological and Pharmaceutical Bulletin* 25, no. 12 2002b: 1647–1650.

Konno, S., D. G. Tortorelis, S. A. Fullerton et al. "A possible hypoglycaemic effect of maitake mushroom on type 2 diabetic patients." *Diabetic Medicine* 18, no. 12 2001: 1010.

Kosty, M. P. "PC-SPES: Hope Or hype?" *Journal of Clinical Oncology: Official Journal of the American Society of Clinical Oncology* 22, no. 18 Sep 15, 2004: 3657–3659. doi:10.1200/JCO.2004.06.920.

Kuhnle, G. G. C., C. Dell"Aquila, S. A. Runswick, and S. A. Bingham. *Variability of Phytoestrogen Content in Foods from Different Sources* 113, 2009: 1184–1187. doi:10.1016/j.foodchem.2008.08.004. http://www.sciencedirect.com/science/article/pii/S0308814608009679.

Lampe, J. W., S. C. Karr, A. M. Hutchins, and J. L. Slavin. "Urinary equol excretion with a soy challenge: Influence of habitual diet." *Proceedings of the Society for Experimental Biology and Medicine. Society for Experimental Biology and Medicine (New York, N.Y.)* 217, no. 3 Mar, 1998: 335–339.

Langley, P. "Why a pomegranate?" *BMJ (Clinical Research Ed.)* 321, no. 7269 Nov 04, 2000: 1153–1154.

Lin, L-C., M-N. Wang, and T-H. Tsai. "Food-drug interaction of (-)-epigallocatechin-3-gallate on the pharmacokinetics of irinotecan and the metabolite SN-38." *Chemico-Biological Interactions* 174, no. 3 Aug 11, 2008: 177–182. doi:10.1016/j.cbi.2008.05.033.

Mahammedi, H., E. Planchat, M. Pouget et al. "The new combination docetaxel, prednisone and curcumin in patients with castrate-resistant prostate cancer: a pilot phase II study. *Oncology* 90, no. 2, 2016: 69–78. doi:10.1159?000441148.

Mahmoud, A. M., W. Yang, and M. C. Bosland. "Soy isoflavones and prostate cancer: A review of molecular mechanisms." *The Journal of Steroid Biochemistry and Molecular Biology* 140, Mar, 2014: 116–132. doi:10.1016/j.jsbmb.2013.12.010.

Malik, A., F. Afaq, S. Sarfaraz, V. M. Adhami, D. N. Syed, and H. Mukhtar. "Pomegranate fruit juice for chemoprevention and chemotherapy of prostate cancer." *Proceedings of the National Academy of Sciences of the United States of America* 102, no. 41 Oct 11, 2005: 14813–14818. doi:10.1073/pnas.0505870102.

Mansky, P. J., J. Grem, D. B. Wallerstedt, B. P. Monahan, and M. R. Blackman. "Mistletoe and gemcitabine in patients with advanced cancer: A model for the phase I study of botanicals and botanical-drug interactions in cancer therapy." *Integrative Cancer Therapies* 2, no. 4 Dec, 2003: 345–352. doi:10.1177/1534735403259061.

Matsui, K., N. Kodama, and H. Nanba. "Effects of maitake (grifola frondosa) D-fraction on the carcinoma angiogenesis." *Cancer Letters* 172, no. 2 2001: 193–198.

Mayell, M. "Maitake extracts and their therapeutic potential." *Alternative Medicine Review* 6, no. 1 2001: 48–60.

Messina, M., C. Nagata, and A. H. Wu. "Estimated asian adult soy protein and isoflavone intakes." *Nutrition and Cancer* 55, no. 1 2006: 1–12. doi:10.1207/s15327914nc5501_1.

Miyanaga, N., H. Akaza, S. Hinotsu et al. "Prostate cancer chemoprevention study: An investigative randomized control study using purified isoflavones in men with rising prostate-specific antigen." *Cancer Science* 103, no. 1 Jan, 2012: 125–130. doi:10.1111/j.1349-7006.2011.02120.x.

Mohamed, M-E. F. and R. F. Frye. "Effects of herbal supplements on drug glucuronidation. Review of clinical, animal, and in vitro studies." *Planta Medica* 77, no. 4 Mar, 2011: 311–321. doi:10.1055/s-0030-1250457.

Myung, S.-K., W. Ju, H. J. Choi, and S. C. Kim. "Soy intake and risk of endocrine-related gynaecological cancer: A meta-analysis." *BJOG: An International Journal of Obstetrics and Gynaecology* 116, no. 13 Dec, 2009: 1697–1705. doi:10.1111/j.1471-0528.2009.02322.x.

Nanba, H. "Maitake D-fraction: Healing and preventing potentials for cancer." *Journal of Orthomolecular Medicine* 12, no. 1 1996: 43–49.

Nechuta, S. J., B. J. Caan, W. Y. Chen et al. "Soy food intake after diagnosis of breast cancer and survival: An in-depth analysis of combined evidence from cohort studies of U.S. and chinese women." *The American Journal of Clinical Nutrition* 96, no. 1 (Jul, 2012): 123–132. doi:10.3945/ajcn.112.035972.

Oh, W. K., P. W. Kantoff, V. Weinberg et al. "Prospective, multicenter, randomized phase II trial of the herbal supplement, PC-SPES, and diethylstilbestrol in patients with androgen-independent prostate cancer." *Journal of Clinical Oncology: Official Journal of the American Society of Clinical Oncology* 22, no. 18 Sep 15, 2004: 3705–3712. doi:10.1200/JCO.2004.10.195.

Oka, S., S. Tanaka, S. Yoshida et al. "A water-soluble extract from culture medium of ganoderma lucidum mycelia suppresses the development of colorectal adenomas." *Hiroshima Journal of Medical Sciences* 59, no. 1 2010: 1–6.

Ostermann, T. and A. Büssing. Retrolective studies on the survival of cancer patients treated with mistletoe extracts: A meta-analysis. *Explore* 8, no. 5 2012: 277–281.

Ostermann, T., C. Raak, and A. Büssing. "Survival of cancer patients treated with mistletoe extract (iscador): A systematic literature review." *BMC Cancer* 9, Dec 18, 2009: 451. doi:10.1186/1471-2407-9-451.

Paller, C. J., A. Pantuck, and M. A. Carducci. "A review of pomegranate in prostate cancer." *Prostate Cancer and Prostatic Diseases* 20, no. 3 Sep, 2017: 265–270. doi:10.1038/pcan.2017.19.

Paller, C. J., X. Ye, P. J. Wozniak et al. "A randomized phase II study of pomegranate extract for men with rising PSA following initial therapy for localized prostate cancer." *Prostate Cancer and Prostatic Diseases* 16, no. 1 Mar, 2013: 50–55. doi:10.1038/pcan.2012.20.

Panahi, Y., A. Saadat, F. Beiraghdar, and A. Sahebkar. "Adjuvant therapy with bioavailability-boosted curcuminoids suppresses systemic inflammation and improves quality of life in patients with solid tumors: A randomized double-blind placebo-controlled trial." *Phytother Res* 28 no 10. Oct, 2014; 1461–1467. doi:10:1002/ptr 5149. Epub 2014 Mar 19.

Pantuck, A. J., C. A. Pettaway, R. Dreicer, J. Corman, A. Katz, A. Ho, W. Aronson, W. Clark, G. Simmons, and D. Heber. "A randomized, double-blind, placebo-controlled study of the effects of pomegranate extract on rising PSA levels in men following primary therapy for prostate cancer." *Prostate Cancer and Prostatic Diseases* 18, no. 3 Sep, 2015: 242–248. doi:10.1038/pcan.2015.32.

Pantuck, A. J., J. T. Leppert, N. Zomorodian et al. "Phase II study of pomegranate juice for men with rising prostate-specific antigen following surgery or radiation for prostate cancer." *Clinical Cancer Research: An Official Journal of the American Association for Cancer Research* 12, no. 13 Jul 01, 2006: 4018–4026. doi:10.1158/1078-0432.CCR-05-2290.

Preuss, H. G. and S. Konno. 2002. *Maitake magic: maitake mushroom fractions: capture the force of nature's amazing powerful immune boosters, cancer protectors, and metabolic activators.* Topanga, CA: Freedom Press.

Ryan, J. L., C. E. Heckler, M. Ling, A. Katz, J. P. Williams, A. P. Pentland, and G. R. Morrow. "Curcumin for radiation dermatitis: A randomized, double-blind, placebo-controlled clinical trial of thirty breast cancer patients." *Radiation Research* 180, no. 1 Jul, 2013: 34–43. doi:10.1667/RR3255.1.

Schad, F., A. Thronicke, A. Merkle, H. Matthes, and M. L. Steele. "Immune-related and adverse drug reactions to low versus high initial doses of *Viscum album L.* in cancer patients." *Phytomedicine* no. 36 Dec 2017: 54–58.

Schimpl, F. C., J. F. da Silva, J. F. Gonçalves, and P. Mazzafera. "Guaraná: Revisiting a highly caffeinated plant from the amazon." *Journal of Ethnopharmacology* 150, no. 1 2013: 14–31.

Seeram, N. P., L. S. Adams, S. M. Henning, Y. Niu, Y. Zhang, M. G. Nair, and D. Heber. "In vitro antiproliferative, apoptotic and antioxidant activities of punicalagin, ellagic acid and a total pomegranate tannin extract are enhanced in combination with other polyphenols as found in pomegranate juice." *The Journal of Nutritional Biochemistry* 16, no. 6 (Jun, 2005): 360–367. doi:10.1016/j.jnutbio.2005.01.006.

Seidi, K., R. Jahanban-Esfahlan, M. Abasi, and M. M. Abbasi. "Anti tumoral properties of punica granatum (pomegranate) seed extract in different human cancer cells." *Asian Pacific Journal of Cancer Prevention: APJCP* 17, no. 3 2016: 1119–1122.

Setchell, K. D. R. and C. Clerici. "Equol: Pharmacokinetics and biological actions." *The Journal of Nutrition* 140, no. 7 Jul, 2010: 8S. doi:10.3945/jn.109.119784.

Setchell, K. D. R., N. M. Brown, and E. Lydeking-Olsen. "The clinical importance of the metabolite equol- A clue to the effectiveness of soy and its isoflavones." *The Journal of Nutrition* 132, no. 12 Dec, 2002: 3577–3584.

Shanafelt, T. D., T. G. Call, C. S. Zent, J. F. Leis, B. LaPlant, D. A. Bowen, et al. Phase 2 trial of daily oral Polyphenon E in patients with asymptomatic Rai stage 0 to II chronic lymphocytic leukemia. *Cancer* 119, no. 2 Jan, 15, 2013: 363–370.

Sharma, P., S. F. McClees, and F. Afaq. "Pomegranate for prevention and treatment of cancer: An update." *Molecules (Basel, Switzerland)* 22, no. 1 Jan 24, 2017. doi:10.3390/molecules22010177.

Shimizu, M., Y. Fukutomi, M. Ninomiya, K. Nagura, T. Kato, H. Araki, M. Suganuma, H. Fujiki, and H. Moriwaki. "Green tea extracts for the prevention of metachronous colorectal adenomas: A pilot study." *Cancer Epidemiology, Biomarkers & Prevention: A Publication of the American Association for Cancer Research, Cosponsored by the American Society of Preventive Oncology* 17, no. 11 Nov, 2008: 3020–3025. doi:10.1158/1055-9965.EPI-08-0528.

Shin, S-C. and J-S Choi. "Effects of epigallocatechin gallate on the oral bioavailability and pharmacokinetics of tamoxifen and its main metabolite, 4-Hydroxytamoxifen, in rats." *Anti-Cancer Drugs* 20, no. 7 Aug, 2009: 584–588. doi:10.1097/CAD.0b013e32832d6834.

Shomori, K., M. Yamamoto, I. Arifuku, K. Teramachi, and H. Ito. "Antitumor effects of a water-soluble extract from maitake (grifola frondosa) on human gastric cancer cell lines." *Oncology Reports* 22, no. 3 2009: 615–620.

Sicherer, S. H., H. A. Sampson, and A. W. Burks. "Peanut and soy allergy: A clinical and therapeutic dilemma." *Allergy* 55, no. 6 Jun, 2000: 515–521.

Small, E. J., M. W. Frohlich, R. Bok, K. Shinohara, G. Grossfeld, Z. Rozenblat, W. K. Kelly, M. Corry, and D. M. Reese. "Prospective trial of the herbal supplement PC-SPES in patients with progressive prostate cancer." *Journal of Clinical Oncology: Official Journal of the American Society of Clinical Oncology* 18, no. 21 Nov 01, 2000: 3595–3603. doi:10.1200/JCO.2000.18.21.3595.

Smith, N. and A. L. Atroch. "Guarana's journey from regional tonic to aphrodisiac and global energy drink." *Evidence-Based Complementary and Alternative Medicine* 7, no. 3 2007: 279–282.

Soares, R., M. Meireles, A. Rocha, A. Pirraco, D. Obiol, E. Alonso, G. Joos, and G. Balogh. "Maitake (D fraction) mushroom extract induces apoptosis in breast cancer cells by BAK-1 gene activation." *Journal of Medicinal Food* 14, no. 6 2011: 563–572.

Somasundaram, S., N. A. Edmund, D. T. Moore, G. W. Small, Y. Y. Shi, and R. Z. Orlowski. "Dietary curcumin inhibits chemotherapy-induced apoptosis in models of human breast cancer." *Cancer Research* 62, no. 13 Jul 01, 2002: 3868–3875.

Sonoda, T., Y. Nagata, M. Mori et al. "A case-control study of diet and prostate cancer in japan: Possible protective effect of traditional japanese diet." *Cancer Science* 95, no. 3 Mar, 2004: 238–242.

Sorokin, A. V., B. Duncan, R. Panetta, and P. D. Thompson. "Rhabdomyolysis associated with pomegranate juice consumption." *The American Journal of Cardiology* 98, no. 5 Sep 01, 2006: 705–706. doi:10.1016/j.amjcard.2006.03.057.

Sovak, M., A. L. Seligson, M. Konas, M. Hajduch, M. Dolezal, M. Machala, and R. Nagourney. "Herbal composition PC-SPES for management of prostate cancer: Identification of active principles." *JNCI: Journal of the National Cancer Institute* 94, no. 17 /09/04, 2002: 1275–1280. doi:10.1093/jnci/94.17.1275.

Srinivas, N. R. "Is pomegranate juice a potential perpetrator of clinical drug-drug interactions? Review of the in vitro, preclinical and clinical evidence." *European Journal of Drug Metabolism and Pharmacokinetics* 38, no. 4 Dec, 2013: 223–229. doi:10.1007/s13318-013-0137-x.

Steele, M. L., J. Axtner, A. Happe, M. Kröz, H. Matthes, and F. Schad. "Adverse drug reactions and expected effects to therapy with subcutaneous mistletoe extracts (viscum album L.) in cancer patients." *Evidence-Based Complementary and Alternative Medicine: ECAM* 2014, 2014: 724258. doi:10.1155/2014/724258.

Tang, N-P., H. Li, Y-L. Qiu, G-M. Zhou, and J. Ma. "Tea consumption and risk of endometrial cancer: A metaanalysis." *American Journal of Obstetrics and Gynecology* 201, no. 6 Dec, 2009: 8. doi:10.1016/j.ajog.2009.07.030.

Thomas, R., M. Williams, H. Sharma, A. Chaudry, and P. Bellamy. "A double-blind, placebo-controlled randomised trial evaluating the effect of a polyphenol-rich whole food supplement on PSA progression in men with prostate cancer--the U.K. NCRN Pomi-T Study." *Prostate Cancer and Prostatic Diseases* 17, no. 2 Jun, 2014: 180–186. doi:10.1038/pcan.2014.6.

Trudel, D., D. Labbe, M. Araya-Farias et al. "A two stage, single arm, phase II study of EGCG-enriched green tea drink as a maintenance therapy in women with advanced stage ovarian cancer. *Gynecologic Oncology* 131, no. 2 Nov, 2013: 357–361. doi:10.1016/j.ygyno.2013.08119.

Tsao, A. S., D. Liu, J. Martin et al. "Phase II randomized, placebo-controlled trial of green tea extract in patients with high-risk oral premalignant lesions." *Cancer Prevention Research (Philadelphia, Pa.)* 2, no. 11 Nov, 2009: 931–941. doi:10.1158/1940-6207.CAPR-09-0121.

Turrini, E., L. Ferruzzi, and C. Fimognari. "Potential effects of pomegranate polyphenols in cancer prevention and therapy." *Oxidative Medicine and Cellular Longevity* 2015, 2015: 938475. doi:10.1155/2015/938475.

Ulbricht, C., W. Weissner, E. Basch, N. Giese, P. Hammerness, E. Rusie-Seamon, M. Varghese, and J. Woods. "Maitake mushroom (grifola frondosa): Systematic review by the natural standard research collaboration." *Journal of the Society for Integrative Oncology* 7, no. 2 2009: 66–72.

van Die, M. D., K. M. Bone, S. G. Williams, and M. V. Pirotta. "Soy and soy isoflavones in prostate cancer: A systematic review and meta-analysis of randomized controlled trials." *BJU International* 113, no. 5b May, 2014: 119. doi:10.1111/bju.12435.

Wanwimolruk, S., K. Wong, and P. Wanwimolruk. "Variable inhibitory effect of different brands of commercial herbal supplements on human cytochrome P-450 CYP3A4." *Drug Metabolism and Drug Interactions* 24, no. 1 2009: 17–35.

Wasser, S. P. 2010. "Reishi." In: P.M. Coates, J. M. Betz, M. R. Blackman et al., eds. *Encyclopedia of Dietary Supplements*, 2nd edn. New York: Informa Healthcare, pp. 680–690.

Weng, X., R. Odouli, and D. K. Li. "Maternal caffeine consumption during pregnancy and the risk of miscarriage: A prospective cohort study." *American Journal of Obstetrics and Gynecology* 198, 3 2008: 279.e1–8.

Wesa K. M., S. Cunningham-Rundles, V. M. Klimek et al. "Maitake mushroom extract in myelodysplastic syndromes (MDS): A phase II study." *Cancer Immunology, Immunotherapy* 64, 2015: 237–247.

Zand, R. S., D. J. Jenkins, and E. P. Diamandis. "Steroid hormone activity of flavonoids and related compounds." *Breast Cancer Research and Treatment* 62, no. 1 Jul, 2000: 35–49.

Zhan, X., J. Wang, S. Pan, and C. Lu. "Tea consumption and the risk of ovarian cancer: A meta-analysis of epidemiological studies." *Oncotarget* 8, no. 23 Jun 06, 2017: 37796–37806.

Zhao, H., Q. Zhang, L. Zhao, X. Huang, J. Wang, and X. Kang. "Spore powder of ganoderma lucidum improves cancer-related fatigue in breast cancer patients undergoing endocrine therapy: A pilot clinical trial." *Evidence-Based Complementary and Alternative Medicine* 2012, 2012: 809614.

Zhang, F. F., D. E. Haslam, M. B. Terry et al. "Dietary isoflavone intake and all-cause mortality in breast cancer survivors: The breast cancer family registry." *Cancer*; 123, 2017: 2070–2079.

Zhang, M., C. W. Binns, and A. H. Lee. "Tea consumption and ovarian cancer risk: A case-control study in china." *Cancer Epidemiology, Biomarkers & Prevention: A Publication of the American Association for Cancer Research, Cosponsored by the American Society of Preventive Oncology* 11, no. 8 Aug, 2002: 713–718.

Zhang, W. and L-Y. Lim. "Effects of spice constituents on p-glycoprotein-mediated transport and CYP3A4-mediated metabolism in vitro." *Drug Metabolism and Disposition* 36, no. 7 Jul, 2008: 1283–1290. doi:10.1124/dmd.107.01

17

Supportive and Palliative Care for Cancer

Mary Chavez, Pedro Chavez, Rachel Ryu, and Britny Rogala

CONTENTS

17.1 Introduction

Patients diagnosed with cancer use botanicals to seek relief from symptoms and also to take control of their disease. Evidence on the efficacy of botanicals in mitigating symptoms of cancer is limited for most agents. As discussed in the Special Populations chapter, concerns exist about the potential effects of botanicals on cancer treatment. Although relief from the adverse effects of treatment is important, the potential that botanicals may alter the benefit of the anticancer treatment should also be carefully considered. This chapter will review the evidence for use of botanicals for supportive and palliative care in cancer patients.

Between 20% and 90% of patients affected by cancer use dietary supplements (Frenkel and Sierpina 2014). A subset analysis of the 2007 National Health Interview Survey conducted by the Centers for Disease Control and Prevention's National Center for Health Statistics compared use of complementary and alternative medicine (CAM) between patients with cancer to those without the condition in the United States (Anderson and Taylor 2012). The investigators compared CAM use by patients who self-reported a diagnosis of cancer (n = 1785) to use in individuals without cancer (n = 21,585). The use of CAM by cancer patients was common and similar to the pattern of use in individuals without cancer, suggesting that the diagnosis of cancer alone may not be the motivation for the use of CAM in cancer patients (Anderson and Taylor 2012). Health care providers should assess the cancer patient's use of dietary supplements in addition to increasing their own knowledge in order to maximize positive patient outcomes. This chapter summarizes current evidence for common botanicals used for supportive and palliative care in cancer.

17.2 Ashwagandha *Withania somnifera* (WS)

17.2.1 Background

Withania somnifera (WS) Dunal, commonly known as Ashwagandha in Sanskrit, or as Indian ginseng and Indian winter cherry, has been used for millennia in Ayurvedic medicine to increase longevity and vitality (Mishra et al. 2000; Palliyaguru et al. 2016). WS is used as a general tonic to increase energy, improve overall health and longevity, and for disease prevention in athletes, elderly and during pregnancy (Mishra et al. 2000, 2016). It grows as a small woody shrub to about 2 feet in height (Mishra et al. 2000; Alam et al. 2016). It can be found in the drier climates including India, Afghanistan, Baluchistan, Sindh, Sri Lanka, regions of Africa, and in the Mediterranean, among other areas.

17.2.2 Pharmacognosy

Withania somnifera is a member of the flowering *Solanaceae* family. More than 35 constituents have been identified including alkaloids, saponins, steroidal lactones which includes the withanolides - withsomine, withaferin A, withanolide A and withanolide D, and several sitoindosides which are withanolides, distinguished by a glucose molecule at carbon 27 (Mishra et al. 2000; Palliyaguru et al. 2016). The bioactive activity has been attributed to the withanolides with studies showing that the distribution of withanolides varies in the different plant parts (Palliyaguru et al. 2016).

17.2.3 Dosing and Preparation

WS is sold in the United States in the form of dried powder capsules and as alcohol extracts (Palliyaguru et al. 2016). The roots are the main part of the plant used medicinally (Alam et al. 2016). The usual dose is 3–6 g daily of dried root, 300–500 mg of an extract standardized to contain 1.5% withanolides, or 6–12 mL of a 1:2 fluid extract daily (Alam et al. 2016).

17.2.4 Safety

Withania somnifera is generally considered safe when taken at the recommended dosage. Large doses have been associated with gastrointestinal upset, diarrhea, and vomiting (Alam et al. 2016). Large doses may have abortifacient properties and its use should be avoided during pregnancy.

WS may produce mild central nervous system (CNS) depressant activity; therefore, patients should avoid alcohol, sedatives, and other CNS depressants while taking this botanical. A study showed no significant interaction between WS and the CYP3A4 or 2D6 enzymes (Savai et al. 2015). WS may modestly interfere with serum digoxin measurements by fluorescent polarization immunoassay (Dasgupta et al. 2008).

17.2.5 Evidence

The botanical has been studied for its effects on chemotherapy-induced fatigue and quality of life (QOL) in patients with breast cancer (Biswal et al. 2013). The open-label, non-randomized, prospective trial enrolled 100 patients to WS extract (50 patients) or to a control group (50 patients). Patients with stage I – IV disease undergoing systemic chemotherapy were eligible to participate. Patients in the WS arm received 2 g of WS root extract as oral capsules every 8 hours throughout six cycles of adjunctive or palliative chemotherapy. QOL and fatigue scores were measured using validated tools. Patients in the WS group had significantly better fatigue scores, along with improved QOL scores compared with control patients (Biswal et al. 2013). A trend toward improved survival was noted in the WS arm which may have potentially affected the QOL and the fatigue scores (Biswal et al. 2013). The results from this study are limited by the unblinded design, the diversity of patient population, which included all stages of cancer, and the range of chemotherapy regimens received. The primary efficacy outcome was not identified, and there were multiple comparisons, with no adjustment made for these. A blinded, randomized trial enrolling a larger patient population receiving similar treatments, with a similar disease at baseline, and a clear primary outcome, is necessary to determine the effects of WS on fatigue and QOL in breast cancer.

17.2.6 Clinical Application

Only one clinical trial has evaluated WS for improved fatigue and QOL in breast cancer patients receiving chemotherapy. Although positive results were reported, evidence is limited for its use in cancer.

17.3 Astragalus

17.3.1 Background

Astragalus membranaceus (Fisch.) Bge. var. mongholicus (Bge.) Hsiao or *Astragalus membranaceus* (Fisch.) Bge., is also known as Astragali Radix, Huang qi in China, Ogi in Japan, and Hwanggi in Korea (Anon 2003; Fu et al. 2014). Astragalus has been used in Traditional Chinese Medicine (TCM) for over 2,000 years according to the classic Shen Nong's Materia Medica, which was written during the Han dynasty (Anon 2003; Fu et al. 2014). Astragalus was used for treatment of general weakness and chronic illness, as well as to increase overall vitality (Auyeung et al. 2009). Astragalus is used to treat allergies, anemia, fever, cardiovascular disorders, and chronic fatigue, among other disorders (Fu et al. 2014).

17.3.2 Pharmacognosy

Astragalus membranaceus is a perennial flowering herb native to northern China, Mongolia and Tibet which grows up to 150 cm in height, with a long, straight cylindrical root. The stems are erect with branches containing small broad elliptical leaves (Fu et al. 2014). The genus *Astragalus*, commonly known as milk-vetch, is large with more than 2,000 species worldwide (Anon 2003).

Astragalus contains over 100 chemical compounds including polysaccharides, amino acids, flavonoids, and triterpenoid saponins (Fu et al. 2014). Other constituents include acrylic acid, amino acids, betaine, caffeic acid, choline, chlorogenic acid, coumarin, daucosterol, fatty acids, ferulic acid, γ- aminobutyric acid, n-hexadecanol, p-hydroxyphenyl, isoferulic acid, L-canavanire, (+)-larciresinol, linoleic acid, lupenone, minerals, phytosterols, and (−)-syringaresinol (Auyeung et al. 2009).

Astragalus has been reported to have immunomodulatory activity, as well antitumor properties (Chu et al. 1990; Wu et al. 2009). Astragalus formulations may increase sensitivity and reduce the adverse effects of conventional chemotherapy (McCulloch et al. 2006).

17.3.3 Dosing and Preparation

Astragalus is commonly used as a dried root, in the form of a decoction or powder usually in combination with other botanicals at variable dosages. Orally the dose of powdered astragalus is from 1–30 g daily, but research suggests that doses greater than 28 grams per day do not offer any benefit and may actually cause immune suppression. The dose of the decoction of astragalus is 0.5–1 L per day, with a maximum 120 grams of whole root per liter of water. As a soup, 30 grams of astragalus is mixed in 3.5 L liquid soup and simmered with other food ingredients (Natural Medicines Comprehensive Database 2016).

17.3.4 Safety

Astragalus appears to be safe with doses as large as 100 mg/kg of the raw botanical given to rats via lavage without adverse effects (Anon 2003). Astragalus may stimulate immune function, therefore its use should be avoided in patients with autoimmune diseases. Similarly, the botanical may decrease the effectiveness of immunosuppressants and its use should be avoided in patients taking these drugs. *Astragalus membranaceus* possesses *in vitro* estrogenic activity and its safety in estrogen -dependent cancers has not been determined (Zhang et al. 2005). *Astragalus membranaceus* can significantly inhibit the metabolism of CYP3A4 (Pao et al. 2012). Recombinant interleukin-2 may be potentiated 10-fold by *Astragalus membranaceus* extract (Zhang et al. 2005). *In vitro* studies have shown that astragalus may interact with antithrombotic agents, which may increase the risk of bleeding (He et al. 2013). Studies have shown that astragalus has natiurectic properties, which may produce additive effects with diuretics (Ai et al. 2008).

17.3.5 Evidence

17.3.5.1 Fatigue

In a phase II randomized double-blind placebo-controlled study, an investigational drug (PG2, PhytoHealth Corp., Taiwan), which is a mixture of polysaccharides extracted from *Astragalus membranaceus*, was administered as an infusion of 500 mg three times weekly for 4 weeks compared to a placebo infusion in patients with advanced cancer as part of standard palliative care (Chen et al. 2012) Fatigue was measured using the Brief Fatigue Inventory – Taiwan (BFI-T) scale, where 0 = no fatigue, and 10 represents extreme fatigue. Improvement in BFI-T was defined as at least a 10% improvement. The number of responders meeting this requirement at any time frame was the study endpoint. A total of 90 patients were enrolled, with 45 in each group, only 35 completed the PG-2 infusion, and 30 patients completed the placebo arm. Cancer-related fatigue improved with

PG2 compared to placebo at the end of week 1 (57.14% improved with PG2 compared to 32.26% in placebo, p = 0.043), but not at the end of week 4 (60% versus 40% respectively, p = 0.108). While the study demonstrated benefit, effects on fatigue appeared to be short lived. The study did include blinding and was powered to identify clinically significant results. The multiple comparisons, short-lived benefit, and the population enrolled with many different cancers, stages and performance status limit interpretation of the study findings.

17.3.5.2 Anorexia

A prospective phase II study administered a botanical decoction with *Astragali radix* to 11 patients with advanced cancer and anorexia, defined as at least a 5% weight loss in the previous 6 months. Patients had a minimum score of 50 on the 0–100 visual analog scale (VAS) with zero representing no anorexia, and 100 indicating maximal anorexia (Lee et al. 2010). The decoction contained 24 g *Astragali radix*, which was administered in three divided doses, 30 minutes after meals for 3 weeks. Appetite, body weight (Kg), various cytokines, and anthropometry were measured. Anorexia was assessed at baseline, and weekly until study termination. All patients were evaluated for analysis. Anorexia VAS improved significantly from baseline to best score (60 versus 40, p = 0.009); however, at end of study no significant difference was observed (60 versus 50, p = 0.082). Weight improved from baseline to best score (54.5–55.6 kg, p = 0.009), but not at end of study (54.5–54.9 kg, p = 0.306) Adverse effects were manageable. The benefits seen were from "best response" times rather than using a controlled design for efficacy endpoints. This study has many flaws in design and lacks adequate power to recommend its use in cancer-related anorexia.

17.3.5.3 Radiation Toxicity

A meta-analysis of 29 randomized controlled studies enrolling 2,547 patients with non-small cell lung cancer concluded that astragalus-containing Chinese combination prescriptions may increase effectiveness and reduce the toxicity of radiation (He et al. 2013). The methodology and reporting in the studies was poor and bias was difficult to determine. For example, most did not describe any blinding, randomization techniques, or methods to evaluate endpoints. Funnel plots and the Eggers Test conducted in the meta-analysis indicated evidence for publication bias. A more rigorous evaluation of the effects of astragalus on radiation effects in non-small cell lung cancer is warranted.

17.3.5.4 Quality of Life

In a randomized, open label Chinese trial, astragalus polysaccharide injection was administered to patients with stage III and IV non-small cell lung cancer receiving vinorelbine and cisplatin to determine its effects on QOL and survival (Guo et al. 2012). This trial enrolled 136 patients, 68 to the astragalus arm and 68 to the control arm. All patients received standard doses of vinorelbine and cisplatin. The study used the European Organization for Research and Treatment of Cancer Quality of Life Questionnaire in Cancer patients (EORTC QLQ-C30) tool to meaure QOL. Patients were evaluated at baseline, and for the first three cycles of chemotherapy. No effect on survival was observed. Parameters that were improved included overall QOL (p = 0.003), physical function (p = 0.01), fatigue (p = 0.001), pain p = 0.007), nausea and vomiting (p = 0.001), and loss of appetite (p = 0.023). Of note, grade III and IV toxicities were similar between the treatment arm and the control group. These results require validation using blinded design before making any recommendation.

17.3.6 Clinical Application

Although *Astragalus membranaceus* appears to be safe, drug interactions may occur. Of particular concern, use may potentially affect hormone sensitive cancers. Additional studies are needed to determine its place as standard adjunct therapy for patients with cancer to alleviate fatigue and anorexia.

17.4 Cat's Claw

17.4.1 Background

The two most common species of Cat's claw are *Uncaria tomentosa* (Willd.) DC and *Uncaria guianensis* (Aublet) J. F. Gmelin, which are members of the *Rubiaceae* family (DerMarderosian and McQueen 2017a,b). Cat's claw are high growing woody vines that wind around and up from the base of tall trees and grows in tropical regions of Southeast Asia, continental Asia, and South America. The thorns are located on the stem at the leaf juncture. *U. guianensis* is commonly collected in South America for the European market and *U. tomentosa* is generally used in America (DerMarderosian and McQueen 2017a,b).

The inner root and bark extracts have been used for abscesses, arthritis, asthma, cancer, among many other conditions. In Peru, a boiled decoction of *U. guianensis* is also used as a contraceptive agent and for treating gonorrhea (DerMarderosian and McQueen 2017a,b).

17.4.2 Pharmacognosy

The healing effects of cat's claw may be attributed to pentacyclic oxindole alkaloids. The principal pentacyclic oxindole alkaloids in cat's claw are pteropodine, isopteropodine, speciophylline, uncarine F, mitraphylline and isomitraphylline (WHO 2007). Tetracyclic oxindoles are also present including isorhynchophylline and rhynchophylline (WHO 2007). Other constituents include alkaloids, catechins, flavonoids, quinovic acid glycosides, steroids, and triterpenes. Different extraction methods, water compared to ethanol at various temperatures, result in extracts with different compositions (DerMarderosian and McQueen 2017a,b).

In vitro studies have shown that constituents in cat's claw extract increase the phagocytic activity of white blood cells, stimulate B and T lymphocytes, decrease production of tumor necrosis factor-α (TNF-α), and decrease cytotoxicity in lipopolysaccharide-stimulated murine macrophages (WHO 2007).

17.4.3 Dosing and Preparation

The roots are used for cat's claw supplements with dosages between 250 and 1,000 mg daily (Erowele and Kalejaiye 2009) and up to 25 g of raw bark used traditionally in decoctions. Cat's claw is available as capsules, extracts, tinctures, decoctions, and teas. Two water-soluble preparations of *U. tomentosa* (AC-11) and Protectagen™ (formerly C-MED-100), are available and are different from many of the previous commercial preparations of cat's claw. The two preparations are extracted for 18 hours by hot water at 95°C and spray dried to contain 8%–10% or 16%–20% carboxy alkyl esters (Erowele and Kalejaiye 2009).

17.4.4 Safety

Anecdotal evidence indicates Cat's claw is well tolerated but can cause diarrhea and abdominal pain (Erowele and Kalejaiye 2009). In a human volunteer study, an aqueous extract of the stem bark was administered to four healthy volunteers at a daily dose of 350 mg for six consecutive weeks (Lemaire et al. 1999). Adverse effects were not reported as judged by hematology laboratory results, body weight changes, lack of diarrhea or constipation, headache, nausea, vomiting, rash, edema, or pain. A significant increase in the number of white blood cells was observed (Lemaire et al. 1999).

Laboratory studies have shown that cat's claw inhibits CYP3A4, which may result in drug interactions. Cat's claw is reported to be an immunostimulant and should be avoided in patients receiving immunosuppressants. Cat's claw may theoretically increase the risk of bleeding, although evidence is limited (DerMarderosian and McQueen 2017a,b).

17.4.5 Evidence

17.4.5.1 Neutropenia

A randomized controlled study evaluated the use of cat's claw extract 300 mg orally daily in patients with invasive ductal carcinoma-stage II, who underwent treatment with 5-fluorouracil, doxorubicin, and cyclophosphamide. After six cycles, the group that received the extract had reduced chemotherapy-associated neutropenia (Santos Araújo et al. 2012).

17.4.5.2 Quality of Life

An uncontrolled prospective phase II study assessed the effects of 100 mg of *U. tomentosa* extract three times daily in 51 patients with advanced solid tumors who had a life expectancy of at least 2 months. The extract significantly improved the patients' overall QOL and social functioning, but did not improve interleukin-1 and -6, C-reactive protein, tumor necrosis factor-α, erythrocyte sedimentation rate, and α-1-acid glycoprotein (dePaula et al. 2015).

Cat's claw was assessed in a trial in 43 patients with colorectal cancer undergoing adjuvant/palliative chemotherapy with 5-fluorouracil/leucovorin plus oxaliplatin and with 300 mg *Uncaria tomentosa* orally daily. At the end of six cycles of chemotherapy plus cat's claw, QOL was not improved (Farias et al. 2012).

17.4.6 Clinical Application

One study that showed improvement in quality of life in terminal cancer patients was small and did not demonstrate an effect on biochemical and inflammatory makers or tumor response. Currently, cat's claw cannot be recommended for supportive care of cancer.

17.5 Essiac

17.5.1 Background

Essiac is a combination of burdock root (*Arctium lappa* L.), Indian rhubarb root which is also known as Turkish rhubarb (*Rheum palmatum* L.), sheep sorrel (*Rumex acetosella* L.), and the inner back of slippery elm (*Ulmus fulva* Michx., synonym *Ulmus rubra* Muhl&) (Cassileth 2011; NCI 2016). The original formulation was developed in the 1920s by Renée Caisse, a Canadian nurse. Essiac is Caisse spelled in reverse (Cassileth 2011). Caisse obtained the formula from a woman who maintained that it healed her breast cancer. The woman had received the formula from an Ontario Ojibwa Native American healer.

Renee Caisse modified the formula several times on the basis of her own experience but the exact formula remained a secret. By 1938, the Royal Cancer Commission, established under the Cancer Remedies Act of Ontario, investigated the clinic because of concerns about the use of Essiac after a death and other reports of toxicity. Members of the Commission were also concerned about the limited evidence of effectiveness (Kaegi 1998).

Between 1959 and 1978, Caisse worked with Dr. Charles Brusch founder of the Brusch Medical Center in Cambridge, Massachusetts. Four other botanicals were added including watercress (*Nasturtium officinal* R.Br.), blessed thistle (*Cnicus benedictus* L.), red clover (*Trifolium pretense* L.), and kelp (*Laminaria digitate* [Hudson] Lamx.). The new formula is known as Flor Essence (NCI 2016). Essiac has also been used to enhance immune function, treat AIDS, appetite stimulant, arthritis, and asthma, among many other conditions (NCI 2016).

17.5.2 Pharmacognosy

In vitro studies using Essiac and Flor Essence have had mixed results. Essiac induced significant antioxidant activity and immunomodulatory effects by stimulating granulocytes, increasing CD8+ cell activation, and moderately inhibiting inflammatory pathways. Essiac showed significant cell-specific cytotoxicity toward ovarian epithelial neoplastic cells (Kaegi 1998). Memorial Sloan-Kettering Cancer Center tested samples of Essiac provided by Caisse on mice to assess immunostimulatory and chemotherapeutic effect of the samples. No immunostimulatory or chemotherapeutic activities were found using the S-180 mouse sarcoma tumor model (NCI 2016).

17.5.3 Dosing and Preparation

The Essiac formulation is a proprietary secret but more than 40 products are available in the United Kingdom, Australia, and North America (Ulbricht et al. 2009). Essiac is primarily administered as an herbal tea, drops, capsules, liquids and dry versions. Limited information is available about the dose and schedule (NCI 2016). The tea is usually administered 1–3 times daily before meals to reduce possible adverse effects.

17.5.4 Safety

Adverse effects from Essiac have not been well studied. Nausea and vomiting has been reported with the use of Essiac (NCI 2016). A 59-year-old woman developed symptoms of anorexia, nausea, myalgia, fatigue, and generalized abdominal pain after consuming Essiac tea for 6 months. Her symptoms resolved after discontinuing the tea (Cassileth 2011). Allergic reactions including skin rashes and anaphylaxis may be possible with Essiac. Reports suggest that both Essiac and Flor-Essence may stimulate *in vitro* growth of human breast cancer cells (Al-Sukhni et al. 2005).

The potential for drug interactions is unclear. Essiac had minimal effects on hepatic microsomal enzymes at a concentration of 9 mcg/mL but inhibited CYP1A2 by 37%, 2C19 by 24%, 2C19 by 24%, 2D6 by 9% and 3A4 by 5% at a concentration of 100 mcg/mL (Kaegi 1998).

17.5.5 Evidence

A retrospective review of 510 Canadian women with primary breast cancer were surveyed to determine the difference in health-related quality of life between those who were new users of Essiac and those who never used the formulation (Zick et al. 2006; Ulbricht et al. 2009). The results did not indicate a significant effect on QOL or mood states with Essiac.

17.5.6 Clinical Application

One cohort study in women found that Essiac did not improve health-related quality of life. The potential effects on human breast cancer cells and the unclear safety are of concern. The available evidence does not support its use for supportive or palliative care.

17.6 Ginger

17.6.1 Background

Ginger (*Zingiber officinale* Rosc.) belongs to the *Zingiberaceae* family and has a long history of use in traditional medicine for gastrointestinal complaints (Ramakrishnan 2013). Ginger is commonly used as adjunctive therapy for patient undergoing chemotherapy.

17.6.2 Pharmacognosy

The exact mechanism of action for the anti-emetic effect of ginger in chemotherapy is unknown (Marx et al. 2017). Multiple mechanisms have been proposed including 5-HT3 receptor antagonism, anti-inflammatory effects, and modulation of gastrointestinal motility (Marx et al. 2017). *See Chapter 7 Gastrointestinal Disease for more discussion.*

17.6.3 Dosing and Preparation

In clinical trials, the typical dosages for nausea and vomiting have been 1–2 g of ginger daily divided into 4–8 capsules and taken for a period of 1–10 days. Most studies used encapsulated, powdered ginger products (Marx et al. 2015). One study evaluating the role of ginger root powder capsules as add-on therapy to ondansetron and dexamethasone in children receiving cisplatin and doxorubicin used 1–2 g daily during the first 3 days of chemotherapy (Pillai et al. 2011).

17.6.4 Safety

See Chapter 7 Gastrointestinal Disease for discussion.

17.6.5 Evidence

A systematic review was conducted of seven randomized controlled trials and/or crossover trials using ginger for prophylaxis or for treatment of chemotherapy-induced nausea and vomiting (CINV) (Marx 2013). Although the results were mixed, the review supported ginger for CINV. Three studies demonstrated positive results, two trials showed ginger to be as effective as metoclopramide, which is no longer routinely used as a stand-alone antiemetic for chemotherapy, and two showed no benefit. The reasons for the mixed results may be due to the various formulations used in the studies.

Newer clinical trials have been published on the use of ginger as an add on therapy for supportive care. In a double-blind, placebo-controlled, multicenter, phase II study, patients receiving moderately to highly emetogenic adjuvant chemotherapy were randomized to 6-gingerol 10 mg (n = 42) or placebo (n = 46) twice daily for 12 weeks (Konmun et al. 2017). Each 5 mg capsule contained 1.4% w/w of ginger extract and all patients received ondansetron, metoclopramide, and dexamethasone. The primary outcome was the rate of complete response (CR), defined as no episodes of emesis or use of rescue treatment during both acute and delayed phases for all chemotherapy cycles. The secondary outcomes included the overall rate of CR for acute and delayed phases, the rates of CR following 1st cycle chemotherapy, the severity of nausea and vomiting, appetite score, health-related QOL and tolerability. Daily measurements were taken for severity of nausea and appetite by the Numerical Rating Scale (NRS) on the Edmonton's Symptom Assessment Scale (ESAS). Episodes for nausea and vomiting were self-reported daily. Quality of life was assessed using the Functional Assessment of Cancer Therapy-General (FACT-G) instrument version four on days 1, 22, 43, and 64 of therapy. Baseline characteristics were similar between the groups, except that patients in the ginger group had presented with an earlier cancer stage at the time of diagnosis. A total of 93% of patients received highly emetogenic chemotherapy. Patients in the ginger group had a significantly higher rate of overall CR compared with the placebo group (77% versus 32%, P < 0.001). The two groups had a significant difference in the mean appetite score (P = 0.001). At 64 days, QOL was higher in the ginger group compared with placebo (86.21 versus 72.36, P < 0.001). Patients given ginger had significantly less grade 3 fatigue (2% versus 20%, P = 0.02). Ginger improved significantly the overall rate of CR in CINV, appetite, and QOL (Konmun et al. 2017).

A randomized, placebo-controlled, double-blind, crossover study administered ginger or placebo to 34 breast cancer patients on Adriamycin and cyclophosphamide who had moderate to severe nausea or vomiting in the first chemotherapy cycle (Thamlikitkul et al. 2017). A 500 mg ginger capsule and placebo were administered twice daily for 5 days beginning on day one of the second cycle. After, patients were crossed over to the other therapy for the third cycle. Ondansetron and dexamethasone were given to all patients. The severity of nausea was recorded daily on days one to five of each cycle. The primary endpoint was the reduction in the nausea score. The mean (±standard error) maximum score for nausea in the ginger and placebo groups were similar 35.36 (±4.43) and 32.17 (±3.71). Ginger did not have a significant benefit in reducing the severity and incidence of vomiting, as well as decreasing the use of rescue medication.

A double-blind trial randomized 65 breast cancer patients receiving chemotherapy to three groups: (1) ginger in addition to dexamethasone, metoclopramide and aprepitant (DMA); (2) chamomile in addition to DMA; and (3) DMA (Sanaati et al. 2016). Ginger and chamomile were administered as a 500 mg capsule twice daily on the 5 days prior to and 5 days following chemotherapy. Patients used a VAS to record CINV and answered questions regarding the use of other antiemetics, missed doses, and side effects. Twenty patients dropped out primarily for weakness, chemotherapy cancellation, and withdrawal. Significant differences were not seen for age, education, chemotherapy drugs, and disease duration among the groups.

Ginger and chamomile did not reduce the severity of nausea (P = 0.238), but both significantly reduced the frequency of vomiting (P < 0.0001). In addition, unlike patients who took chamomile (P = 0.895), those who took ginger had reduced frequency of nausea (P = 0.006).

A phase II-III prospective trial enrolled 150 patients with newly diagnosed breast cancer with planned doxorubicin-containing chemotherapy every 3 weeks (Ansari et al. 2016). Dexamethasone, aprepitant, and granisetron were given in all patients. Participants were randomized to two capsules of 250 mg ginger or placebo, given twice daily for 3 days, although it was not clear which days these were respective to their chemotherapy cycle. After 3 days, patients were required to record the number of vomiting/nausea episodes based on severity. A total of 31 patients were excluded for analysis because they forgot to record their symptoms. After cycle 1 of chemotherapy, the ginger and control groups were similar for mean nausea (1.36 ± 1.31 versus 1.46 ± 1.28). Upon completion of cycle two, the ginger group had a higher nausea score than the placebo group (1.36 versus 1.32). After cycle three, the ginger group had a higher mean nausea severity score than control (1.42 ± 1.30 versus 1.37 ± 1.14). For all patients, the severity of nausea was worse in patients who took ginger. The mean vomiting score following each chemotherapy session was lower in the ginger group compared to the placebo group. For all cycles, the ginger group had reduced severity of vomiting (1.4 ± 1.04 to 0.71 ± 0.86), however the results were not statistically significant.

17.6.6 Clinical Application

A systematic review of randomized control trials for the use of ginger for prophylactic or treatment of chemotherapy-induced nausea and vomiting showed some benefit with more recent clinical trials having mixed results. Most importantly, studies have evaluated ginger in patients receiving antiemetic therapy with standard drugs such as ondansetron and aprepitant.

17.7 Milk Thistle

17.7.1 Background

Milk thistle, *Silybum marianum* (L.) Gaertn., fructus (syn. *Carduus marianus L.*) is a member of *Asteracae* family (PDQ NCI 2017). Milk thistle has been used for aging skin, alcoholic liver diseases, allergic rhinitis, among other conditions, as well as for supportive care for patients with cancer. *See Chapter 7 Gastrointestinal Disease for more discussion.*

17.7.2 Pharmacognosy

Milk thistle seed crude extract contains 65%–80% flavonolignans, termed silymarin, which contains at least seven isomers (silybin A and B, isosilybin A and B, silychristin, isosilychristin, and silydianin) and the flavonoid taxifolin (Green and Kalisch 2015). The seed extract also contains 20%–35% fatty acids, including linoleic acid. A processed form of silymarin, termed silibinin (synonymous with silybin and silybinin), contains the isomers silybin A and B in equal portions (Green and Kalisch 2015).

Silymarin has poor water solubility, low absorption from the gastrointestinal tract, a short half-life, and undergoes phase I and phase II biotransformation in the liver. During phase II biotransformation, silymarin isomers are conjugated by glucuronidation and sulfation, and are primarily eliminated by biliary excretion. Silybin (silibinin) is rapidly absorbed orally and quickly excreted, mainly through the bile as glucuronide or sulfates conjugates. To increase the bioavailability, silybin has been molecularly complexed with phosphatidylcholine (Javed et al. 2011).

Silymarin and/or silybin possess antifibrotic, anti-inflammatory, antioxidant, cell membrane stabilizing, cytotoxic in certain cancer cell lines, among other activities (PDQ NCI 2017).

17.7.3 Dosing and Preparation

Milk thistle is usually given as a standardized extract of 70%–80% silymarin in encapsulated form (Anon 1999). The doses of silymarin in clinical trials ranged from 35 mg three times daily to 1,368 mg daily, and the most commonly used dose was 420 mg daily in divided doses (Tamayo and Diamond 2007). Silibinin phosphatidylcholine was given in a dose escalating study at a dose of 2–12 g daily (Siegel et al. 2014). In children, the dose of milk thistle standardized to 80 mg of silibinin was 5.1 mg/kg/day as an adjunct to chemotherapy (Ladas et al. 2010).

17.7.4 Safety

Adverse effects with milk thistle are uncommon and silymarin is well tolerated at high doses (Green and Kalisch 2015). Clinical trials have found that milk thistle can cause intestinal discomfort, headache, and dizziness. Rare cases of a laxative effect have been reported.

An *in vitro* study demonstrated that silymarin and silybin A and B inhibited the primary intestinal UGT1A isoforms responsible for the glucuronidation of raloxifene. Concomitant administration of raloxifene with silibinin and silymarin may increase the systemic concentration of the drug by four-fold to five-fold (Gufford et al. 2015). Silymarin extracts have minor inhibitory effects on CYP450 isozymes CYP1A2, CYP2A6, CYP2B6, CYP2C8, CYP2C9, CYP2C19, CYP2D6, CYP2E1, and CYP3A4 (Kawaguchi-Suzuki et al. 2014). *See Chapter 2 Pharmacokinetic and Pharmacogenomic Considerations for in-depth discussion of milk thistle's influence on drug metabolism.*

17.7.5 Evidence

17.7.5.1 Oral Mucositis

In a double-blind, placebo-controlled trial, oral silymarin administered over a 6-week period significantly reduced the severity of oral mucositis secondary to radiation in 27 patients with head and neck cancer. The dose used in the study was 420 mg daily in three divided doses starting on the first day of radiotherapy (Elyasi et al. 2016). The authors noted that the study was too small to evaluate any effect silymarin may have specifically on radiation therapy. Since silymarin's proposed mechanism is as an antioxidant, and radiation relies on creating oxidative stress to treat cancer, the evaluation of its effects on radiation is critical.

17.7.5.2 Prevention of Hepatotoxicity

A randomized, double-blind, placebo-controlled study in 50 children between the ages of 1–21 years with grade two or higher hepatic toxicity, who were receiving maintenance therapy for acute lymphoblastic leukemia (ALL), received capsules containing 240 mg of milk thistle, standardized to 80 mg of silibinin, to a target dose of 5.1 mg/kg/day or placebo. After 56 days, the milk thistle group had a significant decrease in mean level of AST and a nonsignificant lower mean ALT level. Of note, milk thistle did not antagonize the effect of methotrexate and vincristine when evaluated using *in vitro* ALL cell line (Ladas et al. 2010).

17.7.5.3 Prevention of Nephrotoxicity

A randomized, double-blind, placebo-controlled study investigated the renoprotective effect of silymarin in 24 patients receiving cisplatin infusions. Silymarin was administrated orally as 140 mg three times daily starting 24–48 hours prior to initiation of cisplatin and continued to the end of three 21-day cycles. The incidence of acute kidney injury and urinary magnesium and potassium wasting did not differ between groups. The study concluded that the administration of silymarin did not prevent cisplatin-induced nephrotoxicity (Shahbazi et al. 2015).

17.7.5.4 Miscellaneous

In a controlled study, use of a silymarin-based cream (Leviaderm®) was compared to standard care for management of postsurgical radiation-associated skin lesions in 101 patients with breast cancer. The median time to toxicity was significantly longer (45 days versus 29 days) in silymarin-based cream group compared to standard care. In addition, the percentage of patients with grade III skin lesions was also reduced significantly (2% versus 28% respectively), and the percentage of patients with no skin lesions during the treatment period was also significantly reduced (23.5% versus 2%) (Becker-Schiebe et al. 2011).

17.7.6 Clinical Application

Milk thistle extract is likely safe at recommended dosages. Laboratory assessments using cell lines or animal models and a small number of clinical human studies have investigated the effect of milk thistle or its primary constituents to increase the efficacy or reduce the toxicity of chemotherapeutic agents. Preliminary data is positive but additional evidence is needed.

17.8 Mistletoe (European)

17.8.1 Background

Mistletoe (*Viscum album* L), or European mistletoe, is a hemiparasitic plant from the *Viscaceae* family that grows on various trees (Bonamin et al. 2017). Mistletoe has yellow-green rounded leaves and white berries that ripen during the winter. Chemical constituents vary depending on the host tree (apple, elm, oak, pine, poplar, and spruce), harvest season, and manufacturing process.

Using mistletoe for cancer treatment began in the 1920 by Rudolf Steiner, the Austrian founder of anthroposophy (Bonamin et al. 2017). Today, mistletoe extracts are commonly used in Europe and marketed as injectable prescription drugs. Mistletoe extract has been used for treatment of arthritis, asthma, dermatitis, epilepsy, and headache, as well as menopausal symptoms (PDQ NCI 2017).

17.8.2 Pharmacognosy

The primary anticancer constituents are lectins and viscotoxins. Other compounds are flanonoids, flavonoids, phenolic acids and phenylpropanoids, which have antioxidant and anti-inflammatory activities. Additional constituents include cytotoxic and apoptotic triterpenes phytosterols, and oligo- and polysaccharides (Nazaruk and Orlikowski 2016).

Mistletoe has the ability to stabilize DNA in mononuclear cells when exposed to DNA-damaging chemotherapeutic agents. It can modulate cytokines, including interleukin-1, interleukin-5, and tumor necrosis factor-α. Mistletoe extract has cytotoxic effects including interfering with protein synthesis in target cells, can induce apoptosis, and bridges the immune system effector cells and tumor cells (PDQ NCI 2017).

17.8.3 Dosing and Preparation

The commercial preparations of mistletoe are made from mixtures of fresh leave shoots that are harvested during the summer and winter when the concentrations of the lectins and viscotoxins are the highest (Bonamin et al. 2017). The extracts may be made as aqueous solutions or solutions of alcohol and water and can be fermented or unfermented (PDQ NCI 2017).

The intravenous infusion dosage of aviscumine, a natural mistletoe lectin-I produced by recombinant DNA, used in a clinical study was 4–5 mcg/kg infused over 24 hours once weekly (Schöffski et al. 2005). The dosage of an aqueous mistletoe extract standardized to lectins administered as intravesicular therapy for bladder cancer was 50 mL weekly for 2 weeks (Elsasser-Beile et al. 2005). The subcutaneous dosage of an aqueous extract of mistletoe containing was 5 mg/mL three times weekly (Deliorman et al. 2001).

17.8.4 Safety

Mistletoe can be classified as a poisonous plant especially the berries (Stirpe 1983). The most common adverse effects in clinical studies were soreness and inflammation at the injection site and flu-like symptoms such as chills, fever, and headache (PDQ NCI 2017). A review of studies also reported increased intracerebral pressure, circulatory problems, lymph node swelling, and thrombophlebitis (Jung et al. 1990). Allergic reactions including anaphylaxis have been reported with its use (PDQ NCI 2017). High doses of mistletoe have been associated with a reversible hepatotoxicity (Kienle et al. 2016).

17.8.5 Evidence

Over 50 clinical trials have evaluated extracts in cancer patients and several systematic reviews have assessed mistletoe for extending cancer survival (PDQ NCI 2017). Patients had breast, colorectal, lung, melanoma, pancreatic and other types of cancer. Although some studies were well designed, many had methodological weaknesses, which made systematic analyses difficult (Ostermann et al. 2010). Six systematic reviews with mistletoe evaluated QOL, survival, and symptom relief in patients with various cancer types who were receiving chemotherapy (Ernst et al. 2003; Horneber et al. 2008). Two quality trials showed a positive effect on QOL and four other trials with good methodology showed no effect on survival (Ernst et al. 2003; Horneber et al. 2008). *See Chapter 16 Cancer Prevention and Treatment for further discussion of mistletoe.*

17.8.6 Clinical Application

Data on mistletoe from high quality clinical trials is lacking. Most evidence is from case reports and unconfirmed evidence. The use of mistletoe cannot be recommended.

17.9 Resveratrol

17.9.1 Background

Resveratrol is a stilbenoid polyphenolic compound found in over 70 different plants such as blueberries, cocoa, coconut, cranberries, grapes, groundnuts, Japanese knotweed, mulberries, pistachio, rhubarb, and tea (DerMarderosian and McQueen 2017a,b). *Darakchasava* is a well-known Ayurvedic preparation that contains resveratrol. Resveratrol was first isolated from the roots of white hellebore (*Veratum grandiflorum* O. Loes) in 1940 by Japanese researchers and from the dried roots of Japanese knotweed (*Polygonum cupsidatum*) in 1963, which is used in traditional Chinese and Japanese medicine (Timmers et al. 2012).

Resveratrol has been used for allergy, age-related macular degeneration, cancer prevention and treatment, cardiovascular disease, chronic obstruction pulmonary disease, diabetes, HIV, hypercholesteremia, inflammation, and menopausal problems, as well as many other conditions (DerMarderosian and McQueen 2017a,b).

17.9.2 Pharmacognosy

Resveratrol is produced by plants in response to stress or traumatic situations such as bacterial or fungal infections and is part of its defensive mechanism (DerMarderosian and McQueen 2017a,b). Resveratrol is synthesized by the plant from p-coumaroyl CoA and malonyl CoA. Black grapes have the highest concentration of resveratrol followed by red grapes which has more than green grapes (Borys et al. 2017). Red wine contains a large amount of resveratrol which is released from grape skins during the fermentation process (Borys et al. 2017; DerMarderosian and McQueen 2017a,b).

Resveratrol is trans-3,5,4′-trihydroxystilbene and is comprised of two phenolic rings connected by an ethylene bridge; the structure exits in two stereoisomers. In nature, the trans form is more common, and is more bioactive and more durable. Under high pH, high temperature, or UV radiation conditions, the trans form is easily isomerized into the cis form (Borys et al. 2017).

A PubMed.gov search of articles about resveratrol resulted in more than 7,400 articles as of Sept 1, 2017 with 1,100 articles specifically on the mechanism of action of resveratrol. The initial excitement about resveratrol has waned due to the growing knowledge that resveratrol affects most of the known biochemical and signaling pathways and that high doses are needed to elicit the desired cellular responses. Resveratrol interferes with the three stages of carcinogenesis, initiation, promotion and progression (Jang et al. 1997).

In vitro studies have demonstrated that resveratrol inhibits cancer cell proliferation (Gehm et al. 1997; Surh et al. 1999; Wang et al. 2008). Researchers demonstrated that resveratrol modulates transcription factor NF-kB (Adhami et al. 2003) transcriptions factors (NF-kB, MAPK), protein kinases (CDK4/6), cell cycle regulatory proteins (SIRT, SAT3) and inhibits angiogenesis (VEGF) in cell and animal models.

Resveratrol acts similarly to selective estrogen receptor modulators by competing with natural estrogens for binding to estrogen receptor α (ERα) and upon binding, resveratrol modulates the receptor as an antagonist (Chakraborty et al. 2013). Resveratrol also inhibits heregulin-beta1-mediated matrix metalloproteinase-9 expression cancer, activates the HER-2 signaling pathway, and inhibits cell invasion in human breast cancer cells (Tang et al. 2008).

Resveratrol has antiandrogenic effects by modulating androgen transcriptional activity in prostate cells (Li et al. 2013). Resveratrol may also reduce prostate tumorigenesis by reducing prostatic levels of mTOR complex 1 activity and increasing the expression of SIRT1 (Zhang et al. 2011).

17.9.3 Dosing and Preparation

In humans, resveratrol is absorbed in the jejunum and ileum but studies have shown that resveratrol has low bioavailability, about 2%, due to rapid biotransformation (Borys et al. 2017). Information is limited on dosing in adults and in children and, therefore, a recommendation cannot be made. The amount of resveratrol in red wine is variable and increasing the consumption of red wine to increase resveratrol poses health risks including liver damage.

17.9.4 Safety

Resveratrol is generally safe even at 1 g daily, although high doses are associated with diarrhea (Howells et al. 2011).

Resveratrol is a substrate of CYP1A1, CYP1A2, and CYP1B1 (Borys et al. 2017). Resveratrol induces CYP2D6 and CYP2C9, and it inhibits CYP3A4 (Howells et al. 2011). Therefore, concurrent use with drugs that are metabolized by these enzymes may be affected.

Resveratrol inhibits platelet aggregation and concurrent use with other antiplatelet drugs may increase the risk of bleeding (Pace-Asciak et al. 1995). Patients with hormone-sensitive cancers should avoid resveratrol since it has estrogen properties and activates both estrogen and androgen receptors (Tang et al. 2008; Li et al. 2013).

17.9.5 Evidence

Despite the theoretical benefits from resveratrol based on *in vitro* studies, clinical trials in supportive and palliative care, as well as in oncology, are not available.

17.9.6 Clinical Applications

Many resveratrol studies have been conducted only *in vitro* due to bioavailability issues. Currently, large well conducted clinical trials using resveratrol for chemoprevention or chemotherapy are needed. Also, in 2012, it was announced that a key resveratrol researcher falsified data and as a result many of his publications were retracted (Callaway 2012). Unfortunately, many of his publications have been cited in other journals.

17.10 Soy

17.10.1 Background

Soy (Glycine max (L.) Merr.), a member of the *Leguminosae* family, is a subtropical legume that is native to southeastern Asia (He and Chen 2013). Other common names are soya, soybean, soyabean, and soy isoflavones. Soy is also known as soy bean curd (dofu, kori-dofu, soybean curds, and tofu), edamame, kinako, kouridofu, miso, hydrolyzed soy protein, natto, nimame, okara, soy protein (isolate/concentrate), soy vegetable protein, and tempeh.

Soy is used orally for asthma, benign prostatic hyperplasia, cardiovascular disease prevention, constipation, type 2 diabetes and diabetic nephropathy, diarrhea, as well as many other conditions. Soy has also been used to prevent or treat breast cancer, colorectal cancer, endometrial cancer, prostate cancer, and thyroid cancer. *See Chapters 6 Endocrine Disorders, 8 Women's Health, and 16 Cancer Prevention and Treatment for additional information.*

17.10.2 Pharmacognosy

Mature dried uncooked soybean usually contains 8.5% moisture, 36.5% protein, 19.9% lipids, and 9.3% dietary fiber (He and Chen 2013). Soybeans also contain phytoestrogens known as isoflavones which function like endogenous estrogen. Soy isoflavones are almost always in the form of low bioavailable glycoside conjugates (Mahmoud et al. 2014). Bioavailability of isoflavones depends on the method they are extracted, processed, and cooked (Mackay 2016). Once absorbed, soy isoflavone glycosides undergo hydrolysis in the small intestine and release the sugar molecule. This makes soy isoflavones more water soluble. Following hydrolysis they are converted to glycones such as genistin, diadzin, and glycetin, or aglycones such as genistein, diadzein, and, to a lesser extent, glycetein (He and Chen 2013). Soybean usually contains approximately 37 mg of diadzein and 24 mg of genistein per kg of dry weight but the amount varies depending on variety, cultivation and geographic location (He and Chen 2013).

The aglycones undergo extensive first pass biotransformation in the colon by bacterial β-glycosidases. Diadzein is further metabolized to equol, which possesses potent estrogenic activity and has a greater affinity for estrogen receptors. The clinical effectiveness of soy isoflavones may be related to the ability to metabolize daidzein to equol. Only 25%–35% of U.S. Caucasians are capable of converting daidzein to equol, whereas 40%–60% of Asians who live in high soy consumption regions are capable of converting daidzein to equol (He and Chen 2013). Hispanics are also more likely to biotransform daidzein to equol (He and Chen 2013). The plasma half-life of genistein and daidzein is approximately 8 hours in adults with peak concentration being reached in 6–8 hours (He and Chen 2013).

Soy isoflavones possess diverse biological functions such as anti-inflammatory, antioxidant, prevention or reduction in bone loss, inhibition of cancer cell proliferation, and prevention of coronary heart disease. Much of the biological activity of isoflavones has been attributed to their structural similarity to 17-β-estradiol (Mahmoud 2014). Research has shown that isoflavones have selective estrogen receptor modulator activity, with preferentially binding for the estrogen receptor-beta rather than the estrogen receptor-α.

17.10.3 Dosing and Preparation

See Chapters 6 Endocrine Disorders, 8 Women's Health, 14 Musculoskeletal Condidtions, and 16 Cancer Prevention and Treatment for additional information.

17.10.4 Safety

Phytoestrogens are well tolerated with primarily gastrointestinal effects. Soy should not be used by individuals who are allergic to soy. The American Cancer Society states that even though animal studies have shown mixed effects on breast cancer with soy supplements, studies in humans have not shown harm from eating soy foods. Moderate consumption of soy foods appears safe for both breast cancer survivors and the general population (McCulloch 2012).

Genistein in combination with sunitinib caused additive cardiotoxicity possibly due to kinase activation leading to intracellular signaling in cardiomyocytes, which produced lethal consequences in mice (Harvey and Leinwand 2015). Concomitant use of soy supplementation in patients receiving tyrosine kinase inhibitors should be monitored closely. *See Chapters 6 Endocrine Disorders, 8 Women's Health, 14 Musculoskeletal Condidtions, and 16 Cancer Prevention and Treatment for additional information.*

17.10.5 Evidence

Hot flashes are a common symptom experienced by breast cancer survivors treated with chemotherapy or tamoxifen, as well as by postmenopausal women not receiving hormone replacement therapy. For many women, hot flashes have a significant effect on their quality of life.

A double-blind, placebo-controlled clinical trial randomized 123 women who were previously treated for breast cancer and had postmenopausal hot flashes to a 250 mL soy beverage with 90 mg isoflavones or a placebo beverage containing rice, both given twice daily for 12 weeks (Van Patten et al. 2002). Women were stratified on concomitant tamoxifen use. The primary endpoint was the difference in the mean 24-hour hot flash score (calculated by frequency x intensity) during the 4-week baseline recordings compared to the last 4 weeks of therapy. Baseline characteristics were similar between the groups. The numbers and severity of hot flashes was similar between the soy and placebo groups. Gastrointestinal adverse effects were similar, although the soy group reported slightly higher severity and frequency.

17.10.6 Clinical Application

Although well tolerated, the effect of soy as a botanical for supportive care has limited evidence, but can be safe to use. Additional information on potential drug interactions is essential.

17.11 Sweet Wormwood

17.11.1 Background

Artemisia annua L. is commonly known as Sweet wormwood, Sweet annie, Sweet sagewort, Annual wormwood and in Chinese as Qīnghāo (Shagar and Garchinski 2014; DerMarderosian and McQueen 2016). It is a different species than wormwood, *Artemisia absinthium*, which is used in the manufacture of the French liqueur absinthe (Shagar and Garchinski 2014). The whole plant *A. absinthium* or its oil can contain high concentrations of thujone which is a hallucinogen and can cause renal failure (Bora and Sharma 2011). There are several species of *Artemisia*, and several are known for their aromatic fragrance and characteristic scent and taste. *A. annua* is a member of the *Asteraceae* (*Compositae*) family which includes chrysanthemums, daisies, marigolds, and ragweed (DerMarderosian and McQueen 2016).

A. annua is indigenous to China but has been widely naturalized throughout the world in temperate, cool temperate and subtropical regions of the world (WHO 2006). The herb is an annual with upright stems and alternate branches. The fern-like leaves, which can measure 2–5 cm in length, are deeply dissected and the flowers are yellow; both the leaves and flowers contain biseriate trichomes. The plant can grow to a height of 30–100 cm naturally and 200 cm when cultivated (WHO 2006).

Sweet wormwood tea and juice has been used for cancer, fever, hepatitis-B, HIV, parasitic infections, worms and malaria (Efferth 2006; Alesaeidi and Miraj 2016). Use of *A. annua* dates back at least 2,000 years, to the first written record devoted to disease treatment, *Wu Shi Er Bing Fang* (DerMarderosian and McQueen 2016). *The Pharmacopoeia of the People's Republic of China includes the dried herb A. annua* (Qinghaosu) for the treatment of chills and fever secondary to malaria and to stop malarial attacks (WHO 2006).

17.11.2 Pharmacognosy

Sesquiterpenoids, flavonoids, coumarins, triterpenoids, steroids, phenolics, purines, lipids and aliphatic compounds, and monoterpenoids have been isolated from different plant parts of *A. annua* (DerMarderosian and McQueen 2016). The plant contains at least 38 amophane and cadinane seesquiterpenes with most of the active constituents found in the flowers, leaves, seeds, and stems. The main active constituent is artemisinin, with the highest concentration located in the leaves prior to flowering. The concentration of artemisinin differs depending on the genotypes and ranges from 0.01% to 0.5% (w/w). Essential oils found in the plant include 1,8-cineol, p-cymene, linalool, thujone, and camphor (DerMarderosian and McQueen 2016). Since the late 1990s, interest has existed in the anticancer properties of artemisinins (Bhaw-Luximon and Jhurry 2017). The mechanism of action may involve a direct effect on stopping tumor cell proliferation through cell cycle arrest mediated by reactive oxygen species (Bhaw-Luximon and Jhurry 2017). In addition, artemisinin derivatives inhibit growth by cell cycle arrest, apoptosis, inhibition of angiogenesis, disruption of cell migration, and modulation of nuclear receptor responsiveness (Firestone and Sundar 2009).

17.11.3 Dosing and Preparation

There is no documented dosage for sweet wormwood for supportive care in cancer.

17.11.4 Safety

Orally sweet wormwood is generally well tolerated. A report of a possible allergic reaction with signs and symptoms of pruritus, rash and urticaria have been reported (DerMarderosian and McQueen 2016). Since sweet wormwood is in the *Asteraceae* family, cross-reactivity may be possible in people sensitive in individuals who are sensitive to ragweed, chrysanthemums, marigolds, and daisies. Two cases of hepatotoxicity associated with the use of dietary supplements containing artemisinin have been reported (Mueller et al. 2004).

A Cochrane review of 23 trials using artemisinin derivatives found that abdominal pain was the most common adverse effect. Pain at the injection site was the most common adverse event with intramuscular artemether. Other adverse effects included bradycardia, prolongation of the QT interval, and hypoglycemia (McIntosh and Olliaro 2000). In a case report, a woman with breast cancer developed symptoms of brainstem encephalopathy which may have been secondary to artemisinin treatment (Panossian et al. 2005).

Animal studies have demonstrated that artemisinin derivatives may be embryotoxic when taken during the first trimester due to depletion of embryonic erythroblasts which may cause miscarriage and congenital malformations, mainly cardiovascular and skeletal (Moore et al. 2016). However, a review of the literature in humans during the first trimester of pregnancy found no evidence of an increased risk of miscarriage or of major congenital malformations associated with treatment with an artemisinin derivative (Moore et al. 2016).

17.11.5 Evidence

Multiple articles have been published on the anticancer effects of artemisinin, dihydroartemisinin, artemether and atermisone *in vitro*. Studies using 55 cancer cell lines have reported inhibitory effects against various cancers such as breast, central nervous system, colon, leukemia, lung, lymphoma, melanoma, ovarian, pancreatic, and prostate cancer (Bhakuni et al. 2001). At present, clinical studies in humans using sweet wormwood for cancer are not available.

17.11.6 Clinical Application

Preliminary *in vitro* and *in vivo* evidence has indicated that artemisinin and artemisinin derivatives have anticancer activities. Currently, evidence is not available on using *A. annua* for the supportive care or treatment of cancer in adults and children.

17.12 Turmeric/Curcumin

17.12.1 Background

See Chapter 14 Musculoskeletal Conditions for discussion.

17.12.2 Pharmacognosy

Curcumin may influence multiple signaling pathways, cytoprotective pathways, metastatic and angiogenetic pathways and various growth factors (Hatcher et al. 2008). Curcumin decreases nuclear factor-kappa B activity, inhibits the activity of activating protein-1, suppresses early growth response gene, decreases nuclear beta-catenin, inhibits epidermal growth factor receptor tyrosine kinase, downregulates polo-like kinase inhibits hypoxia-induced angiogenesis by downregulating hypoxia inducible factor protein and vascular endothelial growth factor expression (Van Erk at al 2004; Siwak et al. 2005; Bae et al. 2006; Ruocco et al. 2007; Abusnina et al. 2015; Starok et al. 2015). In addition, it inhibits cyclin-dependent kinase-2, inhibits metalloproteinase-9, reduces Bcl-2, BCl-XL, COX-2, and IL-8 modulates the p53-E-cadherin pathway, and inhibits cancer-associated fibroblast-driven prostate cancer invasion through MAOA/mTOR/HIF-1α signaling (Woo et al. 2005; Shankar et al. 2008; Zong 2011; Lim et al. 2014; Du et al. 2015; Lee et al. 2015). Curcumin also induced cytoprotective enzymes such as glutamate-cysteine ligase, isoforms of glutathione-S-transferase, heme oxygenase, and NAD(P) H:quinone oxidoreductase. *See Chapters 15 Musculoskeletal and 16 Cancer Prevention and Treatment for additional discussion.*

17.12.3 Dosing and Preparation

See Chapter 14 Musculoskeletal Conditions for discussion.

17.12.4 Safety

Case reports of allergic dermatitis, urticaria, and angioedema have been reported, as well as a documented case of anaphylaxis (DerMarderosian and McQueen 2017). This botanical contains a high concentration of oxalates which may result in increased urinary oxalate excretion, although case reports of kidney oxalate stone formation secondary to turmeric are not available.

See Chapter 14 Musculoskeletal for additional discussion.

17.12.5 Evidence

17.12.5.1 Hand-Foot Syndrome

The use of turmeric has been evaluated in supportive care trials with mixed findings. In a pilot study, 40 patients with gastrointestinal or breast cancer and without prior exposure to capecitabine received two capsules of 1 g turmeric, twice daily, at the start of therapy for 6 weeks (Scontre et al. 2017). Each capsule contained 95% turmeric root extract. The primary outcome was a decrease in the incidence and degree of hand-foot syndrome (HFS) over 6 weeks. Patients were assessed for dermatologic toxicity, and quality of life using the EORTC-QLQC30 and Dermatology Life Quality Index (DLQI) at baseline, and after 3 and 6 weeks. After cycle 1 of capecitabine therapy, 11/40 patients developed HFS. The authors concluded that turmeric reduced the rate and severity of HFS.

17.12.5.2 Radiation Dermatitis

Curcumin use was evaluated in a randomized, double-blind, placebo-controlled trial of 30 patients with breast cancer undergoing radiation (Ryan et al. 2013). Curcumin was administered as a 2-g dose given three times daily with the signs and symptoms of radiation dermatitis evaluated throughout the treatment course. Patients assigned to curcumin were noted to have a significantly decreased Radiation Dermatitis Severity (RDS) score ($P = 0.008$) as well as a significant decrease in moist desquamation by the end of treatment (29% versus 88%, $P = 0.002$). Of note, the RDS score is not a validated tool for assessing radiation dermatitis. No significant differences were noted between arms for demographics, erythema, pain, or symptoms, including diarrhea.

A double-blind, placebo-controlled trial randomized 686 breast cancer patients to curcumin or placebo during radiation therapy (RT) and until 1 week after RT completion (Ryan Wolf et al. 2018). Four capsules, each containing 500 mg of curcumin, was given three times daily. The primary outcome was the RDS score at the end of RT. Secondary outcomes included moist desquamation, pain severity using the McGill Pain Questionnaire-Short Form (SF-MPQ), skin-related quality of life (Skindex-29), and adverse effects. Digital images were taken of the radiation-induced skin changes, and two blinded reviewers, a dermatologist and a radiation oncologist, provided a rating on RDS and moist desquamation. The curcumin group did not have significant reduction of severity in radiation dermatitis at the completion of RT although fewer patients in the curcumin group had more severe RDS.

17.12.5.3 Oral Mucositis

In a single-institution case-control study, a total of 60 patients with treatment-induced oral mucositis received either turmeric powder and honey, applied 5 minutes before and 5 minutes after treatment, or no intervention (Francis and Williams 2014). A statistically significant decrease occurred in the mean World Health Organization Oral Mucositis Assessment Scale (WHO OMAS) and the Modified Patient Judged (MPJ) OMAS scores in the experimental group versus control. Limitations include small sample size, absence of stratification based on treatment type, lack of blinding and absence of a placebo control. Additionally, the formulation used as the intervention was unclear.

A small case series examined the efficacy of Curcumall 10 drops twice per day as a mouthwash in conjunction with chlorhexidine 0.2% mouthwash 30 seconds twice daily for the prevention of oral mucositis in pediatric patients (Francis and Williams 2014). Among the four patients evaluable for response, a reduction was noted in the WHO OMAS and a visual analog pain scale when compared with the incidence previously reported in the literature.

17.12.5.4 Other Adverse Effects

A single-blind, placebo-controlled trial of 160 patients undergoing chemotherapy and radiation suggested that lecithinized curcumin (Meriva®) reduced adverse effects associated with anticancer treatment (Belcaro et al. 2013). Patients taking Meriva® (n = 80) compared with best standard of care for adverse effects (n = 80) had a significantly decreased incidence of nausea and vomiting, diarrhea or constipation, malnutrition/weight loss, memory or cognitive function alteration, infections/sepsis, neutropenia, and cardiotoxicity (p < 0.05). Of concern, the decreased rate of adverse effects with curcumin use, especially neutropenia, might also indicate a decreased chemotherapy or radiation effect and cannot be excluded.

17.12.5.5 Quality of Life

In a randomized, double-blind, placebo-controlled trial, 80 patients were assigned to either curcuminoids 180 mg daily using the Meriva® preparation in a dosage of one capsule three times daily or placebo for 8 weeks (Panahi et al. 2014) in addition to standard of care for solid tumors. The main outcome analyses aimed to determine whether curcumin supplementation could improve quality of life as well as reduce inflammation. The QOL assessment was performed using the validated University of Washington QoL index (UW-QoL). Curcumin supplementation was found to improve these scores (p < 0.001). The curcumin supplementation consistently lowered levels of the inflammatory mediators including TNF-alpha, TGFbeta, IL-6, substance P, hs-CRP, CGRP, and MCP-1, while the placebo group had a greater reduction in IL-8 levels. Due to differences in baseline characteristics such as cancer type, biochemical parameters, and QOL scores, as well as its short duration and the small sample size, strong conclusions could not be drawn from the study. The positive effects on QOL and reduction on inflammatory markers provide a strong rationale for further investigations.

17.12.6 Clinical Application

Turmeric/curcumin has been studied in the supportive care setting and might potentially be of benefit for multiple complications from chemotherapy and radiation. Although larger studies are needed, the evience is interesting. Most importantly, additional evidence that the botanical does not affect the efficacy of standard treatment approaches is needed.

17.13 Cannabis/Medical Marijuana Use in Supportive and Palliative Care

For background information, please refer to Chapter 18 Therapeutic Potential of Cannabis. Using a dataset from the National Health and Examination Survey (NHANES) of adults ages 20–60 years, researchers compared use of marijuana from 2005 to 2014 in patients with cancer (n = 604) to use in non-cancer patients (n = 1650) (Tringale 2017). Patients with cancer were non-significantly more likely to be current marijuana users (40.3%) compared to non-cancer patients (38%) (p = 0.056). Current use of marijuana (defined as use within the past 30 days) increased significantly over the 10 year period (p = 0.028) in cancer patients compared to non-cancer patients. In a 2017 report, 926 out of 2,737 adult cancer patients from the Seattle Cancer Care Alliance completed an anonymous survey on cannabis use (Pergam et al. 2017). The population had a mean age of 58 and was predominantly male, most patients were actively being treated for a solid tumor. Respondents used cannabis for the physical and neuropsychiatric symptoms, especially for pain, nausea and stress from their disease or its treatment. Importantly, few patients had received information on cannabis from their healthcare provider. Among a study of 15 patients with head and neck cancer, cannabis in a variety of dosage forms was reported for weight maintenance, appetite, depression, pain, dysphagia, dry mouth, and "sticky" saliva (Elliott et al. 2016). Given the complexity of the pharmacokinetics and pharmacodynamics of different cannabinoids, research especially comparisons with standard drugs for supportive cancer care has been challenging.

17.13.1 Efficacy

17.13.1.1 Cancer Cachexia Syndrome

A multicenter phase three study by the Cannabis-In-Cachexia Study Group randomized 243 patients with terminal cancer, had at least a 5% unintentional weight loss over the past 6 months, and a life expectancy of 3 months to capsules containing THC (2.5 mg), whole plant cannabis extract (standardized to THC 2.5 mg and cannabidiol 1.0 mg) or placebo (Strasser et al. 2006). The capsule was taken twice daily 1 hour before lunch and dinner or at bedtime. The *Cannabis sativa* plants had been harvested from the same area at the same time. A total of 164 participants with a mean age of 61 years completed the study. One third had over 10% unintentional weight loss at baseline. Patients' anorexia, quality of life, and adverse effects were assessed every 2 weeks for 6 weeks. Of the patients completing the trial, appetite was improved in 73%, 58%, and 69% of individuals receiving the whole plant cannabis extract, THC, or placebo, respectively. The study results indicated no significant between the three interventions in terms of anorexia and QOL with more adverse effects from the whole plant extract. The study limitations included a 20% dropout rate and a large placebo effect.

In addition to the above study, a 2018 systematic review of cannabinoids in palliative care identified four other small trials evaluating cannabinoids on appetite or caloric intake in cancer patients (Mücke 2018). None of the studies identified a benefit with the cannabinoids, but the quality of trials was considered to be low or very low.

17.13.1.2 Cancer Pain

Most of the published evidence on the value of cannabis-containing products for cancer pain have been primarily with the oromucosal spray Sativex that consists of delta-9 THC and cannabidiol, also known as nabiximols. A multicenter randomized study of 177 patients with cancer pain were randomized to the Sativex spray, a THC spray or to a placebo spray (Johnson 2010). Response was defined as a 30% or greater reduction in the mean pain score using the Numerical Rating Scale (NRS). Background opiate therapy remained consistent. In the Sativex group, 43% of patients achieved a response compared to 21% in the placebo group. The THC spray had results similar to placebo. An open-label extension study from this trial followed 43 patients who continued either of the active treatments for between 2 weeks and 1 year. Participants continued to experience pain relief and in insomnia, pain and fatigue (Johnson 2013).

A larger, double-blind phase three study randomized patients with advanced cancer and pain as measured with the NRS between 4 and 8 to either oral mucosal spray (Sativex) containing cannabidiol and 9-delta THC (n = 199) or to placebo (n = 198) (Lichtman 2018). All participants were also on opiates. A 10.7% improvement in pain occurred with the Sativex spray compared with 4.5% with placebo using an intention to treat analysis. With the per protocol analysis, there was a 15.5% and 6.3% improved with Sativex and placebo, respectively. Instruments assessing quality of life showed improvements at 3 and 5 weeks of treatment with the active spray in a posthoc analysis. The study noted that patients in the United States were more likely to demonstrate a response, potentially due to their lower opiate dosages (Lichtman 2018).

17.13.1.3 Chemotherapy-Induced Nausea and Vomiting

One of the most common uses of cannabis in supportive care is for chemotherapy-induced nausea and vomiting. A Cochrane review of studies published from 1975 to 1991, identified 23 trials of cannabis containing product compared either to placebo or to active anti-emetic drugs including prochlorperazine, metoclopramide, domperidone, or chlorpromazine (Smith et al. 2015). Patients were receiving moderately to severely emetogenic chemotherapy and were designed as crossover studies. Compared with placebo, use of the cannabis products had a greater likelihood of a complete absence of nausea and vomiting, as well as feeling high, with an increased risk of withdrawal due to adverse effects. Compared with prochlorperazine, cannabis products did not differ with respect to relief of nausea and vomiting, although again adverse effects were more common. Fewer studies were of cannabis products compared with metoclopramide, domperidone, or chlorpromazine. The quality of the evidence was graded as ranging from very low to moderate with a low to moderate risk of bias. No comparative studies against the first-line current standard of care anti-emetics including serotonin 5-HT3 receptor antagonists such as ondansetron and the neurokinin receptor blocker aprepitant were available. The Cochrane review concluded that cannabis-containing products might have a role in treating refractory nausea and vomiting, although comparisons to the current standard of care are needed.

The 2018 NCCN guidelines recommended the synthetic cannabinoids, dronabinol and nabilone for nausea and vomiting in patients whose symptoms are refractory to conventional antiemetics (NCCN 2018).

17.13.2 Clinical Application

There is no current evidence to support the use of cannabis for anorexia and cachexia in cancer patients. The antiemetic effect of cannabis products may have a role in management of refractory nausea and vomiting. Studies have found that cannabinoids are more effective than placebo for cancer pain control but additional studies are needed.

17.14 Summary

Multiple botanicals have been studied for the supportive and palliative care of patients with cancer. *Withania somnifera* may have benefits for fatigue and quality of life, while astragalus may have short-term effects on fatigue, anorexia and quality of life. Multiple studies have compared ginger as an add-on therapy to standard anti-emetic agents with variable results. Milk thistle has also been evaluated for supportive care in small studies with variable outcomes. Despite its interesting pharmacology, clinical trials of resveratrol have not been conducted in oncology or supportive care. Of the available botanicals for supportive care, turmeric/curcumin may have the most promising role. The potential for interactions with drugs, especially chemotherapy agents, and with radiation should be carefully considered, as clinicians frequently have inadequate information to guide their decision-making with botanicals.

REFERENCES

Abusnina, A., T. Keravis, Q. Zhou, H. Justiniano, A. Lobstein, and C. Lugnier. 2015. Tumour growth inhibition and anti-angiogenic effects using curcumin correspond to combined PDE2 and PDE4 inhibition. *Thrombosis and Haemostasis* 113, no. 02 (Feb): 319–28. doi: 10.1160/th14-05-0454

Adhami, V.M., F. Afaq, and N. Ahmad. 2003. Suppression of ultraviolet B exposure-mediated activation of NF-kappaB in normal human keratinocytes by resveratrol. *Neoplasiam* 5, no. 1 (Jan): 74–82.

Ai, P., G. Yong, G. Dingkun, Z. Qiuyu, Z. Kaiyuan, and L. Shanyan. 2008. Aqueous extract of Astragali Radix induces human natriuresis through enhancement of renal response to atrial natriuretic peptide. *Journal of Ethnopharmacology* 116, no. 3 (March): 413–21. doi: 10.1016/j.jep.2007.12.005

Al-Sukhni, W., A. Grunbaum, and N. Fleshner. 2005. Remission of hormone-refractory prostate cancer attributed to Essiac. *Canadian Journal of Urololgy* 12, no. 5: 2841–2.

Alam, K., O. Hoq, and S. Uddin. 2016. Therapeutic use of withania somnifera. *Asian Journal of Medical and Biological Research* 2, no. 2: 148–55. doi: 10.3329/ajmbr.v2i2.29004

Alesaeidi, S. and S. Miraj. 2016. A systematic review of anti-malarial properties, immunosuppressive properties, anti-inflammatory properties, and anti-cancer properties of *Artemisia annua*. *Electronic Physician* 8, no. 10 (Oct): 3150–55. doi: 10.19082/3150

Anderson, J.G. and A.G. Taylor. 2012. Use of complementary therapies for cancer symptom management: Results of the 2007 national health interview survey. *The Journal of Alternative and Complementary Medicine* 18, no. 3 (Mar): 235–41. doi: 10.1089/acm.2011.0022

Anonymous. 1999. Silybum marianum (Milk Thistle). *Alternative Medicine Review* 4, no. 4: 272–4.

Anonymous. 2003. Astragalus membranaceus. *Alternative Medicine Review* 8, no. 1: 72–7.

Ansari, M., P. Porouhan, M. Mohammadianpanah et al. 2016. Efficacy of ginger in control of chemotherapy induced nausea and vomiting in breast cancer patients receiving doxorubicin-based chemotherapy. *Asian Pacific Journal of Cancer Prevention* 17, no. 8: 3877–80.

Auyeung, K.K., C.H. Cho, and J.K. Ko. 2009. A novel anticancer effect of astragalus saponins: Transcriptional activation of NSAID-activated gene. *International Journal of Cancer* 125, no. 5: 1082–91. doi: 10.1002/ijc.24397

Bae, M.K., S.H. Kim, J.W. Jeong et al. 2006. Curcumin inhibits hypoxia-induced angiogenesis via down-regulation of HIF-1. *Oncology Reports* 15, no. 6 (Jun): 1557–62.

Becker-Schiebe, M., U. Mengs, M. Schaefer, M. Bulitta, and W. Hoffmann. 2011. Topical use of a silymarin-based preparation to prevent radiodermatitis: Results of a prospective study in breast cancer patients. *Strahlentherapie Und Onkologie* 187, no. 8 (Aug): 485–91. doi: 10.1007/s00066-011-2204-z

Belcaro, G., M. Hosoi, L. Pellegrini et al. 2013. A controlled study of a lecithinized delivery system of curcumin (Meriva®) to alleviate the adverse effects of cancer treatment. *Phytotherapy Research* 28, no. 3 (Mar): 444–50. doi: 10.1002/ptr.5014

Bhakuni, R.S., D.C. Jain, R.P. Sharma, and S. Kumar. 2001. Secondary metabolites of Artemisia annua and their biological activity. *Current Science* 80, no. 1: 35–45.

Bhaw-Luximon, A. and D. Jhurry. 2017. Artemisinin and its derivatives in cancer therapy: Status of progress, mechanism of action, and future perspectives. *Cancer Chemotherapy and Pharmacology* 79, no. 3 (Mar): 451–66. doi: 10.1007/s00280-017-3251-7

Biswal, B.M., S.A. Sulaiman, H.C. Ismail, H.I. Zakaria, and K.I. Musa. 2013. Effect of Withania somnifera (Ashwagandha) on the development of chemotherapy-induced fatigue and quality of life in breast cancer patients. *Integrative Cancer Therapies* 12: 312–22. doi: 10.1177/1534735412464551

Bonamin, L.V., A.C. de Carvalho, and S. Waisse. 2017 Jun. Viscum album (L.) in experimental animal tumors: A meta-analysis. *Experimental Therapeutic Medicine* 13, no. 6: 2723–40. doi: 10.3892/etm.2017.437

Bora, K.S. and A. Sharma. 2011. The genus Artemisia: A comprehensive review. *Pharmaceutical Biology* 49, no. 1 (Jan): 101–09. doi: 10.3109/13880209.2010.497815

Borys, S., R. Khozmi, W. Kranc, A. Bryja, M. Jeseta, and B. Kempisty. 2017. Resveratrol and its analogues—Is it a new strategy of anticancer therapy? *Advances in Cell Biology* 5, no. 1: 32–42. doi: 10.1515/acb-2017-0003

Callaway, E. 2012. Red-wine researcher implicated in data misconduct case. *Scientific American*. https://www.scientificamerican.com/article/red-wine-researcher-implicated-misconduct/ (published Jan 12, 2012; Accessed May 31, 2018)

Cassileth, B. 2011. Essiac. *Oncology* 25, no. 11: 1098–9.

Chakraborty, S., A.S. Levenson, and P.K. Biswas. 2013. Structural insights into resveratrol's antagonist and partial agonist actions on estrogen receptor alpha. *BMC Structural Biology* 25, no. 13 (Oct): 27. doi: 10.1186/1472-6807-13-27

Chen, H.W., I.H. Lin, Y.J. Chen et al. 2012. A novel infusible botanically derived drug, PG2, for cancer-related fatigue: A phase II double-bling, randomized placebo-controlled study. *Clinical & Investigative Medicine* 35, no. 1 (Feb): E1–11.

Chu, D., Y. Sun, J. Lin, W. Wong, and G. Mavligit. 1990. [F3, a fractionated extract of Astragalus membranaceus, potentiates lymphokine-activated killer cell cytotoxicity generated by low-dose recombinant interleukin-2]. *Zhong Xi Yi Jie He Za Zhi* 10, no. 1: 34–6.

Dasgupta, A., G. Tso, and A. Wells. 2008. Effect of Asian ginseng, Siberian ginseng, and Indian ayurvedic medicine Ashwagandha on serum digoxin measurement by Digoxin III, a new digoxin immunoassay. *Journal of Clinical Laboratory Analysis* 22, no. 4: 295–301. doi: 10.1002/jcla.20252

Deliorman, D., I. Çalış, and F. Ergun. 2001. A new acyclic monoterpene glucoside from Viscum album ssp. *album. Fitoterapia* 72, no. 2 (Feb): 101–05. doi: 10.1016/s0367-326x(00)00260-4

dePaula, L.C., F. Fonseca, F. Perazzo et al. 2015 Jan. Uncaria tomentosa (cat's claw) improves quality of life in patients with advanced solid tumors. *Journal of Alternative and Complementary Medicine* 21, no. 1: 22–30. doi: 10.1089/acm.2014.0127

DerMarderosian, A. and C.E. McQueen, editors. 2016. Review of Natural Products, The St. Louis, MO. Facts and Comparisons® Publishing Group. ISSN 1089-5302. *STAT!Ref Online Electronic Medical Library*. Accessed July 30, 2017.

DerMarderosian, A. and C.E. McQueen. 2017. Turmeric. In: *The Review of Natural Products. Stat!Ref. Facts and Comparison*, St. Louis, MO. May 13, 2009. Modified July 14, 2017.

DerMarderosian, A. and C.E. McQueen. 2017a. Cat's Claw. In: *The Review of Natural Products. Stat!Ref. Facts and Comparison*, St. Louis, MO. August 11, 2011. Modified, April 13, 2017.

DerMarderosian, A. and C.E. McQueen. 2017b. Resveratrol. In: *The Review of Natural Products. Stat!Ref. Facts and Comparison*, St. Louis, MO. January 2, 2014. Modified, May 26, 2017.

Du, Y., Q. Long, L. Zhang et al. 2015. Curcumin inhibits cancer-associated fibroblast-driven prostate cancer invasion through MAOA/mTOR/HIF-1α signaling. *International Journal of Oncology* 47, no. 6 (Dec): 2064–72.

Efferth, T. 2006. Molecular pharmacology and pharmacogenomics of artemisinin and its derivatives in cancer cells. *Current Drug Targets* 7, no. 4 (Apr): 407–21. doi: 10.2174/138945006776359412

Elliott, D.A., N. Nabavizadeh, J.L. Romer, Y. Chen, and J.M. Holland. 2016. Medical marijuana use in head and neck squamous cell carcinoma patients treated with radiotherapy. *Support Care Cancer* 24, no. 8 (Aug): 3517–24.

Elsasser-Beile, U., C. Leiber, P. Wolf, M. Lucht, U. Mengs, and U. Wetterauer. 2005. Adjuvant intravesical treatment of superficial bladder cancer with a standardized mistletoe extract. *The Journal of Urology* 174, no. 1 (Jul): 76–9. doi: 10.1097/01.ju.0000163261.08619.d0

Elyasi, S., S. Hosseini, M.R. Niazi Moghadam, S.A. Aledavood, and G. Karimi. 2016. Effect of oral silymarin administration on prevention of radiotherapy induced mucositis: A randomized, double-blinded, placebo-controlled clinical trial. *Phytotherapy Research* 30 (Nov): 1879–85. doi: 10.1002/ptr.5704

Ernst, E., K. Schmidt, and M.K. Steuer-Vogt. 2003. Mistletoe for cancer? *International Journal of Cancer* 107, no. 2 (Nov): 262–67. doi: 10.1002/ijc.11386

Erowele, G.I. and A.O. Kalejaiye. 2009. Pharmacology and therapeutic uses of cats claw. *American Journal of Health-System Pharmacy* 66, no. 11 (Jun): 992–95. doi: 10.2146/ajhp080443

Farias, I.L., M.C. Araújo, J.G. Farias et al. 2012. Uncaria tomentosa for reducing side effects caused by chemotherapy in CRC patients: Clinical trial. *Evidence Based Complementary & Alternative Medicine* 2012 (epub Aug 2011): 892182. doi: 10.1155/2012/892182

Firestone, G.L. and S.N. Sundar. 2009. Anticancer activities of artemisinin and its bioactive derivatives. *Expert Reviews in Molecular Medicine* 11, no. e32 (Oct). doi: 10.1017/S1462399409001239

Francis, M. and S. Williams. 2014. Effectiveness of indian turmeric powder with honey as complementary therapy on oral mucositis: A nursing perspective among cancer patients in Mysore. *The Nursing Journal of India* 105, no. 6 (Nov–Dec): 258–60.

Frenkel, M. and V. Sierpina. 2014. The use of dietary supplements in oncology. *Current Oncology Reports* 16, no. 11 (Nov): 411. doi: 10.1007/s11912-014-0411-3

Fu, J., Z. Wang, L. Huang et al. 2014. Review of the botanical characteristics, phytochemistry, and pharmacology of Astragalus membranaceus (Huangqi). *Phytotherapy Research* 28, no. 9: 1275–83. doi: 10.1002/ptr.5188

Gehm, B.D., J.M. McAndrews, P.-Y. Chien, and J.L. Jameson. 1997. Resveratrol, a polyphenolic compound found in grapes and wine, is an agonist for the estrogen receptor. *Proceedings of the National Academy of Sciences* 94, no. 25: 14138–4143. doi: 10.1073/pnas.94.25.14138

Green, J., A. Kalisch, and CAM-Consortium. 2015. Milk thistle (Silybum marianum). CAM-CANCER January, 2015. http://cam-cancer.org/The-Summaries/Herbal-products/Milk-thistle-Silybum-marianum/ (Accessed May 31, 2018).

Gufford, B.T., G. Chen, A.G. Vergara, P. Lazarus, N.H. Oberlies, and M.F. Paine. 2015. Milk thistle constituents inhibit raloxifene intestinal glucuronidation: A potential clinically relevant natural product-drug interaction. *Drug Metabolism and Disposition* 43, no. 9 (Sep): 1353–359. doi: 10.1124/dmd.115.065086

Guo, L., S.P. Bai, L. Zhao, and X.H. Wang. 2012. Astragalus polysaccharide injection integrated with vinorelbine and cisplatin for patients with advanced non-small cell lung cancer: Effects on quality of life and survival. *Medical Oncology* 29, no. 3 (Sep): 1656–662. doi: 10.1007/s12032-011-0068-9

Harvey, P.A. and L.A. Leinwand. 2015. Dietary phytoestrogens present in soy dramatically increase cardiotoxicity in male mice receiving a chemotherapeutic tyrosine kinase inhibitor. *Molecular and Ular Endocrinology* 399 (Jan): 330–5. doi: 10.1016/j.mce.2014.10.011

Hatcher, H., R. Planalp, J. Cho, F.M. Torti, and S.V. Torti. 2008. Curcumin: From ancient medicine to current clinical trials. *Cellular and Molecular Life Sciences* 65, no. 11 (Jun): 1631–652. doi: 10.1007/s00018-008-7452-4

He, F.J. and J.Q. Chen. 2013. Consumption of soybean, soy foods, soy isoflavones and breast cancer incidence: Differences between Chinese women and women in Western countries and possible mechanisms. *Food Science and Human Wellness* 2: 146–61. https://doi.org/10.1016/j.fshw.2013.08.002

He, H., X. Zhou, Q. Wang, and Y. Zhao. 2013. Does the couse of astragalus-containing Chinese herbal prescriptions and radiotherapy benefit to non-small-cell lung cancer treatment: A meta-analysis of randomized trials. *Evidence Based Complementary & Alternative Medicine* 2013: 426207. doi: 10.1155/2013/426207 (Accessed December 1, 2016).

Horneber, M.A., G. Bueschel, R. Huber, K. Linde, and M. Rostock. 2008. Mistletoe therapy in oncology. *Cochrane Database of Systematic Reviews* 2: CD003297. doi: 10.1002/14651858.cd003297.pub2

Howells, L.M., D.P. Berry, P.J. Elliott et al. 2011. Phase I randomized, double-blind pilot study of micronized resveratrol (SRT501) in patients with hepatic metastases—Safety, pharmacokinetics, and pharmacodynamics. *Cancer Prevention and Research* 4, no. 9 (Sep): 1419–25.

Jang, M., L. Cai, G.O. Udeani et al. 1997. Cancer chemopreventive activity of resveratrol, a natural product derived from grapes. *Science* 275, no. 5297 (Jan): 218–20.

Javed, S., K. Kohli, and M. Ali. 2011. Patented bioavailability enhancement techniques of Silymarin. *Recent Patents on Drug Delivery & Formulation* 4, no. 2 (Jun): 145–52.

Johnson, J.R., M. Burnell-Nugent, D. Lossignol, E.D. Ganae-Motan, R. Potts, and M.T. Fallon. 2010. Multicenter, double-blind, randomized, placebo-controlled, parallel-group study of the efficacy, safety, and tolerability of THC: CBD extract and THC extract in patients with intractable cancer-related pain. *J Pain Symptom Manage* 39, no. 2 (Feb): 167–79.

Johnson, J.R., D. Lossignol, M. Burnell-Nugent, and M.T. Fallon. 2013. An open-label extension study to investigate the long-term safety and tolerability of THC/CBD oromucosal spray and oromucosal THC spray in patients with terminal cancer-related pain refractory to strong opioid analgesics. *J Pain Symptom Manage* 46, no. 2 (Aug): 207–18.

Jung, M.L., S. Baudino, G. Ribéreau-Gayon, and J.P. Beck. 1990. Characterization of cytotoxic proteins from mistletoe (Viscum album L.). *Cancer Letters* 51, no. 2 (May): 103–08. doi: 10.1016/0304-3835(90)90044-x

Kaegi, E. 1998. Unconventional therapies for cancer: 1. Essiac. The Task Force on Alternative Therapies of the Canadian Breast Cancer Research Initiative. 1998. *Canadian Medcial Association Journal* 158, no. 7: 897–902.

Kawaguchi-Suzuki, M., R.F. Frye, H.-J. Zhu, B.J. Brinda, K.D. Chavin, H.J. Bernstein, and J.S. Markowitz. 2014. The effects of milk thistle (silybum marianum) on human cytochrome P450 activity. *Drug Metabolism and Disposition* 42, no. 10 (Oct): 1611–616. doi: 10.1124/dmd.114.057232

Kienle, G.S., M. Mussler, D. Fuchs, and H. Kiene. 2016. Intravenous Mistletoe treatment in integrative cancer care: A qualitative study exploring the procedures, concepts, and observations of expert doctors. *Evid Based Complement Alternat Med.* 2016: 4628287. doi: 10.1155/2016/4628287

Konmun, J., K. Danwilai, N. Ngamphaiboon, B. Sripanidkulchai, A. Sookprasert, and S. Subongkot. 2017. A phase II randomized double-blind placebo-controlled study of 6-gingerol as an anti-emetic in solid tumor patients receiving moderately to highly emetogenic chemotherapy. *Medical Oncology* 34, no. 4 (Apr). doi: 10.1007/s12032-017-0931-4

Ladas, E.J., D.J. Kroll, N.H. Oberlies, B. Cheng, D.H. Ndao, S.R. Rheingold, and K.M. Kelly. 2010. A randomized, controlled, double-blind, pilot study of milk thistle for the treatment of hepatotoxicity in childhood acutelymphoblastic leukemia (ALL). *Cancer* 116, no. 2 (Jan): 506–13. doi: 10.1002/cncr.24723

Lee, A.Y., C.C. Fan, Y.A. Chen, C.W. Cheng, Y.J. Sung, C.P. Hsu, and T.Y. Kao. 2015. Curcumin inhibits invasiveness and epithelial-mesenchymal transition in oral squamous cell carcinoma through reducing matrix metalloproteinase 2, 9 and modulating p53-E-cadherin pathway. *Integrative Cancer Therapies* 14, no. 5 (Sep): 484–90. doi: 10.1177/1534735415588930

Lee, J.J. and J.J. Lee. 2010. A phase II study of an herbal decoction that includes Astragali radix for cancer-associated anorexia in patients with advanced cancer. *Integrative Cancer Therapies* 9, no. 1 (Mar): 24–31. doi: 10.1177/1534735409359180

Lemaire, I., V. Assinewe, P. Cano, D.V. Awang, and J. Arnason. 1999. Stimulation of interleukin-1 and -6 production in alveolar macrophages by the neotropical liana, Uncaria tomentosa. *Journal of Ethnopharmacology* 64, no. 2 (Feb): 109–15. doi: 10.1016/s0378-8741(98)00113-5

Li, G., P. Rivas, R. Bedolla, D. Thapa, R.L. Reddick, R. Ghosh, and A.P. Kumar. 2013. Dietary resveratrol prevents development of high-grade prostatic intraepithelial neoplastic lesions: Involvement of SIRT1/S6 K axis. *Cancer Prevention Research* 6, no. 1 (Jan): 27–39. doi: 10.1158/1940-6207.capr-12-0349

Lichtman, A.H., E.A. Laux, R. McQuade et al. 2018. Results of a Double-Blind, Randomized, Placebo-Controlled Study of Nabiximols Oromucosal Spray as an Adjunctive Therapy in Advanced Cancer Patients with Chronic Uncontrolled Pain. *J Pain Symptom Manage* 55, no. 2 (Feb): 179–188.e1. doi: 10.1016/j.jpainsymman.2017.09.001

Lim, T.G., S.Y. Lee, Z. Huang et al. 2014. Curcumin suppresses proliferation of colon cancer cells by targeting CDK2. *Cancer and Prevention Research* 7, no. 4 (Apr): 466–74.

Lopes de Paula, L.C., F. Fonseca, F. Perazzo et al. 2015. *Uncaria tomentosa* (cat's claw) improves quality of life in patients with solid tumors. *Alternative & Complementary Medicine* 21, no. 1 (Jan): 22–30.

Mackay, D. 2016. Soy Isoflavones and other consituents. Chapter 124. In: Pizzorno JE, editor. *Textbook of Natura; Medicine*. 4th ed. St. Louis, Mo: Elsevier Health Sciences.

Mahmoud, A.M., W. Yang, and M.C. Bosland. 2014. Soy isoflavones and prostate cancer: A review of molecular mechanisms. *The Journal of Steroid Biochemisty and Molecular Biology* 140 (Mar): 116–32.

Marx, W., N. Kiss, and L. Isenring. 2015. Is ginger beneficial for nausea and vomiting? An update of the literature. *Current Opinion in Supportive and Palliative Care* 9, no. 2 (Jun): 189–95. doi: 10.1097/spc.0000000000000135

Marx, W., K. Ried, A.L. Mccarthy, L. Vitetta, A. Sali, D. Mckavanagh, and E. Isenring. 2017. Ginger – mechanism of action in chemotherapy-induced nausea and vomiting: A review. *Critical Reviews in Food Science and Nutrition* 57, no. 1: 141–46. doi: 10.1080/10408398.2013.865590

Marx, W.M., L. Teleni, A.L. McCarthy, L. Vitetta, D. McKavanagh, D. Thomson, and E. Isenring. 2013. Ginger (*Zingiber officinale*) and chemotherapy-induced nausea and vomiting: A systematic literature review. *Nutrition Reviews* 71, no. 4: 245–54. doi: 10.1111/nure.12016

McCulloch, M. 2012. *The Bottom Line on Soy and Breast Cancer Risk.* American Cancer Society. http://blogs.cancer.org/expertvoices/2012/08/02/the-bottom-line-on-soy-and-breast-cancer-risk/ (Accessed June 8, 2018).

McCulloch, M., C. See, X.J. Shu et al. 2006. Astragalus-based Chinese herbs and platinum-based chemotherapy for advanced non-small-cell lung cancer: Meta-analysis of randomized trials. *Journal of Clinicial Oncology* 24, no. 3 (Sep): 419–30.

McIntosh, H.M. and P. Olliaro. 2000. Artemisinin derivatives for treating severe malaria. *Cochrane Database of Systematic Reviews* 2: CD000527. doi: 10.1002/14651858.cd000527

Mishra, L.C., B.B. Singh, and S. Dagenais. 2000. Scientific basis for the therapeutic use of Withania somnifera (ashwagandha): A review. *Alternative Medicine Review* 5, no. 4: 334–46.

Moore, K.A., J.A. Simpson, M.K. Paw et al. 2016. Safety of artemisinins in first trimester of prospectively followed pregnancies: An observational study. *The Lancet Infectious Diseases* 16, no. 5 (May): 576–83.

Mueller, M.S., N. Runyambo, I. Wagner, S. Borrmann, K. Dietz, and L. Heide. 2004. Randomized controlled trial of a traditional preparation of Artemisia annua L. (Annual Wormwood) in the treatment of malaria. *Transactions of the Royal Society of Tropical Medicine and Hygiene* 98, no. 5 (May): 318–21.

Mücke, M., M. Weier, C. Carter et al. 2018. Systematic review and meta-analysis of cannabinoids in palliative medicine. *Journal of Cachexia, Sarcopenia and Muscle* 9: 220–34.

National Cancer Institute (NCI). Essiac/Flor Essence (PDQ®) – Health Professional Version. NIH. National Cancer Institute. https://www.cancer.gov/about-cancer/treatment/cam/hp/essiac-pdq#section/all (Accessed April, 11, 2016).

National Comprehensive Cancer Network (NCCN). Antiemesis (Version 3.2018). https://www.nccn.org/professionals/physician_gls/pdf/antiemesis.pdf (Accessed June 14, 2018).

Natural Medicines Comprehensive Database. 2016. www.naturaldatabase.com

Nazaruk, J. and P. Orlikowski. 2016. Phytochemical profile and therapeutic potential of *Viscum album* L. *Natural Product Research* 30, no. 4: 373–85. doi: 10.1080/14786419.2015.1022776

Ostermann, T., C. Raak, and A. Bussing. 2010. Survival of cancer patients treated with mistletoe extract (Iscador): A systematic literature review. *BMC Cancer* 9, no. 451 (Dec). doi: 10.1186/1471-2407-9-451

Pace-Asciak, C.R., S. Hahn, E.P. Diamandis, G. Soleas, and D.M. Goldberg. 1995. The red wine phenolics trans-resveratrol and quercetin block human platelet aggregation and eicosanoid synthesis: Implications for protection against coronary heart disease. *Clinica Chimica Acta* 235, no. 2: 207–19. doi: 10.1016/0009-8981(95)06045-1

Palliyaguru, D.L., S.V. Singh, and T.W. Kensler. 2016. Withania somnifera: From prevention to treatment of cancer. *Molecular Nutrition & Food Research* 60, no. 6: 1342–353. doi: 10.1002/mnfr.201500756

Panahi, Y., A. Saadat, F. Beiraghdar, and A. Sahebkar. 2014. Adjuvant therapy with bioavailability-boosted curcuminoids suppresses systemic inflammation and improves quality of life in patients with solid tumors: A randomized double-blind placebo-controlled trial. *Phytotherapy Research* 28, no. 10 (Oct): 1461–7. doi: 10.1002/ptr.5149

Panossian, L.A., N.I. Garga, and D. Pelletier. 2005. Toxic brainstem encephalopathy after artemisinin treatment for breast cancer. *Annals of Neurology* 58, no. 5 (Nov): 812–13. doi: 10.1002/ana.20620

Pao, L.H., O.Y. Hu, H.Y. Fan, C.C. Lin, L.C. Liu, and P.W. Huang. 2012. Herb-drug interaction of 50 Chinese herbal medicines on CYP3A4 activity *in vitro* and *in vivo*. *The American Journal of Chinese Medicine* 0, no. 01: 57–73. doi: 10.1142/s0192415×1250005x

PDQ® Integrative, Alternative, and Complementary Therapies Editorial Board. PDQ Milk Thistle. Bethesda, MD: National Cancer Institute. Updated June 19, 2017. https://www.cancer.gov/about-cancer/treatment/cam/hp/milk-thistle-pdq (Accessed September 1, 2017). [PMID: 26389223].

PDQ® Integrative, Alternative, and Complementary Therapies Editorial Board. PDQ Mistletoe Extracts. Bethesda, MD: National Cancer Institute. Updated November 6, 2017. https://www.cancer.gov/about-cancer/treatment/cam/hp/mistletoe-pdq (Accessed June 7, 2018).

Pergam, S.A., M.C. Woodfield, C.M. Lee, G.S. Cheng, K.K. Baker, S.R. Marquis, and J.R. Fann. 2017. Cannabis use among patients at a comprehensive cancer center in a state with legalized medicinal and recreational use. *Cancer* 123, no. 22 (Nov): 4488–97. doi: 10.1002/cncr.30879

Pillai, A.K., K.K. Sharma, Y.K. Gupta, and S. Bakhshi. 2011. Anti-emetic effect of ginger powder versus placebo as an add-on therapy in children and young adults receiving high emetogenic chemotherapy. *Pediatric Blood & Cancer* 56, no. 2 (Feb): 234–38. doi: 10.1002/pbc.22778

Ramakrishnan, R. 2013. Anticancer properties of Zingiber officinales – ginger: Review. *International Journal of Medical Research and Pharmaceutical Sciences*: 11–20.

Ruocco, K.M., E.I. Goncharova, M.R. Young et al. 2007. A high-throughput cell-based assay to identify specific inhibitors of transcription factor AP-1. *J Biomol Screen* 12, no. 1 (Feb): 133–39. doi: 10.1177/1087057106296686

Ryan, J.L., C.E. Heckler, M. Ling, A. Katz, J.P. Williams, A.P. Pentland, and G.R. Morrow. 2013. Curcumin for radiation dermatitis: A randomized, double-blind, placebo-controlled clinical trial of thirty breast cancer patients. *Radiation Research* 180, no. 1: 34–43. doi: 10.1667/RR3255.1

Ryan Wolf, J., C.E. Heckler, J.J. Guido et al. 2018. Oral curcumin for radiation dermatitis: A URCC NCORP study of 686 breast cancer patients. *Supportive Care in Cancer*. 26, no. 5 (May): 1543–52. doi: 10.1007/s00520-017-3957-4

Sanaati, F., S. Najafi, Z. Kashaninia, and M. Sadeghi. 2016. Effect of ginger and chamomile on nausea and vomiting caused by chemotherapy in Iranian women with breast cancer. *Asian Pacific Journal of Cancer Prevention* 17, no. 8: 4125–9.

Santos Araújo Mdo, C., I.L. Farias, J. Gutierres et al. 2012. d: Clinical trial. *Evidence Based Complementary & Alternative Medicine* 2012: 676984.

Savai, J., A. Varghese, N. Pandita, and M. Chintamaneni. 2015. Investigation of CYP3A4 and CYP2D6 interactions of Withania somnifera and Centella asiatica in human liver microsomes. *Phytotherapy Research* 29, no. 5: 785–90. doi: 10.1002/ptr.5308

Schöffski, P., I. Breidenbach, J. Krauter et al. 2005. Weekly 24 h infusion of aviscumine (rViscumin): A phase I study in patients with solid tumours. *European Journal of Cancer* 41, no. 10 (Jul): 1431–438. doi: 10.1016/j.ejca.2005.03.019

Scontre, V.A., J.C. Martins, C. Vaz De Melo Sette, H. Mutti, D. Cubero, F. Fonseca, and A. Del Giglio. 2017. Curcuma longa (Turmeric) for prevention of capecitabine-induced hand-foot syndrome: A pilot study. *Journal of Dietary Supplements* 2 (Nov): 1–7. doi: 10.1080/19390211.2017.1366387

Shagar, S.M. and C.M. Garchinski. 2014. Alternative therapies as primary treatments for cancer. Chapter 26. In: Abrams, D.I., and A.T. Weil, editors. *Integrative Oncology*. 2nd ed. New York: Oxford Press, p. 735.

Shahbazi, F., S. Sadighi, S. Dashti-Khavidaki, F. Shahi, M. Mirzania, A. Abdollahi, and M.-H. Ghahremani. 2015. Effect of silymarin administration on cisplatin nephrotoxicity: Report from a pilot, randomized, double-blinded, placebo-controlled clinical trial. *Phytotherapy Research* 29, no. 7: 1046–053. doi: 10.1002/ptr.5345

Shankar, S., S. Ganapathy, Q. Chen, and R.K. Srivastava. 2008. Curcumin sensitizes TRAIL-resistant xenografts: Molecular mechanisms of apoptosis, metastasis and angiogenesis. *Molecular Cancer* 29, no. 7 (Jan): 16. doi: 10.1186/1476-4598-7-16

Siegel, A.B., R. Narayan, R. Rodriguez et al. 2014. A phase I dose-finding study of silybin phosphatidylcholine (milk thistle) in patients with advanced hepatocellular carcinoma. *Integrative Cancer Therapies* 13, no. 1 (Jan): 46–53.

Siwak, D.R., S. Shishodia, B.B. Aggarwal, and R. Kurzrock. 2005. Curcumin-induced antiproliferative and proapoptotic effects in melanoma cells are associated with suppression of IkappaB kinase and nuclear factor kappaB activity and are independent of the B-Raf/mitogen-activated/extracellular signal-regulated protein kinase pathway and the Akt pathway. *Cancer* 104, no. 4 (Aug): 879–90. doi: 10.1002/cncr.21216

Smith, L.A., F. Azariah, V.T. Lavender, N.S. Stoner, and S. Bettiol. 2015. Cannabinoids for nausea and vomiting in adults with cancer receiving chemotherapy. *Cochrane Database Syst Rev* 12, no. 11 (Nov): CD009464. doi: 10.1002/14651858.CD009464.pub2

Starok, M., P. Preira, M. Vayssade, K. Haupt, L. Salomé, and C. Rossi. 2015. EGFR Inhibition by curcumin in cancer cells: A dual mode of action. *Biomacromolecules* 16, no. 5 (May): 1634–42.

Stirpe, F. 1983. Mistletoe Toxicity. *The Lancet* 321, no. 8319 (Feb): 295. doi: 10.1016/s0140-6736(83)91706-3

Strasser, F., D. Luftner, K. Possinger et al. 2006. Comparison of orally administered cannabis extract and delta-9-tetrahydrocannabinol in treating patients with cancer-related anorexia-cachexia syndrome: A multicenter, phase III, randomized, double-blind, placebo-controlled clinical trial from the cannabis-in-cachexia-study-group. *Journal of Clinical Oncology* 24: 3394–400.

Surh, Y.J., Y.J. Hurh, J.Y. Kang, E. Lee, G. Kong, and S.J. Lee. 1999. Resveratrol, an antioxidant present in red wine, induces apoptosis in human promyelocytic leukemia (HL-60) cells. *Cancer Letters* 140, no. 1–2 (Jun): 1–10.

Tamayo, C. and S. Diamond. 2007. Review of clinical trials evaluating safety and efficacy of milk thistle (Silybum marianum [L.] Gaertn.). *Integrative Cancer Therapies* 6, no. 2: 146–57. doi: 10.1177/1534735407301942

Tang, F.Y., S. Yu-Ching, N.C. Chen, H.S. Hsieh, and K.S. Chen. 2008. Resveratrol inhibits migration and invasion of human breast-cancer cells. *Molecular Nutrition & Food Research* 52, no. 6 (Jun): 683–91. doi: 10.1002/mnfr.200700325

Thamlikitkul, L., V. Srimuninnimit, C. Akewanlop et al. 2017. Efficacy of ginger for prophylaxis of chemotherapy-induced nausea and vomiting in breast cancer patients receiving adriamycin-cyclophosphamide regimen: A randomized, double-blind, placebo-controlled, crossover study. *Supportive Care in Cancer* 25, no. 2 (Feb): 459–64. doi: 10.1007/s00520-016-3423-8

Timmers, S., J. Auwerx, and P. Schrauwen. 2012. The journey of resveratrol from yeast to human. *Aging* 4, no. 3 (Mar): 146–58. doi: 10.18632/aging.100445

Tringale, K.R., Y. Shi, and J.A. Hattangadi. 2017. Marijuana utilization in cancer patients: A comprehensive analysis of National Health and Nutrition Examination Survey Data from 2005 to 2014. *International J Radiation Oncol* 99, no. 2 suppl. (Oct.): S11. doi: 10.1016/j.ijrobp.2017.06.042

Ulbricht, C., W. Weissner, S. Hashmi et al. 2009. Essiac: Systematic review by the natural standard research collaboration. *Journal of the Society of Integrative Oncology* 7, no. 2 (Spring): 73–80.

Van Erk, M.J., E. Teuling, Y.C. Staal, S. Huybers, P.J. Van Bladeren, J.C. Aarts, and B. Van Ommen. 2004. Time- and dose-dependent effects of curcumin on gene expression in human colon cancer cells. *Journal of Carcinogenesis* 3, no. 1 (May): 8. doi: 10.1186/1477-3163-3-8

Van Patten, C.L., I.A. Olivotto, G.K. Chambers, K.A. Gelmon, T.G. Hislop, E. Templeton, A. Wattie, and J.C. Prior. 2002. Effect of soy phytoestrogens on hot flashes in postmenopausal women with breast cancer: A randomized, controlled clinical trial. *Journal of Clinical Oncology* 15, no. 6: 1449–55.

Wang, T.T., T.S. Hudson, T.C. Wang et al. 2008. Differential effects of resveratrol on androgen-responsive LNCaP human prostate cancer cells *in vitro* and *in vivo*. *Carcinogenesis* 29, no. 10 (Oct): 2001–10.

Woo, M.S., S.H. Jung, S.Y. Kim, J.W. Hyun, K.H. Ko, W.K. Kim, and H.S. Kim. 2005. Curcumin suppresses phorbol ester-induced matrix metalloproteinase-9 expression by inhibiting the PKC to MAPK signaling pathways in human astroglioma cells. *Biochemical and Biophysical Research Communications* 335, no. 4 (Oct): 1017–025. doi: 10.1016/j.bbrc.2005.07.174

World Health Organization (WHO). 2006. *Monograph on Good Agricultural and Collection Practices (GACP) for Artemisia annua L.* Geneva, Switzerland: World Health Organization Press.

World Health Organization (WHO). 2007. *Corex Uncariae. Monographs on Selected Medicinal Plants.* Vol. 3. Geneva, Switzerland: World Health Organization. http://apps.who.int/medicinedocs/documents/s14213e/s14213e.pdf#page=357 (Accessed March 20, 2007).

Wu, P., J.J. Dugoua, O. Eyawo, and E.J. Mills. 2009. Traditional Chinese medicines in the treatment of hepatocellular cancers: A systematic review and meta-analysis. *Journal of Experimental & Clinical Cancer Research* 12, no. 28 (Aug): 112. doi: 10.1186/1756-9966-28-112

Zhang, C.A., S.X. Wang, Y. Zhang, J.P. Chen, and X.M. Liang. 2005. In vitro estrogenic activities of Chinese medicinal plants traditionally used for the management of menopausal symptoms. *Journal of Ethnopharmacology* 98, no. 3: 295–300. doi: 10.1016/j.jep.2005.01.033

Zhang, C.Z., Y. Feng, S. Qu et al. 2011. Resveratrol attenuates doxorubicin-induced cardiomyocyte apoptosis in mice through SIRT1-mediated deacetylation of p53. *Cardiovascular Research* 90, no. 3 (Jun): 538–45.

Zick, S.M., A. Sen, Y. Feng, J. Green, S. Olatunde, and H. Boon. 2006. Trial of essiac to ascertain its effect in women with breast cancer (TEA-BC). *Journal of Alternative & Complementary Medicine* 12, no. 10: 971–80.

Zong, H., F. Wang, Q.X. Fan, and L.X. Wang. 2011. Curcumin inhibits metastatic progression of breast cancer cell through suppression of urokinase-type plasminogen activator by NF-kappa B signaling pathways. *Molecular Biology Reports* 39, no. 4 (Apr): 4803–808. doi: 10.1007/s11033-011-1273-5

18

The Therapeutic Potential of Cannabis and the Endocannabinoid System

Linda E. Klumpers and Arno Hazekamp

CONTENTS

18.1 History

18.1.1 Origin of Cannabis as Medicine

Cannabis is one of the oldest medicinal plants known to mankind. It is described in almost every ancient handbook on plant medicine, most commonly in the form of a tincture or a tea (Fankhauser 2002; Zuardi 2006). Cannabis most likely originated from Central Asia, as archeological evidence indicates it was cultivated in China and India for food, medicine, and fiber as early as 2700 BCE (Russo 2005; Russo 2007; Russo et al. 2008). Also in ancient Egyptian mummies, clues have been found for the use of cannabis as food or medicine (Balabanova et al. 1992). Cannabis was used for funerary traditions by the Scythians and for medicinal applications by the ancient Greeks (Brunner 1977; Mechoulam 1986). Some religions were closely related with the properties of the cannabis plant. For example, in Hindu legend cannabis (bhang) is believed to be the favorite food of the god Shiva, because of its energizing properties (Chopra and Chopra 1957).

As cannabis spread from Asia toward the West, almost every culture came into contact with this plant. Nowadays, cannabis can be found in all temperate and tropical zones, except in humid, tropical rainforests (Conert et al. 1992). As a fiber plant, cannabis produces some of the best and most durable fibers of natural origin. For centuries these fibers were used to produce sails for sea-ships, paper, banknotes, and even the first Levi's jeans. The oil that can be pressed from the hempseed is nutritious and considered an alternative to fish oil as a source of omega-3 type fatty acids (Oomah et al. 2002).

Even though cannabis was grown for fiber on a large scale in most countries, its abuse as a narcotic remained uncommon in the Western world until relatively recently. People were largely unaware of the psychoactive properties of cannabis and it is unlikely that early cultivars, selected mainly for their fiber qualities, contained significant amounts of the psychoactive compound, delta-9-tetrahydrocannabinol (THC). The medicinal use of cannabis was first introduced in Europe around 1840 by an Irish physician, William O'Shaughnessy, who served for the East India Trading Company in India, where the use of cannabis was widespread (Erkelens and Hazekamp 2014). Compared to the European fiber cannabis, these Indian varieties contained a higher amount of bioactive cannabinoids. In the following decades, the use of cannabis grew in popularity throughout Europe and the United States. At the top of its popularity, dozens of medicinal preparations, including extracts ("drops"), wine hemp and juice of the seeds, were available with cannabis as active ingredient, which were recommended for indications as diverse as menstrual cramps, asthma, insomnia, support of birth labor, migraine, throat infection, and withdrawal from opium use (Grotenhermen and Russo 2002).

However, difficulties with the supply from overseas and varying quality of the plant material made it difficult to prepare a reliable formulation of cannabis. Because no tools yet existed for quality control, it was impossible to prepare a standardized medicine. Moreover, cannabis extract was not water-soluble and could not be injected, whereas oral administration was found to be unreliable because of its slow and erratic absorption. Because of such limitations, the medicinal use of cannabis increasingly disappeared from all Western pharmacopoeias after 1937 (Grotenhermen and Russo 2002). Purified opiates derived from the Opium poppy assumed the role of cannabis.

18.1.2 The Single Convention

In the 1960s, the smoking of cannabis as a recreational drug became a widely-known phenomenon in the Western world, as part of the hippie culture. From then on, the importation of stronger varieties from the tropics, combined with a growing interest in breeding techniques, led to a steady increase in psychoactive potency (Cascini et al. 2012). As early as 1954, the World Health Organization (WHO) began to claim that cannabis and its preparations no longer served any useful medical purpose and were therefore essentially obsolete. This decision was made due to pressure by the newly created U.S. Federal Bureau of Narcotics (later to become the Drug Enforcement Administration) that insisted that cannabis use was a danger to society. Up to that moment, cannabis legislation had been based on a large number of international conventions, causing considerable legal confusion. It was therefore proposed to combine all legislation into a single international convention, the draft of which was accepted by the United Nations in 1961. Under this "Single Convention on Narcotic Drugs," cannabis and its products were defined as "dangerous narcotics with a high potential for abuse and no accepted medicinal value." In following years, several complementary treaties were made to strengthen the convention. These laws would become an important basis for the international "War on Drugs" (Bewley-Taylor and Jelsma 2012).

18.2 The Cannabis Plant

18.2.1 Botanical Description

Cannabis is an annual, usually dioecious (female and male flowers develop on separate plants), more rarely monoecious, wind-pollinated botanical. It can reach more than 5 m (16 feet) in height in a 4–6 months growing season outdoors. It propagates from seed, grows vigorously in brightly lit environments with well drained soils, and has an abundant need for nutrients and water (chapter 4 of Pertwee 2014). In modern breeding and cultivation of recreational cannabis, the preferred way to propagate is by cloning, using cuttings of a so-called "mother plant." Contemporary cannabis has increasingly become a high-tech crop, grown indoors under completely artificial conditions (Elsohly et al. 2016).

Shorter days induce the plant to start flowering (Clarke 1981). The female plant then produces several crowded clusters of individual flowers (flowertops); a large one at the top of the stem and many smaller ones on each branch. The female flowers are the source of a variety of chemical constituents, including *cannabinoids* and *terpenes* which are discussed later in this chapter. Upon fertilization of the flowers, the plant shifts its metabolic energy towards the production of seeds, and away from the biosynthesis of cannabinoids and terpenes. For that reason, male plants are usually removed from indoor growing operations ("sinsemilla" type of cultivation) (Pertwee 2014, chapter 4).

18.2.2 Classification

According to current scientific consensus, cannabis is monotypic and consists of a single species *Cannabis sativa* L. (Erkelens and Hazekamp 2014). Its closest relative in the plant world is Hops (*Humulus lupulus* L.), both species together making up the family of the *Cannabaceae*. Over time, people worldwide have selectively grown cannabis for certain desired characteristics including narcotic effect, plant size, flower yield, smell and taste, etc. As a result of centuries of breeding and selection, a wide range of cannabis varieties have been developed. Over 700 varieties have been described and many more are thought to exist. This has led to extensive discussion on further botanical and chemotaxonomic subclassification (Hazekamp and Fischedick 2012; Erkelens and Hazekamp 2014; Hazekamp et al. 2016).

For forensic and legal purposes, the most important subclassification is that of the "drug type" (marijuana) versus the "fiber type" (hemp), with an emphasis on the total THC content of the plant. In most parts of the world, hemp varieties are not allowed to contain more than about 0.3% by weight of THC in the dried flower tops of the plant (Industrial Hemp Farmers Act of 2015, S. 134).

Until recently, cannabis products used for medicinal purposes in official programs all belonged to the drug type, because of their high content of delta-9-tetrahydrocannabinol-acid (THCA) that is transformed to the biologically more active THC by heat. However, increasingly cannabis medication is offered based on cannabidiol (CBD)-rich extracts from hemp type cannabis that contains cannabidiolic acid (CBDA). The constituents THC, THCA, CBD, and CBDA belong to a group of chemical structures called cannabinoids, discussed in more detail later in this chapter.

18.2.3 Sativa and Indica

Another commonly used subclassification, based more on phenotypic traits, distinguishes *sativa* from *indica* types of cannabis, both regarded as a subspecies of *Cannabis sativa* L. (Erkelens and Hazekamp 2014). According to the botanical description of cannabis, sativa types were originally grown in the Western world on an industrial scale for fiber, seed oil, and animal feedstuff. They are phenotypically characterized by tall growth with few widely-spaced branches and long, thin leaves. In contrast, plants of the indica type originated in South Asia and were known historically as Indian hemp. They are characterized by shorter bushy plants and broader leaves, typically maturing relatively fast. Most cannabis plants that are currently used as drug or medicine are a hybrid (cross-breed) of sativa and indica ancestors. By some researchers, cannabis-type *ruderalis* is also recognized as a separate subspecies. It is a smaller and "weedy" plant originally from Central Russia (Erkelens and Hazekamp 2014).

Besides the botanical distinction between sativa and indica types of cannabis, a parallel vernacular system of classifying cannabis varieties has developed among experienced (recreational) growers and users of cannabis. Users often talk about "strains" instead of using the botanically more proper term "varieties." This vernacular distinction between *sativa* and *indica* strains is an important guide for recreational users and patients alike, and is mainly based on the physical effects the strains cause. Sativa strains are typically characterized as uplifting and energetic. The effects are mostly cerebral ("head-high"), also described as spacey or hallucinogenic. This type gives a feeling of optimism and well-being. In contrast, indica strains are primarily described as calming and grounding ("body-high"). This type is said to cause relaxation, stress relief, and an overall sense of serenity (Pearce et al. 2014).

It is currently unclear to what extent the *botanical* and the *vernacular* use of the terms sativa and indica are overlapping (McPartland and Guy 2015; Hazekamp et al. 2016; Piomelli and Russo 2016). Sativa and indica strains tend to have a different smell, which may reflect a different terpene profile. Indeed, a recent study identified terpenes, and not cannabinoids, to explain the major chemical differences between the two types. The study suggested that hydroxylated terpenes in the cannabis plant, including linalool, guaiol, eudesmol, and alpha-terpineol, could be considered as markers for indica strains of cannabis (Hazekamp et al. 2016).

18.2.4 Cannabinoids and Terpenes

Cannabis plants contain glandular hairs, also called trichomes, which are particularly concentrated around the female inflorescence (flowers). These trichomes excrete a sticky resin that accumulates in little droplets at the tip of each hair (Potter 2014). The resin contains the compounds that are considered pharmacologically most valuable, particularly cannabinoids and terpenes.

Cannabinoids are considered to be the main biologically active constituents of the cannabis plant, and they are found, with few exceptions (Gertsch et al. 2010) nowhere else in nature. The naturally occurring cannabinoids form a complex group of closely related terpeno-phenolic compounds of which currently about 100 are known (Elsohly and Slade 2005; Andre et al. 2016). The most well-known cannabinoids are THC and CBD. THC is the pharmacologically and toxicologically most relevant constituent of the cannabis plant, producing a myriad of effects in animals and humans. Through activation of the CB_1 receptor, higher doses of THC may cause a feeling of intoxication known as being "high." Additional cannabinoids are also making their appearance in new products, despite the fact almost nothing is known about the pharmacology and toxicology of these compounds (Uchiyama et al. 2010; Kim and Monte 2016). The biological activities of the most important cannabinoids are described under Section 18.5.

Terpenes are volatile compounds that commonly occur in many plant species and these molecules have been of great interest to various industries (food, perfume, cosmetics, and aromatherapy) mainly due to their pleasant odors (Bohlmann and Keeling 2008). To date more than 120 different terpenes have been identified in cannabis, mainly of the mono- and sesquiterpene type. Most notably, terpenes are responsible for the distinct smell of specific cannabis varieties (Hazekamp et al. 2016). However, these compounds also display a wide range of biological activities and hence may play a role in some of the pharmacological effects of various cannabis preparations. Some of the terpenes may work in tandem with the cannabinoids to enhance or modify the biological activities of these compounds in a synergistic manner, such as enhancement of cannabinoid uptake in the intestines, lungs, or skin and influencing receptor binding or metabolism (for reviews, see McPartland and Pruitt 1999; Russo 2011). Individual terpenes have also been shown to produce their own pharmacological effects (Maffei et al. 2011).

An obvious question is whether the wide range of cannabis varieties reflect an actual difference in medicinal properties. And if so, what cannabinoids and/or terpenes are responsible for the major differences in claimed therapeutic effects between varieties. With a better understanding of cannabis constituents, it may be possible to move away from the current system of cannabis classification, dominated by sativa/indica and hemp/marijuana labeling, toward a more comprehensive classification based on a well-defined and reproducible chemical profile or phenotype.

18.3 Cannabis Products and Administration Forms

18.3.1 Extraction Techniques and Products

To experience the therapeutic or the intoxicating effects of cannabis, the botanical material can be consumed directly, or the compounds of interest can be separated from the plant. Traditionally, the dried flowers and/or larger leaves of female cannabis plants are usually smoked or ingested without modification (Russo 2007). Nowadays, cannabis is available to consumers in various forms, ranging from the manicured dried flowers (also known as *buds* or *flos*) to more refined products such as *hash*, *kief* or extracts. The extraction process reduces the consumption of excess herbal material by increasing the concentration of the biologically active components. Several techniques that are commonly applied for this separation are discussed below, and listed in Table 18.1.

18.3.1.1 Dry Processing

Dry processing methods typically refers to rubbing cannabis plant matter over a fine mesh screen, thereby capturing the trichomes that fall through. This yields a concentrate of trichomes called *kief* or *dry sift* (Clarke and Frank 2012). A modification of this process uses liquid nitrogen or dry ice, to freeze the trichomes to make them more brittle (*dry-ice kief*). In contrast, *finger hashish* is prepared by rubbing the plant between the fingers, thereby creating a sticky ball of resin. Variations of this method use other materials to collect the sticky resin known as *hashish* or *hash*. Dry-processed oils called *rosin* are obtained by putting buds under high pressure in order to squeeze out the resin. Rosin can also be

TABLE 18.1

Overview of Production Techniques, Products and Their Most Common Administration Forms

Production Method	Product	Main Administration Forms
Dried, herbal material	Flower, bud, flos	Intrapulmonary (vaping, smoking), oral (eating, tea)
Dry processes	Kief or dry sift	Intrapulmonary (vaping, dabbing, smoking)
Dry processes	Dry-ice kief	Intrapulmonary (vaping, smoking)
Dry processes	Finger hash	Intrapulmonary (vaping, smoking)
Dry processes (can also be made from ice water extracted material)	Rosin	Intrapulmonary (dabbing)
Ice water extraction	Bubble hash	Intrapulmonary (vaping, dabbing, smoking)
Solvent-based processes	Butane honey oil or butane hash oil (BHO)	Intrapulmonary (vaping, dabbing), oral
Solvent-based processes	Organic solvent extract	Intrapulmonary (vaping, dabbing), oral
Solvent-based processes	CO_2 oil	Intrapulmonary (vaping, dabbing), oral

Note: Smoking: smoking cannabis products by burning; vaping: vaporizing cannabis products, which does not require burning; dabbing: a type of vaporization that is typically done with high-THC concentration products at higher temperatures than conventional vaporization.

produced by putting extracts that are obtained from other processing techniques under high pressure, thereby separating the oils from the waxes.

18.3.1.2 Water-Based Processing

Ice cold conditions make the trichomes more brittle, thereby making it easier to separate them from plant matter. *Ice water hash* or *bubble hash* is made by using ice cold water to break off the trichomes (Clarke and Frank 2012). Cannabinoids and terpenes are virtually insoluble in water, so the trichomes will not dissolve during this procedure (Thomas et al. 1990).

18.3.1.3 Solvent-Based Extraction

Solvent-based concentrates are made by macerating cannabis plant material in non-polar organic solvents that allow for the lipophilic cannabinoids to dissolve. Commonly used solvents include acetone, ethanol, hexane, isopropanol, and naphtha. After the cannabis material is soaked in, or rinsed with, the solvent, the latter is removed by boiling, by applying a vacuum and by other methods. If the concentrates are not further processed, this method creates a viscous dark-colored oil, which may still contain significant amounts of residual solvents (Romano and Hazekamp 2013). Because of their high volatility, terpenes are generally not well captured using solvent-based methods (Romano and Hazekamp 2013). Supercritical CO_2 or butane, where a fluid state of the gas is held at its critical temperature and pressure, can also be used as a solvent for cannabinoids and terpenes (Raber et al. 2015). For supercritical extraction, however, specialized equipment set-ups are needed.

18.3.1.4 Other Products

Additional products may be derived from the extraction techniques above by further processing the extracts. These products include for example *shatter*, *budder* and *wax*.

18.3.2 Methods of Intake

Cannabis products can be consumed in various ways. Smoking cannabis, with or without tobacco, is the most common method of intake. Table 18.2 presents an overview of the methods most commonly tried by medicinal users of cannabis. It should be noted that for some methods of administration extensive scientific data is available (e.g., smoking, sublingual), while others have hardly been studied at all (raw juicing, edibles).

18.3.3 Decarboxylation

Depending on the method of intake used, various changes to the original chemical profile of the plant material may occur. For instance, a common factor of most administration forms is a heating step, which is essential for a chemical conversion known as *decarboxylation*. THC and CBD are the two most well-known cannabinoids, but contrary to popular belief they are not actually present in fresh cannabis plants: metabolically, the plant produces all its cannabinoids in a carboxylic acid form known as cannabinoid-acids. When sufficient heat is applied, for example when cannabis is burned for smoking, baked for edibles, or boiled for tea, THC-acid (or THCA) quickly converts into THC, CBD-acid (or CBDA) turns into CBD, and so on for all other cannabinoids (Veress et al. 1990; Wang et al. 2016). The carboxylic acid group is thereby released in the form of carbon dioxide. It should be noted that cannabinoid-acids may have important medical properties of their own. For example, CBD-acid has promising anti-inflammatory effects (Takeda et al. 2008), while THC-acid was found to have a potent effect on the human immune system (Verhoeckx et al. 2006; Burstein 2014).

Although heat is needed for decarboxylation, overheating may lead to the formation of degradation products such as cannabinol (CBN; an oxidation product of THC) and delta-8-THC (Δ^8-THC; an isomer of THC), both of which have potential pharmacological properties of their own (for a review

TABLE 18.2

Common Administration Forms of Cannabis and Their Pharmacological Characteristics

Administration Forms	Different Administration Methods	Pharmacology		
		Onset	Peak Effect	Duration
Intrapulmonary	Smoking of herbal cannabis with the use of for example cigarette-paper (smoking) Inhalation of herbal cannabis or extract with the use of a special vaporizing device (vaping) Inhalation of THC-rich oil with the use of a dab rig (dabbing)	Instantly or within about 5 minutes (Ohlsson et al. 1980, Huestis et al. 1992, for review see Grotenhermen 2003b)	20–30 minutes (Ohlsson et al. 1980, for review see Grotenhermen 2004)	Around 3-4 hours (Ohlsson et al. 1980, for review see Grotenhermen 2004 or Grotenhermen 2003b)
Sublingual or oromucosal	Sublingual (under the tongue) administration, for example with tinctures or sprays Note that the most pharmacological studies on oromucosal administration have been done with Sativex, a spray containing THC and CBD	30–45 minutes, moderate psychiatric effects (Karschner et al. 2011)	Between 3 and 4 hours post dose for THC:CBD (Karschner et al. 2011)	2.5 h (Klumpers et al. 2012) to 10.5 h (Karschner et al. 2011) in healthy volunteers, and about 4 h in patients (Tomida et al. 2006)
Oral	Preparing tea or cookies containing herbal cannabis or extract (eating/drinking) Ingesting concentrated extracts (cannabis oil) Ingesting unheated herbal cannabis as a vegetable, or by juicing it (raw juicing) Note that several edibles, except for capsules or tables that do not disintegrate in the mouth, can have partial oromucosal absorption when taken orally.	15 min (Klumpers et al. 2012) to 30 min (Karschner et al. 2011) but can start as late as 2.5 h (Karschner et al. 2011, for review, see Grotenhermen 2004), depending on the oral formulation and the effect measured	1–3 hours for THC (Klumpers et al. 2012, for review, see Grotenhermen 2004); as well as 4.5 h (Karschner et al. 2011) have been reported	4-8 hours (Klumpers et al. 2012, for review see Grotenhermen 2004), whereas effects can last for 10.5 h (Karschner et al. 2011)

of *in vitro* pharmacological properties, see Chapter 6 of Pertwee 2014). Volatile components such as the terpenes may easily evaporate, for example during the boiling of tea, or while evaporating an organic solvent during the preparation of a concentrated extract (Hazekamp et al. 2007; Romano and Hazekamp 2013).

18.3.4 Pharmacological Implications of Administration Forms

As a result of the chemical conversions listed above, each administration form will essentially deliver a different subset of active constituents to the user. Moreover, each cannabis preparation comes with its own efficiency of uptake (e.g., intestines, lungs, oral mucosa) and its own set of specific metabolites formed upon consumption, as described under Section 18.5. Particularly the difference between oral (ingested) and intrapulmonary (inhaled) preparations is of importance here. The main reason is that inhaled cannabinoids and terpenes enter directly and virtually unaltered through the lungs into the bloodstream, whereas orally ingested compounds are significantly delayed and altered by the digestive system before it reaches the systemic circulation, also called first pass effect (Grotenhermen 2003a,b). The combination of these factors may result in a different type and duration of effects for various administration forms, even when the same type and dose of cannabis are used. In general, inhaling cannabinoids leads to higher cannabinoid plasma levels, more rapid onset of effect, and shorter total duration of effect compared to ingesting cannabinoids.

18.4 Analytical Aspects

18.4.1 Quality Control

A clearly defined composition is an essential requirement for medicines, because it prevents unexpected surprises regarding its effects, potency or purity. For a botanical medicine, such as cannabis, this starts with tightly controlling and monitoring the conditions under which the plants are cultivated. Besides obvious differences in plant shape and appearance of different varieties, cannabis plants may differ by their specific content of cannabinoids and terpenes. The synergistic combination of these active components present in a cannabis product defines its ultimate medical effect (McPartland and Russo 2014). This means that relatively small changes in cannabis composition may have significant effects on the medical properties of cannabis.

In general, two sets of tests are applied to determine the quality of cannabis. One set is performed to verify that products have the proper chemical composition of desired constituents including cannabinoids, terpenes, and moisture content. Another set of tests is applied to ensure that unwanted elements are absent, such as adulterants, microbes, heavy metals, or pesticides. Cannabis can be called *standardized*, and therefore acceptable for pharmaceutical use, when produced batches are consistently shown to be of the same high quality over a longer period of time. The cannabinoid composition is the most important aspect to measure for therapeutically used cannabis. When referring to cannabis as a medicine, as opposed to a narcotic drug, THC is usually not considered the sole active component. There is mounting scientific evidence that CBD, and lesser-known cannabinoids such as tetrahydrocannabivarin (THCV), cannabigerol (CBG) or cannabichromene (CBC) or their acids may play a role as well (chapter 6 of Pertwee 2014). Also, interest is growing in the pharmacological activity of terpenes and their interaction with cannabinoids. Although currently no official pharmaceutical monograph exists for medicinal cannabis, general requirements can be learned from the World Health Organization (WHO 2011) and European Pharmacopoeia (EP 2016) guidelines for herbal drugs or the American Herbal Pharmacopoeia (AHP).

18.4.2 Contamination

Cannabis samples obtained from uncontrolled sources may be contaminated with various harmful substances. The most important contaminants are described below.

Because cannabis is grown under very warm and humid conditions, this creates the perfect conditions for microbes to develop. Manure-based fertilizers or poor hygiene standards may infect plants with intestinal (*E. coli*) bacteria, while contamination with molds of *Aspergillus* or *Penicillium* species, for example, may lead to life-threatening infections especially in immune-compromised patients (Hazekamp 2016). Some microbes produce spores or toxic compounds such as aflatoxins and ochratoxins that may be resistant to heat and can be inhaled during the smoking of a cannabis cigarette or while using a vaporizer (Raters and Matissek 2008). Gamma-irradiation treatment may be used to decontaminate cannabis, without significant effects on the chemical composition or appearance of the product (Hazekamp 2016).

Although pesticides are widely applied in agriculture, their use is always restricted to specific crops in limited quantities. In the case of cannabis, it is unclear which pesticides, if any, pose a threat to the health of patients. An important consideration is that cannabis is often consumed in different ways than other crops that are typically orally ingested. For example, research has shown that many pesticides are inhaled intact when contaminated cannabis is smoked (Sullivan et al. 2013).

Heavy metals such as mercury, arsenic, cadmium, or lead are usually not applied to cannabis on purpose. However, they may be present in materials that come into contact with the plant during cultivation, such as soil, water, or fertilizers. The cannabis plant efficiently absorbs heavy metals through its roots (Shi et al. 2012). Upon consumption of cannabis, these heavy metals may accumulate in a patient's tissues causing harm over time (Busse et al. 2008).

Cannabis is typically sold by weight (per gram), and demands a higher price with increased potency. Therefore, to increase weight, *adulterants* such as fine sand or metal particles such as lead and iron have been found in herbal cannabis samples in various countries. To increase the appearance of potency, finely ground-up glass or talcum powder has been added to mimic the presence of glandular hairs (Scheel et al. 2012).

A recent trend is the addition of *synthetic cannabinoids* to plant material by soaking or spraying. These compounds are often used as recreational drugs to avoid positive cannabis drug testing and are sold under various brand names. They are commonly referred to as spice or K2, and are relatively cheap to produce. Synthetic cannabinoid products are highly potent and can be toxic (CNN 2016; Kim and Monte 2016).

Inhalation or ingestion of any of the substances listed above may lead to harmful situations such as infection, poisoning, psychosis or organ failure. Consequently, the proper analytical methods should be developed and validated for identifying and quantifying their presence in all legally available medicinal cannabis products.

18.4.3 Available Analysis Methods

For single, purified cannabinoid compounds, for example, present in a pharmaceutical preparation, specific analytical procedures can be developed in a straightforward manner. However, modern studies with herbal cannabis require accurate identification of the whole chemical profile in a complex (plant) matrix. Consequently, analytical methods must be available to identify and quantify neutral and acidic cannabinoids, and perhaps also terpenes present in the plant materials used.

Advanced instrumental methods are most often used for the identification and classification (e.g., fiber type versus drug type) of cannabis plants and products. Because of the complex chemistry of cannabis, separation techniques, such as gas chromatography (GC) or high-performance liquid chromatography (HPLC), often coupled with mass spectroscopy (MS), are necessary for the acquisition of the typical chemical profiles that may consist of dozens of compounds of interest. The most commonly used separation technique for cannabinoids and their acid forms has been HPLC while for terpenes mainly GC is used. The chromatographic and spectroscopic properties of the cannabinoids have been extensively reviewed (Hazekamp et al. 2005), and various analytical methods have been published (e.g., Upton et al. 2013; OMC 2016).

For rapid screening purposes and for on-site field testing, non-instrumental techniques such as thin-layer chromatography (TLC) (Fischedick et al. 2009) and chemical color reactions (Bailey 1979) may be helpful. These methods are mainly effective for qualitative analysis identifying presence of specific compounds above a certain threshold level and are not meant to be used for quantitative analysis determining the exact concentration present.

In the end, the only way researchers and medical professionals can communicate about the pros and cons of cannabis in a consistent manner is by using validated and standardized methods to understand the composition of various cannabis preparations. Unfortunately, this has been a problem with professional laboratories showing inconsistent analytical results, even when analyzing the exact same samples (Gieringer and Hazekamp 2011). Ideally, a comprehensive overview of the cannabinoid content (i.e., the chemical fingerprint) of cannabis preparations used in studies should be a standard part of scientific reports on the effects of cannabis (Hazekamp 2016; Hazekamp et al. 2016).

18.5 Cannabinoid Pharmacology and the Endocannabinoid System

18.5.1 Physiology and Function of the Endocannabinoid System

The endogenous cannabinoid signalling system, or endocannabinoid system (ECS), is a ubiquitous neuromodulatory system with wide-ranging physiological actions. It comprises of cannabinoid receptors, their endogenous ligands, and enzymes responsible for the production, transport, and degradation of those ligands. Regulation of feeding was believed to be the initial function of the ECS in primitive organisms (De Petrocellis et al. 1999). In more complex organisms, such as humans, it is thought that the primary function of the ECS evolved into controlling homeostasis, or a physiological balance in the body, especially during a state of illness (Ligresti et al. 2016).

The cannabinoid receptors belong to the large family of the G-protein coupled receptors (GPCRs). Two types of receptors have been identified and cloned (Matsuda et al. 1990; Munro et al. 1993), while there is speculation about additional types (Fonseca et al. 2011; Laprairie et al. 2017). The cannabinoid receptor type 1 (CB_1) is predominantly present in the central nervous system, particularly in those brain regions that regulate functions that typically become disturbed when under the influence of cannabis including sleep, appetite, perception of time, short term memory, and coordination, among others (Fattore and Fratta 2010). In fact, CB_1 is the most abundant GPCR known to be present in the brain (Nogueras-Ortiz and Yudowski 2016).

The cannabinoid receptor type 2 (CB_2) is mainly present on cells of the immune system where it can influence pain, inflammation, and tissue damage (for a review, see Chapter 8 of Pertwee 2014). It should be noted that not all cannabinoid effects can be explained by receptor-binding alone, and it is believed that at least some effects are caused through other mechanisms (Pertwee 2014; Mallipeddi et al. 2017).

Endocannabinoids are the endogenous compounds that bind to the cannabinoid receptors. A variety of compounds with endocannabinoid activity have been isolated, typically having an eicosanoid-related structure, or synthesized. The best studied endogenous ones are called anandamide (Devane et al. 1992) and 2-arachidonylglycerol (2-AG) (Mechoulam et al. 1995; Sugiura et al. 1995). Endocannabinoids are described as *retrograde* transmitters because they commonly travel backwards against the usual synaptic transmitter flow, that is, they are released from the postsynaptic cell and act on the presynaptic cell, where the target receptors are densely concentrated.

Several pathways are known for the synthesis and degradation of endocannabinoids, and there appears to be a high redundancy. Basically, endocannabinoids exist intracellularly as precursors in the plasma membrane of neurons as part of certain phospholipids. They are released on demand by distinct biochemical pathways involving enzymes that include phospholipases C and D. Endocannabinoid degradation involves reuptake into the presynaptic cell, followed by rapid hydrolysis of the amide- or ester-bonds by specialized enzymes, including fatty acid amide hydrolase (FAAH) and monoacylglycerol lipase (MAGL) (Iannotti et al. 2016).

18.5.2 The Cannabis Mode of Action

Several plant cannabinoids may interact with the ECS through binding with one or more of the cannabinoid receptors. In some cases, the resulting effects may be therapeutic, while under other conditions unwanted effects may occur. The most well-known effect is caused by THC: consumption of cannabis rich in THC leads to stimulation of central CB_1 receptors resulting in the user feeling intoxicated or "high." Besides THC, various other cannabinoids have affinity for CB_1 and/or CB_2. Some of these, like THC, act as partial agonists (e.g., CBN, Δ^8-THC) while others can show an antagonist effect (e.g., THCV) (Izzo et al. 2009; McPartland et al. 2015). Stimulation of the cannabinoid receptors by exogenous plant cannabinoids, or phytocannabinoids, may have an effect on any of the physiological systems normally regulated by the endocannabinoid system, including pain, sleep, appetite, and inflammation (Robson 2014; Kowal et al. 2016).

Cannabis terpenes may influence the therapeutic effect in several possible ways, for example by helping cannabinoids to penetrate the blood brain barrier or by altering liver metabolism of cannabinoids (McPartland and Russo 2014). Some terpenes may even compete with cannabinoids at the receptor level.

For example, β-caryophyllene is one of the major terpenes found in cannabis, and it selectively binds to the CB_2 receptor at nanomolar concentrations, acting as a full agonist (Gertsch et al. 2008). Some terpenes also have their own effects independent of the cannabinoid receptors (Park et al. 2011). Perhaps as a result, some studies show that whole plant preparations of cannabis containing various cannabinoids and terpenes have superior therapeutic effects compared to purified cannabinoids alone (McPartland and Russo 2014). This indicates that, at least for some therapeutic uses, cannabis constituents may work in a synergistic manner.

18.5.3 Cannabinoid Pharmacology

The pharmacokinetics of medicinal drugs describes their absorption, distribution, metabolism and elimination. Although the pharmacokinetics of THC is well-known, only limited data have been reported on other cannabinoids. The pharmacokinetics of THC is described in the following sections.

18.5.3.1 Absorption

The rate at which THC enters the bloodstream is dependent on the methods of administration. In general, cannabinoids are almost instantly absorbed after inhalation (minutes) while oral ingestion may take an hour or more before significant absorption occurs through the gastrointestinal tract. Figure 18.1 shows typical plasma concentration profiles for the main administration routes.

18.5.3.2 Distribution

Due to its lipophilic nature, THC and its metabolites are extensively protein bound, around 97%, and rapidly distributed to fatty tissues and highly vascularized organs, such as the brain, lungs, adipose tissue and intestines (Wall 1983; Peat 1989).

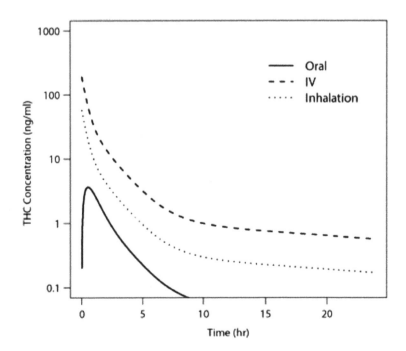

FIGURE 18.1 Simulations of plasma concentration profiles of 5 mg THC after inhalation, intravenous and oral absorption. The THC plasma profile after inhalation of pure THC is comparable to the profile after intravenous administration, with a rapid peak plasma concentration and a steep decline of plasma concentration. (From Klumpers, L. E. 2014. Novel approaches in clinical development of cannabinoid drugs. Phd, Centre for Human Drug Research, Faculty of Medicine/ Leiden University Medical Center (LUMC), Leiden University.)

18.5.3.3 Metabolism

In humans, THC is predominantly metabolized by hydroxylation and oxidation via cytochrome P450 (CYP) enzymes, including CYP2C9, and to a lesser extent CYP2C19 (Dinis-Oliveira 2016). Metabolism mainly takes place in the liver, and to lesser extent in other organs, such as the heart and lungs (Dinis-Oliveira 2016). Particularly the metabolite 11-hydroxy-THC (11-OH-THC) should be noted; its psychotropic potential (feeling "high") may be equipotent to or even larger than its parent molecule THC, while having a similar pharmacokinetic profile (Lemberger et al. 1971). In contrast, the subsequent metabolite 11-carboxy-THC (11-COOH-THC) has no psychotropic activity. Most of 11-COOH-THC is finally converted into its glucuronide form. When THC is inhaled through smoking or vaporizing, it largely avoids first-pass metabolism by the liver, and metabolism takes place much slower as compared to oral administration. As a result, the ratios at which THC metabolites occur after administration, is largely dependent on the administration route.

Of the other cannabinoids, only the metabolism of CBD has been described in some detail (for a review, see Ujváry and Hanuš 2016). An important aspect of CBD is that it inhibits certain CYP450 enzymes which may be important because of drug-drug interactions that could occur in the case that CBD is co-administered with drugs that share the same metabolic enzymes. *In vitro* studies showed that the main CYP450 enzymes for CBD metabolism include CYP1A1, CYP1A2, CYP2D6, CYP3A4, and CYP3A5, while CYP2A9 plays a minor role.

18.5.3.4 Elimination

Metabolism is the major route for the elimination of THC from the body. As a result, only negligible amounts of THC are excreted in unchanged form. Of an oral dose, about 15%–30% of THC is excreted in urine with less than 0.05% of unchanged THC, and about 30%–65% is excreted in feces with less than 5% as unchanged drug. Among the metabolites, 11-COOH-THC is a major one identified in both urine and feces, in its native as well as in its glucuronidated form (Kelly and Jones 1992).

The half-life of THC and its metabolites consists of multiple phases, is dependent on the detection method, and can be several days. The slow elimination from the plasma could be explained by redistribution from peripheral tissues, such as adipose tissue, into the bloodstream. Following single dose administration, low levels of THC metabolites have been detected for more than 5 weeks in the urine and feces (Lemberger et al. 1971; for a review, see Verstraete 2004).

18.5.4 Cannabinoid Toxicology and Tolerability

Although cannabinoids might exert both euphoric and therapeutic effects, several studies have indicated that cannabis use may also induce schizophrenia, psychosis, anxiety, bipolar disorders, and major depression in healthy individuals who are at risk of these conditions (Andrade 2016; Feeney and Kampman 2016). In contrast to opioids, which may cause respiratory depression leading to death when overdosed, lethal overdosing with cannabinoids has never been established (Walker and Huang 2002; Calabria et al. 2010). The reason is that, different from opioid receptors that are abundantly expressed on the brainstem thereby regulating vital signs, cannabinoid receptors are only sparsely found in brain areas of vital importance (Hu and Mackie 2015). Long-term cannabis use has been associated with cognitive decline although abstinence of use for a few days reverses this decline (Solowij 1995; Pope et al. 2002).

18.5.5 Clinical Applications

The main physiological function of the ECS is believed to be controlling homeostasis throughout the human body. In many pathologies, the ECS is involved in compensating for the disruption caused by the illness (Lutz et al. 2015; Tasker et al. 2015), and as a result it is pushed out of its natural balance.

TABLE 18.3

Overview of the Major Cannabis and Cannabinoid Effects in Humans (the Oncological and Genetic Effects Have Been Found *In Vitro*), Inspired by Grotenhermen and Russo (2002)

System	Effects
Neurologic	Analgesia (Abrams et al. 2011; Cooper and Haney 2016); muscle relaxation (Carter and Rosen 2001); appetite stimulation (Farrimond et al. 2011; Le Foll et al. 2013); vomiting (Traver et al. 2009); anti-emetic effects (Söderpalm et al. 2001); fragmented thinking (Radhakrishnan et al. 2014); perception of enhanced creativity and impaired divergent thinking (Kowal et al. 2015); disturbed memory (Dornbush 1974; Ranganathan and D'Souza 2006); unsteady gait (Broyd et al. 2013); ataxia (Viana et al. 2009); slurred speech (Chase et al. 2016); deterioration or amelioration of motor coordination (Dervaux et al. 2013); drowsiness (Hollister 1986; Kaufmann 2010)
Psychiatric	Fatigue (Patton et al. 2002; Kaufmann 2010); euphoria (Purnell and Gregg 1975; Lukas et al. 1995); enhanced well-being (Schmid et al. 2010); dysphoria (Martin-Santos et al. 2012); anxiety (Jurkus et al. 2016); anxiolytic effects (Zuardi et al. 1982; Berrendero and Maldonado 2002); depersonalization (Hürlimann et al. 2012); increased sensory perception (Broyd et al. 2013); hallucinations (Naz 2016); alteration of time perception (Sewell et al. 2013); psychotic states (Thacore and Shukla 1976; Moore et al. 2007)
Hormonal	Prolactin decrease (Block et al. 1991); glucose metabolism (Volkow et al. 1996); reduced sperm count and sperm motility (du Plessis et al. 2015); suppressed ovulation (Jukic et al. 2007)
Cardiovascular	Tachycardia (Weil et al. 1968); vasodilation (Aversa et al. 2008); orthostatic hypotension (Robertson and Robertson 1994); *in vitro* inhibition of platelet aggregation (Formukong et al. 1989)
Respiratory	Bronchodilation (Williams et al. 1976; Hartley et al. 1978; Grassin-Delyle et al. 2014); short-term hyposalivation (Schulz-Katterbach et al. 2009); dry mouth (Darling and Arendorf 1993)
Eye	Injected (reddened) conjunctivae (Green 1982; Green and Roth 1982); reduced tear flow (Tomida et al. 2006); decrease of intraocular pressure (Purnell and Gregg 1975; Green 1982; Tomida et al. 2006)
Gastrointestinal	Reduced bowel movements and delayed gastric emptying (Hejazi et al. 2010; Naftali et al. 2014; Weiss and Friedenberg 2015; Ahmed and Katz 2016)
Immunological	Impairment of cell-mediated and humoral immunity (Specter et al. 1986); anti-inflammatory and immune-stimulating effects (Klein et al. 1998; Nagarkatti et al. 2009; Rajan et al. 2016)
Oncological and genetic	Antineoplastic activity *in vitro* and *in vivo* in preclinical studies (Rocha et al. 2014; Lukhele and Motadi 2016); inhibition of synthesis of DNA, RNA, and proteins *in vitro* (Blevins and Regan 1976)
Embryologic	Malformations (Linn et al. 1983; Jaques et al. 2014); growth retardation (El Marroun et al. 2009); impairment to fetal and postnatal cerebral development (Fried 1980; Fried and Watkinson 1988; Calvigioni et al. 2014; Huizink 2014); impairment of cognitive functions (Fried 1980; Fried and Watkinson 1988; Calvigioni et al. 2014; Huizink 2014)

This phenomenon is mainly reactionary and should not be considered as a causal relationship with the pathology. There are speculations, however, about the existence of an endocannabinoid deficiency syndrome (Smith and Wagner 2014). The administration of plant-based cannabinoids, perhaps with the aid of terpenes, may help to return the ECS back towards a healthy state.

Based on the available clinical data, cannabinoids are believed to exhibit a therapeutic potential mainly as an analgesic for chronic neuropathic pain, as an appetite stimulant and anti-emetic for debilitating diseases such as cancer, AIDS, and hepatitis C, as well as in the symptomatic treatment of multiple sclerosis. Additionally, cannabinoids show promising results in the symptomatic treatment of spinal cord injuries, intestinal dysfunction, Tourette's syndrome, hyperactivity and anxiety disorders, and epilepsy (Ben Amar 2006; Hazekamp and Grotenhermen 2010; Kowal et al. 2016).

Animal studies and isolated cancer cells indicate possible involvement of the ECS in the development and spreading of various cancers, opening up the exciting possibility of cannabinoids as a future treatment of cancer (Suárez et al. 2014). These effects have not yet been replicated in human studies. Table 18.3 is an overview of the most important effects of cannabis that have been demonstrated in humans *in vivo*.

Cannabis may also enhance the efficacy of other medications, such as the analgesic effects of opioids (Nielsen et al. 2017), and/or reduce harmful side effects associated with them, such as nausea and vomiting, or sleeping problems (Turgeman and Bar-Sela 2017).

18.6 Global Perspectives

18.6.1 Cannabis Programs in Different Countries

In recent years, the medicinal use of cannabis has rapidly gained acceptance worldwide. Several countries already have government-supervised programs, in which quality-controlled herbal cannabis, as well as derived products such as cannabis oil (Section 18.3), are supplied by specialized and licensed companies. Other countries are in the process of setting up their own programs, or import products from such as the Dutch program. The large regulatory shifts in these countries signal that the Single Convention, discussed earlier in this chapter, and the punishment-based prohibition that goes with it, may have reached its expiry date. Below is an overview of some of the most relevant countries and their regulations (in alphabetical order).

18.6.1.1 Australia

In 2016, Australia amended its Narcotics Drug Act at the State level to permit the cultivation of cannabis and its manufacture to pharmaceutical finished dose forms intended for medicinal purposes. These legislative changes are currently being interpreted by individual States and Territories, which may result in different regulatory approaches adopted across the country. Patient access is generally approached through a Special Access Scheme, typically requiring evidence that other, conventional, treatments have failed. The permitted indications vary by individual States and Territories, meaning there is inequitable access regarding the types of diseases that can be treated. The recreational use of cannabis is illegal in Australia, with formal criminal charges from illegal cannabis use varying across the country.

18.6.1.2 Canada

In Canada, cannabis is regulated under the Canadian Controlled Drugs and Substances Act (CDSA) as a Schedule II controlled substance. As such, all activities associated with it are illegal except those under authorized federal regulations. The conditions for possessing, consuming or growing cannabis for medicinal purposes have been outlined in the "Marihuana for Medical Purposes Regulations" (MMPR) issued by Health Canada that was first created in 2011 and came into force in 2013. On October 17, 2018, the Cannabis Act came into effect, which legalized recreational cannabis in Canada (Justice Laws Website). At the time of this book going to press, about 75 cannabis producers had been licensed so far (Health Canada 2018).

18.6.1.3 Germany

Germany started a medicinal cannabis program on March 10, 2017 and medicinal cannabis cultivation is overseen by the Cannabisagentur, or Cannabis Agency (Germany, BFARM). Patients receive reimbursement by health insurance companies of the products used.

18.6.1.4 Israel

Already in 1992, the Ministry of Health in Israel approved marijuana for medical use, but it took until 2007 before the Ministry established a formal medical marijuana program that has been updated several times since then (Ministry of Health, Medical Cannabis Unit). The program is regulated by the Israel Medical Cannabis Agency (IMCA) and registered patients receive either cannabis oil or cannabis flowers through a dispensary or directly from the medicinal cannabis growers.

18.6.1.5 The Netherlands

Whereas most countries have followed an approach of punishment-based prohibition on cannabis and other drugs, the Netherlands have traditionally focused on harm-reduction. Cannabis has not been legalized, but small-scale sales through outlets known as *coffeeshop* and personal use are tolerated. In 2001, this approach became the basis of creating the Dutch Medicinal Cannabis program, under supervision of the Ministry of Health (OMC 2016). Various cannabis varieties are available on prescription from pharmacies around the country. Cannabis is typically prescribed when other, conventional medicines, have proven ineffective, or too many adverse effects occurred. In some cases, health insurance companies reimburse the expense to the patient. Currently, The Netherlands legally export pharmaceutical grade cannabis to a range of countries.

18.6.1.6 New Zealand

New Zealand adopted clinical guidelines for the use of medicinal cannabis in 2007, but initially very few patients were able to access cannabis-based medicines. Non-registered, pharmaceutical grade cannabis-based medicines are now permitted for use in named patients only, under the oversight of a specialist, when all other traditional treatment options have failed. The recreational use of cannabis is illegal in New Zealand; however, a police cannabis diversion scheme exists which removes first time offenders from formal criminal charges resulting from illegal cannabis use.

18.6.1.7 United States

In the United States, the use, sale, and possession of all forms of cannabis is illegal at a Federal level. Cannabis is a Schedule I drug under the federal Controlled Substances Act, (FDA, Controlled substances act, Title 21, Chapter 13). Despite this fact, California was the first U.S. state to allow the so-called medical marijuana, by referendum in 1996 (California Department of Public Health, Proposition 215). As of early 2019, almost every state in the U.S. has introduced laws that allow the medicinal use of cannabis, and close to a dozen have fully legalized all use including recreational or "adult use." Also, each state where cannabis is allowed has their own regulatory landscape. In 2011, (updated in 2013) the U.S. Department of Justice announced a memorandum to its federal marijuana enforcement policy (Cole memorandum) that says that based on assurances that states will impose an appropriately strict regulatory system, the U.S. Department of Justice defers its right to challenge their legalization laws at this time (United States Department of Justice, Office of Public Affairs). The Cole memorandum was rescinded by a memo signed by Attorney General Jeff Sessions in January 2018. https://www.documentcloud.org/documents/4343764-Sessions-marijuana-memo.html

18.6.2 Regulatory Issues

An increasing number of countries have taken steps to decriminalize the use and possession of cannabis, and recently the first few territories have fully legalized the drug (Uruguay, Canada, some U.S. states). At the same time, with the exception of GW Pharmaceutical's cannabis extracts Sativex and Epidiolex, no country has yet formally acknowledged cannabis as conventional, registered medication, mainly due to the lack of solid clinical proof on the safety and efficacy of these products in systematic reviews (e.g., Whiting et al. 2015; Walitt et al. 2016). This has created confusing and sometimes contrasting situations. Below, we outline the regulatory issues that are relevant to the most important stakeholders in the production, prescribing and use of medicinal cannabis products, that is, producers, patients, prescribers and researchers.

18.6.2.1 Producers

The making of cannabis products consists of series of steps, including the processes around the *growers* (cultivation, harvest and packaging of the herbal material) and further steps by *product manufacturers* where raw material is processed into products such as extracts, oils, edibles, or vaping pens (see Section 18.3). To enhance safety and reliability of cannabis products, it may be recommended to adopt international guidelines for cultivation such as Good Agricultural Practice (GAP) and guidelines for herbal drugs for growers, and (pharmaceutical) Good Manufacturing Practice (GMP) for product manufacturers. Quality testing should be performed by independent, certified labs that follow international standardization guidelines, such as ISO and Good Laboratory Practice (GLP). This should prevent inaccurate or false label claims, which currently seems to be a common problem (Vandrey et al. 2015; FDA 2016). The goal would be to remove questionable sources of plant material and products from the legal market, and to focus on standardized, quality controlled products only.

18.6.2.2 Prescribers

Prescribers are the bottleneck in any medicinal cannabis program; without the signature of a prescribing health care professional, a patient cannot receive a prescription and therefore could not use cannabis legally. However, many physicians do not feel comfortable prescribing an unregistered botanical drug with abuse potential, or to engage in informed discussions with patients about cannabis (Ziemianski et al. 2015). Priority should therefore be given, in all countries where legal medicinal cannabis products are available, to developing continued medical education programs, preferably within the existing medical training environment. In some countries, medical associations have already started formulating general guidelines for the responsible use of cannabis (e.g., Kahan et al. 2014). Also, more attention should be given to the endocannabinoid system and its therapeutic potential in medical school. It would make sense that cannabis can only be prescribed by physicians who received a proper basic training, equivalent to the guidelines that govern the prescription of opioids and other controlled substances (Webster and Grabois 2015).

18.6.2.3 Patients

Providing proper information on different levels is of great importance to the main stakeholders in the medicinal cannabis debate: patients. Firstly, governments and medical and patient organizations should clearly inform the public about the legality, the medical benefits and the adverse effects of cannabis, thereby helping to change patient's perceptions from cannabis as an *illegal drug* to cannabis as an *accepted medicinal product*. This is of particular importance as many patients are unsure about these aspects and therefore might avoid using cannabis unjustly. Proper and consistent information can cause a rapid social change (Gallup 2015). Secondly, in regulated markets, patients should be able to fully rely on the quality of products offered, by proper labeling of such products. This will avoid patients getting into contact with unregulated, illegal cannabis markets with the potential risks of receiving ineffective or unsafe products. These proposed changes will require a pro-active attitude by governments and regulatory bodies, not only by actively providing fact-based information, but also by responding promptly to false or unsupported medical claims on any cannabis-related product.

18.6.2.4 Researchers

Over the past decades, academic and pharmaceutical research on the endocannabinoid system has lagged compared to the research field of other physiological systems such as the opioid system (with ligands from poppy plants, and involved in e.g., pain regulation), the serotonergic system (with a ligand such as LSD, and involved in e.g., depression) or the dopaminergic system (with ligands such as cocaine and methamphetamine, and involved in e.g., psychoses and vomiting). The reason for this lag cannot be found in the rich historical literature on cannabis effects (Russo 2007) and numerous anecdotal patient recordings. However, more likely, clinical researchers who strive to better understand the therapeutic potential of cannabinoids encounter complex legal obstructions (Andreae et al. 2016). Removing these, mainly administrative, barriers would enable scientists to gain access to crucial elements for research, such as pharmaceutical grade cannabis with standardized cannabinoid and terpene content, international exchange of cannabis products, and chemical reference standards. Furthermore, it would facilitate research collaborations, including more (public) funding spent on addressing the most pressing research questions. This will result in faster progress in understanding the pharmacological characteristics, toxicity and tolerability, and medicinal value of the cannabis plant.

18.7 General Conclusion

As of 2019, the classification of cannabis as a narcotic drug around the world is based on historical conventions rather than on the current state of scientific knowledge. This situation is seriously obstructing cannabis' development into modern medicines. Although cannabis products and cannabis constituents have so far not proven to be definite cures for any disease state, studies have shown therapeutic effects with regard to symptom treatment in several diseases, as described in this chapter. Therefore, the authors believe that, firstly, international conventions and regulations on a national level should be updated to the current state of knowledge with regards to facilitating availability of this medicinal product for patients that benefit from its therapeutic values (in agreement with Nutt et al. 2007). Setting up such medicinal cannabis programs requires optimal regulations to safeguard product quality and safety for patients.

Our scientific understanding of the potential of cannabis has increased significantly over the past decade or so; however, these insights are only slowly incorporated into new legislation. Therefore, secondly, an expansion of the options for performing research is needed. Creating a clear regulatory environment, for example related to efficiently obtaining research permits for the study of cannabis and its unique cannabinoids, will provide an immediate boost to a wide range of research fields, ranging from cultivation and chemical analysis, to product development and, ultimately, clinical trials. Only the prospect of more and better research (areas of essential research can, e.g., be found in the 2017 publication on cannabis medicine by the National Academies of Sciences, Engineering and Medicine, 2017) will improve our understanding of the benefits and risks of applying cannabis and its constituents in contemporary medicine.

REFERENCES

Abrams, D. I., P. Couey, S. B. Shade, M. E. Kelly, and N. L. Benowitz. 2011. Cannabinoid-opioid interaction in chronic pain. *Clinical Pharmacology & Therapeutics* 90 (6):844–851.

Ahmed, W., and S. Katz. 2016. Therapeutic use of cannabis in inflammatory bowel disease. *Gastroenterology & Hepatology* 12 (11):668.

Andrade, C. 2016. Cannabis and neuropsychiatry, 1: Benefits and risks. *Journal of Clinical Psychiatry* 77 (5):e551–e664.

Andre, C. M., J. F. Hausman, and G. Guerriero. 2016. Cannabis sativa: The plant of the thousand and one molecules. *Front Plant Science* 7:19.

Andreae, M. H., E. Rhodes, T. Bourgoise, G. M. Carter, R. S. White, D. Indyk, H. Sacks, and R. Rhodes. 2016. An ethical exploration of barriers to research on controlled drugs. *American Journal of Bioethics* 16 (4):36–47.

Aversa, A., F. Rossi, D. Francomano, R. Bruzziches, C. Bertone, V. Santiemma, and G. Spera. 2008. Early endothelial dysfunction as a marker of vasculogenic erectile dysfunction in young habitual cannabis users. *International Journal of Impotence Research* 20 (6):566–573.

Bailey, K. 1979. The value of the Duquenois test for cannabis—A survey. *Journal of Forensic Sciences* 24 (4):817–841.

Balabanova, S., F. Parsche, and W. Pirsig. 1992. First identification of drugs in Egyptian mummies. *Naturwissenschaften* 79 (8):358.

Ben Amar, M. 2006. Cannabinoids in medicine: A review of their therapeutic potential. *Journal of Ethnopharmacology* 105 (1–2):1–325.

Berrendero, F., and R. Maldonado. 2002. Involvement of the opioid system in the anxiolytic-like effects induced by Delta(9)-tetrahydrocannabinol. *Psychopharmacology* 163 (1):111–117.

Bewley-Taylor, D., and M. Jelsma. 2012. Regime change: Re-visiting the 1961 single convention on narcotic drugs. *The International Journal on Drug Policy* 23 (1):72–81.

Blevins, R. D., and J. D. Regan. 1976. Δ-9-Tetrahydrocannabinol: Effect on macromolecular synthesis in human and other mammalian cells. *Archives of Toxicology* 35 (2):127–135.

Block, R. I., R. Farinpour, and J. A. Schlechte. 1991. Effects of chronic marijuana use on testosterone, luteinizing hormone, follicle stimulating hormone, prolactin and cortisol in men and women. *Drug and Alcohol Dependence* 28 (2):121–128.

Bohlmann, J., and C. I. Keeling. 2008. Terpenoid biomaterials. *Plant Journal* 54 (4):656–669.

Broyd, S. J., L. M. Greenwood, R. J. Croft, A. Dalecki, J. Todd, P. T. Michie, S. J. Johnstone, and N. Solowij. 2013. Chronic effects of cannabis on sensory gating. *International Journal of Psychophysiology* 89 (3):381–389.

Brunner, T. F. 1977. Marijuana in ancient Greece and Rome? The literary evidence. *Journal of Psychedelic Drugs* 9 (3):221–225.

Burstein, S. H. 2014. The cannabinoid acids, analogs and endogenous counterparts. *Bioorganic & Medicinal Chemistry* 22 (10):2830–2843.

Busse, F., L. Omidi, A. Leichtle, M. Windgassen, E. Kluge, and M. Stumvoll. 2008. Lead poisoning due to adulterated marijuana. *New England Journal of Medicine* 358 (15):1641–1642.

Calabria, B., L. Degenhardt, W. Hall, and M. Lynskey. 2010. Does cannabis use increase the risk of death? Systematic review of epidemiological evidence on adverse effects of cannabis use. *Drug and Alcohol Review* 29 (3):318–330.

California Department of Public Health Proposition 215. https://www.cdph.ca.gov/programs/MMP/Pages/CompassionateUseact.aspx

Calvigioni, D., Y. L. Hurd, T. Harkany, and E. Keimpema. 2014. Neuronal substrates and functional consequences of prenatal cannabis exposure. *European Child & Adolescent Psychiatry* 23 (10):931–941.

Canada, Health Canada. 2018. Authorized Licensed Producers for Medical Purposes. http://www.hc-sc.gc.ca/dhp-mps/marihuana/info/list-eng.php

Canada, Justice Laws Website, Cannabis Act, https://laws-lois.justice.gc.ca/eng/acts/C-24.5/

Carter, G. T., and B. S. Rosen. 2001. Marijuana in the management of amyotrophic lateral sclerosis. *The American Journal of Hospice & Palliative Care* 18 (4):264–270.

Cascini, F., C. Aiello, and G. Di Tanna. 2012. Increasing delta-9-tetrahydrocannabinol (Delta-9-THC) content in herbal cannabis over time: Systematic review and meta-analysis. *Curr Drug Abuse Rev* 5 (1):32–40.

Chase, P. B., J. Hawkins, J. Mosier, E. Jimenez, K. Boesen, B. K. Logan, and F. G. Walter. 2016. Differential physiological and behavioral cues observed in individuals smoking botanical marijuana versus synthetic cannabinoid drugs. *Clin Toxicol (Phila)* 54 (1):14–19.

Chopra, I. C., and R. N. Chopra. 1957. The use of cannabis drugs in India. *Bulletin on Narcotics*: 4–29.

Clarke, R. C. 1981. *Marijuana Botany: An Advanced Study, the Propagation and Breeding of Distinctive Cannabis.* Berkeley, Calif.: And/Or Press.

Clarke, R. C., and M. Frank. 2012. *Hashish!: Updated Second Edition.* Red Eye Press.

CNN. 2016. "Fake pot" causing zombielike effects is 85 times more potent than marijuana. http://edition.cnn.com/2016/12/16/health/zombie-synthetic-marijuana/

Conert, H. J., E. J. Jäger, J. W. Kadereit, W. Schultze-Motel, G. Wagenitz, H. E. Weber, and G. Hegi. 1992. Illustrierte Flora von Mitteleuropa. In *Illustrierte Flora von Mitteleuropa*, edited by Hegi, G, 283–295, 473–474. Berlin/Hamburg.

Cooper, Z. D., and M. Haney. 2016. Sex-dependent effects of cannabis-induced analgesia. *Drug and Alcohol Dependence* 167:112–120.

Darling, M. R., and T. M. Arendorf. 1993. Effects of cannabis smoking on oral soft tissues. *Community Dentistry and Oral Epidemiology* 21 (2):78–81.

De Petrocellis, L., D. Melck, T. Bisogno, A. Milone, and V. Di Marzo. 1999. Finding of the endocannabinoid signalling system in Hydra, a very primitive organism: Possible role in the feeding response. *Neuroscience* 92 (1):377–387.

Dervaux, A., X. Laqueille, M. C. Bourdel, and M. O. Krebs. 2013. Neurological soft signs in non-psychotic patients with cannabis dependence. *Addiction Biology* 18 (2):214–221.

Devane, W. A., L. Hanus, A. Breuer, R. G. Pertwee, L. A. Stevenson, G. Griffin, D. Gibson, A. Mandelbaum, A. Etinger, and R. Mechoulam. 1992. Isolation and structure of a brain constituent that binds to the cannabinoid receptor. *Science* 258 (5090):1946–1949.

Dinis-Oliveira, R. J. 2016. Metabolomics of Delta9-tetrahydrocannabinol: Implications in toxicity. *Drug Metabolism Reviews* 48 (1):80–87.

Dornbush, R. L. 1974. Marijuana and memory: Effects of smoking on storage. *Trans N Y Acad Sci* 36 (1):94–100.

El Marroun, H., H. Tiemeier, E. A. P. Steegers, V. W. V. Jaddoe, A. Hofman, F. C. Verhulst, W. van den Brink, and A. C. Huizink. 2009. New research: Intrauterine cannabis exposure affects fetal growth trajectories: The generation R study. *Journal of the American Academy of Child & Adolescent Psychiatry* 48:1173–1181.

ElSohly, M. A., Z. Mehmedic, S. Foster, C. Gon, S. Chandra, and J. C. Church. 2016. Changes in cannabis potency over the last 2 decades (1995–2014): Analysis of current data in the United States. *Biological Psychiatry* 79 (7):613–619.

Elsohly, M. A., and D. Slade. 2005. Chemical constituents of marijuana: The complex mixture of natural cannabinoids. *Life Sciences* 78 (5):539–548.

Erkelens, J. L., and A. Hazekamp. 2014. That which we call Indica, by any other name would smell as sweet. An essay on the history of the term Indica and the taxonomical conflict between the monotypic and polytypic views of Cannabis. *Cannabinoids* 9 (1):9–15.

European Directorate for the Quality of Medicines. 2016. *European Pharmacopoeia 8.0*. Strasbourg, France.

Fankhauser, M. 2002. Cannabis and cannabinoids : Pharmacology, toxicology, and therapeutic potential. In *Cannabis and Cannabinoids : Pharmacology, Toxicology, and Therapeutic Potential*, edited by Grotenhermen, F., and E. Russo, 37–51. New York: Haworth Integrative Healing Press.

Farrimond, J. A., M. S. Mercier, B. J. Whalley, and C. M. Williams. 2011. Cannabis sativa and the endogenous cannabinoid system: Therapeutic potential for appetite regulation. *Phytotherapy Research* 25 (2):170–188.

Fattore, L., and W. Fratta. 2010. How important are sex differences in cannabinoid action? *British Journal of Pharmacology* 160 (3):544–548.

FDA. Controlled substances act, Title 21, Chapter 13. http://www.fda.gov/regulatoryinformation/legislation/ucm148726.htm

FDA. 2016 Warning Letters and Test Results for Cannabidiol-Related Products. http://www.fda.gov/NewsEvents/PublicHealthFocus/ucm484109.htm

Feeney, K. E., and K. M. Kampman. 2016. Adverse effects of marijuana use. *The Linacre Quarterly* 83 (2):174–178.

Fischedick, J. T., R. Glas, A. Hazekamp, and R. Verpoorte. 2009. A qualitative and quantitative HPTLC densitometry method for the analysis of cannabinoids in Cannabis sativa L. *Phytochemical Analysis* 20 (5):421–426.

Le Foll, B., J. M. Trigo, K. A. Sharkey, and Y. Le Strat. 2013. Cannabis and Delta9-tetrahydrocannabinol (THC) for weight loss? *Medical Hypotheses* 80 (5):564–567.

Fonseca, B. M., N. A. Teixeira, M. Almada, A. H. Taylor, J. C. Konje, and G. Correia-da-Silva. 2011. Modulation of the novel cannabinoid receptor—GPR55—during rat fetoplacental development. *Placenta* 32 (6):462–469.

Formukong, E. A., A. T. Evans, and F. J. Evans. 1989. The inhibitory effects of cannabinoids, the active constituents of Cannabis sativa L. on human and rabbit platelet aggregation. *Journal of Pharmacy and Pharmacology* 41 (10):705–709.

Fried, P. A. 1980. Marihuana use by pregnant women: Neurobehavioral effects in neonates. *Drug and Alcohol Dependence* 6 (6):415–424.

Fried, P. A., and B. Watkinson. 1988. 12- and 24-month neurobehavioural follow-up of children prenatally exposed to marihuana, cigarettes and alcohol. *Neurotoxicology and Teratology* 10 (4):305–313.

Gallup. 2015. Gallup Marijuana polls. http://www.gallup.com/poll/186260/back-legal-marijuana.aspx

Germany, Federal Institute for Drugs and Medical Devices (BFARM), 2018 https://www.bfarm.de/DE/Bundesopiumstelle/Cannabis/Cannabisagentur/_node.html

Gertsch, J., M. Leonti, S. Raduner, I. Racz, J. Z. Chen, X. Q. Xie, K. H. Altmann, M. Karsak, and A. Zimmer. 2008. Beta-caryophyllene is a dietary cannabinoid. *Proceedings of the National Academy of Sciences of the United States of America* 105 (26):9099–9104.

Gertsch, J., R. G. Pertwee, and V. D. Marzo. 2010. Phytocannabinoids beyond the Cannabis plant – do they exist? *British Journal of Pharmacology* 160 (3):523–529.

Gieringer, D., and A. Hazekamp. 2011. How accurate is potency testing. *O'Shaugnessy's Online Journal* 17.

Grassin-Delyle, S., E. Naline, A. Buenestado, C. Faisy, J. C. Alvarez, H. Salvator, C. Abrial, C. Advenier, L. Zemoura, and P. Devillier. 2014. Cannabinoids inhibit cholinergic contraction in human airways through prejunctional CB1 receptors. *British Journal of Pharmacology* 171 (11):2767–2777.

Green, K. 1982. Marijuana and the eye—A review. *Journal of Toxicology: Cutaneous and Ocular Toxicology* 1 (1):3–32.

Green, K., and M. Roth. 1982. Ocular effects of topical administration of δ9-tetrahydrocannabinol in man. *Archives of Ophthalmology* 100 (2):265–267.

Grotenhermen, F. 2003a. Clinical pharmacokinetics of cannabinoids. *Journal of Cannabis Therapeutics* 3 (1):3–51.

Grotenhermen, F. 2003b. Pharmacokinetics and pharmacodynamics of cannabinoids. *Clinical Pharmacokinetics* 42 (4):327–360.

Grotenhermen, F. 2004. Cannabinoids for therapeutic use. *American Journal of Drug Delivery*, 2 (4):229–240.

Grotenhermen, F., and E. Russo. 2002. *Cannabis and Cannabinoids. Pharmacology, Toxicology, and Therapeutic Potential.* Binghamton/New York: Haworth Press.

Hartley, J. P., S. G. Nogrady, and A. Seaton. 1978. Bronchodilator effect of delta1-tetrahydrocannabinol. *British Journal of Clinical Pharmacology* 5 (6):523–525.

Hazekamp, A. 2016. Evaluating the effects of gamma-irradiation for decontamination of medicinal cannabis. *Front Pharmacol* 7:108.

Hazekamp, A., K. Bastola, H. Rashidi, J. Bender, and R. Verpoorte. 2007. Cannabis tea revisited: A systematic evaluation of the cannabinoid composition of cannabis tea. *Journal of Ethnopharmacology* 113 (1):85–190.

Hazekamp, A., and J. T. Fischedick. 2012. Cannabis—From cultivar to chemovar. *Drug Test Anal* 4 (7–8):660–667.

Hazekamp, A., and F. Grotenhermen. 2010. Review on clinical studies with cannabis and cannabinoids 2005-2009. *Cannabinoids* 5 (Special Issue):1–21.

Hazekamp, A., A. Peltenburg, R. Verpoorte, and C. Giroud. 2005. Chromatographic and spectroscopic data of cannabinoids from cannabis sativa L. *Journal of Liquid Chromatography & Related Technologies* 28 (15):2361–2382.

Hazekamp, A., K. Tejkalová, and S. Papadimitriou. 2016. Cannabis: From cultivar to chemovar II—A metabolomics approach to cannabis classification. *Cannabis and Cannabinoid Research* 1 (1):202–215.

Hejazi, R. A., T. H. Lavenbarg, and R. W. McCallum. 2010. Spectrum of gastric emptying patterns in adult patients with cyclic vomiting syndrome. *Neurogastroenterology and Motility: The Official Journal of the European Gastrointestinal Motility Society* 22 (12):1298.

Hollister, L. E. 1986. Health aspects of cannabis. *Pharmacological Reviews* 38 (1):1–1220.

Hu, S. S., and K. Mackie. 2015. Distribution of the endocannabinoid system in the central nervous system. *Handbook of Experimental Pharmacology* 231:59–93.

Huestis, M. A., A. H. Sampson, B. J. Holicky, J. E. Henningfield, and E. J. Cone. 1992. Characterization of the absorption phase of marijuana smoking. *Clinical Pharmacology & Therapeutics* 52 (1):31–41.

Huizink, A. C. 2014. Prenatal cannabis exposure and infant outcomes: Overview of studies. *Progress in Neuro-Psychopharmacology & Biological Psychiatry* 52:45–52.

Hürlimann, F., S. Kupferschmid, and A. E. Simon. 2012. Cannabis-induced depersonalization disorder in adolescence. *Neuropsychobiology* 65 (3):141–146.

Iannotti, F. A., V. Di Marzo, and S. Petrosino. 2016. Endocannabinoids and endocannabinoid-related mediators: Targets, metabolism and role in neurological disorders. *Progress in Lipid Research* 62:107–128.

Industrial Hemp Farmers Act of 2015. https://www.congress.gov/bill/114th-congress/senate-bill/134

Izzo, A. A., F. Borrelli, R. Capasso, V. Di Marzo, and R. Mechoulam. 2009. Non-psychotropic plant cannabinoids: New therapeutic opportunities from an ancient herb. *Trends in Pharmacological Sciences* 30 (10):515–527.

Jaques, S. C., A. Kingsbury, P. Henshcke, C. Chomchai, S. Clews, J. Falconer, M. E. Abdel-Latif, J. M. Feller, and J. L. Oei. 2014. Cannabis, the pregnant woman and her child: Weeding out the myths. *Journal of Perinatology* 34 (6):417–424.

Jukic, A. M. Z., C. R. Weinberg, D. D. Baird, and A. J. Wilcox. 2007. Lifestyle and reproductive factors associated with follicular phase length. *Journal of Women's Health (15409996)* 16 (9):1340–1347.

Jurkus, R., H. L. L. Day, F. S. Guimarães, J. L. C. Lee, L. J. Bertoglio, and C. W. Stevenson. 2016. Cannabidiol regulation of learned fear: Implications for treating anxiety-related disorders. *Frontiers in Pharmacology* 7:454.

Kahan, M., A. Srivastava, S. Spithoff, and L. Bromley. 2014. Prescribing smoked cannabis for chronic noncancer pain: Preliminary recommendations. *Canadian Family Physician Medecin de Famille Canadien* 60 (12):1083–490.

Karschner, E. L., W. D. Darwin, R. P. McMahon, F. Liu, S. Wright, R. S. Goodwin, and M. A. Huestis. 2011. Subjective and physiological effects after controlled Sativex and oral THC administration. *Clinical Pharmacology & Therapeutics* 89 (3):400–407.

Kaufmann, R. M. 2010. Acute psychotropic effects of oral cannabis extract with a defined content of Delta9-Tetrahydrocannabinol (THC) in healthy volunteers. *Pharmacopsychiatry* 43 (1):24–32.

Kelly, P., and R. T. Jones. 1992. Metabolism of tetrahydrocannabinol in frequent and infrequent marijuana users. *Journal of Analytical Toxicology* 16 (4):228–235.

Kim, H. S., and A. A. Monte. 2016. Colorado cannabis legalization and its effect on emergency care. *Annals of Emergency Medicine* 68 (1):71–75.

Klein, T. W., H. Friedman, and S. Specter. 1998. Marijuana, immunity and infection. *Journal of Neuroimmunology* 83 (1–2):102–115.

Klumpers, L. E. 2014. Novel approaches in clinical development of cannabinoid drugs. *Phd*, Centre for Human Drug Research, Faculty of Medicine/Leiden University Medical Center (LUMC), Leiden University.

Klumpers, L. E., T. L. Beumer, J. G. van Hasselt, … and J. van Gerven. 2012. Novel Δ9-tetrahydrocannabinol formulation Namisol® has beneficial pharmacokinetics and promising pharmacodynamic effects. *British Journal of Clinical Pharmacology* 74 (1):42–53.

Kowal, M., A. Hazekamp, and F. Grotenhermen. 2016. Review on clinical studies with cannabis and cannabinoids 2010-2014. *Cannabinoids* 11 (Special Issue):1–18.

Kowal, M. A., A. Hazekamp, L. S. Colzato, H. van Steenbergen, N. J. van der Wee, J. Durieux, M. Manai, and B. Hommel. 2015. Cannabis and creativity: Highly potent cannabis impairs divergent thinking in regular cannabis users. *Psychopharmacology* 232 (6):1123–1134.

Laprairie, R. B., A. M. Bagher, and E. M. Denovan-Wright. 2017. Cannabinoid receptor ligand bias: Implications in the central nervous system. *Current Opinion in Pharmacology* 32:32–43.

Lemberger, L., N. R. Tamarkin, J. Axelrod, and I. J. Kopin. 1971. Delta-9-tetrahydrocannabinol: Metabolism and disposition in long-term marihuana smokers. *Science* 173 (3991):72–74.

Ligresti, A., L. De Petrocellis, and V. Di Marzo. 2016. From phytocannabinoids to cannabinoid receptors and endocannabinoids: Pleiotropic physiological and pathological roles through complex pharmacology. *Physiological Reviews* 96 (4):1593–1659.

Linn, S., S. C. Schoenbaum, R. R. Monson, R. Rosner, P. C. Stubblefield, and K. J. Ryan. 1983. The association of marijuana use with outcome of pregnancy. *American Journal of Public Health* 73 (10):1161–1164.

Lukas, S. E., J. H. Mendelson, and R. Benedikt. 1995. Electroencephalographic correlates of marihuana-induced euphoria. *Drug and Alcohol Dependence* 37 (2):131–140.

Lukhele, S. T., and L. R. Motadi. 2016. Cannabidiol rather than Cannabis sativa extracts inhibit cell growth and induce apoptosis in cervical cancer cells. *BMC Complementary and Alternative Medicine* 16 (1).

Lutz, B., G. Marsicano, R. Maldonado, and C. J. Hillard. 2015. The endocannabinoid system in guarding against fear, anxiety and stress. *Nature Reviews Neuroscience* 16 (12):705–718.

Maffei, M. E., J. Gertsch, and G. Appendino. 2011. Plant volatiles: Production, function and pharmacology. *Natural Product Reports* 28 (8):1359–1380.

Mallipeddi, S., D. R. Janero, N. Zvonok, and A. Makriyannis. 2017. Functional selectivity at G-protein coupled receptors: Advancing cannabinoid receptors as drug targets. *Biochemical Pharmacology* 128:1–11.

Martin-Santos, R., J. A. Crippa, A. Batalla et al. 2012. Acute effects of a single, oral dose of d9-tetrahydrocannabinol (THC) and cannabidiol (CBD) administration in healthy volunteers. *Current Pharmaceutical Design* 18 (32):4966–4979.

Matsuda, L. A., S. J. Lolait, M. J. Brownstein, A. C. Young, and T. I. Bonner. 1990. Structure of a cannabinoid receptor and functional expression of the cloned cDNA. *Nature* 346 (6284):561–564.

McPartland, J., and G. Guy. 2015. Correct(ed) vernacular nomenclature of Cannabis. *O'Shaugnessy's Online Journal Edition* 4.

McPartland, J. M., M. Duncan, V. Di Marzo, and R. G. Pertwee. 2015. Are cannabidiol and Delta(9)-tetrahydrocannabivarin negative modulators of the endocannabinoid system? A systematic review. *British Journal of Pharmacology* 172 (3):737–753.

McPartland, J. M., and P. L. Pruitt. 1999. Side effects of pharmaceuticals not elicited by comparable herbal medicines: The case of tetrahydrocannabinol and marijuana. *Alternative Therapies in Health and Medicine* 5 (4):57.

McPartland, J. M., and E. B. Russo. 2014. Non-phytocannabinoid constituents of cannabis and herbal synergy. In *Handbooks in Psychopharmacology*, edited by Pertwee, R. G., 280–295. Oxford, United Kingdom; New York, NY: Oxford University Press.

Mechoulam, R. 1986. The pharmacohistory of Cannabis sativa. In *Cannabinoids as Therapeutic Agents*, edited by Mechoulam, R., 1–19. Boca Raton, Fla.: CRC Press.

Mechoulam, R., S. Ben-Shabat, L. Hanus et al. 1995. Identification of an endogenous 2-monoglyceride, present in canine gut, that binds to cannabinoid receptors. *Biochemical Pharmacology* 50 (1):83–90.

Moore, T. H. M., S. Zammit, A. Lingford-Hughes, T. R. E. Barnes, P. B. Jones, M. Burke, and G. Lewis. 2007. Cannabis use and risk of psychotic or affective mental health outcomes: A systematic review. *The Lancet* 370 (9584):319–328.

Munro, S., K. L. Thomas, and M. Abu-Shaar. 1993. Molecular characterization of a peripheral receptor for cannabinoids. *Nature* 365 (6441):61–65.

Naftali, T., R. Mechulam, L. B. Lev, and F. M. Konikoff. 2014. Cannabis for inflammatory bowel disease. *Digestive Diseases* 32 (4):468–474.

Nagarkatti, P., R. Pandey, S. A. Rieder, V. L. Hegde, and M. Nagarkatti. 2009. Cannabinoids as novel anti-inflammatory drugs. *Future Medicinal Chemistry* 1 (7):1333–1349.

National Academies of Sciences, Engineering, and Medicine. 2017. *The Health Effects of Cannabis and Cannabinoids: The Current State of Evidence and Recommendations for Research.* Washington (DC).

Naz, F. 2016. Cannabis (bhang, charas) consumption. *Professional Medical Journal* 23 (5):597–602.

Nielsen, S., P. Sabioni, J. M. Trigo et al. 2017. Opioid-sparing effect of cannabinoids: A systematic review and meta-analysis. *Neuropsychopharmacology* Apr 5 [Epub ahead of print].

Nogueras-Ortiz, C., and G. A. Yudowski. 2016. The multiple waves of cannabinoid 1 receptor signaling. *Molecular Pharmacology* 90 (5):620–626.

Nutt, D., L. A. King, W. Saulsbury, and C. Blakemore. 2007. Development of a rational scale to assess the harm of drugs of potential misuse. *Lancet* 369 (9566):1047–1053. doi: 10.1016/S0140-6736(07)60464-4

Ohlsson, A., J. E. Lindgren, A. Wahlen, S. Agurell, L. E. Hollister, and H. K. Gillespie. 1980. Plasma delta-9-tetrahydrocannabinol concentrations and clinical effects after oral and intravenous administration and smoking. *Clinical Pharmacology & Therapeutics* 28 (3):409–416.

OMC. 2016. Dutch Office of Medicinal Cannabis. www.cannabisbureau.nl

Oomah, B., M. B. Dave, D. V. Godfrey, and J. C. G. Drover. 2002. Characteristics of hemp (Cannabis sativa L.) seed oil. *Food Chemistry* 76 (1):33–43.

Park, H. M., J. H. Lee, J. Yaoyao, H. J. Jun, and S. J. Lee. 2011. Limonene, a natural cyclic terpene, is an agonistic ligand for adenosine A(2A) receptors. *Biochemical and Biophysical Research Communications* 404 (1):345–348.

Patton, G. C., C. Coffey, J. B. Carlin, L. Degenhardt, M. Lynskey, and W. Hall. 2002. Cannabis use and mental health in young people: Cohort study. *BMJ* 325 (7374):1195.

Pearce, D. D., K. Mitsouras, and K. J. Irizarry. 2014. Discriminating the effects of Cannabis sativa and Cannabis indica: A web survey of medical cannabis users. *Journal of Alternative and Complementary Medicine* 20 (10):787–1191.

Peat, M. A. 1989. Distribution of delta-9-tetrahydrocannabinol and its metabolites. In *Advances in Analytical Toxicology*, edited by Baselt, R. C., 186–217. Mosby.

Pertwee, R. G. 2014. *Handbook of Cannabis. 1st Ed, Handbooks in Psychopharmacology.* Oxford, United Kingdom; New York, NY: Oxford University Press.

Piomelli, D., and E. B. Russo. 2016. The cannabis sativa versus cannabis indica debate: An interview with Ethan Russo, MD. *Cannabis and Cannabinoid Research* 1 (1):44–46.

du Plessis, S. S., A. Agarwal, and A. Syriac. 2015. Marijuana, phytocannabinoids, the endocannabinoid system, and male fertility. *Journal of Assisted Reproduction and Genetics* 32 (11):1575–1588.

Pope, H. G., Jr., A. J. Gruber, J. I. Hudson, M. A. Huestis, and D. Yurgelun-Todd. 2002. Cognitive measures in long-term cannabis users. *Journal of Clinical Pharmacology* 42 (11 Suppl.):41S–47S.

Potter, D. J. 2014. A review of the cultivation and processing of cannabis (Cannabis sativa L.) for production of prescription medicines in the UK. *Drug Testing and Analysis* 6 (1–2):31–38.

Purnell, W. D., and J. M. Gregg. 1975. Delta(9)-tetrahydrocannabinol,, euphoria and intraocular pressure in man. *Annals of Ophthalmology* 7 (7):921–923.

Raber, J. C., S. Elzinga, and C. Kaplan. 2015. Understanding dabs: Contamination concerns of cannabis concentrates and cannabinoid transfer during the act of dabbing. *Journal of Toxicological Sciences* 40 (6):797–803.

Radhakrishnan, R., S. T. Wilkinson, and D. C. D'Souza. 2014. Gone to pot—A review of the association between cannabis and psychosis. *Frontiers in Psychiatry* 5:54.

Rajan, T. S., S. Giacoppo, R. Iori, G. R. De Nicola, G. Grassi, F. Pollastro, P. Bramanti, and E. Mazzon. 2016. Anti-inflammatory and antioxidant effects of a combination of cannabidiol and moringin in LPS-stimulated macrophages. *Fitoterapia* 112:104–115.

Ranganathan, M., and D. C. D'Souza. 2006. The acute effects of cannabinoids on memory in humans: A review. *Psychopharmacology* 188 (4):425–444.

Raters, M., and R. Matissek. 2008. Thermal stability of aflatoxin B1 and ochratoxin A. *Mycotoxin Res* 24 (3):130–134.

Robertson, D., and R. Robertson. 1994. Causes of chronic orthostatic hypotension. *Archives of Internal Medicine* 154 (14):1620–1624.

Robson, P. J. 2014. Therapeutic potential of cannabinoid medicines. *Drug Test Anal* 6 (1–2):24–30.

Rocha, F. C. M., J. G. dos Santos Júnior, S. C. Stefano, and D. X. da Silveira. 2014. Systematic review of the literature on clinical and experimental trials on the antitumor effects of cannabinoids in gliomas. *Journal of Neuro-Oncology* 116 (1):11–24.

Romano, L. L., and A. Hazekamp. 2013. Cannabis Oil: Chemical evaluation of an upcoming cannabis-based medicine. *Cannabinoids* 1 (1):1–11.

Russo, E. B. 2005. Cannabis in India: Ancient lore and modern medicine. In *Cannabinoids as Therapeutics*, edited by Mechoulam, R., 272 p. Basel; Boston: Birkhäuser.

Russo, E. B. 2007. History of cannabis and its preparations in saga, science, and sobriquet. *Chemistry & Biodiversity* 4 (8):1614–1648.

Russo, E. B. 2011. Taming THC: Potential cannabis synergy and phytocannabinoid-terpenoid entourage effects. *British Journal of Pharmacology* 163 (7):1344–1364.

Russo, E. B., H. E. Jiang, X. Li et al. 2008. Phytochemical and genetic analyses of ancient cannabis from Central Asia. *Journal of Experimental Botany* 59 (15):4171–4182.

Scheel, A. H., D. Krause, H. Haars, I. Schmitz, and K. Junker. 2012. Talcum induced pneumoconiosis following inhalation of adulterated marijuana, a case report. *Diagn Pathol* 7:26.

Schmid, K., J. Schonlebe, H. Drexler, and M. Mueck-Weymann. 2010. The effects of cannabis on heart rate variability and well-being in young men. *Pharmacopsychiatry* 43 (4):147–150.

Schulz-Katterbach, M., T. Imfeld, and C. Imfeld. 2009. Cannabis and caries--does regular cannabis use increase the risk of caries in cigarette smokers? *Schweizer Monatsschrift FüR Zahnmedizin = Revue Mensuelle Suisse D'odonto-Stomatologie = Rivista Mensile Svizzera Di Odontologia E Stomatologia/SSO* 119 (6):576–583.

Sewell, R. A., A. Schnakenberg, J. Elander, R. Radhakrishnan, A. Williams, P. D. Skosnik, B. Pittman, M. Ranganathan, and D. C. D'Souza. 2013. Acute effects of THC on time perception in frequent and infrequent cannabis users. *Psychopharmacology* 226 (2):401–413.

Shi, G., C. Liu, M. Cui, Y. Ma, and Q. Cai. 2012. Cadmium tolerance and bioaccumulation of 18 hemp accessions. *Applied Biochemistry and Biotechnology* 168 (1):163–173.

Smith, S. C., and M. S. Wagner. 2014. Clinical endocannabinoid deficiency (CECD) revisited: Can this concept explain the therapeutic benefits of cannabis in migraine, fibromyalgia, irritable bowel syndrome and other treatment-resistant conditions? *Neuro Endocrinology Letters* 35 (3):198–201.

Solowij, N. 1995. Do cognitive impairments recover following cessation of cannabis use? *Life Sciences* 56 (23-24):2119–2126.

Specter, S. C., T. W. Klein, C. Newton, M. Mondragon, R. Widen, and H. Friedman. 1986. Marijuana effects on immunity: Suppression of human natural killer cell activity of delta-9-tetrahydrocannabinol. *International Journal Of Immunopharmacology* 8 (7):741–745.

State of Israel, Ministry of Health, Medical Cannabis Unit. https://www.health.gov.il/UnitsOffice/HD/cannabis/Documents/canabis_medical.pdf

Sugiura, T., S. Kondo, A. Sukagawa, S. Nakane, A. Shinoda, K. Itoh, A. Yamashita, and K. Waku. 1995. 2-Arachidonoylglycerol: A possible endogenous cannabinoid receptor ligand in brain. *Biochemical and Biophysical Research Communications* 215 (1):89–97.

Sullivan, N., S. Elzinga, and J. C. Raber. 2013. Determination of pesticide residues in cannabis smoke. *J Toxicol* 2013:378168.

Suárez, A. I. T., A. I. F. Sánchez, and A. Fernández-Carballido. 2014. Cannabinoides: una prometedora herramienta para el desarrollo de nuevas terapias. *Anales de la Real Academia Nacional de Farmacia* 80 (3):1.

Söderpalm, A. H., A. Schuster, and H. de Wit. 2001. Antiemetic efficacy of smoked marijuana: Subjective and behavioral effects on nausea induced by syrup of ipecac. *Pharmacology Biochemistry and Behavior* 69 (3-4):343–350.

Takeda, S., K. Misawa, I. Yamamoto, and K. Watanabe. 2008. Cannabidiolic acid as a selective cyclooxygenase-2 inhibitory component in cannabis. *Drug Metabolism and Disposition* 36 (9):1917–1921.

Tasker, J. G., C. Chen, M. O. Fisher, X. Fu, J. R. Rainville, and G. L. Weiss. 2015. Endocannabinoid regulation of neuroendocrine systems. *International Review of Neurobiology* 125:163–201.

Thacore, V., and S. P. Shukla. 1976. Cannabis psychosis and paranoid schizophrenia. *Archives of General Psychiatry* 33 (3):383–386.

Thomas, B. F., D. R. Compton, and B. R. Martin. 1990. Characterization of the lipophilicity of natural and synthetic analogs of delta 9-tetrahydrocannabinol and its relationship to pharmacological potency. *Journal of Pharmacology and Experimental Therapeutics* 255 (2):624–630.

Tomida, I., A. Azuara-Blanco, H. House, M. Flint, R. G. Pertwee, and P. J. Robson. 2006. Effect of sublingual application of cannabinoids on intraocular pressure: A pilot study. *Journal of Glaucoma* 15 (5):349–353.

Traver, F., S. Edo, and G. Haro. 2009. Cyclic hyperemesis secondary to chronic consumption of cannabis: A reconceptualization of psychogenic vomiting. *Addictive Disorders & Their Treatment* 8 (4):175–184.

Turgeman, I., and G. Bar-Sela. 2017. Cannabis use in palliative oncology: A review of the evidence for popular indications. *Israel Medical Association Journal* 19 (2):85–88.

Uchiyama, N., R. Kikura-Hanajiri, J. Ogata, and Y. Goda. 2010. Chemical analysis of synthetic cannabinoids as designer drugs in herbal products. *Forensic Science International* 198 (1):31–38.

Ujváry, I., and L. Hanuš. 2016. Human metabolites of cannabidiol: A review on their formation, biological activity, and relevance in therapy. *Cannabis and Cannabinoid Research* 1 (1):90–101.

United States Department of Justice, Office of Public Affairs. https://www.justice.gov/opa/pr/justice-department-announces-update-marijuana-enforcement-policy

Upton, R., L. Craker, M. ElSohly, A. Romm, E. Russo, and M. Sexton. 2013. *"Cannabis Inflorescence: Cannabis spp." Standards of Identity, Analysis and Quality Control.* Scotts Valley, CA: American Herbal Pharmacopoeia.

Vandrey, R., J. C. Raber, M. E. Raber, B. Douglass, C. Miller, and M. O. Bonn-Miller. 2015. Cannabinoid Dose and Label Accuracy in Edible Medical Cannabis Products. *JAMA* 313 (24):2491–2493.

Veress, T., J. I. Szanto, and L. Leisztner. 1990. Determination of cannabinoid acids by high-performance liquid chromatography of their neutral derivatives formed by thermal decarboxylation. *Journal of Chromatography A* 520:339–347.

Verhoeckx, K. C., H. A. Korthout, A. P. van Meeteren-Kreikamp, K. A. Ehlert, M. Wang, J. van der Greef, R. J. Rodenburg, and R. F. Witkamp. 2006. Unheated Cannabis sativa extracts and its major compound THC-acid have potential immuno-modulating properties not mediated by CB1 and CB2 receptor coupled pathways. *International Immunopharmacology* 6 (4):656–665.

Verstraete, A. G. 2004. Detection times of drugs of abuse in blood, urine, and oral fluid. *Therapeutic Drug Monitoring* 26 (2):200–205.

Viana, B. d. M., A. de Souza Moura, J. M. Moreira, H. A. C. Prais, and F. Cardoso. 2009. Ataxia and dementia due to thinner abuse. *Movement Disorders: Official Journal Of The Movement Disorder Society* 24 (12):1850–1852.

Volkow, N. D., H. Gillespie, N. Mullani, L. Tancredi, C. Grant, A. Valentine, and L. Hollister. 1996. Brain glucose metabolism in chronic marijuana users at baseline and during marijuana intoxication. *Psychiatry Research: Neuroimaging* 67 (1):29–38.

Walitt, B., P. Klose, M. A. Fitzcharles, T. Phillips, and W. Hauser. 2016. Cannabinoids for fibromyalgia. *Cochrane Database of Systematic Reviews* 7:CD011694.

Walker, J. M., and S. M. Huang. 2002. Cannabinoid analgesia. *Pharmacology & Therapeutics* 95 (2):127–135.

Wall, M. E. 1983. Metabolism, disposition, and kinetics of delta-9-tetrahydrocannabinol in men and women. *Clinical Pharmacology and Therapeutics* 34:352–363.

Wang, M., Y.-H. Wang, B. Avula, M. M. Radwan, A. S. Wanas, J. v. Antwerp, J. F. Parcher, M. A. ElSohly, and I. A. Khan. 2016. Decarboxylation study of acidic cannabinoids: A novel approach using ultra-high-performance supercritical fluid chromatography/photodiode array-mass spectrometry. *Cannabis and Cannabinoid Research* 1 (1):262–271.

Webster, L. R., and M. Grabois. 2015. Current Regulations Related to Opioid Prescribing. *PM R* 7 (11 Suppl.):S236–S247.

Weil, A. T., N. E. Zinberg, and J. M. Nelsen. 1968. Clinical and psychological effects of marihuana in man. *Science.*

Weiss, A., and F. Friedenberg. 2015. Full length article: Patterns of cannabis use in patients with inflammatory bowel disease: A population based analysis. *Drug and Alcohol Dependence* 156:84–89.

Whiting, P. F., R. F. Wolff, S. Deshpande et al. 2015. Cannabinoids for medical use: A systematic review and meta-analysis. *JAMA* 313 (24):2456–2473.

Williams, S. J., J. P. Hartley, and J. D. Graham. 1976. Bronchodilator effect of delta1-tetrahydrocannabinol administered by aerosol of asthmatic patients. *Thorax* 31 (6):720–723.

World Health Organization. 2011. *Quality Control Methods for Herbal Materials.* Geneva, Switzerland: WHO Press.

Ziemianski, D., R. Capler, R. Tekanoff, A. Lacasse, F. Luconi, and M. A. Ware. 2015. Cannabis in medicine: A national educational needs assessment among Canadian physicians. *BMC Medical Education* 15:52.

Zuardi, A. W. 2006. History of cannabis as a medicine: A review. *Revista Brasileira de Psiquiatria* 28:153–157.

Zuardi, A. W., I. Shirakawa, E. Finkelfarb, and I. G. Karniol. 1982. Action of cannabidiol on the anxiety and other effects produced by delta 9-THC in normal subjects. *Psychopharmacology* 76 (3):245–250.

Index

W

Wal-Mart, 40
Warehouse buying clubs, 40
Warfarin, 15, 55
Water-based processing, 398
Watercress (*Nasturtium officinal*), 370
Water hyssop, *see* Bacopa (*Bacopa monnieri*)
Websites/online databases, 4–5
Weight loss
    appetite suppressants, 316–319
    botanical products in treatment of obesity, 316
    digestion inhibitors, 319–322
    miscellaneous agents, 326–332
    supplements, 315
    thermogenic agents, 322–326
Weight mean differences (WMD), 274
Western Ontario and McMaster Universities Osteoarthritis
        Index (WOMAC), 297
Wheatgrass (*Triticum aestivum*), 146–147
White hellebore roots (*Veratum grandiflorum*), 376
WHO, *see* World Health Organization
WHO OMAS, *see* World Health Organization Oral
        Mucositis Assessment Scale
Wiklund menopause symptom score, 174
Wild chamomile, *see* Feverfew (*Tanacetum parthenium*)
Wild cucumber, *see* Bitter melon (*Momordica charantia*)
Wild yam (*Dioscorea villosa*), 181
Willow bark, 40, 258–259
Witch hazel (*Hamamelis virginiana*), 287
Withania somnifera (WS), 365
    supportive and palliative care for cancer, 365–366

WMD, *see* Weight mean differences
Wolf's bane, *see Arnica montana*
WOMAC-VAS, *see* WOMAC-visual analogue
WOMAC-visual analogue (WOMAC-VAS), 297
WOMAC, *see* Western Ontario and McMaster Universities
        Osteoarthritis Index
Women's health
    menstrual problems, 161–166
    perimenopause/menopause, 173–183
    pregnancy and lactation, 167–173
World Health Organization (WHO), 39, 53, 245, 296,
        395, 400
World Health Organization Oral Mucositis Assessment
        Scale (WHO OMAS), 382
Wound healing, 280
WS, *see Withania somnifera*
WS® 1442 extracts, 80

X

Xerosis, 275–276

Y

Yohimbe (*Pausinystalia yohimbine*), 41, 198–199
Yohimbine, 40, 42
    for ED, 199

Z

Zingerone, 139
Zingiber officinale, see Ginger

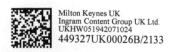

Milton Keynes UK
Ingram Content Group UK Ltd.
UKHW051942071024
449327UK00026B/2133